Therapeutic Programs
for Musculoskeletal Disorders

Therapeutic Programs for Musculoskeletal Disorders

EDITED BY

James F. Wyss, MD, PT

Assistant Attending Physiatrist
Assistant Fellowship Director
Hospital for Special Surgery
Physiatry Department
New York, NY

Amrish D. Patel, MD, PT

Sports and Spine Physiatrist
Ortho Georgia
Macon, GA

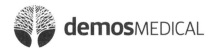 demosMEDICAL

Visit our website at www.demosmedpub.com

ISBN: 9781936287406
e-book ISBN: 9781617050794

Acquisitions Editor: Beth Barry
Compositor: Newgen Imaging

Medicine is an ever-changing science. Research and clinical experience are continually expanding our knowledge, in particular our understanding of proper treatment and drug therapy. The authors, editors, and publisher have made every effort to ensure that all information in this book is in accordance with the state of knowledge at the time of production of the book. Nevertheless, the authors, editors, and publisher are not responsible for errors or omissions or for any consequences from application of the information in this book and make no warranty, express or implied, with respect to the contents of the publication. Every reader should examine carefully the package inserts accompanying each drug and should carefully check whether the dosage schedules mentioned therein or the contraindications stated by the manufacturer differ from the statements made in this book. Such examination is particularly important with drugs that are either rarely used or have been newly released on the market.

Library of Congress Cataloging-in-Publication Data

Therapeutic programs for musculoskeletal disorders / edited by James Wyss, Amrish Patel.
     p. ; cm.
  Includes bibliographical references and index.
  ISBN 978-1-936287-40-6 (alk. paper) — ISBN 978-1-61705-079-4 (e-book)
  I. Wyss, James. II. Patel, Amrish.
  [DNLM: 1. Musculoskeletal Diseases—therapy. 2. Patient Care Planning. WE 140]

  616.7'06—dc23

                                                                    2012033213

Special discounts on bulk quantities of Demos Medical Publishing books are available to corporations, professional associations, pharmaceutical companies, health care organizations, and other qualifying groups. For details, please contact:
Special Sales Department
Demos Medical Publishing, LLC
11 West 42nd Street, 15th Floor
New York, NY 10036
Phone: 800–532-8663 or 212–683-0072
Fax: 212–941-7842
E-mail: rsantana@demosmedpub.com

Printed in the United States of America by Bradford & Bigelow Printing.

12 13 14 15 / 5 4 3 2 1

Contents

Contributors

Giselle Aerni, MD
Primary Care Sports Medicine Fellow
University of Connecticut
St. Francis Hospital
Hartford, CT

Neeti Bathia, MD
Physiatrist; Sports and Spine Fellow
Hospital for Special Surgery
New York, NY

Curtis W. Bazemore, PT, ATC
Director of Physical Therapy
Sports Medicine South
Lawrenceville, GA

Scott Becker, MPT, MDT
Staff Physical Therapist
Good Shepherd Penn Partners
Pennsylvania Hospital
Philadelphia, PA

Gina M. Benaquista DeSipio, DO
Attending Physician
Physical Medicine and Rehabilitation
MossRehab at Elkins Park
Elkins Park, PA

Anna-Christina Bevelaqua, MD
Chief Resident
New York Presbyterian Hospital
Department of Rehabilitation Medicine
New York, NY

Joanne P. Borg-Stein, MD
Associate Professor of Physical Medicine and Rehabilitation
Harvard Medical School
Director
Harvard/Spaulding Sports Medicine Fellowship
Medical Director
Spaulding-Wellesley Rehab Center
Medical Director
NWH Spine Center
Newton, MA

Erik S. Brand, MD, MSc
Sports Medicine Fellow
Harvard Medical School/Spaulding Rehabilitation Hospital
Boston, MA

Meredith B. Brazell, PA-S
Emory University Physician Assistant Program
Research Assistant
Sports Medicine South
Lawrenceville, GA

Edward R. Calem, PT
Advanced Clinician Orthopaedic Physical Therapy
Department of Rehabilitation and Regenerative Medicine
New York Presbyterian Hospital
Columbia Presbyterian Medical Center
Clinical Instructor
Program in Physical Therapy
College of Physicians and Surgeons
Columbia University
New York, NY

Jose Santiago Campos, MD
Sports and Spine Fellow
Hospital for Special Surgery
New York, NY

Brite Chalunkal, DO, DPT
NYPH Columbia and Cornell University Medical Center
Resident, Department of Physical Medicine and Rehabilitation
New York, NY

Theresa A. Chiaia, PT, DPT
Section Manager
Sports Rehabilitation and Performance Center
Department of Rehabilitation
Hospital for Special Surgery
New York, NY

Gary P. Chimes, MD, PhD
Sports and Spine Rehabilitation
Fellowship Director
Musculoskeletal Sports and Spine Fellowship
University of Pittsburgh Medical Center
Department of Physical Medicine and Rehabilitation
Pittsburgh, PA

Larry H. Chou, MD
Medical Director
Sports and Spine Rehabilitation Division
Premier Orthopaedic and Sports Medicine Associates
Havertown, PA

Kim Cohee, MS, PT, DPT, OCS
Manager
Therapy Services
University of Utah Orthopaedic Center
Salt Lake City, UT

Jeffrey L. Cole, MD
Director
Electrodiagnostic Medicine and Musculoskeletal
Rehabilitation
Kessler Institute for Rehabilitation
West Orange, NJ

Paul M. Cooke, MD
Assistant Attending Physiatrist
Department of Physiatry
Hospital for Special Surgery
New York, NY

Eduardo J. Cruz-Colón, MD
Physical Medicine and Rehabilitation
Resident UMDNJ-NJMS
Newark, NJ

Carly Day, MD
Staff Physician
Department of Orthopaedic Surgery
Cleveland Clinic
Cleveland, OH

D. Nicole Deal, MD
Assistant Professor of Hand Surgery
Department of Orthopaedic Surgery
University of Virginia
Charlottesville, VA

Robert DePorto, DO
Attending Physician
Clinical Assistant Professor
Physical Medicine and Rehabilitation
NYU Medical Center
Rusk Institute for Rehabilitation
New York, NY

Robert DeStefano, DC
Certified Chiropractic Sports Physician
ART Instructor
Hackenstack, NJ and New York, NY

Mirielle Diaz, MD, MPH
Board Certified Physical Medicine and Rehabilitation
New York Physical Rehabilitation and Wellness
New York, NY

Pete Draovitch MS, ATC, PT, CSCS
Clinical Supervisor
Sports Rehabilitation and Performance Center
Center for Hip Preservation
Hospital for Special Surgery
New York, NY

Stacia Dyer, OTR, CHT
Hand Therapy Services
St Clare's Hospital
Denville, NJ

Jaime Edelstein, PT, DScPT, COMT, CSCS
Site Manager
Physical Therapy
Affiliated with Hospital for Special Surgery at Goldman Sachs
New York, NY

Trasey D. Falcone, DO
Resident Physician
Department of Physical Medicine and Rehabilitation
University of Pittsburgh Medical Center
Pittsburgh, PA

Joseph Feinberg, MD
Chief of Physiatry
Department of Physical Medicine and Rehabilitation
Hospital for Special Surgery
New York, NY

David E. Fish, MD, MPH
Associate Clinical Professor
Department of Orthopaedics
Physical Medicine and Rehabilitation
The UCLA Spine Center David Geffen School of Medicine
Los Angeles, CA

Stacey Franz, DO, PT
Interventional Physiatrist/Medical Director
Northeast Spine and Sports Medicine
Jackson, NJ

Marilyn Freedman, DPT
Essential Physical Therapy
Great Neck, NY

Annemarie E. Gallagher, MD
Chief Resident
New York Presbyterian Hospital
The University Hospital of Columbia and Cornell
Department of Physical Medicine and Rehabilitation
New York, NY

Susan Garstang, MD
Staff Physician
Physical Medicine and Rehabilitation Service
Clinical Associate Professor
UMDNJ-NJMS
Residency Program Director
UMDNJ-NJMS/Kessler Institute
Newark, NJ

Brett A Gerstman, MD
Pain Medicine Fellow
UCLA/WLA VA
PM&R Pain Medicine Fellowship Program
David Geffen School of Medicine
Los Angeles, CA

Stephanie L. Griggs, ATC
Head Athletic Trainer
Sports Medicine South
Lawrenceville, GA

Andrew Hall, MD
Resident Physician
Physical Medicine and Rehabilitation
Johns Hopkins University
Baltimore, MD

Sean Hampton, MPT
Director
ADI Rehab Inc
Los Angeles, CA

Jo A. Hannafin, MD, PhD
Attending Orthopedic Surgeon
Director of Orthopedic Research
Professor of Orthopaedic Surgery
Weill Cornell Medical College of Cornell University
Hospital for Special Surgery
New York, NY

Mark A. Harrast, MD
Director, Sports Medicine Fellowship
Clinical Associate Professor
Department of Rehabilitation Medicine
Department of Orthopedics and Sports Medicine
University of Washington

Daniel C. Herman, MD, PhD
Resident Physician
University of Virginia
Department of Physical Medicine and Rehabilitation
Charlottesville, VA

Jay Hertel, PhD, ATC, FNATA
Joe Gieck Professor of Sports Medicine
University of Virginia
Department of Human Services
Charlottesville, VA

Mark S. Hopkins, PT, CPO, MBA
Clinical Director
Dankmeyer, Inc.
Linthicum, MD

Debra Ibrahim, DO
Physical Medicine and Rehabilitation Resident
UMDNJ/Kessler Institute for Rehabilitation
West Orange, NJ

Neil N. Jasey, MD
Clinical Assistant Professor
Kessler Institute for Rehabilitation
West Orange, NJ

Prathap Jayaram, MD
Department Physical Medicine and Rehabilitation
UMDNJ
Newark, NJ

Anjan P. Kaushik, MD
Resident Physician
University of Virginia Department of Orthopaedic Surgery
Charlottesville, VA

Elizabeth Kennedy, ATC
Fort Myers, FL

Phong Kieu, MD
Resident Physician
Physical Medicine and Rehabilitation
Johns Hopkins University
Baltimore, MD

Monika Krzyzek, DO, CPT (MC)
UMDNJ-NJMS
Kessler Institute for Rehabilitation
Physical Medicine and Rehabilitation
Newark, NJ

Paul H. Lento, MD
Associate Professor
Temple University School of Medicine
Philadelphia, PA

Gary A. Levengood, MD
Board Certified Orthopedic Surgeon
Medical Director/Owner
Sports Medicine South
Lawrenceville, GA

Benjamin D. Levy, MD
Musculoskeletal/Interventional Spine Fellow
Department of Physical Medicine and Rehabilitation
New Jersey Medical School
UMDNJ
Newark, NJ

Rex Ma, MD
Clinical Assistant Professor
Department of Physical Medicine and Rehabilitation
UMDNJ
Staff Physician
VA NJ Healthcare System
East Orange, NJ

Eric Magrum, PT, OCS, FAAOMPT
Physical Therapist
UVA-Healthsouth Outpatient Sports Medicine Center
Charlottesville, VA

Gerard A. Malanga, MD
New Jersey Sports and Spine
Cedar Knolls, NJ

Gautam Malhotra, MD
Clinical Assistant Professor
Department of Physical Medicine and Rehabilitation
University of Medicine and Dentistry
New Jersey Medical School
Attending Physician
Physical Medicine and Rehabilitation Service
Veterans Affairs New Jersey Health Care System
East Orange, NJ

Robert Maschi, PT, DPT, OCS, CSCS
Assistant Clinical Professor
Drexel University
Department of Physical Therapy and Rehabilitation Sciences
Physical Therapist
Drexel University Physical Therapy Services
Clinical Practice Patient Education
Philadelphia, PA

Stephen Massimi, MD
Resident
Physical Medicine and Rehabilitation
New York Presbyterian Hospital—Columbia and Cornell
New York, NY

Steve Matta, DO, MBA
Primary Care Sports Medicine Fellow
Mountainside Sports Medicine
Montclair, NJ

Jill May, PT, DPT, OCS
Physical Therapist
Johns Hopkins Medicine
Lutherville, MD

Terrence G. McGee, PT, DScPT, FAAOMPT
Clinical Specialist
The Johns Hopkins Outpatient Rehabilitation Facility
Director
The Johns Hopkins Orthopedic Physical Therapy Residency
Lutherville, MD

John McMurtry, BS
Medical Student
University of Virginia School of Medicine
Charlottesville, VA

Kim Middleton, MD
Resident Physician
Department of Rehabilitation
University of Washington
Seattle, WA

Peter J. Moley, MD
Assistant Attending Physiatrist
Hospital for Special Surgery
Assistant Professor of Rehabilitation Medicine
Weill Cornell Medical College
Center for Hip Preservation
New York, NY

Rosalyn T. Nguyen, MD
Attending Physiatrist
Department of Physical Medicine and Rehabilitation
Spaulding Rehabilitation Hospital and Massachusetts General
    Hospital
Clinical Instructor
Harvard Medical School
Boston, MA

Elizabeth T. Nguyen, MD
Resident
Department of Physical Medicine and Rehabilitation
New York Presbyterian Hospital/Columbia-Cornell
New York, NY

Michael R. Nicoletti, MD
Resident
Physical Medicine and Rehabilitation
SUNY Downstate Medical Center
New York, NY

Jeremiah Nieves, MD
Attending Physician
Kessler Institute for Rehabilitation
West Orange, NJ

Kambiz Nooryani, MD
UMDNJ
Department Physical Medicine and Rehabilitation
Newark, NJ

Oluseun A. Olufade, MD
Chief Resident
Physical Medicine and Rehabilitation
Temple University Hospital/Moss Rehab
Philadelphia, PA

Brian Owens, PT, DPT, CSCS
Lead Physical Therapist
Mountainside Hospital
Montclair, NJ

Amrish D. Patel, MD, PT
Sports and Spine Physiatrist
Ortho Georgia
Macon, GA

Shounuck I. Patel, DO
Director of Sports Medicine
Sports Medicine South
Lawrenceville, GA

Harris A. Patel, PA-C, ATC
Director of Sports Medicine
Sports Medicine South
Lawrenceville, GA

Deena Petrocelli, MD
Attending Physician
Primary Care Sports Medicine
Long Island Jewish Medical Center
North Shore University Hospital
Team Physician New York Islanders
Team Physician USA Rugby
Team Physician Hofstra University
Team Physician Molloy College
New York, NY

Christine Pfisterer, DO
Resident
UMDNJ/Kessler PM&R Residency Program
Newark, NJ

Christopher Plastaras, MD
Director
Penn Spine Center
Department of Physical Medicine and Rehabilitation
University of Pennsylvania
Hospital of the University of Pennsylvania
Philadelphia, PA

Smita Rao, PT, PhD
Assistant Professor
Department of Physical Therapy
New York University
New York, NY

Heather Roehrs Galgon, DO
Physical Medicine and Rehabilitation Resident
Temple University Health System
Havertown, PA

Christine Roque-Dang, MD
Physical Medicine and Rehabilitation
Resident UMDNJ-NJMS
Newark, NJ

Lee Rosenzweig, PT, DPT, CHT
Physical Therapist
Hospital for Special Surgery
New York, NY

Lynn A. Ryan, MS, OTR
Chief of Occupational Therapy
Physical Medicine and Rehabilitation Service
Veterans Affairs New Jersey Health Care System
East Orange, NJ

Lori Sabado, BS, PT
Department of Rehabilitation Medicine Clinical Faculty
University of Washington
Seattle, WA

Marcello Sarrica, PT, DPT, OCS, CSCS
Physical Therapist
New York Physical Rehabilitation and Wellness
New York, NY

Kelly Scollon-Grieve, MD
Sports and Spine Fellow
Sports and Spine Rehabilitation Division
Premier Orthopaedic and Sports Medicine Associates
Havertown, PA

Meredith K. Sena, MSPT
Physical Therapist
Kingman Regional Medical Center
Kingman, AZ

Heather Sleece, PT, DPT
Certified in Vestibular Therapy
Kessler Institute for Rehabilitation
West Orange, NJ

Jeffrey T. Smith, OTR/CHT
Occupational Therapist
UVA-Healthsouth Hand Rehabilitation Center
Charlottesville, VA

Jennifer L. Solomon, MD
Assistant Attending Physiatrist
Hospital for Special Surgery
New York, NY

Todd Stitik, MD
Director
Musculoskeletal/Occupational Medicine
Associate Professor of Physical Medicine and Rehabilitation
Department of Physical Medicine and Rehabilitation
UMDNJ, Newark, NJ

Suzanne Gutiérrez Teissonniere, MD
Spine and Sports Medicine Fellow
Hospital for Special Surgery
New York, NY

Gaurav Raj Telhan, MD
Resident
Department of Rehabilitation and Regenerative Medicine
NYPH/Columbia and Cornell University Medical Centers
New York, NY

Alon Terry, MD
Resident in Department of Physical Medicine and Rehabilitation
UMDNJ/Kessler Institute for Rehabilitation
West Orange, NJ

Jiaxin Tran, MD
Resident
Department of Physical Medicine and Rehabilitation
UMDNJ
Newark, NJ

Daniel Tufaro, OTR/L
Senior Occupational Therapy Specialist
New York Presbyterian Hospital-Weill Cornell Medical Center
Department of Rehabilitation Medicine
Inpatient Rehabilitation Unit
New York, NY

Ashley Varughese, DPT
Physical Therapist
Department of Physical Therapy
New York-Presbyterian Hospital
New York, NY

John M. Vasudevan, MD
Education Chief Resident
Department of Rehabilitation Medicine
Thomas Jefferson University Hospital
Philadelphia, PA

Tracey A. Viola, DO
Primary Care Sports Medicine Fellow
University of Connecticut
St. Francis Hospital
Hartford, CT

Christopher J. Visco, MD
Assistant Professor of Clinical Rehabilitation
Department of Rehabilitation and Regenerative Medicine
Columbia University College of Physicians and Surgeons
Assistant Attending Physician
New York-Presbyterian Hospital
New York, NY

John Walker, DPT, MDT
Senior Physical Therapist
Certified McKenzie Practitioner
Temple University Orthopaedics and Sports Medicine
Philadelphia, PA

Ian Wendel, DO
Department of Physical Medicine and Rehabilitation
UMDNJ-NJMS
Newark, NJ

Stuart Willick, MD, FASCM
Associate Professor
Department of Physical Medicine and Rehabilitation
University of Utah
Salt Lake City, UT

Brian Domenic Wishart, MMS
Undergraduate Teaching Fellow, OMS VI
Philadelphia College of Osteopathic Medicine
Philadelphia, PA

Eric Wisotzky, MD
Associate Director of Cancer Rehabilitation
National Rehabilitation Hospital
Washington, DC

James F. Wyss, MD, PT
Assistant Attending Physiatrist
Assistant Fellowship Director
Hospital for Special Surgery
Physiatry Department
New York, NY

Peter P. Yonclas, MD, BS
Director
Trauma Rehabilitation
Assistant Professor
Physical Medicine and Rehabilitation
Newark, NJ

Foreword

Amrish and James both trained and served as chief residents at my residency program at UMDNJ. Both were excellent residents and served locally and nationally to improve residency education. They share strong interests in musculoskeletal, sports, and academic medicine; and both had prior careers as physical therapists before entering training programs in physical medicine and rehabilitation. This background has provided them with a unique perspective on the role of various health care professionals in musculoskeletal medicine, and on the value of exceptional nonoperative care to treat and prevent the recurrence of these conditions. For this reason they discussed this book proposal with me and have set out to fill a perceived gap in the literature.

Their primary goal has been to provide guidance to musculoskeletal medicine trainees (including but not exclusive to physical medicine & rehabilitation, sports medicine, family medicine, internal medicine, rheumatology, orthopedics, and neurology) for writing prescriptions and developing individualized therapeutic programs with the help of allied health care practitioners (including but not exclusive to physical therapists, occupational therapists, certified athletic trainers, and chiropractors).

Their secondary goal, which they are well suited to advance, is to enhance the collaborative effort between the prescribing physicians and the allied health care practitioners providing the treatments. Their vision includes a health care setting where physicians from various specialties and allied health care professionals work collectively and communicate effectively for the benefit of the patient and their musculoskeletal health. This book is a reflection of that vision.

Joel A. DeLisa, MD, MS
Professor and Chair
Department of Physical Medicine and Rehabilitation
UMDNJ—New Jersey Medical School

Preface

Amrish and I met in 2008 during his first rotation at the UMDNJ-Kessler Institute for Rehabilitation training program. I was a second year physical medicine and rehabilitation resident, foolishly confident of my knowledge of musculoskeletal medicine and expecting to share my knowledge with a junior resident. When he answered all my questions and told me he had no questions for me prior to seeing his first patient, I was a little surprised and disappointed. He smoothly ran through his first busy day at the DOC. I asked him how he managed everything so well and he told me that he practiced as a physical therapist prior to medical school, just as I had, and was comfortable evaluating and treating patients with routine musculoskeletal conditions. We had a lot in common, shared a lot of experiences, he even shared his apartment when my commute grew to 2 hours each way and we became very good friends along the way. We worked together on many projects and I was more than happy to pass the administrative chief resident responsibilities to him approximately one and a half years later.

One project we both enjoyed was putting together a therapy-based educational curriculum for the residents at UMDNJ. We discussed and demonstrated common therapeutic exercises used for the treatment of musculoskeletal conditions. We were frequently asked to explain to junior residents "how to write a physical therapy prescription (Rx)." We explained this to the best of our ability and tried to withhold personal biases. We would explain that while an Rx that states "Back pain: evaluate and treat" can be liberating for a physical therapist (PT) compared to an Rx that requests specific treatment modalities only, somewhere in the middle is the perfect Rx that provides a specific and accurate diagnosis with recommendations for treatment and freedom for the therapist to utilize his or her skill set to further individualize the treatment program. We further explained that this type of Rx establishes a team approach to patient care with open communication between the physician and the provider of therapy services. Due to this frequently asked question, we eventually gave an impromptu lecture on the topic to our residency program.

Our attendings, specifically Nigel Shenoy and Gautam Malhotra, encouraged us to expand this teaching into a manual for internal use. After speaking with Beth Barry from Demos Medical Publishing at the AAP conference in 2010, we decided to broaden our objectives and put our ideas into a book. *Therapeutic Programs for Musculoskeletal Disorders* is intended to fill some of the gaps in the training of physicians who practice musculoskeletal medicine by focusing on how to write evidence-based therapy prescriptions that guide effective conservative management of common conditions. We hope we have accomplished our goal, and our readers will find the collaborative information they need to design individualized programs that improve outcomes for patients with musculoskeletal problems.

We would like to thank Gary Chimes and Christopher Visco, who mentored us through the book proposal process, and Gerard Malanga, who gave us his support throughout this project and assisted with writing several important chapters. Dr. Malanga also provided tremendous mentorship during our residency training and reinforced the need to follow the fundamental principles of rehabilitation (e.g., the phases of rehabilitation), which we have tried to further reinforce throughout this book.

CONTENT

The introductory section of this book addresses basic principles in musculoskeletal rehabilitation, including phases of rehabilitation, physical modalities, manual therapy, therapeutic exercise, patient education, and how to write effective therapy prescriptions.

The remainder of the book is broken into ten anatomical sections covering the conservative treatment of common musculoskeletal disorders. The majority of these condition-specific chapters are written collaboratively by musculoskeletal physicians, allied health professionals, and trainees to foster a team approach to treating these conditions. Each chapter includes:

- Background information on the condition, including description of the pathology/pathoanatomy, clinical presentation, physical examination, and relevant diagnostics
- Introduction to rehabilitation of the specific condition
- Therapeutic modalities
- Manual therapy
- Therapeutic exercises with illustrations to highlight the most important exercises
- Specialized approaches
- Case example
- Detailed sample therapy prescription
- Printable patient handout with home modalities and therapeutic exercises (on DVD)

PURPOSE

Our primary goal in initiating this book is to provide guidance to musculoskeletal medicine trainees and practitioners for writing effective therapy prescriptions and developing individualized, evidence-based treatment plans with the help of allied health care practitioners.

Our secondary goal, as practicing physicians and physical therapists, is to enhance the collaborative effort between the prescribing physicians and the allied health care practitioners, who are providing the treatments, to improve patient outcomes.

We strongly believe that the type of therapeutic program implemented greatly influences the patient's response. We are hopeful that by providing a concise, evidence-based guide to comprehensive therapeutic programs, our patients with musculoskeletal disorders will receive an optimal, individualized, and evidence-based program and, when possible, will be able to prevent the need for more invasive treatment options and avoid re-injury.

James F. Wyss
Amrish D. Patel

Acknowledgments

To all our contributing authors, thank you for your time, effort, and dedication to this project. Your hard work has given us the opportunity to put forth ideas that we think can improve patient care and medical education. We would especially like to thank those who have made a substantial contribution to this project: Gerard Malanga, Daniel Herman, Peter Moley, Gautam Malhotra, Gary Chimes, and Christopher Visco. Bella Shah for her dedication to the artwork included in this book, Jessica Hettler for her contributions to the introductory chapters, and Beth Barry and Demos Publishing for their continued support.

James F. Wyss
Amrish D. Patel

I would like to thank the following individuals, but realize there are many others who are not specifically listed who have provided great support during my life and career. I would like to thank my entire family, especially my beautiful wife Tonya who is my best friend, my initial editor and reviewer of all my ideas and writing projects. Without her, this book would not be possible. I would like to thank her and our children Emmariah and Jackson who together have supported me and understood the time commitment that this book project required. My mother, Angelina Wyss, who has supported me every step of my life and is the reason why I am a physician today. My grandparents and I am blessed to have two living grandparents, Mildred Cairo and Frank Wyss. My sister Jackie and her family, who have always encouraged me to share my ideas. And, last but certainly not least, my mentors—Dr. Joel DeLisa and Dr. Gerard Malanga, and my coeditor and close friend Amrish Patel.

James F. Wyss

I can only give my deepest gratitude and thanks to those who constantly supported me in the pursuit of my career and all endeavors in my life. Specifically, my deepest heartfelt thanks goes to my family, who have supported me through all my dreams, my greatest supporter and motivator, Kimberly, who has supported me through all the time and energy to make this project come to fruition. My parents, Dinu and Meena Patel, who have been my role models for life, supported and encouraged me not to give up on my dreams, which is why I became a physician, and taught me to always do what was right. Both of my sisters, Anita and Heena Patel, and their families who have taught me about life, balance, and supporting me in this project to share our thoughts and ideas. And to some of the most influential people in my life and career, my mentors Dr. Gerard Malanga, Dr. Gary Chimes, Dr. Jose Ramirez-Del Toro, and my coeditor and good friend James Wyss, without whom this project would still just be an idea that two friends and colleagues had talked about.

Amrish D. Patel

Introduction to Musculoskeletal Rehabilitation

James F. Wyss and Amrish D. Patel

Sports and musculoskeletal (MSK) medicine continues to advance at a rapid pace and currently includes more advanced imaging tools, minimally invasive surgeries, and biological therapies (e.g., platelet rich plasma) that *potentially* offer restoration or even regeneration of pathological tissues. The key word in the previous sentence is *potentially*. Therefore, we all must remember and continue to optimize the foundation of sports and MSK medicine: *the rehabilitation program.*

The rehabilitation program is designed to restore function and quality of life through the use of therapeutic modalities, manual therapies, therapeutic exercises, and patient education. When these therapies are chosen correctly, initiated at the right time, individualized to the patient, and implemented in a way to ensure patient compliance, then they offer significant potential benefit with usually minimal risk.

It is our opinion that many basic principles of MSK rehabilitation aren't always adhered to and, therefore, patient outcomes are negatively impacted. On the other hand, we are quite certain that the outcome can be positively impacted by following these basic principles. Effective communication between prescriber and provider, selection of interventions based on good clinical reasoning and support from the literature, adherence to the phases of rehabilitation, individualized treatment, and patient education that encourages compliance are a few principles that can dramatically influence patient outcome.

Effective communication between physicians and providers of rehabilitation services should occur via a detailed prescription followed by written or verbal communication after the therapists' evaluation. This creates a team or multidisciplinary approach to care and has been proven beneficial across other specialties (1,2). If this doesn't occur, many potential benefits of team care are lost. For example, the physician can often share details of the imaging findings such as the disc extrusion being foraminal in location at L4-5 as opposed to paracentral and this will influence the therapists' approach to an individualized therapeutic program.

Selection of treatment or intervention should be based on sound clinical judgment and the use of the best available evidence to support the choice. Selection of intervention can be influenced by the available resources, personal biases, and many other factors. As a result many treatments are underutilized, misused, or even abused. Freburger et al recently looked at the types of treatments provided by physical therapists to treat chronic lower back pain (CLBP) in North Carolina and they concluded that individuals who saw a physical therapist did not always receive evidence-based treatments (3).

The phases of rehabilitation are designed to gradually progress the patient from an episode of acute pain and inflammation to full range of motion (ROM), normal biomechanics and strength, and eventually restoration of function. These phases provide a stepwise approach to treatment and a way to measure progress (4). When followed properly, the patient can more predictably progress through each phase. When neglected it becomes difficult to restore ROM before swelling is reduced and strength can't be adequately restored unless pain decreases and ROM improves.

Patient education is the link between good intentions and actual success. Patient education ensures the proper use of home modalities, the safe performance of home exercises, and the prevention of reinjury. Patient education often needs to be addressed at each visit through verbal, visual, and written instruction to ensure safety and compliance. When utilized properly, patient education can improve the duration of benefit and even reduce health care costs (5). Without adequate patient education, noncompliance can occur and lead to treatment failure, even when the other principles are followed.

In the subsequent chapters of this section, we will review in further detail the basic principles of MSK rehabilitation, including the phases of MSK rehabilitation, modalities, manual therapy, therapeutic exercise, and patient education. Finally, we will conclude this section with a *guide to the principles of therapy prescription writing.* In the end, we hope that these therapeutic programs will be better designed and individualized to the patient, as prescriber and provider scientifically and artfully incorporate modalities, manual therapy, and therapeutic exercise to not only restore and optimize function, but also to prevent future injury.

REFERENCES

1. Larsson J, Stenström A, Apelqvist J, Agardh C-D. Decreasing incidence of major amputation in diabetic patients: a consequence of a multidisciplinary foot care team approach? *Diabet Med.* 1995;12:770–776. doi: 10.1111/j.1464–5491.1995.tb02078.x
2. Grady KL, Dracup K, Kennedy G, Moser DK, Piano M, Stevenson LW, et al. Team management of patients with heart failure: a statement for healthcare professionals from The Cardiovascular Nursing Council of the American Heart Association. *Circulation.* 2000;102(19):2443–2456.
3. Freburger JK, Carey TS, Holmes GM. Physical therapy for chronic low back pain in North Carolina: overuse, underuse, or misuse? *Phys Ther.* 2011;91(4):484–495.
4. Malanga GA, Ramirez-Del Toro JA, Bowen JE, Feinberg JH, Hyman GS. Sports medicine. In: Frontera RW, DeLisa JA, Gans BM, Walsh NE, Robinson LE, eds. *Delisa's Physical Medicine & Rehabilitation: Principles and Practice.* 5th ed. Philadelphia, PA: Lippincott Williams & Wilkins; 2010:1413–1436.
5. Lorig KR, Mazonson PD, Holman HR. Evidence suggesting that health education for self-management in patients with chronic arthritis has sustained health benefits while reducing health care costs. *Arthr Rheumat.* 1993;36(4):439–446.

Phases of Musculoskeletal Rehabilitation

James F. Wyss, Amrish D. Patel, and Gerard A. Malanga

INTRODUCTION

There are many examples in the literature regarding the phases of rehabilitation. There is a great deal of variability regarding the number of phases and terminology used to describe each phase. They have been applied to various medical conditions, including cardio-pulmonary and orthopedic conditions. Usually 3 to 5 phases of rehabilitation have been described in the literature. Orthopedic rehabilitation programs occasionally refer to the following three phases of tissue healing to guide rehabilitation: inflammatory, proliferative, and maturation phases. Wilk et al described four phases for rehabilitating the overhead throwing athlete. He named them acute, intermediate, advanced strengthening, and the return to activity phase (1). Paulos et al described five phases of knee rehabilitation after ACL reconstruction. In this chapter, they were named the maximum protection, moderate protection, minimum protection, return to activity, and activity/maintenance phase (2).

One fact is constant, their purpose doesn't change. They have been established to provide a safe and logical way to progress through the rehabilitation program in an attempt to restore function. The phases that we prefer using are from the chapter on Sports Medicine in Dr. Delisa's textbook of *Physical Medicine & Rehabilitation* (3). We have found them to be logical, step-wise, and clinically applicable. They are described as the phases of sports rehabilitation but they can be applied to musculoskeletal (MSK) conditions in all patient populations. We have made minor modifications to these phases (Table 2.1) and we will describe, detail, and demonstrate their clinical applicability in the remainder of this chapter.

TABLE 2.1: Phases of Rehabilitation

Phase I: Decrease pain and swelling (PRICE protocol)
Phase II: Restore ROM and normal arthrokinematics
Phase III: Strength training
Phase IV: Neuromuscular control and proprioceptive training
Phase V: Functional or sport specific training

We recommend following these phases in a fairly stepwise fashion. However, we do acknowledge the need for addressing components of overlapping phases during the rehabilitation program, but progression through a more advanced phase shouldn't supersede work on the initial phases of rehabilitation (e.g., pain control, ROM restoration). When good clinical reasoning is applied, it often makes sense to overlap parts of each phase without disregard for the overall goal of stepwise progression through the phases of MSK rehabilitation. In certain conditions, for example grade I-II lateral ankle sprains, the literature supports an early and accelerated rehabilitation program that rapidly progresses through the phases of rehabilitation (4).

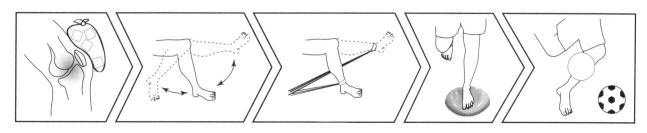

PHASE I: DECREASE PAIN AND SWELLING (PRICE PROTOCOL)

The initial phase of treatment focuses on reducing pain associated with the acute inflammatory response to injury. As far as the patient is concerned, this is often the most important phase, because pain is the reason why most seek treatment from a physician. Although a goal of decreased pain is important, the patient should be explained the full treatment program and the need to progress through all five phases of rehabilitation to prevent recurrent injuries.

During this phase, reduction of pain is important for patient comfort. Proper treatment of acute pain may in theory prevent the development of chronic pain syndromes. Inflammation needs to be controlled as opposed to eliminated, because the inflammatory response is necessary for adequate tissue healing. Inhibition of the inflammatory cascade may lead to inadequate healing of muscle tissues (5), with increased fibrosis and decreased tensile strength. The traditional way to control pain and inflammation is by applying the PRICE (protection, rest, ice, compression, and elevation) protocol. Analgesics, nonsteroidal antiinflammatory medications, electrical stimulation, or acupuncture are often used as adjunctive treatments if the PRICE protocol alone isn't sufficient.

Protection can be accomplished by methods of bracing, taping, splinting, or even in some cases casting. Protected weight bearing with an assistive device or a controlled ankle movement (CAM) walker can also be very helpful. Subsequent injury is prevented as well as significant deconditioning, because ambulation is permitted as long as the injured structure is protected. Elimination of gait aides, such as crutches, can be considered once the athlete is able to ambulate without pain and without alteration in gait.

Rest should really be approached as a period of *relative rest*. Relative rest refers to resting the injured area while allowing exercise for the remainder of the body. This can often be accomplished by utilizing aquatic therapy and/or arm cycle ergometry during lower limb injuries. As a result, cardiovascular conditioning is maintained during this period of relative rest. Prolonged immobilization of the injured area, if not required for adequate healing, should be avoided to prevent detrimental effects to muscle, tendon, and joints, such as muscle atrophy and soft tissue contracture to name a few of the negative effects that can occur with prolonged immobilization.

Ice or cryotherapy is utilized to control the inflammatory response, as well as control the pain associated with this initial inflammatory response. Examples include gel ice packs, crushed ice applications, ice baths, ice immersion, and what has become very popular are combined methods of ice and compression (e.g., Cryo cuff, Game Ready®, etc.). These methods and their rationale for use will be discussed in further detail in the chapter on Therapeutic Modalities. Initial applications are applied for 15 to 20 minutes and can be repeated every 1 to 2 hours. Expert opinion suggests application of ice for at least 48 to 72 hours post-acute soft tissue injuries, although systematic reviews have not provided definitive support for its use (6).

Compression applications are utilized to control local edema at the site of injury. Examples include Tubigrip™, ace wraps, air splints, and elastic sleeves. Local compression not only controls local edema but also provides pain control, possibly by the gate control theory.

Elevation is the remaining step in the PRICE protocol. Elevation of the injured limb above the level of the heart enhances both venous and lymphatic drainage.

Successful completion of this initial phase will allow for progression through the next two phases. Inflamed tissues or joint effusions will prevent the restoration of normal ROM in phase II. Likewise, along with inflammation, pain will inhibit muscle function and prevent the restoration of strength in phase III. Therefore, these issues must be addressed during the initial phase to allow for successful completion of the next two phases.

PHASE II: RESTORE ROM AND NORMAL BIOMECHANICS

ROM exercises and controlled mobility are initiated early to prevent the secondary effects of immobilization, including contracture formation and atrophy. Dramatic decreases in muscle mass and strength have been shown with short term bed rest (7); therefore, early motion should be encouraged to prevent these detrimental secondary effects.

Early ROM should be gentle and pain free and gradually progressed as tolerated. As the patient's pain decreases they will tolerate more aggressive ROM and stretching, which will eventually allow for full restoration of motion. Full ROM will allow for better results during the strength training phase. Strengthening can only occur within the available ROM; therefore, if ROM is restricted strength gains will be limited, which may affect the functional outcome. Restricted ROM may lead to increased joint forces across specific parts of the articulating surfaces, and in theory may lead to focal degenerative changes.

Biomechanical analysis is another important component of this phase. Pain and restricted joint motions will alter normal movement patterns. For example, subacromial impingement syndromes may lead to decreased shoulder abduction and altered scapulothoracic joint motion (8), including increased upward rotation and elevation of the scapula. If these abnormal movement patterns are not corrected during this phase, it may lead to abnormal movement patterns and abnormal tissue loading that becomes very difficult to correct via neuromuscular reeducation exercises. Persistence of these altered movement patterns can lead to muscle imbalances, recurrent injury, or a different MSK condition.

PHASE III: STRENGTH TRAINING

We strongly discourage any aggressive strength training prior to significant improvements in pain and inflammation control. Persistent pain can lead to altered movement patterns, muscle inhibition, and will reinforce abnormal biomechanics. Restricted ROM will only allow for strengthening within this limited range. This will prevent full return of strength and may lead to decreased muscle length further preventing full restoration of ROM. For these reasons, strength training is usually limited to isometric exercises during the early rehabilitation phases. The primary goal of isometric exercise is to prevent extensive muscle atrophy (9) without aggravating the existing condition. Some authors have suggested the use of electrical stimulation with or without isometrics to prevent muscle atrophy during periods of rest (10). Progression to isotonic strengthening exercises within a pain free range, usually mid-range, is an appropriate choice early on in phase III. Isotonic resistance training throughout the full ROM begins when it is well tolerated. The exercises are also performed in a single plane and only progressed to multiple planes when the patient has made strength gains. Usually low weight, high repetition isotonic strengthening is recommended initially, stressing proper technique throughout the entire range of motion.

Closed kinetic chain (CKC) exercises often begin early during phase III, often before open chain exercises (OKC) (11). Once weight bearing is permitted and tolerated, CKC exercises mimic functional tasks and are a more functional way to rehabilitate lower limb injuries. Some studies have shown that CKC exercises produce less shear forces across specific joints, such as the knee (12); therefore, minisquats are usually begun prior to OKC knee extensions. CKC exercises also mimic functional tasks because they can provide resistance training in multiple planes of motion and activate multiple muscle groups along the entire limb. Upper limb injuries are more commonly rehabilitated through OKC exercises but CKC exercises have gained popularity. CKC exercises

appear to be good choices for scapular stability (13) and provide needed proprioceptive input following injury. As strength gains occur, a gradual shift in the rehabilitation focus toward neuromuscular control, proprioceptive exercises, and progressive functional exercises should occur.

PHASE IV: NEUROMUSCULAR CONTROL AND PROPRIOCEPTIVE TRAINING

Neuromuscular training exercises are designed to restore the normal timing patterns of muscular recruitment and to provide adequate control or coordination of muscle activation across the joint. For example, proprioceptive neuromuscular facilitation (PNF) principles recommend the development of proximal stability prior to distal mobility (14). In the rehabilitation of an upper limb injury, this means that trunk and scapular control must be accomplished prior to the practice of upper limb tasks, such as throwing. This component of rehabilitation requires hands on treatment and patient instruction using multiple sensory cues to accomplish improved neuromuscular control. Sensory cues include visual (e.g., mirror) and tactile (e.g., muscle tapping) cues. Occasionally physical modalities such as neuromuscular electrical stimulation and biofeedback are utilized to accomplish this goal.

The definition of proprioception is often debated, but in this textbook we will define it as a subcortical control of joint movement and positioning. Proprioceptive abilities become impaired after joint injuries and with degenerative joint conditions (15). Rehabilitation of this system should be restored in an attempt to decrease the risk of reinjury. This can be accomplished through the use of balance training exercises, such as wobble board training, single leg stance activities, or "ball on wall" activities for the upper limb. As neuromuscular control and proprioception improves, the rehabilitation program can shift toward the final phase: functional or sport specific training.

PHASE V: FUNCTIONAL OR SPORT SPECIFIC TRAINING

The final phase begins when all prior phases have been successfully completed. Then in a gradual, stepwise fashion parts of the patient's functional activities (ADL's, work or sports activities) are recreated in the gym environment. Tasks are broken down into specific components, and then put together as the patient masters each part of the task. For example, the ability to stair climb can start with achieving balance with single leg stance activities, weight shift in single leg stance, then progress to advancing the contralateral limb while balancing on the ipsilateral lower limb. Finally as these movement patterns are put together, the patient will be able to complete the functional task of ascending a flight of steps. This task is then practiced until it is mastered. Descending the stairs is an entirely different task, requiring significant eccentric muscle activation. Therefore, it too must be broken down into similar smaller movements, then combined and then practiced. If the functional activity the patient is returning to is a sport, then plyometric exercises are often essential to mimic components of the sport, such as line or box jumping to mimic defensive tasks and rebounding in basketball.

When the patient has completed all five phases of rehabilitation and their functional tasks are pain free, then they have completed their rehabilitation program. Return to play criteria should also be considered and would include no pain, full and symmetric ROM; normal and symmetric strength and ability to perform the tasks required for the patient's activities or sport in the controlled environment. Patient education on the importance of a continued home exercise program (HEP) becomes very important for maintenance and prevention of reinjury. This topic will be discussed in a subsequent chapter on Patient Education.

SUMMARY

The phases of MSK, sports or functional rehabilitation, as outlined in the chapter, are one of the most important principles in the nonoperative treatment of orthopedic conditions and injuries. These phases must be clearly understood prior to supervising a rehabilitation program. Treatment success is far more likely if they are followed in this stepwise logical approach. Therapists, athletic trainers, and physicians should monitor progress and expect progression through these phases to guide patients during their recovery from injury. Although a stepwise approach is recommended, we acknowledge the need for addressing components in overlapping phases during rehabilitation, such as the use of isometric strengthening exercises to prevent extensive muscle atrophy during phase II or the introduction of low level proprioceptive and neuromuscular control exercises during phase III. If the clinician applies sound reasoning and a solid understanding of the tissue healing response, it often makes sense to overlap certain phases while appreciating the patient's stepwise progression through the phases of this suggested functional rehabilitation approach.

REFERENCES

1. Wilk KE, Meister K, Andrews JR. Current concepts in the rehabilitation of the overhead throwing athlete. *Am J Sports Med.* 2002;30(1):136–151.
2. Paulos L, Noyes FR, Grood E, Butler DL. Knee rehabilitation after anterior cruciate ligament reconstruction and repair. *Am J Sports Med.* 1981;9(3):140–149.
3. Malanga GA, Ramirez-Del Toro JA, Bowen JE, Feinberg JH, Hyman GS. Sports medicine. In: Frontera RW, DeLisa JA, Gans BM, Walsh NE, Robinson LE, eds. *Delisa's Physical Medicine & Rehabilitation: Principles and Practice.* 5th ed. Philadelphia, PA: Lippincott Williams & Wilkins, 2010:1413–1436.
4. Bleakley CM, O'Connor SR, Tully MA, Rocke LG, Macauley DC, Bradbury, I et al. Effect of accelerated rehabilitation on function after ankle sprain: randomised controlled trial. *BMJ.* 2010;340:c1964. doi: 10.1136/bmj.c1964
5. Shen W, Li Y, Tang YY, Cummins J, Huard J. NS-398, a cyclooxygenase-2-specific inhibitor, delays skeletal muscle healing by decreasing regeneration and promoting fibrosis. *Am J Pathol.* 2005;167(4):1105–1117.
6. Bleakley C, McDonough S, MacAuley D. The use of ice in the treatment of acute soft-tissue injury: a systematic review of randomized controlled trials. *Am J Sports Med.* 2004;32(1):251–261.
7. Bloomfield SA. Changes in musculoskeletal structure and function with prolonged bed rest. *Med Sci Sports Exerc.* 1997;29(2):197–206.
8. Graichen H, Stammberger T, Bonél H, Wiedemann E, Englmeier KH, Reiser M, et al. Three-dimensional analysis of shoulder girdle and supraspinatus motion patterns in patients with impingement syndrome. *J Orthop Res.* 2001;19(6):1192–1198.
9. Akima H, Kubo K, Imai M, Kanehisa H, Suzuki Y, Gunji A, et al. Inactivity and muscle: effect of resistance training during bed rest on muscle size in the lower limb. *Acta Physiol Scand.* 2001;172(4):269–278.
10. Gibson JN, Smith K, Rennie MJ. Prevention of disuse muscle atrophy by means of electrical stimulation: maintenance of protein synthesis. *Lancet.* 1988;2(8614):767–770.
11. Karandikar N, Vargas O. Kinetic Chains: A review of the concept and its clinical application. *PMR.* 2011;3(8):739-745.
12. Lutz GE, Palmitier RA, An KN, Chao EY. Comparison of tibiofemoral joint forces during open-kinetic-chain and closed-kinetic-chain exercises. *J Bone Joint Surg Am.* 1993;75(5):732–739.
13. Kibler WB, McMullen J. Scapular dyskinesis and its relation to shoulder pain. *J Am Acad Orthop Surg.* 2003;11(2):142–151.
14. Voss DE. Proprioceptive neuromuscular facilitation. *Am J Phys Med.* 1967;46(1):838–899.
15. Jerosch J, Prymka M. Proprioception and joint stability. *Knee Surg Sports Traumatol Arthrosc.* 1996;4(3):171–179.

Therapeutic Modalities

Brite Chalunkal, Ashey Varughese, and Joseph Feinberg

INTRODUCTION

Therapeutic or physical modalities are agents used to create a therapeutic response in tissues. Modalities can serve as an integral part of a comprehensive treatment plan for any musculoskeletal (MSK) disorder. This chapter will briefly review several modalities commonly utilized in MSK rehabilitation along with their associated indications, precautions, and contraindications. Thermotherapy, hydrotherapy, electrotherapy, and light therapy will be the major types of modalities reviewed. In addition, some new and emerging modalities will be briefly discussed.

MODALITY PRESCRIPTION

Prescriptions for the use of any modality should include the following information: patient's identifying factors (e.g., name, date of birth), diagnosis, relevant past medical history (PMH) and associated precautions, specific modality, location, intensity, duration, and frequency of use. These components of therapeutic modalities should be included when prescribed as part of a comprehensive therapeutic prescription. Therapy based prescription writing is explained in further detail in the chapter titled Guide to Therapy Prescription Writing.

Thermotherapy

A common question that will be posed to a clinician treating MSK pain will be whether to use ice or heat at the site of pain. A general rule to apply is that any acute injury (24–72 hours) would benefit from cold applications to decrease inflammation, and pain; while heat would be beneficial to promote extensibility of tissues and to treat chronic pain after the inflammation and pain associated with the initial injury has resolved (1). This clinical rule is based on expert opinion and the knowledge of the inflammatory cascade that results from tissue injury.

Cryotherapy

Most types of cryotherapy, also known as the therapeutic use of cold modalities, are superficial in nature and usually transfer thermal energy via the principle of conduction. The most common types of cold modalities include cold packs, ice massage, cold water immersion, cryotherapy compression units, vapocoolant spray, and whirlpool baths (2). Relative contraindications or precautions for cryotherapy include impaired sensation, Raynaud's disease and other cryopathies, arterial insufficiency, cognitive or communication deficits, and cold hypersensitivity (3,4). Cryotherapy should be used acutely after injury or posttherapeutic exercise to reduce tissue inflammation and swelling. Cryotherapy can also be used in myofascial pain syndrome, postsurgically, and in the management of spasticity (5). Monitoring the skin closely with application of cryotherapy is a must, especially in patients who may suffer from sensory deficits.

Cold Packs

Ice packs, endothermic chemical gel packs, and hydrocollator packs are all types of cold packs. Ice packs are easily used at home and are reasonably priced. Endothermic chemical gel packs have compounds of water and ammonium nitrate that when mixed undertake a heat absorbing reaction. Hydrocollator packs are cooled in the freezer to −12°C and applied with a towel as the barrier between the area of skin and the hydrocollator pack. Cold packs and ice packs can cool skin to 5°C at 2 cm of depth (6).

Treatment application typically lasts 20 to 30 minutes and can be repeated every 1 to 2 hours for management of acute pain and swelling.

Ice Massage

Ice massage is the direct application of ice to the affected area of the skin using tender stroking motions. This treatment includes the therapeutic effects of cooling combined with the mechanical effects of massage. Ice massage is generally used for localized symptoms and applied for 5 to 10 minutes per site. Initially the patient will feel coolness followed by burning or aching and finally numbness. This type of cryotherapy is commonly used by athletes post-training after sustaining local injury or tissue inflammation. This technique has been demonstrated to be *not* effective for the treatment of postexercise delayed onset muscle soreness (DOMS) (7).

Cold Water Immersion

Immersion in cold water is best suited for circumferential cooling of the limbs. Cold water immersion is believed to boost immune function, decrease inflammation and pain, and increase blood flow and metabolic rate. Typically temperatures from 5 to 13°C help attain these results. Cold water immersion is utilized in athletic settings as well but studies to date are poor to determine if cold water immersion prevents postexercise DOMS (8).

Cryotherapy Compression Units

Cryotherapy compression units include a cuff through which water is circulated and can be pneumatically compressed statically or in a sequential, distal to proximal pumping action (9). This type of therapy combines the use of ice and compression and is typically used in the treatment of acute MSK injury with soft tissue swelling, and occasionally after a number of surgical procedures. Temperatures of 7°C and pressures up to 60 mmHg are used (10). This modality may play a very important role in the early phases of rehabilitation to reduce pain and swelling.

Vapocoolant Spray

Vapocoolant spray can be used to treat myofascial and MSK pain syndromes, although it remains an unproven treatment modality for these conditions. The technique includes a series of unidirectional applications of Fluori-Methane spray. Treatment is initiated at the "trigger area" and expands over the area of referred pain while passively stretching the involved muscle. The precautions of vapocoolant spray include general cold precautions and avoidance of skin freezing (11).

HEAT MODALITIES

Heat can be classified by depth of penetration and by form of heat transfer. Superficial heating modalities include hot packs, heating pads, paraffin baths, fluidotherapy, whirlpool baths, and radiant heat. Deep heating modalities include ultrasound, short wave, and microwave diathermy. Mechanisms of heat transfer include conduction, convection, radiation, evaporation, and conversion (12). Caution should be advised when using heat modalities on those with vascular insufficiency or decreased sensation. General precaution for heat therapy must be taken in pregnant, pediatric, and geriatric populations. Also, precaution must be taken when using heat in proximity to metal implants or open wounds. General contraindications for heat therapy include ischemia of the extremity, bleeding disorders, impaired sensation, malignancy, dementia, poor thermal regulation, and acute inflammation (5).

Superficial Heating Modalities

Superficial heating modalities achieve their greatest tissue temperatures in the skin and subcutaneous fat, usually 1 to 2 cm in depth and are usually utilized in the setting of subacute and chronic injuries to treat pain, muscle spasm, and joint stiffness. Heat applications dilate the blood vessels causing vasodilatation; this process increases the flow of oxygen and nutrients to the desired area, theoretically helping to heal and restore the damaged tissue. Hydrocollator packs, heating pads, chemical packs, radiant heat, fluidotherapy, and paraffin baths are all examples of superficial heating agents (13).

This type of heat is used most often in patients who suffer from arthritis (especially osteoarthritis), neck pain, low back pain, myofascial pain syndromes, and an assortment of other MSK disorders (14). They may allow for muscle relaxation and help with joint stiffness that can allow patients to better participate in their therapeutic exercise program. Additional precautions and advice include allowing patients to lie on the hot pack because these modalities may also lead to sedation, prolonged treatment, and subsequent burns.

Hydrocollator Packs

Hydrocollator packs are traditionally silica filled packs that are heated by immersing them into a hydrocollator at which the temperature is approximately 75°C. They are then applied to the desired body part with a cover and appropriate number of towels for insulation and to prevent burns to the treated tissues. After several minutes of heating, the superficial skin must be inspected to ensure that the temperature is suitable for the individual patient. Total heating treatment time is generally between 15 to 30 minutes depending on the body part, patient's tolerance, and depth of desired penetration. Patients should always be supervised when the hot pack is being used, due to common causes of burns from improper usage, limited sensation, and increase in treatment time (15). Hot packs can be prescribed prior to initiation of therapy to allow for improved joint and soft tissue mobility and improved participation in the therapeutic exercise program.

Heating Pads

There are two main types of heating pads: circulating and electric fluid pads. Circulating fluid heating pads usually control heat output thermostatically, whereas an electric heating pad typically controls heat output by regulating current flow. When using heating pads, general heat precautions must be observed as with all forms of heat therapy.

Fluidotherapy

Fluidotherapy is a dry and superficial heating agent that uses convection heating. The desired extremity is placed in a fluidotherapy machine while the solid-gas system behaves like a heterogeneous fluid of low viscosity, allowing the freedom to perform range of motion (ROM) exercises (16). The typical temperatures range from 46°C to 49°C. Both the agitation and temperature can be adjusted. Appropriate length of treatment and observation by a therapist is important to avoid any heat related injuries. A contraindication to this type of therapy would be an open or infected wound (17).

Paraffin Baths

With this method, paraffin wax and mineral oil are mixed in a 6:1 ratio. The treatment temperatures typically range from 52°C to 54°C and heat transfer occurs by conduction. Paraffin baths are typically indicated to decrease pain, relax muscle, and stimulate blood circulation and is commonly used to treat individuals who suffer from osteoarthritis (OA), especially of the hand, rheumatoid arthritis, scleroderma, and/or stretching a scar or adhesion prior to performing a mobilization technique. The different methods of application include dipping, immersion, and brushing. Immersion provides the greatest quantity and duration of temperature increase, while brushing can be especially useful in areas that are difficult to immerse. Exercise in combination with this therapy will augment its effectiveness. Contraindications to this therapy include: impaired skin sensation, open skin/wounds, infections, cancerous regions, circulatory dysfunction, and lack of comprehension.

DEEP HEATING MODALITIES

Examples of deep heating modalities include ultrasound, microwave, and shortwave diathermy. They provide a greater depth of heating, reported to be up to 3 to 5 cm, which may improve the extensibility of deeper structures like joint capsule and ligaments.

Ultrasound

Ultrasound is a treatment modality which utilizes low and high frequency sound waves to promote tissue healing and/or relief in painful joints and muscles. The frequencies used for treatment range from 1 MHz (deeper) to 3 MHz (more superficial heating effects), while the intensity ranges from 0.5 to 2.0 W/cm^2 (18). A simple rule of thumb is the greater the frequency, the shallower the depth of penetration and heat development.

Temperatures of up to 46°C can be achieved in deep tissues with ultrasound therapy. Ultrasound should be administered using gentle, circular motions, and the treatment typically lasts 5 to 10 minutes per treatment area. The patient will often report feeling a tingling sensation and/or mild heat production. If the ultrasound head is not moved during treatment, intense heating will be felt and there is potential to develop a burn injury. As with other heating modalities, ultrasound can potentially help relieve pain and inflammation, reduce muscle spasms, and accelerate healing. The treatment can also improve connective tissue extensibility, but for a short duration, therefore, ROM and stretching exercises should be performed immediately after treatment. Precautions for ultrasound include: general heat precautions and avoidance of use near a pacemaker, brain, spine, eyes (or any hollow organ), or reproductive organs, malignancy, and skeletal immaturity (19).

Phonophoresis is another way to utilize ultrasound to improve the delivery of topically applied medications such as analgesics and antiinflammatory agents. Conditions commonly treated with phonophoresis include bursitis and tendonitis. Evidence for use of this modality is very limited in the literature.

Diathermy

Shortwave or microwave diathermy are rarely utilized in current clinical practice, but they deserve historical mention and description. Both shortwave and microwave diathermy utilize conversion as its principal form of heat production. Shortwave diathermy commonly uses a frequency of 27.12 MHz while microwave diathermy ranges from 915 MHz and 2456 MHz. The lower frequency has the advantage of increased depth of penetration; however, it also has the disadvantage of greater beam distribution and the requirement of larger applicators (20). General heat precautions apply for this modality and use must be avoided over metal implants, pacemakers, skeletal immaturity, brain and reproductive organs, and fluid-filled cavities (21). Microwave has also been linked to the development of cataracts and is no longer being sold as a therapeutic modality, whereas shortwave diathermy is occasionally found in clinics.

Hydrotherapy

Hydrotherapy is the external application of hot or cold water, in any form, in order to treat an illness. Whirlpool baths, Hubbard tanks, shower cart, and contrast baths are the major forms of hydrotherapy. Primarily, these therapies are used in the treatment of arthritis, an assortment of MSK conditions, as well as in the cleaning and debridement of burns and further dermal injuries (22). Hydrotherapy use in therapy

clinics has been limited secondary to lack of evidence in the literature and potential for cross contamination with patient use.

Whirlpool baths and Hubbard tanks

The whirlpool is most frequently used to accomplish a superficial change in tissue temperature by manipulating water temperature and agitation by aeration, dispersing thermal energy by convection. Whirlpool baths are produced in a variety of sizes and are utilized for treating a limb or localized lesion. Hubbard tanks are larger and can accommodate entire body immersion (22). Both the whirlpool and the Hubbard tank can provide relief of pain, increase in ROM, as well as relaxation. As a general rule, the water temperature should not surpass 38°C, nor should the temperature be less than 10°C. Cross contamination and auto contamination are some of the risks involved when using a whirlpool bath and/or Hubbard tank (22).

Contrast baths

Contrast baths entail alternating immersion of the distal limb in cold and then hot water, with a gradual increase in the temperature gradient that is guided by patient tolerance. Cold temperatures vary from 8°C to 12°C, whereas hot temperatures vary from 42°C to 45°C. Cyclic vasoconstriction and vasodilatation is produced by the temperature extremes. On average the treatment session lasts approximately 30 minutes. This treatment is beneficial in individuals suffering from neuropathic pain, rheumatologic disease, complex regional pain syndrome, and other chronic pain syndromes (22).

ELECTROTHERAPY

Introduction

Although the details of the physiology of electrical current are beyond the scope of this chapter, it is important to understand a couple of key concepts that will be discussed in this section. The modality of electrical stimulation is commonly applied in four different ways: the peripheral nerve can be stimulated for muscle activity, the central nerves can be stimulated for muscle activity, the skin can be stimulated to promote wound healing, and finally the central and peripheral fibers can be stimulated to modify the sensory pain fibers (23).

Neuromuscular Electrical Stimulation

Activating muscles using the peripheral nerve stimulation is also known as neuromuscular electrical stimulation (NMES). In order for NMES to work, the axon of the peripheral nerve must be intact. Unlike physiological nerve fiber stimulation, external induction of muscle contraction requires 100 to 1000 times the stimulation to reach threshold. It is also important to note that the threshold to reach stimulation with an externally applied current is inversely proportional to the nerve fiber diameter (24).

NMES systems are composed of a power source, electrodes, and a stimulator (25). The system typically utilizes a pulsed wave form setting, which can be adjusted for amplitude and duration. The electrodes are either placed externally on the skin, or internally near the target nerve structure. The NMES system has been shown to be effective in the upper limb as a neuroprosthesis, improving motor recovery by enhancing cortical plasticity, and in treatment of poststroke shoulder pain. NMES has also been used in the lower limbs to primarily enhance standing and walking (10).

Transcutaneous Electrical Nerve Stimulation

A transcutaneous electrical nerve stimulation (TENS) unit consists of signal generators, a battery, and a set of electrodes. The TENS unit can produce variable stimuli with adjustments of strengths, pulse rates, and pulse widths. The waveform is generally biphasic and the typical pulse rate is set between 70 to 100 Hertz, or as low as 1 to 10 Hertz if the stimulus is set high. The amplitude and current are set at a low intensity level, just above sensory threshold and to comfort. The pulse width is set between 10 to 1000 microseconds (26).

Patients are instructed to adjust the TENS at different frequencies and intensities to determine the best pain control. Although the optimal settings are subjective and are determined by trial and error, electrode positioning is quite important. The leads are most effective when placed surrounding the site of pain (27).

TENS can be utilized under two different settings: conventional or burst mode, also known as acupuncture like TENS. In a conventional TENS setting, the frequency is set high (50–120 Hz), with low intensity and short pulse duration (50 microseconds). In patients who do not respond to conventional setting, another option is the acupuncture setting. This setting involves producing a low frequency stimulus at 5 to 10 Hz at a high intensity, close to the patient's tolerance. With the burst or pulsed TENS setting high frequency bursts of low-intensity stimuli are used. The frequency of impulses within each burst is at 100 Hz, with recurrent bursts discharge at 2 to 3 Hz. This setting may be trialed when someone accommodates to and no longer experiences significant pain relief with conventional TENS.

Indications for TENS include treatment of neurogenic pain, pain from reflex sympathetic dystrophy, postherpetic neuralgia, trigeminal neuralgia, atypical facial pain, and pain after spinal cord injury (SCI). It can also be used to treat MSK pain such as joint pain from rheumatoid arthritis and OA, as well as acute postoperative pain. Studies have shown that TENS is effective in treating diabetic neuropathy (28). Reports have shown that TENS treatment can also assist patients in regaining motor function following a stroke, decrease nausea, and is effective treating post fracture pain (23).

Contraindications to TENS or electrical stimulation include avoiding use in patients with a pacemaker, automated internal cardiac defibrillator, or during pregnancy as it is theorized to possibly induce premature labor. The TENS leads should *not* be placed over the following areas: the carotid sinuses due to the risk of acute hypotension through a vasovagal reflex; over the anterior neck because of risk of laryngospasm; nor over an area of sensory impairment, where the possibility of sustaining a burn exists. Particular caution must be used when using TENS units in patients with a spinal cord stimulator or any intrathecal pump (29).

Interferential Current Therapy

Interferential current therapy (IFC) is a modality that utilizes two alternating current signals of slightly different frequencies and is presumed to create an "interference" or summated wave pattern at the intersection of the two sinusoidal waveforms. IFC has been used in the treatment of neurologic and MSK conditions, and the management of urinary incontinence, though limited evidence is available. Precautions include not using IFC close to or around implanted stimulators, understand the potential for vascular responses when used near the sympathetic ganglia or the carotid sinus. IFC should not be used near any open incisions or abrasions, in the presence of venous thrombosis, near the gravid uterus, insensate areas, or on a patient cognitively impaired (30).

Iontophoresis

Iontophoresis treatments are utilized to deliver medications directly to the patient through their skin with the use of an electric current (31). This modality is known as a transdermal delivery system in which a substance bearing a charge is driven through the skin by a low electrical current (32). Local anesthetics, corticosteroids, analgesics, and antibiotics are some of the medications that are used in conjunction with iontophoresis. Treatment involves use of a controller as well as an electrode that is applied to the patient's affected skin region (33). The ionic solution is placed on the electrode of the identical polarity, and then the negative, positive, and ground electrodes are then applied to the skin. A direct current typically between 10 to 30 mA is applied to force the solution away from the electrode and into adjacent tissues. Bursitis and tendonitis are conditions commonly treated with iontophoresis in PT clinics and plantar fasciitis has been shown to respond favorably to iontophoresis with or without other modalities (34).

LIGHT THERAPY

Low-Energy Laser Therapy

Low-energy laser therapy, also known as low power, low level, or cold laser therapy, involves light amplification by stimulated production of radiation. It is a form of concentrated focal light therapy that delivers nominal energies between 1 and 4 Joules (35). This modality does not produce significant tissue temperature changes and therefore the physiological effects are nonthermal. Laser therapy has been utilized clinically to enhance would healing, bone healing, and soft tissue healing. Further research is required to determine the most appropriate clinical uses for laser therapy.

EMERGING MODALITIES

Besides laser therapy, other modalities have gained increased clinical use and interest. One example is extracorporeal shockwave therapy.

Extracorporeal Shockwave Therapy

This treatment can now be applied in a low energy form, in the office without anesthesia. Extracorporeal shockwave therapy (ESWT) had been clinically applied to common MSK conditions such as Achilles tendinopathy and plantar fasciitis. Studies have revealed mixed results and will be further discussed in certain condition specific chapters of this book.

SUMMARY

Therapeutic or physical modalities are an integral part of the treatment of MSK disorders, even though evidence to support their use is limited. It is, however, widely accepted (expert opinion) that therapeutic modalities can provide significant symptomatic relief and allow patients to participate more effectively in their therapeutic exercise program. There is a critical need for well-designed randomized controlled studies to determine the quantitative effects and to provide evidence-based support for their routine use in clinical practice. Future research will hopefully guide the appropriate use of these therapeutic modalities.

REFERENCES

1. Abramson DI, Chu LSW, Tuck S, et al. Effect of tissue temperatures and blood flow on motor nerve conduction velocity. *JAMA.* 1966;198:1082–1088.
2. Bell KR, Lehmann JF. Effect of cooling on H- and T-reflexes in normal subjects. *Arch Phys Med Rehabil.* 1987;68:490–493.
3. Clarke DH, Stelmach GE. Muscular fatigue and recovery curve parameters at various temperatures. *Res Q.* 1966;37:468–479.
4. Melzack R, Jeans ME, Stratford JG, et al. Ice massage and transcutaneous electrical stimulation: comparison of treatment for low-back pain. *Pain.* 1980;9:209–217.
5. Ciolek JJ. Cryotherapy. Review of physiological effects and clinical application. *Cleve Clin Q.* 1985;52(2):193–201.
6. Elliott J. New technique measures depth, extent of cryotherapy *JAMA.* 1979;242(6):505.
7. Howatson G, Van Someren KA. Ice massage. Effects on exercise-induced muscle damage. *J Sports Med Phys Fitness.* 2003;43(4):500-505.
8. Bleakley C, McDonough S, Gardner E, Baxter GD, Hopkins JT, Davison GW. Cold-water immersion (cryotherapy) for preventing and treating muscle soreness after exercise. *Cochrane Database Syst Rev.* 2012;2:CD008262.
9. Ritzmann SE, Levin WC. Cryopathies: a review. *Arch Intern Med.* 1961;107:186–204.
10. Sheffler LR, Chae J. Neuromuscular electrical stimulation in neurorehabilitation. *Muscle Nerve.* 2007;35(5):562–590.
11. Lowdon BJ, Moore RJ. Determinants and nature of intramuscular temperature changes during cold therapy. *Am J Phys Med.* 1975;54:223–233.

12. Borell RM, Henley EJ, Ho P, et al. Fluidotherapy: evaluation of a new heat modality. *Arch Phys Med Rehabil.* 1977;58:69–71.

13. Lehmann JF, Masock AJ, Warren CG, et al. Effect of therapeutic temperatures on tendon extensibility. *Arch Phys Med Rehabil.* 1970;51:481–487.

14. Robertson V, Ward A, Jung P. The effect of heat on tissue extensibility: a comparison of deep and superficial heating. *Arch Phys Med Rehabil.* 2005;86:819–825.

15. Lehmann JF, DeLateur BJ, Warren CG, et al. Therapeutic temperature distribution produced by ultrasound as modified by dosage and volume of tissue exposed. *Arch Phys Med Rehabil.* 1967;48:662–666.

16. Henley E. Fluidotherapy. *Crit Rev Phys Med Rehabil.* 1991;3:173–195.

17. Shulman AG. Ice water as primary treatment of burns. *JAMA.* 1960;173:96–99.

18. Hekkenberg RT, Oosterbaan WA, vanBeekum WT. Evaluation of ultrasound therapy devices. *Physiotherapy.* 1986;72:390–394.

19. Thornton KL. Principles of ultrasound. *J Reprod Med.* 1992;37:27–32.

20. Docker M, Bazin S, Dyson M, et al. Guidelines for the safe use of continuous shortwave therapy equipment. *Physiotherapy.* 1992;78:755–757.

21. Draper D, Castro J, Feland B, et al. Shortwave diathermy and prolonged stretching increase hamstring flexibility more than prolonged stretching alone. *J Orthop Sports Phys Ther.* 2004;34:13–20.

22. Woodmansey A, Collins DH, Ernst MM. Vascular reactions to the contrast bath in health and in rheumatoid arthritis. *Lancet.* 1938;2:1350–1353.

23. Ada L, Foonghchomcheay A. Efficacy of electrical stimulation in preventing or reducing subluxation of the shoulder after stroke: a meta-analysis. *Aust J Physiother.* 2002;48:257–267.

24. Gedes LA, Baker LE, ed. *Principles of Applied Biomedical Instrumentation,* 3rd ed. New York, NY: John Wiley and Sons; 1989.

25. Jones DA, Bigland-Ritchie B, Edwards RH. Excitation frequency and muscle fatigue: mechanical responses during voluntary and stimulated contractions. *Exp Neurol.* 1979;64(2):401–413.

26. Shribner WJ, ed. *A Manual of Electrotherapy.* 4th ed. Philadelphia, PA: Lea and Febiger; 1975.

27. Solomonow M. External control of the neuromuscular system. *IEEE Trans Biomed Eng.* 1984;31(12):752–763.

28. Hamza MA, White PF, Craig WF, et al. Percutaneous electrical nerve stimulation: a novel analgesic therapy for diabetic neuropathic pain. *Diabetes Care.* 2000;23(3):365–370.

29. Howson DC. Peripheral neural excitability. Implications for transcutaneous electrical nerve stimulation. *Phys Ther.* 1978;58(12):1467–1473.

30. Kloth LC. Interference current. In: Nelson RM, Currier DP, ed. *Clinical electrotherapy,* 2nd ed. Norwalk, CT: Appleton & Lange; 1991:34–35.

31. Li LC, Scudds RA. Iontophoresis: an overview of the mechanisms and clinical application. *Arthritis Care Res.* 1995;8(1):51–61.

32. Costello CT, Jeske AH. Iontophoresis: application in transdermal medication delivery. *Phys Ther.* 1995;75(6):554–563.

33. Banga A, Panus P. Clinical applications of ionophoretic devices in rehabilitation medicine. *Crit Rev Phys Med Rehabil.* 1998;10:147–179.

34. Gudeman SD, Eisele SA, Heidt RS Jr, Colosimo AJ, Stroupe AL. Treatment of plantar fasciitis by iontophoresis of 0.4% dexamethasone. A randomized, double-blind, placebo-controlled study. *Am J Sports Med.* 1997;25(3):312–316.

35. Schindl A, Schindl M, Pernerstofer-Schon H, et al. Low-intensity laser therapy: a review. *J Invest Med.* 2000;48:312–326.

Manual Therapy

Phong Kieu and Terrence G. McGee

OVERVIEW OF MANUAL THERAPY

The most simplistic definition of manual therapy is the use of hands to apply a force with a therapeutic intent (1). The common uses of manual therapy are to treat a variety of musculoskeletal conditions. The therapeutic force may be applied using various techniques described in this chapter and includes manipulations, massage, and traction. The specific techniques used and the philosophies behind them vary according to the different professions who use manual therapy including, but not limited to, chiropractors, osteopathic physicians, and physical therapists.

Historically, the origins of manual therapy can be traced back to parallel developments in many different civilizations during ancient times. The Old Testament was the first to describe it as "the laying of hands" to heal. Hippocrates (BC 460–385), the father of modern medicine, was the first to describe the use of prone traction to treat scoliosis (2). Manual therapy expanded and became a cornerstone in the treatment of musculoskeletal disorders through the centuries. In the late 18th century, practitioners of manual therapy and contemporary medicine began emphasizing pharmacological approaches (2,3). Bonesetters and other practitioners of manual therapy clashed with contemporary allopathic medicine leading to a separation of the two.

During the late 19th century in the United States of America, Dr. Andrew Still and Daniel David Palmer founded osteopathic and chiropractic medicine respectively. In the 1920s Dr. James Mennell and physiotherapist Edgar Cyriax became engrossed in the use of manual therapy in orthopedic medicine (1–3). Later, their sons would be instrumental in establishing manipulation of joints and soft tissues as a foundational skill for physical therapists (1–3). Today, there are diverse specialists who have incorporated manual therapy into their practice with different techniques employing various philosophies. For the purposes of this chapter, we will focus on techniques commonly used by physical therapists, although the following techniques are commonly utilized by others who practice manual medicine (e.g., chiropractors, osteopathic physicians, massage therapists).

JOINT MOBILIZATIONS

Joint mobilization techniques include a broad spectrum, from the general passive motions performed in the physiologic cardinal planes at any point in the range, to the semi-specific and specific accessory (arthrokinematic) joint glides, or joint distractions, initiated from the open-packed position of the joint (4). Considered to be the "cornerstone" of most rehabilitation programs, these techniques can be used to improve tissue extensibility, increase range of motion (ROM), induce relaxation, mobilize/manipulate soft tissue and joints, modulate pain, and to reduce swelling and inflammation.

Different grading systems exist for joint mobilizations and include those for traction, sustained holds, and oscillatory techniques; however, the most widespread system is that used for describing the oscillatory technique proposed by Maitland. This system has five grades (4,5):

- Grade I—slow, small amplitude movements performed at the beginning of the range (pain relieving)
- Grade II—slow, large amplitude movements performed that do not reach the limit of the range (pain relieving)
- Grade III—slow, large amplitude movements performed up to the limit of the range (stretch)
- Grade IV—slow, small amplitude movements performed at the limit of the range (stretch)
- Grade V—high velocity, small amplitude (thrust) movements performed beyond the pathologic limit. (*Joint Manipulation or HVLA*)

Much attention as of late has been made to the immediate effects of *joint manipulation*, and as such, this section will focus primarily on the proposed effects, indications, contraindications, and literature review of this technique.

Although Grade V or joint manipulation techniques share similarities with Grade IV in terms of amplitude and direction, it is the velocity at which the technique is employed that sets them apart. There are several proposed effects by which joint manipulations are thought to aid in the restoration of joint play or gliding. Mechanical effects include the restoration of joint play, the snapping of adhesions, and altering of positional relationships. Neurophysiologic effects on pain have also been proposed. Type III mechanoreceptors are stimulated by joint manipulation, which in turn provides reflex inhibition of muscles. Additionally, joint manipulations are thought to modulate pain via the Gate Control Theory. Finally, as mentioned earlier in describing manual therapy, the "laying of hands" provides confidence and assurance to the patient that something good will result. The psychological effects are not why manipulations are performed, but they should be considered (6–8).

Joint manipulations are indicated in the presence of a dysfunction (e.g., joint restriction) as well as for the neurophysiological effects on pain but yet contraindicated in the absence of a dysfunction, relative to the skill/experience of the practitioner, and in the presence of a more serious pathology that may be adversely affected by a manipulation. There are several regional contraindications as well which include vertebral artery syndrome, traumatized transverse ligament of C1-2, Cauda Equina syndrome, and postoperatively. Absolute contraindications include any condition that could weaken bone (osteoporosis, neoplasm, and infection), fracture, ligament rupture, excessive pain or resistance, and empty end-feel and or severe multidirectional spasm to name a few (7,9). General guidelines for joint manipulation or mobilization suggest these techniques should be utilized in the setting of joint hypomobility and avoided in the setting of joint multidirectional hypermobility.

There is mounting evidence to support the use of spinal manipulative therapy (SMT) for the treatment of acute neck and low back pain (LBP). Bronfort et al found that spinal manipulation provides either similar or better pain outcomes in the short and long term when compared to placebo as well as other treatments including McKenzie based therapy, medical care provided by the primary care physician (PCP), soft tissue treatment, and "back school" (10). Another randomized clinical trial compared SMT to

exercise and to SMT and exercise combined. The results indicate that SMT followed by exercise is more beneficial in the treatment of LBP (11). Additionally, there is moderate evidence to support the use of manual therapy when combined with exercise for the treatment of low back and neck pain as well as osteoarthritis of the hip and knee (11–15). Childs et al validated a clinical prediction rule that demonstrated that clinicians can accurately identify patients with LBP who are likely to benefit from SMT. The probability of successful outcome among patients who met at least four of the five criteria in the rule increased from 45% to 95% (16).

The evidence further suggests that manual therapy directed to the neck, particularly when combined with exercise, is effective for patients with mechanical neck pain without radicular symptoms. There is also mounting evidence to support the use of SMT of the thoracic spine for the treatment of acute neck pain. It is theorized that the biomechanical relationship between the cervical spine and thoracic spine make it possible that disturbances in joint mobility in the thoracic spine may contribute to movement restrictions and pain in the cervical region (17). A clinical prediction rule was also developed to determine the likely success for patients with neck pain who may benefit from thoracic SMT. Although improvements were noted, the rule could not be validated.

MUSCLE ENERGY TECHNIQUES

Muscle energy technique (MET) was developed between 1945 and 1950 by the osteopathic physician, Dr. Fred Mitchell. MET is a manual medicine treatment procedure that involves the voluntary contraction of a muscle by the patient in a precisely controlled direction, at varying levels of intensity, against a distinctly executed counterforce applied by the operator. METs can be used to restore joint mobility, retrain global movement patterns, reduce tissue edema, stretch fibrotic tissues, and to retrain the stabilizing function of the intersegmental muscles. Contraindications include fracture, trauma, significant pain, severe sprain/strain, muscle rupture, and an uncooperative patient (4,7,18).

Unfortunately, few studies have assessed the effectiveness of METs. Previous research has found that MET of the low back improved self-reported disability; however, its effect as an isolated treatment has not been investigated. Schenk et al found an increase in cervical ROM after seven sessions, and an increase in lumbar extension after two sessions (19). Roberts et al indicated that the short-term effects of MET include decreased pain, increased ROM, decreased muscle tension and spasm, and increased strength. However, these effects were only transient; indicating that MET would have to be applied several times throughout the day (20).

STRAIN-COUNTERSTRAIN

Strain-Counterstrain (SCS) utilizes passive positioning of the patient to place the joint or body part in a position of greatest comfort to relieve pain by relaxing myofascial or ligamentous soft tissues. It may occasionally be referred to as "positional release techniques" (21). Dr. Lawrence Jones, DO, originally developed SCS in 1955 to treat recalcitrant LBP (22). He theorized that muscles which are strained are inappropriately shortened. SCS positions the restricted muscle in a shortened position and its antagonist muscle in an overly stretched position. By doing so, one allows the inappropriately shortened muscle to "reset" their spindles and arrest the inappropriate proprioceptor activity to the spinal cord (22). This technique is occasionally referred to as an indirect technique as positioning occurs opposite the restricted barrier.

SCS is typically performed by first identifying a tender point via palpation. The patient is then positioned until the tender area is at least 80% improved. This position is then maintained for 90 seconds with the exception of the ribs which are held for 120 seconds. There is then a slow passive return to a neutral position to avoid inappropriate firing of the muscle. The tender point is then reevaluated, and the technique may be repeated as needed (22).

The indications for SCS are tension, local edema, joint hypomobility, and muscle spasms (22). Several studies have shown decreased pain with use of SCS. Wong and Schauer showed that when treating patients with hip tender points, SCS decreased pain more than exercise alone (23). Perreault performed a blinded randomized study using SCS versus sham for upper trapezius pain, and the results showed significant decrease in pain with both techniques and no difference after 24 hours (24). Despite limited data, SCS is considered to be safe and effective, and may be used in the very young and the elderly patients. There are no absolute contraindications for SCS, but open wounds, sutures, healing fractures, hematoma, hypersensitivity of the skin, and local infections may prevent the practitioner from achieving adequate positioning to perform SCS appropriately (23).

MYOFASCIAL RELEASE

Myofascial release (MFR) is a relatively new technique popularized and expanded by physical therapist John Barnes during the 1980s. MFR is a hands on soft tissue technique that facilitates a stretching of fascia which has become a restricted barrier (25). Fascia is a tough connective tissue that surrounds and supports muscles, blood vessels, organs, bones, and nerves throughout the body. Tightening of the fascia is believed to occur after trauma and is thought to be a protective phenomenon. Due to this tightening or loss of pliability, the fascial network becomes restricted, increases tension, and ultimately leads to altered structural alignment. Poor muscular biomechanics results from this cycle of events presenting as pain and impaired functioning. By releasing or restoring the length of the myofascial tissue, the pressure will be taken off pain sensitive structures, allowing correct alignment of muscles and joints (26).

MFR is specific for different regions of the body. After identifying a restrictive tissue barrier, a sustained pressure is applied for 90 to 120 seconds until palpable release is felt. This is repeated in surrounding directions until the tissue becomes soft and pliable (27).

General indications for MFR are LBP, fibromyalgia, plantar fasciitis, headaches, and painful scars (26). Ajimshaw has demonstrated that MFR improves tension headaches when compared to standard massage (28). Grieve, Clarke, Pearson et al showed that MFR can improve ROM in patients with restricted ankle dorsiflexion (29). However limited, the data for MFR looks promising. MFR appears to be a safe and effective soft tissue technique without any absolute contraindications. Some relative contraindications are febrile states, acute circulatory conditions, sutures, healing fractures, cellulitis, obstructive edema, and open wounds (26).

SOFT TISSUE MOBILIZATION

The term *soft tissue mobilization* (STM) has been applied to various different techniques including massage, but has evolved over time. Today, the term STM is used for a direct therapy maneuver to elongate fascial fibers that surround muscles. This may be performed using manual manipulation or assistive devices (30). STM originated from the various manipulation techniques including Dr. Andrew Still's osteopathic manipulations and Ida Pauline Rolf's Rolfing technique, but has evolved most notably in the 1980s from many parallel institutions (31).

There are many different individualized techniques that exist today, but the concept is uniform and continues to be refined.

Early research showed that manipulation of soft tissues can improve circulation, decrease spasms, and reduce pain (32). The underlying cause of tissue restriction was determined to be fibrotic adhesions or scar tissues which form after tissue damage by trauma, acute or repetitive (33). STM is performed by locating adhesions in the muscles, tendon, or fascia which is causing pain or restricting joint ROM (33). The affected muscle is trapped by applying manual pressure or tools in the direction of the muscle fiber. The patient is then asked to actively move the body part, taking the affected muscle from a shortened position to an elongated position. The therapist continues to apply pressure until the tension in the tissue is improved. This maneuver is typically repeated several times until there is significant improvement.

As this treatment is becoming more defined and the evidence is being developed, there are no formal indications for treatment. It can be used on any number of joints for painful and restricted ROM, chronic tendinopathy, lymphedema, and acute muscle spasms. Christenson demonstrated that STM improved pain and ROM in a single case study of Achilles tendinopathy (34). Another study showed that STM improved hamstring flexibility in a normal population in a randomized control study (35). There are no absolute contraindications for STM, but treatments can be uncomfortable and even painful. Therefore, practitioners must carefully choose the patient who can both tolerate and benefit from the treatment. Some relative contraindications include an active infection, inflammatory conditions, and unstable joints.

ACTIVE RELEASE TECHNIQUES

Active release technique (ART) is a soft tissue technique developed by P. Michael Leahy in the late 1980s utilizing a combination of active movement and massage (36). Similar to STM and MFR, the technique focuses on releasing adhesions or scar between muscles, tendons, ligaments, fascia, and nerves which arise from overuse trauma. The adhesions lead to decreased blood supply, increased pain, poor mobility, and subsequent functional limitations (37).

ARTs are specific to the affected area in regard to amount of pressure, placement of hands, and the movement of the limb. The provider evaluates the affected tissue for adhesions by palpation (36). The provider then performs treatments similar to deep-tissue massage to break up the scar tissue while the patient is actively moving the area of interest in prescribed motions.

This technique is new and evidence is being developed to expand its uses, but preliminary data has shown that it is useful for shin splints, carpal tunnel syndrome, and various tendinopathies (38). No absolute contraindications have been cited, but use in cases of blunt trauma or active inflammation has been advised against.

MASSAGE

Massage can be defined as the systematic, therapeutic, and functional stroking and kneading of the soft tissues. The French have been credited with the introduction of massage into Europe. Studies have demonstrated that deep massage increases circulation and skin temperature as a result of vasodilation of capillaries in the treated area (39). Traditional massage techniques employed in clinical practice include (40):

▪ Effleurage: general stroking technique applied to the muscles and soft tissues in a centripetal direction to enhance relaxation and venous/lymphatic drainage
▪ Pétrissage: a term used to describe a group of techniques that involve the compression of soft tissues and include kneading, wringing, rolling, and picking-up to release muscle fibrosis and to "milk" the muscles of waste products that collect after trauma
▪ Tapotement: movements generally include rapid, rhythmic movements of the hands, originating from a relaxed wrist, which strikes the body briskly and alternately, usually at a rate between 4 to 10 strikes per second. Differences in the part of the therapist's hand utilized as well as the depth of pressure applied are what differentiate the techniques of tapotement from one another
▪ Acupressure: based on the ancient arts of shiatsu and acupuncture, it involves manual pressure over the acupuncture points of the body to improve the flow of the body's energy or chi. Western scientific research has proposed several mechanisms for the effect of acupressure in pain relief, which include the gate control theory of pain, diffuse noxious inhibitory control, and the stimulation of endorphins, serotonin, and acetylcholine which enhance analgesia

Indications of massage include relief from stress, reduction of headaches, decrease edema, strengthen the immune system, improve mental function, increase ROM and an adjunctive treatment for chronic LBP. Massage is contraindicated in the presence of high fever, contagious diseases, open wounds, burns, as well as individuals suspected to be under the influence of drugs and/or alcohol. Additionally, approval from a primary care physician should be obtained in the presence of conditions such as cancer, neurological disorders such as Parkinson's disease, cerebral palsy, and epilepsy, and in cases of extreme fatigue and elderly patients (40).

The effects of massage have been discussed in the literature. Many have advocated for massage to boost the immune system; however, Birk et al concluded that there was no significant improvement (41). Bass et al investigated the effect of massage on lymphatic drainage in breast cancer and concluded that massage did significantly improve uptake into the lymph nodes (42). Massage has also been found to alleviate depression in pregnant women, generate pain relief, as well as increase blood flow (43). However, massage had no effect on sports performance including blood lactate concentration, heart rate, and maximum or mean power (44).

Another commonly employed form of massage performed by physical therapists is transverse friction massage (TFM). Its purpose is to provide movement to the muscle, tendon, or ligaments while inducing traumatic hyperemia in order to stimulate healing. Additionally, TFM has been used to increase mobility and extensibility of muscles, tendons, and ligaments, and to treat scar tissue (4,45). However, no high quality studies have shown histologic support of this premise. Walker investigated the use of TFM on the medial collateral ligaments of rabbits and found no difference between massaged and control rabbits. However, the experimentally induced sprain may have been insufficient to demonstrate a healing response (45). TFM is contraindicated for acute inflammation, hematomas, open skin, peripheral nerves, and in patients who have diminished sensation in the affected area (4).

TRACTION

Traction is the use of a force to separate two objects by pulling one end away from another (3). The first descriptions of its use in medicine are from Hippocrates as he was using traction in an attempt to correct scoliosis (46). Traction is used in various orthopedic conditions acutely including fracture fixation and joint relocation. Physical therapists use traction as a form of manual therapy for cervical and lumbar disorders to separate the

vertebral bodies in order to relieve pressure off the joints and nerves. It can also be used in peripheral joints with restricted ROM to promote joint distraction that can lead to muscle relaxation or in arthritic joints to help alleviate joint related discomfort. There are various types of traction that exist which include manual, mechanical, and autotraction (47). The differences are related to the source of the traction force. Manual traction is dependent on the therapist, mechanical traction typically involves a hydraulic or motorized system, and autotraction utilizes the forces of gravity (the patient's body weight) and harnesses which the patient can control.

The amount of force used to separate the vertebral joint spaces has been studied extensively in the literature. Studies have shown that the optimum weight for cervical traction is 25 pounds to elongate the cervical spine 2 to 20 mm and in 30° of cervical flexion (47). For the lumbar spine, investigators have reported 3 mm widening at one intervertebral level with 70 to 300 pounds of force. Typical treatments are 10 to 30 minutes, but the optimum length of time is still indeterminate. Theories behind traction suggest that stimulation of proprioceptive receptors within the vertebral complex will inhibit abnormal input (48). Cyriax suggested that abnormally shortened paraspinal muscles will fatigue and relax (46). Ultimately, the goal would be to create a prolonged elongation to assist abnormal disk, joint, or nerves to heal. Unfortunately, there is little empirical evidence to support these claims.

Although traction is the oldest form of manual therapy, there are few scientifically robust studies that can distinguish the effects of traction from natural history of pathology. Clarke, van Tulder, and Blomberg performed a rigorous review of literature in 2006 and found traction as a sole treatment for acute, subacute, or chronic LBP with or without sciatica was not effective (48). The Agency for Health Care Policy and Research (AHCPR) published a statement in 1994 stating "spinal traction is not recommended in the treatment of acute low back problems" (49). The evidence for cervical traction is less robust than that for lumbar traction.

There are no formal indications for the use of traction, but it is most commonly used for subacute or chronic LBP with or without leg pain. A 2008 review by Gay and Brault found the available evidence does not define an ideal patient for traction therapy (50). No scientific reports delineate clear contraindications for traction therapy, but commonly listed contraindications include spinal malignancy, spinal cord compression, local infection, osteoporosis, inflammatory spondyloarthritis, acute fracture, aortic or iliac aneurysm, uncontrolled hypertension, or severe cardiovascular disease (51). Specific to cervical traction, patients with ligamentous instability due to advanced rheumatoid arthritis or connective tissue disease and vertebral basilar insufficiency should not be treated.

SUMMARY

Manual therapy techniques are considered one of medicine's oldest treatments and practiced worldwide. Despite quality medical evidence supporting their isolated use, specific treatments include manipulation, massage, and traction are being used and requested by patients. However, some literature does exist for each of these techniques for specific conditions. More literature is being published demonstrating the role of manual therapy in combination with other treatments. The risks appear to be minimal with the potential for significant benefits to the patient. As a prescribing physician who is treating musculoskeletal conditions, it is prudent to become familiar with these techniques and treatment strategies.

REFERENCES

1. Smith AR Jr. Manual therapy: The historical, current, and future role in the treatment of pain. *ScientificWorldJournal*. 2007;7:109–120.
2. Pettman E. A history of manipulative therapy. *J Man Manip Ther*. 2007;15(3):165–174.
3. Wieting M, Andary M, Holmes T, Rechtien J, Zimmerman G. Manipulation, massage, and traction. In: Frontera W, Delisa J, eds. *Physical Medicine & Rehabilitation: Principles and Practice*. 5th ed. Philadelphia, PA: Wolters Kluwer/Lippincott Williams & Wilkins Health; 2010:285–309.
4. Dutton M. *Orthopaedic Examination, Evaluation, and Intervention*. New York, NY: McGraw-Hill; 2004.
5. Maitland GD. *Maitland's Vertebral Manipulation,* 7th ed. Philadelphia, PA: Elsevier; 2005.
6. Gibbons P, Tehan P. *Manipulation of the Spine, Thorax, and Pelvis. An Osteopathic Perspective,* 3rd ed. New York, NY: Elsevier; 2010.
7. Kruchowsky T, Kroon P. *Course notes, MTI manual therapy residency and fellowship program*; 2007.
8. Schmid A, Brunner F, Wright A, Bachmann LM. Paradigm shift in manual therapy? Evidence for a central nervous system component in the response to passive cervical joint mobilization. *Man Ther*. 2008;13:387–396.
9. Vautravers P, Isner ME, Blaes C. Professional practices and recommendations. Manual Medicine—Osteopathy in France—organization, education, field of expertise. *Ann. Phys Med Rehab*. 2010;53:342–351.
10. Bronfort G, Hass M, Evans RL, Bouter RL. Efficacy of spinal manipulation and mobilization for low back pain and neck pain: a systematic review and best evidence synthesis. *Spine*. 2004;4:335–356.
11. Deyle GD, Henderson NE, Matekel RL, Ryder MG, Garber MB, Allison SC. Effectiveness of manual physical therapy and exercise in osteoarthritis of the knee: a randomized, controlled trial. *Ann Intern Med*. 2000;132:173–181.
12. Hoeksma HL, Dekker J, Ronday HK, et al. Comparison of manual therapy and exercise therapy in osteoarthritis of the hip: a randomized clinical trial. *Arthr Rheum*. 2004;51:722–729.
13. Jull G, Trott P, Potter H, et al. A randomized controlled trial of exercise and manipulative therapy for cervicogenic headache. *Spine*. 2002;27:1835–1843.
14. UK BEAM Trial Team. United Kingdom back pain exercise and manipulation (UK BEAM) randomized trial: effectiveness of physical treatments for back pain in primary care. *BMJ*. 2004;329:1377.
15. Bang MD, Deyle GD. Comparison of supervised exercise with and without manual physical therapy for patients with shoulder impingement syndrome. *J Orthop Sports Phys Ther*. 2000;30:126-137.
16. Childs JD. A clinical prediction rule to identify patients with low back pain most likely to benefit from spinal manipulation: a validation study. *Ann Intern Med*. 2004;141:920–928.
17. Cleland JA, Childs JD, McRae M, Palmer JA, Stowell T. Immediate effects of thoracic manipulation in patients with neck pain: a randomized clinical trial. *Man Ther*. 2005;10:127–135.
18. Goodridge JP. Muscle energy technique: Definition, explanation, methods of procedure. *J AM Osteopath Assoc*. 1981;81:249–254.
19. Schenk R. The effects of muscle energy technique on cervical range of motion. *J Man Manip Ther*. 1994;2:149–155.
20. Roberts BL. Soft tissue manipulation: Neuromuscular and muscle energy techniques. *J Neurosci Nurs*. 1997;29:123–127.
21. McClain R. Counterstrain technique In: Karageanes SJ, ed. *Principles of Manual Sports Medicine*. Philadelphia, PA: Lippincott Williams & Wilkins; 2005:21–26.
22. Wong CK. Strain counterstrain: Current concepts and clinical evidence. *Man Ther*. 2012;17(1):2–8.
23. Wong C, Schauer-Alvarez C. The effect of strain counterstrain on pain and strength. *J Man Manip Ther*. 2004;12(4):215–224.
24. Perreault A, Kelln B, Hertel J, Pugh K, Saliba S. Short-term effects of strain counterstrain in reducing pain in upper trapezius tender points. *ATSHC*. 2009;1(5):214–221.
25. Nagrale AV, Glynn P, Joshi A, Ramteke G. The efficacy of an integrated neuromuscular inhibition technique on upper trapezius trigger points in subjects with non-specific neck pain: A randomized controlled trial. *J Man Manip Ther*. 2010;18(1):37–43.
26. Barnes MF. The basic science of myofascial release: Morphologic change in connective tissue. *J Bodyw Mov Ther*. 1997;1(4):231–238.

27. Barnes J. Myofascial release. In: Hammer WI, ed. *Functional Soft Tissue Examination and Treatment by Manual Methods: New Perspectives.* Gaithersburg, MD: Aspen; 2005:533–548.

28. Ajimsha MS. Effectiveness of direct vs indirect technique myofascial release in the management of tension-type headache. *J Bodyw Mov Ther.* 2011;15(4):431–435.

29. Grieve R, Clark J, Pearson E, Bullock S, Boyer C, Jarrett A. The immediate effect of soleus trigger point pressure release on restricted ankle joint dorsiflexion: A pilot randomised controlled trial. *J Bodyw Mov Ther.* 2011;15(1):42–49.

30. Hunter G. Specific soft tissue mobilization in the management of soft tissue dysfunction. *Man Ther.* 1998;3(1):2–11.

31. Cottingham JT, Maitland J. A three-paradigm treatment model using soft tissue mobilization and guided movement-awareness techniques for a patient with chronic low back pain: A case study. *J Orthop Sports Phys Ther.* 1997;26(3):155–167.

32. Sutton GS, Bartel MR. Soft-tissue mobilization techniques for the hand therapist. *J Hand Ther.* 1994;7(3):185-192.

33. Prentice WE, Voight ML. *Techniques in Musculoskeletal Rehabilitation.* New York, NY: McGraw-Hill, Medical Pub. Division; 2001:780.

34. Christenson RE. Effectiveness of specific soft tissue mobilizations for the management of achilles tendinosis: Single case study—experimental design. *Man Ther.* 2007;12(1):63–71.

35. Hopper D, Deacon S, Das S, et al. Dynamic soft tissue mobilisation increases hamstring flexibility in healthy male subjects. *Br J Sports Med.* 2005;39(9):594–598; discussion 598.

36. Leahy PM. Active release techniques soft tissue management system, manual. In: *Active release techniques.* Colorado, CO: LLC; 2000:3–15.

37. Schiottz-Christensen B, Mooney V, Azad S, Selstad D, Gulick J, Bracker M. The role of active release manual therapy for upper extremity overuse Syndromes—A preliminary report. *J Occup Rehabil.* 1999;9(3):201-211.

38. Drover JM, Forand DR, Herzog W. Influence of active release technique on quadriceps inhibition and strength: A pilot study. *J Manipulative Physiol Ther.* 2004;27(6):408–413.

39. Drust B, Atkinson G, Gregson W, French D, Binningsley D. The effects of massage on intramuscular temperature in the vastus lateralis in humans. *Int J Sports Med.* 2003; 24:395–399.

40. Tappan FM, Benjamin PJ. *Tappan's Handbook of Healing Massage Techniques: Classic, Holistic, and Emerging Methods.* Norwalk, CT: Appleton & Lange. 1998.

41. Birk TJ, McGrady A, MacArthur RD, Khuder S. The effects of massage therapy alone and in combination with other complementary therapies on immune system measures and quality of life in human immunodeficiency virus. *J Altern Complement Med.* 2000;6:405–414.

42. Bass SS, Cox CE, Salud CJ, et al. The effects postinjection massage on the sensitivity of lymphatic mapping in breast cancer. *J Am Coll Surg.* 2001;192:9–16.

43. Field T, Diego MA, Hernandez-Reif M, Schanberg S, Kuhn C. Massage therapy effects on depressed women. *J Psychosomatic Obstet Gynaecol.* 2004;25:115-121.

44. Hemmings B, Smith JM, Graydon J, Dyson R. Effects of massage on physiological restoration, perceived recovery, and repeated sports performance. *Br J Sports Med*; 34;109–114.

45. Walker JM. Deep transverse frictions in ligament healing. *J Orthop Sci Phys Ther.* 1984; 6:89–94.

46. Cyriax JH, Coldham M. *Textbook of Orthopaedic Medicine, v. 2: Treatment by Manipulation Massage and Injection.* 11th ed. London, UK: Philadelphia: Baillière Tindall; 1984:266.

47. Wieting M. *Massage, Traction, and Manipulation.* Retrieved from http://emedicine.medscape.com/article/324694. Accessed October 01, 2012.

48. Clarke J, van Tulder M, Blomberg S, de Vet H, van der Heijden G, Bronfort G. Traction for low back pain with or without sciatica: An updated systematic review within the framework of the cochrane collaboration. *Spine (Phila Pa 1976).* 2006; 31(14):1591–1599.

49. Susman J. AHCPR guideline on acute low back problems. *Am Fam Physician.* 1995;51(2):334, 339–340.

50. Gay RE, Brault JS. Evidence-informed management of chronic low back pain with traction therapy. *Spine J.* 2008;8(1):234–242.

51. Pellecchia GL. Lumbar traction: A review of the literature. *J Orthop Sports Phys Ther.* 1994;20(5):262–267.

Therapeutic Exercise

Andrew Hall and Amrish D. Patel

Therapeutic exercise (Therex) is the utilization of voluntary muscle contraction and/or body movement with the specific goal of relieving symptoms, improving function or improving, retaining, or slowing deterioration of health. It encompasses the treatment, rehabilitation, and prevention of pathological conditions. It is often regarded as the key element of the rehabilitation program since it requires active participation by the patient along with performance of a home exercise program (HEP) to further rehabilitation and prevent recurrent musculoskeletal injuries. Exercise in general has many benefits and is shown to improve all-cause mortality, prevent cardiovascular disease, regulate blood pressure, lipid management and weight control, and many others (1).

The Therex program must be individualized to the patient and their diagnosis. The most important factor in designing the Therex program is to base it on an accurate and specific medical diagnosis as well as impairments and functional limitations of the patient. This will guide the development of an appropriate exercise program for the musculoskeletal condition that is presented to the treating physician and therapist. Other important factors in designing a Therex program include but are not limited to consider: exercise history, current fitness level past medical/surgical history, current medications, along with the patient's and clinician's rehabilitation goals.

Fundamentals exist to any therapy program as they do for most interventions. Therapeutic exercise prescriptions should specify a diagnosis, precautions, frequency, duration, and specific exercise types. There are also many dimensions to therapeutic exercise including: range of motion (ROM: passive, active assisted, and active), flexibility and stretching, strengthening (including core strengthening and stabilization programs), and proprioceptive exercise and functional activities. Each of these groups of activities has several different methods of obtaining the desired outcomes which will be discussed in greater detail throughout this chapter. Further details on exercise prescription writing can be found in the chapter titled Guide to Therapy Prescription Writing.

Various aspects of therapeutic exercise (ROM, stretching, strengthening, proprioceptive exercises, neuromuscular reeducation and functional training) will be reviewed in detail in the remainder of this chapter. In our opinion the most important aspect of the therapeutic exercise program is the patient's ability and commitment to perform the exercises on a regular basis at home. This requires the therapist to educate the patient on appropriate exercises and expected outcomes. The patient's ability to perform the exercises, and adjust them based on their response to performing a movement, allows them further independence in their care. It is the job of the therapist and the physician to guide patients with musculoskeletal injuries toward independence. Patient education and instruction will, in our opinion, affect the overall outcome of therapy programs. Education is the key factor to patient compliance.

RANGE OF MOTION

ROM can be obtained by any activity that addresses restriction in normal motion at a joint or tissue interface. Exercises can be done through the application of passive, active assisted, or active ROM. Motion should be assessed in both an active (AROM) and passive (PROM) manner to distinguish if limitations in motion are secondary to restriction in contractile and/or noncontractile elements, which can help guide the most appropriate forms of exercise (e.g., AROM, PROM, stretching).

The three ROM modalities can be defined as:
PROM (passive): The examiner moves the joint or limb without assistance from the patient (external force applied)

AROM (active): Patient initiates the movement of the joint or limb (internal force), without any assistance

AAROM (active-assisted): Movement of the joint or limb is the result of the patient's efforts with assistance from an external source (a health care provider or the unaffected limb).

ROM can be utilized to provide controlled stress to a joint and can be modulated by a number of factors including injury to muscle, tendon, ligament, joint capsule, and soft tissue structures (1). For example, injury to the surrounding soft tissue at the elbow due to blunt trauma can cause excessive fluid buildup and swelling leading to impaired ROM. In any case of restricted ROM it is imperative to continue with the above mentioned ROM modalities in order to limit long term consequences of restricted ROM and to prevent joint contracture. When connective tissues are not stretched, a gradual shortening of the soft tissue ensues leading to impaired ROM and disuse impairments. Therefore, gentle A/AA/PROM should be initiated to avoid the vicious cycle of pain, immobility, contracture, and overall impaired function.

One of the most effective modalities for acute injury is stretching within a pain-free ROM. Stretching is generally incorporated during ROM exercises to facilitate improvements in mobility.

Common types of stretching include:

Static stretching, which involves holding a stretch for certain time period, often 15 to 30 seconds, and is considered to be relatively safe

Passive stretching (a form of static stretching), which is a relaxed stretching where the person assumes a position and holds it with another part of the body or with the assistance of a partner (2)

Dynamic stretching, which utilizes momentum to engage end ROM while incorporating controlled movements during the stretch. Dynamic stretching engages the contractile elements and maintains them at the end of their available range (2). Dynamic stretching is used most often during sport-specific warm ups. It is not effective for mobilizing noncontractile tissues when end ROM is unable to be achieved

Basic guidelines for stretching include the duration of the hold, the number of repetitions, and the need for the stretching to be pain-free. Holding a stretch for 15 to 30 seconds at the point of tightness or slight discomfort enhances joint ROM; older patients may experience greater improvements in ROM with longer durations (60 seconds) of stretching (3). Common recommendations are primarily based on expert opinion and include stretching twice a day with 3 to 5 repetitions for each muscle or muscle group being targeted.

Other methods of stretching include ballistic and variations of contract-relax stretching described by the proprioceptive neuromuscular facilitation (PNF) literature. Ballistic stretching has fallen out of favor in the injured population. PNF is used clinically by physical and/or occupational therapists when performing comprehensive treatment regimens. PNF is performed in certain diagonal patterns (D1 and D2) for both the upper and lower limbs. PNF patterns have been shown to be the most effective method of obtaining ROM for a short duration (4). It is thought that PNF patterns improve ROM by reciprocal inhibition, however this is not proven in the literature (5).

Specialized ROM programs exist for certain conditions, such as for low back pain (LBP), which continues to be a common reason for primary care visits, disability, and a substantial economic burden. Examples include the William's flexion program or the McKenzie method. William's flexion exercises are a set of related physical exercises intended to enhance lumbar flexion, avoid lumbar extension, and strengthen the core in an effort to manage LBP. McKenzie method is a standardized assessment tool utilized by physiotherapists to treat musculoskeletal disorders of the spine and extremities. Classification directs an individualized treatment program. The McKenzie classification system was developed to be inclusive of the majority of patients with mechanical LBP syndromes (6). The centralization phenomenon is the most important pattern of pain response observed in McKenzie's assessment, defined as the situation in which referred pain arising from the spine is reduced and transferred to a more central position where movements in specific directions are performed (7,8). The technique is primarily a self-treatment strategies, and minimizes manual therapy procedures to restore pain-free ROM and function.

STRENGTHENING

The concept of strengthening exercises involves moving any resistance or weight through the ROM of a muscle to enhance contractility and force generation. The determinants of muscle strength include size, shape, insertion site, torque curves, number of involved joints, and neural factors. Muscle strength can be defined as the maximal force generated by a muscle group at a specified velocity. Functionally, strength training has been shown to be beneficial in the elderly and has been associated with better walking speed, balance, and stair climbing and has demonstrated a decrease in risk factors associated with falls (9,10).

Two main types of muscle contractions are concentric and eccentric contractions. Concentric muscle contraction is when the muscle action results in the origin and insertion of a muscle moving closer together, or a shortening action of the muscle fibers. When the action results in the origin and the insertion moving further apart from each other this is called eccentric contraction, or a lengthening action of the muscle (11). Typically concentric contractions occur against gravity and eccentric contractions occur with gravity. Eccentric contractions increase control of the lengthening action resulting in greater muscle tension, higher potential for tissue injury, and greater potential for muscle hypertrophy. Eccentric exercise programs have also been shown to provide benefit in treatment of chronic tendinopathy/tendinosis (12).

Three basic components to strengthening programs are isometric, isotonic, and isokinetic. Isometric movement is a type of strengthening when the joint angle or muscle length does not change during the contraction, such as pushing on a wall. This is neither concentric nor eccentric and is often thought of as a third type of muscle contraction. Isometric activities in theory have the lowest risk for injury but also offer lowest potential for strength gains. Isotonic movement is when the tone remains the same throughout the full ROM (muscle length changes) and contains eccentric and concentric contractions if done properly. Isotonic exercises have a higher risk for injury as compared to isometric contractions but also offer a higher potential for strength gains (2). An example of an isotonic contraction would be an unweighted squat. The tone in the quadriceps and gluteal muscles remains constant but involves both concentric and eccentric contractions. Lastly, isokinetic movement is a dynamic action where there is equal speed and resistance throughout the ROM as muscle length changes (2). This activity requires specialized equipment and is often found in rehabilitation settings.

Another important concept of therapeutic exercise is closed versus open kinetic chain exercises. The kinetic chain refers to the body segment as a series of linked mobile segments. When exercising in an open kinetic chain the distal or mobile segment is not fixed and in the closed kinetic chain the distal segment is fixed. Closed kinetic chain exercises tend to coactivate agonist and antagonist muscle groups and tend to simulate functional movements. Both open and closed chain exercises produce significant functional improvements (11). Strengthening in a functional closed chain position has been shown to provide performance benefits greater than those of open chain strengthening exercises (13). Exercising in closed kinetic chain reduces the shear forces generated across the joint (refer to Chapter 2 on Phases of Musculoskeletal Rehabilitation for further details).

The use of strengthening exercises, also known as resistance exercise or training, involves anabolic building of muscle through various pathways. Progressive resistance exercises (PREs) is a term used to describe a strength training program that gradually challenges the patient in a safe manner. When physicians and therapists initiate a strengthening program one must consider the individual and the goals that are to be accomplished to design a safe and effective program. Many different strengthening modalities exist and may include elastic or resistance bands, body weight and/or gravity based resistance, manual resistance, and weights in the form of dumbbells, bars, or machines to name a few. PNF augmentation with tapping, brushing, stroking, and biofeedback are utilized to achieve the desired neuromuscular control in addition to strength training. One of the most well known modalities for strength training is weight lifting, in which a person lifts a maximum amount of weight for a set number of repetitions until fatigued; in essence lifting with low repetitions and high resistance (14). Two of the most common methods for strength training with weights are the DeLorme and Oxford methods, which are both based on a 10 repetition maximum [10 RM]). With the DeLorme method, also known as ascending pyramids, the individual starts with 10 repetitions at 50% of 10 RM, then 10 repetitions at 75% 10 RM, finally 10 repetitions at 100% 10 RM. Whereas the Oxford method, also known as descending pyramids, begins with 10 repetitions at 100% 10 RM, then the next two sets of 10 repetitions are performed at a lower percentage of the 10 RM. Both methods produce strength gains, but neither has been proven to be more effective than the other (15).

When evaluating which strengthening modality would be most effective for a certain population it is important to consider:

1. The muscle groups being targeted
2. Basic energy sources to be trained (anaerobic vs. aerobic)
3. Muscle action and movement desired

4. The patient's medical history, including prior musculoskeletal (MSK) injuries, past exercise experience, and current hobbies
5. Specific needs (program tailored to the individual) for the program to be successful (1)

The goal should be an effective program that produces strength gains in a safe and controlled manner. Once a strengthening program is developed and implemented, the patient should be monitored to assess progress and evaluate for functional gains. Adjustments to the program should be based on the individual's pain, progress, and functional goals.

Specialized strengthening programs include core strengthening and stability training. Core strengthening targets the trunk muscles, including abdominal muscles (specifically transverse abdominis and obliques), back, and pelvic musculature which significantly improves balance, stability, and posture of the trunk and pelvis. Core strengthening is incorporated into musculoskeletal rehabilitation programs for upper limb, lower limb, and spinal conditions. A strong core provides a stable base in which the arms and legs move. Core strengthening is utilized with good clinical rationale but still requires further investigation to confirm its role and best applications. Stabilization programs may be applied to the scapula, pelvis, and spine. They utilize similar concepts as core strengthening by teaching the patient to maintain improved and pain-free posture/alignment while performing progressively challenging exercises of the upper and lower limbs. Muscle imbalances are the focus of scapular stabilization programs. Restoration of mobility and stability involves stretching of the tight pectorals and upper trapezius and strengthening of the weakened serratus anterior, lower trapezius, and rhomboids. Lumbar stabilization programs have been studied and have demonstrated reductions in LBP and improved multifidus muscle function and bulk (16). The muscles often targeted in lumbar stabilization programs include stretching of tight hip flexors and erector spinae and strengthening of the multifidus, hip extensors, and core stabilizers as discussed above.

PROPRIOCEPTION AND NEUROMUSCULAR CONTROL

Neuromotor exercise training, sometimes called functional fitness training, incorporates motor skills such as balance, coordination, gait, agility, and proprioceptive training. Studies have shown that proprioception is affected in multiple medical conditions including osteoarthritis, diabetes mellitus, rheumatological disease, and aging (1). Progressive therapeutic interventions must include proprioceptive exercises that can improve agility, balance, and coordination and reduce fall risks. There are many modalities by which one can challenge and improve overall balance. In the elderly, Tai chi has been shown to improve balance and reduce the risk of falls (17). In female athletes, there are ACL injury prevention programs that focus on functional strength, balance, and neuromuscular control (18). The use of BOSU balls, foam pads, and unstable surfaces can be used to progressively challenge balance while performing functional activities to train the integrated balance system, therefore potentially reducing the risk of lower limb injury (19).

PNF methods, a neuromotor exercise, take several forms and commonly includes contract-relax stretching, which includes taking a muscle to its fullest extent and then an isometric contraction of the selected muscle tendon group followed by stretching of the same group (2). However, PNF techniques are much more than stretching and functional movements; they help develop muscular strength and endurance, joint stability, mobility, neuromuscular control, and coordination, all of which are aimed at improving the overall functional ability of patients. The proprioceptive system must be challenged in order to reeducate movement patterns resulting in a decreased likelihood of reinjury.

Neuromuscular training exercises are designed to restore the normal timing patterns of muscular recruitment and to provide adequate control or coordination of muscle activation across the joint. For further details on this topic please refer to the chapter on the Phases of Musculoskeletal Rehabilitation. As stated in prior chapters, as neuromuscular control and proprioception improve, the rehabilitation program can shift toward the final phase of rehabilitation: functional or sport-specific training.

FUNCTIONAL ACTIVITIES

The earlier goals of therapeutic exercise are to improve flexibility, strength, ROM, and perceived health but the most important goals are to restore function and prevent injury. A number of functional exercises may be utilized such as plyometrics, occupational and sport-specific training, aquatic exercise, and even yoga, Pilates, or Tai chi may be considered as functional activities to complete the therapeutic exercise. All of these exercise options can be progressed and designed to fit into a HEP and can be performed a few times per week. Yoga and Pilates may be used for those with chronic LBP to improve flexibility and core strength through a mind and body approach (20).

Aquatic exercises may be utilized for those who are unable to tolerate land-based therapy. The water may assist in unloading a patient to assist in gait training while maintaining appropriate weight bearing status to ensure safety and proper healing. Resistance of the water also provides multidirectional resistance throughout movement patterns, assisting in strengthening (21). In addition, the warmth of the water may improve the patient's exercise tolerance. Aquatic exercise allows the performance of functional activities (running, jumping, etc.) in a supportive environment before the progression to performance of these same activities on land.

Plyometric exercises have also been shown to improve an athlete's performance in speed, agility, and endurance (22). Interval training has been utilized in sports and now for recreational training and has shown changes in muscle at the cellular level with carbohydrate metabolism (23) and improved endurance in a shorter duration of treatment time than traditional endurance training (24). For those looking to return to work or sport, occupational, and sport-related activities, ergonomic training and a specific movement analysis with correction of any remaining biomechanical errors should be targeted to allow safe return to activity.

When prescribing these exercises and completing the therapeutic exercise program, maintenance via a HEP is extremely important and care should be taken to limit the exacerbation of current musculoskeletal or health problems such as cardiovascular, pulmonary, and other systemic disease processes. Currently exercise guidelines, per the 2011 American College of Sports Medicine, recommend most adults should engage in moderate-intensity cardiorespiratory exercise training for 30 minutes per day (or greater), 5 days/week (or greater) for a total of 150 min/wk. On 2 to 3 days/week (or greater), adults should also perform resistance exercises for each of the major muscle groups, and neuromotor exercise involving balance, agility, and coordination. Crucial to maintaining joint ROM, completing a series of flexibility exercises for each the major muscle tendon groups (a total of 60 seconds per exercise) on 2 days/week (or

greater) is recommended (5). All physicians and therapists should consider these guidelines when designing a HEP and advocate for patients to follow them. Exercise prescription, specifically HEP prescription, can also be a fundamental part of all therapy plans as a goal to motivate patients to maintain a healthy lifestyle after recovering from injury.

PATIENT EDUCATION

Patient education is another integral part of the Therex program as the patient must learn how to correctly perform the exercises, how to self-monitor response to the exercises, and how to progress with the exercises in a safe and efficient manner. By teaching the patient how to constantly reassess their symptoms and response to exercises, it will give them the ability to self-manage their condition. This ability to help improve or control their symptoms will hopefully increase their "buy in" to the treatment program and improve compliance. Simply giving exercises and handouts without proper instruction does not afford this "buy in" that results in the patient taking an active role in their healthcare and in our opinion better overall outcomes. Utilization of patient education to improve patient compliance is an extremely important topic and, therefore, will be discussed in greater detail in the chapter titled Patient Education.

SUMMARY

Therapeutic exercise is often regarded as the key element to any rehabilitation program since it requires active participation by the patient along with the performance of a HEP to advance rehabilitation and prevent recurrence of their musculoskeletal condition. The therapeutic exercise program is tailored to the individual and the diagnosis helps to serve as a guide to appropriate activities. Therapeutic exercises include ROM, stretching, strengthening, neuromuscular reeducation, and proprioceptive exercises. These types of exercises are strategically chosen to reduce pain, rebuild strength, and restore function in an active way.

REFERENCES

1. Hoffman MD, Sheldahl LM, Kraemer WJ. Therapeutic exercise. In: Delisa J, ed. *Physical Medicine and Rehabilitation. Principles and Practice*: 4th ed. Philadelphia, PA: Lippincott Williams & Wilkins; 2005:389–433.
2. Dave SJ, Buschbacher RM, Strock G, et al. Therapeutic exercise: essentials. In: Young BJ, Young MA, Stiens SA, eds. *Physical Medicine and Rehabilitation Secrets*. 3rd ed. Philadelphia, PA: Mosby; 2008:179–186.
3. Feland JB, Myrer JW, Schulthies SS, Fellingham GW, Measom GW. The effect of duration of stretching of the hamstring muscle group for increasing range of motion in people aged 65 years or older. *Phys Ther*. 2001;81(5):1110–1117.
4. Sharman MJ, Cresswell AG, Riek S. Proprioceptive neuromuscular facilitation stretching: mechanisms and clinical implications. *Sports Med*. 2006;36(11):929–939.
5. Garber CE, Blissmer B, Deschenes MR, et al. Quantity and quality of exercise for developing and maintaining cardiorespiratory, musculoskeletal, and neuromotor fitness in apparently healthy adults: guidance for prescribing exercise. *Med Sci Sports Exerc*. 2011;43:1334–1359.
6. Werneke MW, Hart D, Oliver D, et al. Prevalence of classification methods for patients with lumbar impairments using the McKenzie syndromes, pain pattern, manipulation, and stabilization clinical prediction rules. *J Man Manip Ther*. 2010;18(4):197–204.
7. Clare HA, Adams R, Maher CG. A systematic review of efficacy of McKenzie therapy for spinal pain. *Aust J Physiother*. 2004;50:209–216.
8. Machado LA, Souza MS, Ferriera PH, et al. The McKenzie method for low back pain: a systematic review of the literature with a meta-analysis approach. *Spine*, 2006;31(9): E254–E262.
9. Hurley BF, Roth SM Strength training in the elderly: effects on risk factors for age-related diseases. *Sports Med*. 2000;30(4):249–268.
10. Frontera WR, Bigard X. The benefits of strength training in the elderly. *Science & Sports*. 2002;17:109–116.
11. Frontera WR, Lexell J. Assessment of human muscle function. In: Delisa J, ed. *Physical Medicine and Rehabilitation. Principles and Practice*. 4th ed. Philadelphia, PA: Lippincott Williams & Wilkins; 2005:139–154.
12. Visnes H, Bahr R. The evolution of eccentric training as treatment for patellar tendinopathy (jumper's knee): a critical review of exercise programmes. *Br J Sports Med*. 2007;41(4):217–223.
13. Augustsson J, Esko A, Thomeé R, et al. Weight training of the thigh muscles using closed vs. open kinetic chain exercises: a comparison of performance enhancement. *J Orthop Sports Phys Ther*. 1998;1:3–8.
14. Bloodworth D. Cardiovascular conditioning exercise and cardiac rehabilitation. In: Garrison SJ, ed. *Handbook Of Physical Medicine and Rehabilitation*. 2nd ed. Philadelphia, PA: Lippincott Williams & Wilkins; 2003:86–104.
15. Fish DE, Krabak BJ, Johnson-Greene D, DeLateur BJ. Optimal resistance training: comparison of DeLorme with Oxford techniques. *Am J Phys Med Rehabil*. 2003;82(12):903–909.
16. Hides JA, Stanton WR, McMahon S, Sims K, Richardson CA. Effect of stabilization training on multifidus muscle cross-sectional area among young elite cricketers with low back pain. *J Orthop Sports Phys Ther*. 2008;38(3):101–108.
17. Li F, Harmer P, Fisher KJ, McAuley E. Tai Chi: improving functional balance and predicting subsequent falls in older persons. *Med Sci Sports Exerc*. 2004;36(12):2046–2052.
18. Sadoghi P, von Keudell A, Vavken P. Effectiveness of anterior cruciate ligament injury prevention training programs [published online ahead of print March 28, 2012]. *J Bone Joint Surg Am*.
19. Willardson JM. Core stability training: applications to sports conditioning programs. *J Strength Cond Res*. 2007;21(3):979–985.
20. Sorosky S, Stilp S, Akuthota V. Yoga and pilates in the management of low back pain. *Curr Rev Musculoskelet Med*. 2008;1(1):39–47.
21. Becker BE. Aquatic therapy: scientific foundations and clinical rehabilitation applications. *PMR*. 2009;1(9):859–872.
22. Chelly MS, Ghenem MA, Abid K, Hermassi S, Tabka Z, Shephard RJ. Effects of in-season short-term plyometric training program on leg power, jump- and sprint performance of soccer players. *J Strength Cond Res*. 2010;24(10):2670–2676.
23. Burgomaster KA, Heigenhauser GJ, Gibala MJ. Effect of short-term sprint interval training on human skeletal muscle carbohydrate metabolism during exercise and time-trial performance. *J Appl Physiol*. 2006;100(6):2041–2047.
24. Gibala MJ, Little JP, van Essen M, et al. Short-term sprint interval versus traditional endurance training: similar initial adaptations in human skeletal muscle and exercise performance. *J Physiol*. 2006;575(Pt 3):901–911.

Patient Education

Robert Maschi

INTRODUCTION

Patient education is recognized by health professionals as an important tool for effective management of patients. These strategies can be used to improve outcomes, increase compliance, decrease pain, improve patient satisfaction, and reduce health care cost (1–4). For these reasons inclusion of patient education has been mandated recently by health care accrediting agencies and insurance companies who reimburse for healthcare. Patient education can be defined as the process by which health care professionals and others impart information to patients that will alter their health behaviors or improve their health status (5).

The degree of integration of patient education principles by healthcare providers has evolved throughout history. Early medical models viewed the patient in a passive role. Patients were given little information and were essentially told what to do. Today it is preferred that the patient should be an active participant in the delivery of his or her healthcare, and, therefore, needs to be educated in order to make informed decisions. Also with diminishing reimbursement benefits, a larger burden may fall on patients as they will be responsible to do more on their own, without supervision of therapist or physician. Given the trend toward greater patient responsibility in their healthcare, patients need to be educated and empowered in order to participate effectively.

Patient education has continued to grow as an important role of the physical therapist. During World War I, the influx of a large volume of patients forced reconstruction aides (the predecessors of modern physical therapists) to educate injured soldiers to self administer exercise (6). During the 1950s and 1960s physical therapy (PT) curriculum began to increase emphasis on the physical therapist's role as a teacher (7) and in the late 1970s the American Physical Therapy Association (APTA) began to require, as part of their accreditation

process for schools granting the PT degree, inclusion of curriculum addressing educational skills and teaching theory (8). A large majority of physical therapists embrace the role of educator and report using patient education as a tool during their treatments. Chase et al discovered that 87% of physical therapists responding to a survey report using patient education with 80% to 100% of patients (9). The respondents most often teach patients about treatment rationale and home exercise programs (HEPs) and use verbal discussion and demonstration as the preferred method for patient education (9). Information regarding their condition and prognosis is highly valued by patients (10–14). At the same time, it has been shown that healthcare professionals tend to underestimate their patients' need for information (11,14).

METHODS OF PATIENT EDUCATION

There are many ways that the clinician can use patient education to foster improved outcomes and to facilitate the process of delivering patient care. Patient education can occur through the use of verbal, visual, or written instruction. Examples include providing educational materials in various media such as written information, pictures, video, and website formatted information. This material can address the patients' condition, prognosis, and management options. Physical therapists routinely prescribe HEPs for patients to complement clinic visits. Description of exercises can be given in the form of a list, pictures with specific directions, or with the use of video, smart phone applications, and other emerging technologies. Patient education can also address issues such as ergonomics, posture, body mechanics, injury prevention, and advice regarding activity modification.

Activity modification instruction is focused on changing patient behavior. These strategies should address both behaviors that are beneficial and those that are potentially harmful. Strategies should be developed to overcome barriers to changing harmful behaviors and to adopting those behaviors that will improve outcome and overall health status. For example the patient who had ACL reconstruction surgery must be instructed in a HEP and wound care, but also needs to be advised about activities to avoid. Inappropriate behavior such as prolonged standing or ambulation during the early post operative period may lead to increased edema and pain, and subsequently an inability to make progress in therapy. This must be clearly explained to the patient. Then if the patient identifies barriers to compliance, a solution (or many potential solutions) to the barrier should be offered as well as explanation of the effect that not changing the behavior may have on long-term outcome.

Patient education often requires ongoing interaction to create a fluid exchange of ideas between patient and clinician. Suggestions may be made that are implemented, reassessed, and then changed again to meet the patient's needs. It is important to realize that there is a difference between teaching and telling. Simply telling a patient what to do is not the full extent of patient education. One must understand the patient's perspective and investigate how the information will be integrated as well as the impact of this change on the patient's life. Teaching involves providing information that enables patients to understand their illness or condition. Importantly, there is also an expectation that education will lead to a change in behavior, whether it is performing an exercise correctly or refraining from harmful activity. The ability of the patient to change behavior is also a component that the therapist and physician must assess. The transtheoretical model of behavior change while controversial, attempts to describe a patients' ability to change health behaviors. This theory identifies stages of readiness to accept and initiate change. It is composed of six stages: precontemplation, contemplation, preparation, action, maintenance, and termination. It may be useful to identify which stage the patient is in to address barriers to change. It has been demonstrated in behavioral health that stage matched interventions can help with progress toward behavior change (15).

PATIENT COMPLIANCE

Patient compliance with HEP or activity modification behaviors will have a direct impact on the outcome of PT. A review of the literature regarding compliance to a HEP that supplements a clinic based program is discouragingly low. Adherence to unsupervised HEPs and splinting home programs ranged from 18% to 57% (16–18). In a specific population, patients with arthritis do not follow prescribed exercise programs 45% to 60% of the time (19). It is difficult to measure compliance objectively because there is a spectrum of compliance. Patients may adhere to advice in varying degrees. Although difficult to measure, clinicians should strive to maximize compliance given its impact on outcome.

For this reason it is important to understand the factors influencing adherence to patient education strategies and the techniques utilized in patient education. Certain techniques can increase the likelihood that the patient education strategy will be effective. Mayo reviewed the literature on patient compliance and found that education may increase patient's knowledge about a condition or regimen without necessarily improving compliance (20). The literature did indicate that, among other factors, the patient's attitude toward the illness or disability, the complexity of the program, and the degree of lifestyle disruption had a significant effect on compliance (20). She recommended that therapists become more knowledgeable about their patients' individual barriers to compliance.

This is true because compliance is often affected by what the client believes about his or her disability. A patient's belief that they have the ability to change their situation and improve their condition affects compliance. The therapist and physician play an integral role in educating and empowering the patient with the knowledge that they can change their situation. Those with the belief that health and illness are beyond their control (external locus of control) tend to be less compliant than those with internal locus of control (21). Additionally, patient beliefs about their prognosis impacts compliance. Those who believed that they had a good prognosis and their complaints would go away exercised more than those with a poor prognosis (22). Those individuals who showed low compliance were also less likely to believe that the exercise intervention was likely to help (23). Perhaps more time and/or effort should be devoted to educating patients about the physiological benefits of exercise and the relationship between therapeutic exercise and improved outcomes. The importance of the patient "buy in" may be undervalued in the overall treatment plan and may need to be moved up the treatment paradigm.

FEEDBACK

Patient feedback also appears to be related to compliance. Patients who reported that their therapist was very satisfied with their compliance to the exercise program were more compliant than patients who did not know if their therapist was satisfied with their adherence to the program (22). Simply giving patients acknowledgement and positive feedback does seem to improve their compliance. In these same patients there was a difference between two groups of therapists. In one group, patients were more compliant and in the other group patients were relatively less compliant. Therapists in the more compliant group asked the patients more questions regarding performance, monitored patients more often, and more frequently motivated their patients to exercise at home (22). Being persistent with feedback seems to improve compliance.

Lorish points out that frequently asking about treatment adherence communicates the importance of these issues to the patient and that the patient's behavior will be monitored. This accountability and/or the desire to please the therapist can motivate patients initially and can help sustain the behavior once it is initiated (24). Monitoring compliance on a regular basis and resolving problems the patient encounters or barriers to adherence improves compliance (14,25–28). In addition to monitoring, providing positive or motivating feedback also improved compliance (10,14,25). Providing immediate feedback and making adjustments to treatments can also improve the patient's "buy in," especially if they feel improved symptoms during the treatment.

BARRIERS

There are many potential barriers to patient education. The therapist or physician may believe that a specific piece of information is important for the patient to understand. However, the patient may have a different perception about what is important or specific to their condition. The patient will have multiple factors that influence motivation to comply or barriers that discourage compliance. These can include their occupation, family role, and cultural influences. Motivation is a complex construct and understanding what influences a patient's motivation is not always obvious.

The motivation to change a behavior, such as starting and maintaining an exercise program, involves a series of decisions. The Health Belief Model asserts that in order to make a behavioral change, the motivation to do so comes from several criteria being met (29). The patient must believe that they are susceptible to a disease or condition, believe that there are serious consequences,

believe that making a change in behavior can reduce the threat or improve their condition, believe that the benefits of making a change in behavior are greater than the costs or barriers of changing, and believe that one is able to successfully make the change (29).

Patients weigh these options when making decisions; therefore, it is prudent to make sure they have the correct information. Patients may get information from various sources, which may not be correct or may be based on inaccurate beliefs. Therefore, it is important to ask patients what they see as the barriers to change and what they perceive as their costs and benefits to see if they are realistic. Provide patients with trusted sources so that they may evaluate the correct information themselves. Patients may also need education regarding these issues and decisions. They should also have realistic awareness of consequences of action or inaction. If a patient does not believe that the treatment is likely to help or that there are too many barriers and "costs" to the treatment, then attempts to modify any and all of those beliefs should be initiated (29).

PATIENT RELATIONSHIP

A productive working relationship between patient and healthcare provider is important. A good relationship leads to greater satisfaction, better retention of information, and better compliance with the therapy program (11,14,25,30). Sluijs describes several verbal and nonverbal behaviors that contribute to a good therapist–patient relationship such as reinforcing the patient's performance, showing concern for pain, showing interest in the patient, showing involvement in the treatment, and facilitating patient participation (14). Hall et al reported on the positive associations found between patient outcomes and the degree of patient–therapist alliance. This alliance was determined by three factors: (a) the therapist–patient agreement on goals of treatment, (b) the therapist–patient agreement on interventions, and (c) the affective bond between patient and therapist. Significant positive associations were found between the alliance and the patient's global perceived effect of treatment, change in pain, physical function, patient satisfaction with treatment, depression, and general health status (31).

Sluijs found that patients are more willing to participate when they have a clearly described plan of care. This approach has the clinician utilize a planned and systematic treatment approach. Patients recognize this as an indicator of quality of care, and are more likely to be motivated to participate in this situation (14). The approach involves working according to four-stage procedure: (a) identifying the problem, (b) setting a treatment goal, (c) making a rational treatment plan, and (d) assessing goal achievement (14). This information, including the planned and systematic treatment approach, should be shared with the patient.

PRACTICAL APPLICATION

Patients are less likely to adhere to a HEP when it is not tailored to the individuals' situation or daily routine (32,33). The more inconvenient a program is, the less likely the patient will comply. Finding a way to incorporate the HEP into their daily routine will decrease the time commitment and hopefully improve compliance. One strategy to do this is to advise patients to perform the HEP at the same time and the most convenient time every day. Finding a time that works best and making it a permanent part of their daily routine will help improve compliance. In our experience, providing short duration exercises that can be repeated several times throughout the day can also be beneficial. Breaking up the exercises also makes the HEP more manageable and may increase compliance.

Make sure to individualize their HEP to the environment where they are most likely to perform it. For the patient who doesn't go to a gym or exercise regularly, prescribing an exercise program that can be performed at home and without equipment will facilitate more regular participation with a smaller cost to overcome. Utilizing resistance bands and household objects such as a can of soup or bottle of water for light resistance, rather than having to buy weights or dumbbells will make the program more accessible. For patients who travel often, resistance bands are easy to travel with and may increase compliance to their HEP while away from home.

With respect to numbers of exercises and directions, it appears best to keep it simple. Complex regimens lead to greater noncompliance than simple ones (34). The number of exercises in a program or the time it takes to complete the program may affect compliance. This may be more important in patients who are elderly. Henry found in her study of patients aged 65 and older that they performed better with fewer exercises. The group with two exercises had significantly better compliance than the group with eight (35). Also consider the complexity of wording and language in your instructions. In order to be effective, educational information should be presented

in simple everyday language, meaningful to patients, and tailored to suit their needs (36).

USE OF HOME EXERCISE PROGRAMS

Use of home-based exercises versus clinic-based therapy has been investigated in the literature. Friedrich et al examined outcomes for patients with neck and low back pain who received instruction from either a therapist or from an educational brochure. Patients receiving instructions from a therapist performed the exercises more accurately and had a greater decrease in pain as compared with the patients receiving instructions from a brochure (37). This study demonstrates that patients have improved outcomes with therapist supervision versus patient education alone. In the ideal case, patient education will supplement the PT intervention rather than replace it.

In the case of declining insurance reimbursements and limited therapy visits, it appears that patient education can improve patient outcomes. There have been studies that examine the use of HEP versus clinic-based program with therapist supervision for rotator cuff repair and ACL reconstruction (38,39). In both of these patient populations investigators compared a group that had less clinic visits but were supplemented with significant patient education materials against those with more clinic sessions. The authors report similar outcomes with respect to functional levels at follow up.

Basset demonstrated that using a home-based program for treating ankle sprains with the use of adherence enhancement strategies resulted in equivalent recovery in that population versus patients coming into the clinic (40). The home-based exercises were supplemented with a significant amount of equipment and educational and cognitive behavioral adjuncts, such as strapping tape, resistance bands, wobble boards, an information booklet on their condition, and many others. It may be used for patients who are unable to attend PT in the clinic or have issues with insurance coverage.

Lo examined the use of computer-aided learning programs and found this method was able to increase favorable patient outcomes in a class for diabetes care education. This suggests that for some individuals this may be a beneficial learning medium (41). As people become more electronic media and digitally oriented this type of learning may prove to be preferable to traditional media such as booklets and paper handouts. The therapist must consider what method and media work best for each individual patient.

MANAGING INFORMATION

At one time physicians were the sole providers of patient education and information regarding their medical condition. Today patients have too much information available via Internet websites, health club blogs and forums, television programs and advertising by pharmaceutical companies, surgical implant manufacturers, and athletic shoe companies. Some of this information is accurate and some is not in varying degrees. Many times the information may not be applicable or equivalent to the patient's situation. Also, there is often confusing and conflicting information. Part of the physician's and therapist's role in patient education today may be to educate the consumer to select appropriate information, find reliable resources, and differentiate between advertisement and factual data (42).

SUMMARY

Patient education is a valuable tool in patient care. It has been shown to increase patient satisfaction and improve outcomes. The physical therapist is in a unique position to provide education regarding a patient's condition, prognosis, and management. There are tools that therapists can utilize to improve patient education and thereby create positive changes in behavior directed at improving the health status of their patients. The physician and physical therapist together play a key role in providing accurate information and credible resources for patients to make informed decisions regarding their care and to become actively involved in the management of their own health.

REFERENCES

1. Superio-Cabuslay E, Ward MM, Lorig KR. Patient education interventions in osteoarthritis and rheumatoid arthritis: a meta-analytic comparison with non steroidal anti inflammatory drug treatment. *Arthr Rheum.* 1996;9(4):292–301.
2. Lorig KR, Mazonson PD, Holman HR. Evidence suggesting that health education for self-management in patients with chronic arthritis has sustained health benefits while reducing health care costs. *Arthr Rheum.* 1993;36(4):439–446.
3. Leslie M, Schuster PA. The effect of contingency contracting on adherence and knowledge of exercise regimens. *Purienr Educurion und Counseling.* 1991;18:231–241.
4. Sluijs EM, Knibbe JJ. Patient compliance with exercise: different theoretical approaches to short-term and long-term compliance. *Patient Education and Counseling.* 1991;11:191–204.
5. Koongstvedt PR. *The Managed Health Care Handbook.* 4th ed. Gaithersburg, MD: Aspen Publishers; 2001:788.
6. Murphy W. *Healing the Generations: A History of Physical Therapy and the American Physical Therapy.* Lyme, CT: Greenwich Publishing Therapy Association; 1995.
7. Scully RM, Rames MR, eds. *Physical Therapy.* Philadelphia, PA: JB Lippincott Co; 1989.
8. Commission on Accreditation in Physical Therapy Education. *Accreditation Handbook, 1997-1998,* Alexandria, VA: American Physical Therapy Association; 1997:70.
9. Chase L, Elkins J, Readinger J, et al. Perceptions of physical therapists towards patient education. *Phys Ther.* 1993;73:787–796.
10. Ice R. Long-term compliance. *Phys Ther.* 1985;65:1832-1839.
11. Ley PH. Giving information to patients. In: Eiser JR, ed. *Social Psychology and Behavioural Medicine.* New York, NY: John Wiley & Sons; 1982:339–373.
12. Kindelan Y, Kent G. Patients' preferences for information. *J R Coll Gen Pract.* 1986;36:461–463.
13. Simonds SK. Individual health counseling and education: emerging directions from current theory, research, and practice. *Patient Counselling and Health Education.* 1983;4(17):181.
14. Sluijs EM. A checklist to assess patient education in physical therapy practice. *Phys Ther.* 991;71(8):561–569.
15. Prochaska JO, Velicer WF. The transtheoretical model of health behavior change. *Am J Health Promot.* 1997;12(1):38–48.
16. Taal E, Rasker J, Seydel E, Wiegman O. Health status, adherence with health recommendations, self-efficacy, and social support in patients with rheumatoid arthritis. *Patient Education and Counseling.* 1993;20:63–76.
17. Moon MH, Moon BA, Black WA. Compliance in splint-wearing behavior of patients with rheumatoid arthritis [abstract]. *N Z Med J.* 1976;83:360–365.
18. Feinberg J, Brandt KD. Use of resting splints by patients with rheumatoid arthritis. *Am J Occup Ther.* 1981;135:173–178.
19. Jette AM. Improving patient cooperation with arthritis treatment regimens. *Arthri Rheum.* 1982;25:447–445.
20. Mayo NE. Patient compliance: practical implications for physical therapists. *Phys Ther.* 1978;58:1083–1090.
21. Becker MH. Patient adherence to prescribed therapies. *Med Care.* 1985;23:539–555.
22. Sluijs EM Kok GJ, van der Zee J. Correlates of exercise compliance in physical therapy. *Phys Ther.* 1993;73(11):771–782.
23. Engström OL, Öberg EB. Patient adherence in an individualized rehabilitation programme: A clinical follow-up. *Scand J Public Health.* 2005;33:11–18.
24. Lorish C. Facilitating behavior change: Strategies for education and practice. *J Phys Ther Ed.* 1999;13(2):1–11.
25. DiMatteo MR, DiNicola DD. *Achieving Patient Compliance.* Elmsford, NY: Pergamon Press Inc; 1982.
26. Bartlett EE. Behavioral diagnosis: a practical approach to patient education. *Patient Counselling and Health Education.* 1982;4:29–35.
27. Strecher VJ. Improving physician-patient interactions: a review. *Patient Counselling and Health Education.* 1983;4:129–136.
28. Stone GC. Patient compliance and the role of the expert. *J Soc Issues.* 1979;35:35–59.

29. Maiman LA, Becker MR. The Health Belief Model: origins and correlates in psychological theory. *Health Education Monographs*. 1974;2:336–353.

30. Feinberg J. The effect of patient practitioner interaction on compliance: a review of the literature and application to rheumatoid arthritis. *Patient Education and Counselling*. 1988;11:171–187.

31. Hall A, Ferreira PH, Maher CG, Latimer J, Ferreira ML. The influence of the therapist-patient relationship on treatment outcome in physical rehabilitation: a systematic review. *Phys Ther*. 2010;90(8):1099–1110.

32. Posavac El, Sinacore JM, Brotherton SE, et al. Increasing compliance to medical treatment regimens: a meta-analysis of program evaluation. *Evaluation and the Health Professions*. 1985;8:7–22.

33. Bartlett EE. Behavioral diagnosis: a practical approach to patient education. *Patient Counseling and Health Education*. 1982;4:29–35.

34. Becker MH. Patient adherence to prescribed therapies. *Med Care*. 1985;23:539–555.

35. Henry KD, Rosemond D, Eckert LB. Effect of number of home exercises on compliance and performance in adults over 65 years of age. *Phys Ther*. 1990;70(3):270–276.

36. Raynor DK. The influence of written information on patient knowledge and adherence to treatment. In: Myers LB, Midence K, eds. *Adherence to Treatment in Medical Conditions*. Reading, United Kingdom: Harwood Academic Publishers; 1998: 83–111.

37. Friedrich M, Cermak I, Maderbacher R. The effect of brochure use versus therapist teaching on patients performing therapeutic exercises and on changes in impairment status. *Phys Ther*. 1996;76:1082–1088.

38. Roddey TS, Olson SL, Gartsman GM, Hanten WP, Cook KF. A randomized controlled trial comparing 2 instructional approaches to home exercise instruction following arthroscopic full-thickness rotator cuff repair surgery. *J Orthop Sports Phys Ther*. 2002;32(11):548–559.

39. Grant JA, Mohtadi NG, Maitland ME, Zernicke RF. Comparison of home versus physical therapy-supervised rehabilitation programs after anterior cruciate ligament reconstruction: a randomized clinical trial. *Am J Sports Med*. 2005;33(9):1288–1297.

40. Bassett SF, Prapavessis H. Home-based physical therapy intervention with adherence-enhancing strategies versus clinic-based management for patients with ankle sprains. *Phys Ther*. 2007;87(9):1132–1143.

41. Tu K, Lo D, Wells E, et al. The development and evaluation of a computer-aided diabetes education program. *Aust J Adv Nurs*. 1996;13(4):19–27.

42. May BJ. Patient education: past and present. *J Phys The Ed*. 1999;13(2):1–7.

Guide to Therapy Prescription Writing

Gautam Malhotra, James F. Wyss, and Amrish D. Patel

INTRODUCTION: A FAREWELL TO "PLEASE EVALUATE AND TREAT"

When "please evaluate and treat" is the entire prescription, it puts the entire responsibility of developing a treatment plan on the therapist. Although some therapists have grown to enjoy the autonomy that this type of practice has engendered, in the end, this situation results in the patient losing the benefits of an interdisciplinary approach to care. In the authors' experiences the answer is quite clear: If you were to ask any patient whether they would prefer to be treated by multiple separate clinicians (multidisciplinary approach) or a team of clinicians who work together on developing a diagnosis and treatment plan (interdisciplinary approach), they would prefer the interdisciplinary team approach.

Like many residents and fellows, the authors quickly realized that they would never be equally proficient to a therapist at delivering hands-on modalities, functional training, or exercise education. Also, the therapist tends to spend hours with the patient while their interactions with patients are much shorter and less frequent encounters. As the prescribing clinicians, this was a humbling realization and has resulted in the practice of genuinely seeking and honoring the feedback, advice, evaluations, and outcomes delivered by therapists. This in turn builds respect and lines of communication from the therapist back to the prescribing physician. In the end, the patient reaps a more comprehensive yet expeditious experience derived from such an interdisciplinary team approach.

If you are reading this book, it means you are a clinician who is interested in taking an active role in the rehabilitation of your patients. Whether you are a physiatrist, family physician, sports medicine specialist, rheumatologist, internist, or surgeon, this book is an attempt to bridge some of the gaps between the prescribing physician and the therapist. It is *not* meant to be a cookbook with recipes for a dogmatic cookie-cutter approach to prescriptions. Templates can be useful starting points to ensure all

options are considered and to streamline the delivery of a prescription. However, in their experience, therapists do not respond as well to long lists that are not individualized to the patient's particular situation. Patients do not recover or rehabilitate productively with this approach either.

APPROACH TO THERAPY PRESCRIPTION WRITING

In addition to the thoughts above, here are some specific thoughts to consider as you work to individualize your prescriptions:

- You will prescribe therapy much like you would a medication. You have to know the patient, the problem that you are addressing, concurrent problems that could affect your prescription, and most important, what the goal is
- Use therapy like it's your bag of tricks to accomplish treatment goals. The prescription requires a thoughtful goal-oriented approach rather than a mindless cookbook recipe approach. (Do *not* just copy and paste)
- It is helpful to think about the following questions:
  What therapeutic modalities are safe and beneficial for my patient?
  What types of manual therapy techniques would be beneficial?
  What structures are weak and need to be strengthened? What structures are tight and need to be stretched or lengthened?
  What movements are poorly coordinated or have biomechanical faults that need to be retrained and corrected?
  What other impairments (e.g., poor balance, impaired proprioception) exist?

What activities or positions should be avoided due to their detrimental effects versus what activities or positions should be encouraged to promote recovery? What educational training and resources would be helpful for my patient?

▪ Some components of the prescription may require detailed specificity to ensure that the therapist understands it to be important in your thought process. Flexibility in other components of the prescription will be appreciated by your therapist as it will allow some personalization at the time of therapy. So be careful to consider every word in your prescriptions in order to avoid over-writing as well. The balance of writing enough but not too much is more like an art that takes years of experience with the therapists and patient populations in your community

COMPONENTS OF A THERAPY PRESCRIPTION

The prescription may incorporate the following fields (see sample Rx at the end of the chapter).

Identifying Information

Including the patient's name, date of birth, medical record numbers etc… along with the date the prescription was written.

Discipline

Indicate physical therapy (PT) or occupational therapy (OT). Although these are the main disciplines considered in this textbook other disciplines may need to be included as well: athletic training, exercise physiology, massage therapy, recreational therapy, even speech and language pathology.

Diagnosis

Begin with your primary diagnosis, then secondary diagnoses if relevant. Identify contributing factors to the diagnosis (e.g., tight hamstrings in the setting of mechanical low back pain). Also identify relevant past medical and surgical history to effectively communicate with the therapist.

Problem List (Optional)

This section provides an additional way to communicate mechanical and functional deficits that may be contributing factors to the development of the diagnosis or that may lead to delayed rehabilitation of the condition if not properly addressed. An example would include decreased passive and active ankle dorsiflexion following acute lateral ankle sprain. Failure to restore this range of motion (ROM) may lead to incomplete functional recovery or recurrent ankle sprains.

Precautions

Spend time detailing precautions for the patient's therapy program; examples include weight bearing restrictions, ROM restrictions, and specific exertion to avoid. Precautions will be dictated by information elicited on history and physical examination. Does the patient have a history of falls or are they at significant risk of future falls? Cardiac or pulmonary disease? Seizures? Is there a history of severe osteoporosis necessitating fracture risk precautions? Are they insensate in areas that may burn if heat is used or develop pressure ulcers if unchecked? Do they have any breaks or openings in the skin? Are there issues that need to be resolved/clarified/cleared by other physicians (e.g., surgeon, cardiologist, internist) before therapy can be initiated?

Frequency of Visits

Most prescriptions are written "2-3x/week," but please take the time to consider the needs of the specific patient. An athletic patient with good body awareness may adequately progress with weekly visits and a daily home exercise program. Whereas patients with acute injuries or postsurgical cases may initially require more frequent visits. The burdens of being a sole caregiver, sole provider, or difficulty with travel or financial limitations may play a part in the decision on frequency of treatment. Every effort must be made to consider these practical impediments to participation.

Duration of Treatment

The most common length of treatment is 4 to 6 weeks, but take the time to individualize the duration as well. Based on known natural history or acuity of the condition, shorter (1–2 weeks) or longer (> 6 weeks) may be anticipated for improvement or resolution.

Treatment

This part of the Rx is the most challenging and may be overwhelming the first time you do it. It is useful to approach it systematically with the list in the text box and by applying the concepts or questions discussed in the "*approach to therapy prescription writing*" section.

Therapeutic Modalities

- **Thermotherapy**:
  - Cryotherapy: (ice pack, ice bath, ice massage) for inflammation/swelling/pain
  - Superficial heat therapy: (hot packs, warm bath, paraffin, fluidotherapy, whirlpool, contrast baths) for pain relief and to enhance recovery
  - Deep heat therapy: ultrasound, short wave diathermy, laser therapy
- **Phototherapy**: laser therapy, UV light
- **Electrical stimulation**: transcutaneous electrical nerve stimulation (TENS), interferential current (IFC), functional electrical stimulation (FES), neuromuscular stimulation (NMES), Iontophoresis

Manual Therapy

- Massage, joint mobilization, myofascial release (MFR), soft-tissue mobilization, acupressure, transverse friction massage, positional release or counter-strain, traction (manual, mechanical) are some techniques to consider for your patient

Therapeutic Exercise

- ROM exercises: passive, active assisted, active
- Stretching: self-stretching, therapist-assisted stretching, contract-relax stretching
- Strengthening: generalized strengthening or identify the need to strengthen specific muscle groups, isotonic (eccentric/concentric) versus isometric, closed versus open kinetic chain progressive resistive exercise (PRE), core strengthening or stabilization programs
- Balance/proprioceptive training, neuromuscular reeducation
- Conditioning exercises: this may be indicated as general conditioning exercises (GCEs) or if necessary, specific programs with a warm-up/cool down, duration and type of exercise may be considered. Examples include: Upper body ergometry (UBE), treadmill, upright or recumbent stationary bike, or ambulation training with or without assistive devices (e.g., parallel bars)

Specialized Treatments

- Some examples include the use of aquatic therapy or kinesiology taping
- Other examples include analysis of the kinetic chain, functional movement screen, or even a running analysis could be considered here
- The prescribing physician may also request a specific therapeutic approach in this section, such as mechanical diagnosis and therapy (MDT), also known as the McKenzie method
- Other examples are related to task specific functions, such as:
  - **Mobility training:** kinetic chain or biomechanical analysis and training, gait analysis and training, transfer training, postural analysis and training
  - **Activities of Daily Living (ADL) training:** Personal care activities with or without adaptive equipment such as dressing, eating, or personal hygiene
  - **Instrumental ADL:** These activities are related to independent living but not necessary for fundamental functioning (e.g., food preparation, accounting, housework, etc.)
  - **Equipment:** Use of specific supportive or assistive devices, orthotic training, and durable medical equipment to aid in all of the above categories

Patient Education

Patient education is provided to the patient and possibly their family in the form of verbal, visual, and written instruction; or digital media. Examples of patient education include an explanation of their specific condition and associated prognosis, home exercise program, and postural education. Joint protection and energy conservation techniques are other examples. In addition, all of the therapeutic exercises discussed above have an educational component and require carryover by the patient to change posture, correct movement patterns, and eliminate causative factors of pain.

Reevaluation

Time until physician reevaluation should be clearly communicated with the patient and the therapist. Communicating with the providing therapist is crucial. Therapists vary in their training, experience, skill sets, biases, philosophies on healthcare delivery, and even bedside manner, just as physicians do. We recommend getting to know the therapists at your hospital and in your local community. Knowing their strengths and weaknesses in these fields will be a crucial step in correctly pairing patients and therapists to successfully obtain favorable outcomes. In addition, you will need to communicate (written or verbally) with the therapist to make sure they are following the therapeutic program you have prescribed and what the outcomes have been, just as you would with a nurse regarding a prescribed medication.

We recommend requesting formal feedback on patient progress to help guide your reevaluation. Read the therapist's notes or call them to clarify the patient's progress and tolerance to the therapeutic program. Their feedback is vital when reassessing the patient's condition, when deciding to continue or discontinue your patient's therapy program, and when deciding if additional diagnostic studies or treatments are necessary. If therapy is to be continued, the prescription should change at follow-up to incorporate the progress and/or changes in symptomatology.

SUMMARY

Therapy prescription writing is more of an art than a science. If you invest time and effort into this part of your practice we do believe it will influence patient outcomes. In this chapter, we have presented a "guide to therapy prescription writing" that can be utilized for the overall framework, concepts, and systematic approach. As you become more comfortable with your practice and develop relationships with therapists at your hospital and in your community, your style of writing will evolve, but always remember to utilize it to establish a team approach to care that provides all the necessary medical information to the treating therapist and treatment recommendations that are evidence based and individualized to your patient.

 SAMPLE THERAPY PRESCRIPTION

Name with identifying factors: (e.g., DOB)

Date:

Discipline: PT, OT, or other

Diagnosis or diagnoses:

Problem list:

Precautions:

Frequency of visits: such as 2 to 3x/week.

Duration of treatment: such as 3 to 4 weeks; or 8 to 12 total visits used at the therapist's discretion

Treatment:

1. *Therapeutic modalities:* such as heat or cold packs, electrical stimulation

2. *Manual therapy:* such as MFR, massage, or joint mobilization

3. *Therapeutic exercise:* such as active, active assisted, and passive range of motion (A/AA/PROM), stretching, strengthening/PREs, balance/proprioceptive training, neuromuscular reeducation, or conditioning exercises

4. *Specialized treatments:* kinesiology taping, aquatic therapy, or kinetic chain analysis

5. *Patient education:* such as written home exercise program

Goals: such as decrease pain and swelling, restore ROM/flexibility then strength, or safely return to functional activities (e.g., sport, hobbies, and work)

Reevaluation: such as 3 to 4 weeks by referring physician.

Shoulder Impingement Syndromes

Rex Ma, Debra Ibrahim, Jose Santiago Campos, and Lynn A. Ryan

INTRODUCTION

There are four types of impingement that have been described in the literature. Impingement has been described as primary versus secondary and/or internal versus external impingement. Primary or external impingement is an irritation at the bursal side of rotator cuff tendons. Multiple factors can contribute to external impingement including: shape of the acromion process, acromioclavicular (AC) joint arthropathy, subacromial spur, rotator cuff weakness, or scapular dyskinesia (1,2). Secondary impingement is described as microinstability leading to difficulty keeping the humeral head centered on the glenoid fossa during movement (2). This can be due to impairment of the static stabilizers (labrum, capsular ligaments), dynamic stabilizers (weakness of the rotator cuff muscles), and scapular stabilizers.

Internal impingement is the most common cause of posterior shoulder pain in overhead athletes (3,4). Impingement occurs at the articular surface of the rotator cuff against the posterior superior glenoid and the glenoid labrum, hence it is often termed posterior superior glenoid impingement (PSGI) (3,4). The correct diagnosis is important to determine the underlying cause and to guide proper treatment.

The focus of this chapter will look at primary or external rotator cuff impingement by the acromion or coracoacromial arch, which is a common condition that has been well described in the literature. This condition is thought to arise from repetitive or excessive contact of the rotator cuff tendons with other anatomic structures in the shoulder, and usually results in functional loss and disability. The spectrum of problems caused by impingement can range from subacromial bursitis to full thickness rotator cuff tears. Cadaveric studies have shown there to be an incidence of 5% to 30% of rotator cuff tears, with a large proportion being attributed to preexisting rotator

cuff impingement (5,6). The supraspinatus tendon is generally the first involved among the rotator cuff, often attributed to the tendon's relative avascularity, age-related changes in collagen, and mechanical trauma as it courses under the acromion (1,3,7,8). Neer previously described the mechanical impingement of the rotator cuff tendon beneath the anteroinferior portion of the acromion, attributing the morphology of the acromion (flat, curved, hooked) on the incidence of rotator cuff impingement. He also described three stages of impingement: Stage 1 injuries involve edema and hemorrhage related to overactivity, generally within a younger, athletic population (< 25 years old). Stage 2 injuries have been related to recurrent injuries and inflammation, leading to fibrotic changes and tendinitis (25–40 years old). Stage 3 injuries have been described to occur in an older population (> 40 years old), resulting in bone spur formation and incomplete/complete rotator cuff tears (4,9).

A comprehensive history and physical examination plays a vital role in the management of patients with shoulder impingement. It helps to confirm the diagnosis as well as identify risk factors and altered shoulder biomechanics that may contribute to or even cause the problem. From these physical findings, the clinician can develop an evaluation-based treatment plan. This section highlights important aspects of the history and physical examination in the development of the program. Important physical examination maneuvers are described below and the reader is encouraged to seek out additional resources (2,10) for information on a more detailed shoulder exam.

History should include age, occupation, as well as mechanism of injury. Quantifying and qualifying the pain are also important considerations. This will include the type, onset, location, severity, duration, exacerbating and ameliorating factors, and frequency of the pain. Patients usually present with an insidious onset of worsening shoulder pain exacerbated by overhead activities. Night time pain while lying on the shoulder, as well as weakness with shoulder elevation can develop (11). Although this syndrome more commonly affects the older population, it is frequently seen in athletes or workers who participate in repetitive overhead activities as well.

Key elements of the physical examination include inspection, palpation range of motion (ROM) testing, neurovascular examination, clearance of the cervical spine, strength assessment especially of the rotator cuff, and special tests. The physical examination is useful in confirming or ruling out the diagnosis of shoulder impingement. Ideally the test should be sensitive and specific or in other words, accurate for this diagnosis. One study evaluated various physical examination maneuvers on 913 patients and reported the accuracy of these tests in the diagnosis of shoulder impingement (12). The most accurate test for patients with any type of impingement was reported to be the painful arc sign (76%). If these patients were divided into subgroups, then the cross body adduction test was the most accurate for impingement patients with bursitis (73%) and partial RTC tear (71%). The supraspinatus and infraspinatus strength tests were the most accurate test for impingement patients with full thickness RTC (rotator cuff) tear (both 70%). A combination of positive tests will increase the probability of making the correct diagnosis. For example, with a positive painful arc sign, infraspinatus muscle strength test and Hawkins-Kennedy impingement sign, there is a posttest probability of >95% for impingement syndrome. If the painful arc sign and infraspinatus muscle strength test is combined with the drop arm sign instead, this can help diagnose the subgroup of impingement patients with full thickness RTC tear with a posttest probability of >91%. On the other hand, there is a posttest probability of <9% for a full thickness tear if none of these tests were positive. This information will be very useful for the clinician to help choose between conservative management versus referral to an orthopedist for surgical evaluation.

Besides establishing the diagnosis of shoulder impingement, the physical examination can help identify contributing biomechanical factors to be addressed by the rehabilitation program. The following elements are important to include: postural assessment, ROM, flexibility and strength testing, and scapular motion. Postural dysfunctions to look for include forward head (decreased cervical lordosis), forward-rounded shoulders (scapular protraction), thoracic kyphosis, or scoliosis, which can alter both shoulder and scapular mechanics. Improper posture can result in decreased outlet space of the coracoacromial arch as well as altering scapular mechanics, both of which can predispose patients to impingement. Then an evaluation and comparison of shoulder ROM, including flexion, abduction, and scaption as well as internal and external rotation. For flexibility testing, the key is to have a working knowledge of muscles around the shoulder that are prone to tightness and focus the examination on these muscles. These muscles include the upper trapezius (UT), levator scapulae, pectoralis major, pectoralis minor, scalenes, latissimus dorsi, and teres major (2). Generally speaking, when deficits are seen, treatment should be directed to restore ROM, flexibility, or movement for any musculoskeletal complaint. Two important problems to look for are pectoralis minor tightness and glenohumeral internal rotation deficit (GIRD) (13), both of which can predispose patients to impingement syndromes and other upper limb MSK conditions.

RTC weakness is often present in patients with shoulder impingement (14–17), if detected on physical examination, then in theory RTC strengthening should be included in the rehabilitation program. Unfortunately, it is unclear whether traditional manual muscle testing or isometric assessment of shoulder weakness is sensitive enough to detect weakness that can be seen with use of a dynamometer. To maximize the detection of subtle RTC weakness, it is helpful to use tests that isolate the targeted muscles. The full can test (18) (for isolation of the supraspinatus), infraspinatus strength test at 45° IR (18), the bear hug test, and the belly press test (19) (for isolation of the subscapularis) are physical examination maneuvers that have been shown to be useful for isolation of the specific RTC muscles indicated above. Even with specialized tests our examination doesn't assess for functional strength, such as muscular endurance with occupational tasks.

Scapular examination for signs of dyskinesis should always be performed in patients with suspected impingement since there is growing literature that correlates dysfunction with shoulder impingement (20–23). Scapular dyskinesis is generally characterized by a lack of upward rotation, lack of posterior tilting, and increased internal or medial rotation of the scapula. There are many tests to evaluate the scapula. One test with good interrater reliability that may be helpful for guiding treatments is the modified scapular assistance test (24). This maneuver may help with impingement symptoms by increasing the subacromial space (25). When performing the test, a decrease or abolishment of symptoms with this maneuver is thought to be positive for a patient with poor scapular control. In theory, emphasizing scapular stabilization and strengthening for this patient would be helpful.

Other important parts of the physical examination with suspected impingement include testing for glenohumeral joint (GHJ) instability, since instability can cause secondary impingement due to increased humeral head translation. Additional physical examination maneuvers would be necessary to rule out injuries to surrounding structures in the neck and shoulder. These include cervical spine and upper limb inspection, postural assessment, palpation, flexibility, ROM, and neurovascular examination.

Plain radiographs are not very sensitive or specific for impingement syndromes, but can be obtained to identify traumatic injuries, arthritic changes, tendon or bursal calcifications, humeral head subluxation that may suggest a rotator cuff tear, or to assess shape of the acromion. Further imaging may consist of an MRI to evaluate for partial or full thickness tears of the rotator cuff. Ultrasound examination is gaining increasing acceptance as an imaging modality for assessment of the rotator cuff and impingement syndromes. Once the diagnosis is confirmed and concomitant injuries (e.g., fracture, dislocation, or neurovascular injury) have been ruled out, a comprehensive rehabilitation program is planned based on the severity of the injury.

SHOULDER IMPINGEMENT SYNDROMES

▪ This condition has a very high prevalence, often among the elderly population, but may be related to athletes performing repetitive overhead activities as well

▪ Patients typically present with shoulder pain exacerbated by overhead activities and night time discomfort

▪ Key physical examination maneuvers, such as Neer's and Hawkins-Kennedy test are used to confirm the diagnosis

▪ Assessment of biomechanical factors that contribute to impingement syndrome include postural assessment, RTC strength, and scapular motion

▪ Additional physical examination maneuvers, such as inspection of the neck and upper limb, cervical spine ROM, and neurological examination, should be performed to rule out injuries to surrounding structures

▪ MRI evaluation should be obtained if significant rotator cuff tears are suspected

THE REHABILITATION PROGRAM

Multiple systematic reviews concluded that a comprehensive therapy program is beneficial for shoulder impingement syndromes (26–30). The specifics of the program typically involve patient education, use of modalities, manual therapy, and therapeutic exercise. This section highlights important aspects of each of these areas.

Therapeutic Modalities

Various therapeutic modalities are often used for the treatment of shoulder impingement. They include moist heat, cryotherapy, therapeutic ultrasound (thermal and nonthermal), low level laser, and transcutaneous electrical nerve stimulation (TENS). Literature supporting the use of these modalities is limited at best. Therapeutic ultrasound and low level laser have been theorized to help with pain relief as well as healing of the damaged tendon. However, based on the available research for the treatment of shoulder impingement, most studies and reviews showed no effective benefit with either low level laser or therapeutic ultrasound (31–36). With regards to moist heat, cryotherapy, and TENS, there is no significant data for or against their use. Therefore, the use of these modalities should be optional and individualized to the patient. One practical approach is to utilize modalities such as moist heat prior to manual or exercise therapy and cryotherapy after exercise to minimize the pain that may occur during a therapy session.

Manual Therapy

Manual therapy, when combined with an exercise program, has been shown to be effective for treatment in patients with shoulder impingement (37–39). The treatment typically involves soft tissue and/or joint mobilizations with the goal of releasing tight soft tissue and restoring better scapular mechanics and glenohumeral ROM. This is indicated for patients with joint or soft tissue hypomobility, which is often seen with primary impingement. Depending upon the findings, scapular mobilizations to consider include scapular distraction, inferior glide to assist scapular depression, and medial glide to assist retraction. Caudal and cranial rotations of the scapula assist with extension/adduction and flexion/abduction, respectively. GHJ mobilizations can also be considered in patients with hypomobility. Typical treatments include inferior and posterior glides, or distraction to assist with shoulder elevation, abduction, and flexion. As a word of caution, when a patient has signs of glenohumeral instability on physical examination, mobilization to that joint would contraindicated while stabilization exercises would be emphasized.

Therapeutic Exercise

It is without a doubt that a rehabilitation program, with the focus being therapeutic exercise, is beneficial for patients with shoulder impingement (26–30). However, there is no standard protocol for exercise in patients with impingement; therefore, a logical approach is to design a rehabilitation program based on the patient's examination findings (30,40). This section highlights important exercises that can be incorporated into an evaluation-based rehabilitation program. Remember to follow the phases of rehabilitation and the major exercise categories including ROM/flexibility, RTC strengthening, and scapular strengthening/stabilization. Keep in mind that depending upon the patient's level of fitness, he/she may be unable to participate in certain exercises. In addition, for patients whose goal is to return to a high level of activity with the shoulder, additional exercises may be required. In general this will include kinetic chain movements that integrate the entire body into the movement patterns. Other exercises can include isokinetic strengthening, plyometrics, and sports specific exercises. The specific details of these exercises are beyond the scope of this chapter.

ROM and flexibility exercises are initiated in phase II of rehabilitation. The patient is initially instructed to limit shoulder movement to a pain-free range which is usually below shoulder level, therefore, the program can start with Codman's pendulum exercises (Figure 8.1) and wand exercises without elevation. ROM with elevation can be added as tolerated by pain. Stretches should also be introduced early in the exercise program and can be added by instructing the patient to apply slight pressure at the end range during the wand exercises. Two areas where tightness can predispose patients to shoulder impingement include the pectoralis minor muscle and posterior/inferior capsule resulting in GIRD. For the pectoralis minor muscle, the most effective stretch has been shown to be the unilateral self stretch (Figure 8.2) (41) while for patients with GIRD, two particularly good stretches include the cross body adduction (Figure 8.3) and the sleeper stretch (Figure 8.4). A study compared these two stretches and concluded that both improve internal rotation (IR) IR ROM of the shoulder but the cross adduction stretch resulted in more IR ROM and caused less pain than the sleeper stretch (42). All stretches should be performed daily and should be held between 15 to 30 seconds repeating at least three to five times. Keep in mind that these stretches should not reproduce subacromial pain and should be deferred if there is significant pain. Other areas to consider for stretching, based upon physical findings, include the UT, levator scapulae, scalenes, and suboccipital muscles.

Strengthening of the RTC is clearly an important part of the exercise program as improvement is seen in multiple studies that involve RTC strengthening (37–39,43–46). At this time, there is no consensus on the best strengthening exercises but it would make sense to advance the exercises based on pain tolerance. Strengthening can start with isometrics without shoulder elevation. Isometric strengthening for internal and external rotators can be performed

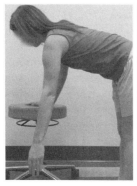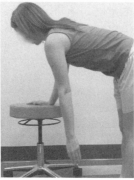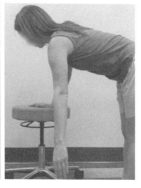

FIGURE 8.1: Codman's pendulum exercises.

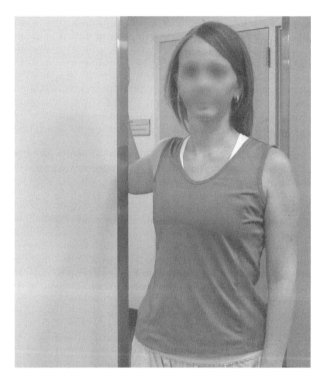

FIGURE 8.2: Unilateral self stretch of the pectoralis muscle group, including the pectoralis miinor.

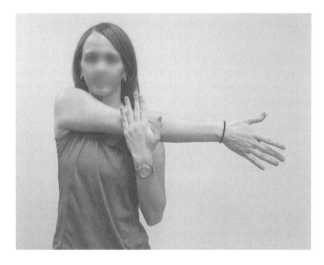

FIGURE 8.3: Cross body adduction.

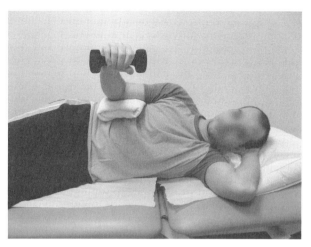

FIGURE 8.4: Resisted external rotation for rotator cuff strengthening.

against a static body. Once ROM has improved and pain decreased, isotonic RTC strengthening can be added. This phase of strengthening can be done with the use of either dumbbells or resistance tubing or bands. Initial isotonic RTC strengthening should emphasize cuff function without elevation to minimize discomfort. With the shoulder on the side and elbows flexed to 90 degrees, the rotator cuff can be strengthened in external rotation, internal rotation, and extension (Figure 8.4). A pillow or rolled up towel should be placed underneath the arm to minimize adduction. RTC strengthening with elevation can be added when there is minimal to no pain. This can include flexion (Figure 8.5a), abduction (Figure 8.5b) as well as scaption. These exercises can be performed in 3 sets of 10 repetitions and repetitions or intensity can increase as tolerated.

Scapular rehabilitation addresses impaired scapular mechanics early in the rehabilitation program. The initial goal is to normalize the resting position of the scapula without putting high demands on the shoulder joint. Various exercises have been shown to be helpful during this phase, including inferior glide, low row, lawnmower, and robbery exercises (47). The next phase of scapular stabilization involves correcting muscle imbalances of the scapular stabilizers. These imbalances occur as a result of weaker scapular stabilizers, namely the middle trapezius (MT), lower trapezius (LT), and serratus anterior (SA) along with overactivity of the UT (20,48–50). Forward flexion in side lying and side lying external rotation exercises (51) are optimal for restoration of UT/MT and UT/LT imbalance whereas the push up plus exercise (Figure 8.6) (48) is optimal for restoration of UT/SA imbalance. The side lying external rotation exercise is an especially good exercise since it has the added advantage of strengthening the supraspinatus, infraspinatus, teres minor, and posterior deltoid muscles (52,53). Once muscle balance is restored, general scapular strengthening exercises may be used to

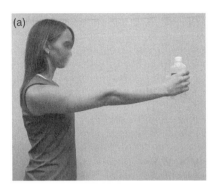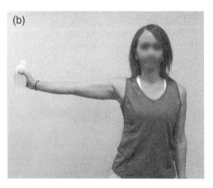

FIGURE 8.5: (a) Resisted flexion and (b) abduction.

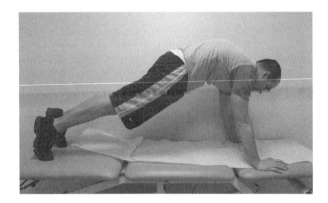

FIGURE 8.6: Push up plus exercise.

increase muscle strength. During this phase, exercises that maximally activate the targeted muscles can be used. They include overhead arm raise in line with the LT with dumbbell, which maximally activates MT and LT, and a diagonal exercise with a combination of shoulder flexion, horizontal flexion, and external rotation with dumbbell or rubber tubing bands that maximally activates SA (54).

Specialized Techniques

The Kinesio Taping® Method for the treatment of shoulder impingement is often used to reeducate movement patterns, reduce pain, and decrease inflammation by targeting receptors in the somatosensory system. This method has been shown to have positive results in patients with impingement (55,56). Clinical experience has shown a benefit in taping the pectoralis, rhomboids, biceps brachii, trapezius, and supraspinatus muscles as well as the use of a mechanical correction to promote external rotation of the humerus in the GHJ. Selection of which applications to use is based on the patient's presentation.

Education

Patient education has been shown to improve shoulder function and pain when combined with a therapeutic exercise program (39,40,57). Education should begin with patient understanding of his/her condition and instructions in the modification of daily activities that cause shoulder pain including self-care, work tasks, and leisure activities. Whenever possible, the patient should avoid repetitive motion and positions of the arm known to exacerbate pain. However, this recommendation is often difficult for the patient to accept based on job demands for overhead tasks and task performance habits. Therefore, assistance in identifying alternative positions to decrease pain is helpful. One practical recommendation for the patient is to work and exercise the shoulder using a "*thumbs up*" position in the scapular plane. In addition, the importance of posture needs to be emphasized to the patient. These two recommendations can help maximize the outlet space during shoulder motion, which in turn can minimize symptoms of impingement. Another important area to address is positioning during sleep. Strategies that can be helpful include not sleeping directly on the affected shoulder to avoid pressure over the painful area and putting a pillow or towel underneath the arm to minimize adduction of the shoulder. The adducted position increases tension of the supraspinatus tendon resulting in decreased vascularity (58). This is known as the "wringing out" phenomenon and is thought to contribute to degeneration of the tendon. This position also decreases the subacromial space which may contribute to impingement (59).

Home Exercise Program

Home exercise program (HEP) is an integral part of the rehabilitation program. Almost all the studies that demonstrated improvement with supervised therapeutic exercise included a HEP (38,39,43–46,60,61). Typically, a HEP starts early in the rehabilitation program and the progression of the HEP should mirror the exercises performed during supervised therapy program. The details of the program should be based on the evaluation and include the elements that have been discussed in the previous sections, including stretching, ROM, RTC strengthening, scapular stabilization, and postural training. A patient can be discharged to a HEP once supervised exercise and manual therapy are no longer indicated. If a patient is unable to come for regular supervised therapy, prior literature has shown that a guided self-training program without a supervised exercise program can result in improvements for patients with shoulder impingement (45,46).

SUMMARY

Shoulder pain associated with impingement is one of the most common conditions seen in both general and musculoskeletal practices. The history and physical examination help confirm the diagnosis as well as identify factors, such as altered shoulder biomechanics, that may contribute to this problem. A comprehensive rehabilitation program has clearly demonstrated benefits for these patients in multiple studies. The details of the program will depend on the physical findings and can include education, manual therapy, and therapeutic exercises that emphasize posture, flexibility, RTC strength, and scapular motion. Eventually, the patient can be discharged to a HEP once supervised therapy is no longer indicated. With proper rehabilitation, these patients can expect good outcomes and return to their sport, work, or leisure activity with minimal to no shoulder discomfort.

SAMPLE CASE

A 46-year-old male handyman with a history of hypertension (HTN) and hyperlipidemia presents with complaint of right posterolateral shoulder pain that has been present on/off for the past 6 months and has been worse during the past 10 days after painting. He describes a dull, aching pain that is exacerbated by reaching overhead and while lying on his right side while sleeping at night. He denies any radiation of pain, numbness/tingling through right upper limb. ROS is unremarkable and he denies any significant prior musculoskeletal or sports injuries. On examination, cervical ROM was within normal limits, Spurling's was negative, and had limited ROM in right shoulder abduction and flexion with a painful arc. Tight pectoralis minor was noted on the symptomatic side. The following special tests were positive: Hawkin's impingement test, painful arc sign, and infraspinatus strength test. Scapular dyskinesis was also noted that was improved with the modified scapular assistance test. No significant instability of the shoulder is noted. Neurovascular examination is unremarkable.

 SAMPLE THERAPY PRESCRIPTION

Discipline: Physical or occupational therapy.

Diagnosis: Right shoulder pain secondary to RTC impingement.

Problem list: Tight pec minor, scapular dyskinesis as evidenced by reduced impingement symptoms with scapular assistance test.

Frequency of visits: 2 to 3x/week

Duration of treatment: 3 to 4 weeks; or an alternative would be to provide a total of 8 to 12 visits used at the therapist's discretion

Treatment:

1. *Modalities:* cryotherapy (ice pack, ice bath, ice massage), moist heat

2. *Manual therapy:*
   - Soft tissue mobilization
   - Glenohumeral and scapulothoracic mobilization to restore shoulder ROM

3. *Specialized techniques:* Trial of Kinesio Taping®

4. *Therapeutic exercise:*

- ROM: start with pendulum, Codman, and wall climbing exercises in pain-free ROM, P/A/AAROM at shoulder in all planes

- Stretching: especially pectoralis minor

- Strengthening:

  i. Scapular stabilizers including lower trapezius, middle trapezius, and SA should be initial focus of strengthening program

  ii. RTC strengthening: Start without elevation and advance with elevation as tolerated

- Postural training

5. *Patient education:*

- Teach HEP and transition to the program once patient is independent with HEP and manual therapy is no longer necessary

- Strategies on proper technique for using the shoulder to minimize pain

Goals: Decrease pain and swelling, restore shoulder ROM/flexibility then restore strength, safely return to functional activities (e.g., sport, hobbies, work), and educate effective HEP.

Reevaluation: in 4 weeks by referring physician.

REFERENCES

1. Meyer AW. Chronic functional lesions of the shoulder. *Arch Surg*. 1937;35:646–674.
2. Dutton M. The shoulder complex. In: Johnson C, Naglieri C, eds. *Orthopaedic Examination, Evaluation, and Intervention*. McGraw-Hill, Medical Publishing Division; 2008:489-652.
3. Valadie AL III, Jobe CM, Pink MM, Ekman EF, Jobe FW. Anatomy of provocative tests for impingement syndrome of the shoulder. *J Shoulder Elbow Surg*. 2000;9(1):36–46.
4. Neer CS. Impingement lesions. *Clinical Orthop*. 1983;173:70–77.
5. Bokor DJ, Hawkins RJ, Huckell GH, Angelo RL, Schickendantz MS. Results of nonoperative management of full-thickness tears of the rotator cuff. *Clin Orthop Relat Res*. 1993;294:103–110.
6. Chard MD, Hazleman R, Hazleman BL, King RH, Reiss BB. Shoulder disorders in the elderly: a community survey. *Arthritis Rheum*. 1991;34(6):766–769.
7. Clark JM, Harryman DT. Tendons, ligaments, and capsules of the rotator cuff. *J Bone Joint Surg Am*. 1992;74(5):713–725.
8. Brewer BJ. Aging of the rotator cuff. *Am J Sports Med*. 1979;2:102–110.
9. Neer CS. Anterior acromioplasty of the chronic impingement syndrome in the shoulder. *J Bone JointSurg Am*. 1972;54:41–50.
10. Magee D. *Orthopedic Physical Assessment*. 5th ed. Philadelphia, PA: Saunders Elsevier; 2008.

TABLE 8.1: Description of Important Physical Exam Maneuvers

TEST	DESCRIPTION
Hawkin's impingement test (62)	Position shoulder and elbow in 90° of flexion. Passively internally rotate the arm with the shoulder stabilized. Positive if pain is present in the shoulder
Supraspinatus strength/Jobe/ empty can test (63)	Position extended arm in 90° scapular plane and internally or neutrally rotated. Examiner applies downward force while patient attempts to resist. Positive if pain or weakness in the shoulder
Infraspinatus strength test (64)	Position the arm at the side with the elbow flexed to 90°. Position the arm in either neutral (Leroux) rotation or 45° of IR (Kelly). Examiner then applies an internal rotation force to the arm while the patient resist in external rotation. Positive if the patient gave way because of weakness or pain
Full can test (18)	Position extended arm in 90° scapular plane and externally rotated. Examiner applies downward force while patient attempts to resist. Positive if pain or weakness is noted
Belly press test (19)	Patient is asked to press maximally into the abdomen by internal rotation of the shoulder. Positive if patient compensates with flexion at the wrist and shoulder adduction and arm extension
Modified scapular assistance test (24)	Patient actively flexes and abducts the affected arm as tolerated. If scapular tilting and winging is noted, the patient is asked to repeat the motion while the examiner pushes the inferior medial scapular border in an anterior, lateral and upward direction. Positive if there is a decrease or abolishment of symptoms

11. Kernwein GA, Rosenberg B, Sneed WR Jr. Aids in the differential diagnosis of the painful shoulder syndrome. *Clin Orthop*. 1961;20:11–20.

12. Park L, Yokota A, Gill H, El Rassi G, McFarland E, Diagnostic accuracy of clinical tests for the different degrees of subacromial impingement syndrome. *J Bone Joint Surg Am*. 2005;87(7):1446–1455.

13. Burkhart SS, Morgan CD, Kibler WB. The disabled throwing shoulder: spectrum of pathology Part I: pathoanatomy and biomechanics. *Arthroscopy*. 2003;19(4):404–420.

14. Erol O, Ozçakar L, Celiker R. Shoulder rotator strength in patients with stage I-II subacromial impingement: relationship to pain, disability, and quality of life. *J Shoulder Elbow Surg*. 2008;17:893–897.

15. Reddy AS, Mohr KJ, Pink MM, et al. Electromyographic analysis of the deltoid and rotator cuff muscles in persons with subacromial impingement. *J Shoulder Elbow Surg*. 2000;9:519–523.

16. Kibler WB, Sciascia A, Dome D. Evaluation of apparent and absolute supraspinatus strength in patients with shoulder injury using the scapular retraction test. *Am J Sports Med*. 2006;34:1643–1647.

17. Tate AR, McClure PW, Kareha S, Irwin D. Effect of scapula reposition test on shoulder impingement symptoms and elevation strength in overhead athletes. *J Ortho Sports Phys Ther*. 2008;38(1):4–11.

18. Kelly BT, Kadrmas WR, Speer KP. The manual muscle examination for rotator cuff strength. An electromyographic investigation. *Am J Sports Med*. 1996;24:581–588.

19. Tokish JM, Decker MJ, Ellis HB, Torry MR, Hawkins RJ. The belly press test for the physical examination of the subscapularis muscle: electromyographic validation and comparison to the lift-off test. *J Shoulder Elbow Surg*. 2003;12:427–430.

20. Ludewig PM, Cook TM. Alterations in shoulder kinematics and associated muscle activity in people with symptoms of shoulder impingement. *Phys Ther*. 2000;80:276–291.

21. Warner JJ, Micheli LJ, Arslanian LE, et al. Scapulothoracic motion in normal shoulders and shoulders with glenohumeral instability and impingement syndrome. A study using Moire topographic analysis. *Clin Orthop Relat Res*. 1992;285:191–199.

22. Hébert LJ, Moffet H, McFadyen BJ, et al. Scapular behavior in shoulder impingement syndrome. *Arch Phys Med Rehabil*. 2002;83:60–69.

23. McClure PW, Michener LA, Karduna AR. Shoulder function and 3-dimensional scapular kinematics in people with and without shoulder impingement syndrome. *Phys Ther*. 2006;86:1075–1090.

24. Rabin A, Irrgang JJ, Fitzgerald GK, Eubanks A. The intertester reliability of the Scapular Assistance Test. *J Orthop Sports Ther*. 2006;36(9):653–660.

25. Seitz AL, McClure PW, Lynch SS, Ketchum JM, Michener LA. Effects of scapular dyskinesis and scapular assistance test on subacromial space during static arm elevation. *J Shoulder Elbow Surg*. 2012;21:631–640.

26. Desmeules F, Cote CH, Fremont P. Therapeutic exercise and orthopaedic manual therapy for impingement syndrome. A systematic review. *Clin J Sports Med*. 2003;13:176–182.

27. Grant HJ, Arthur A, Pichora DR. Evaluation of interventions for rotator cuff pathology: a systematic review. *J Hand Ther*. 2004;17:274–299.

28. Green S, Buchbinder R, Hetrick S. Physiotherapy interventions for shoulder pain. *Cochrane Database Syst Rev*. 2003;2:CD004258.

29. Kuhn J. Exercise in the treatment of rotator cuff impingement: a systematic review and a synthesized evidence-based rehabilitation protocol. *J Shoulder Elbow Surg*. 2009;18:138–160.

30. Ellenbecker TS, Cools A. Rehabilitation of shoulder impingement syndrome and rotator cuff injuries: an evidence based review. *Br J Sports Med*. 2010;44:319–327.

31. Michener LA, Walsworth MK, Burnet EN. Effectiveness of rehabilitation for patients with subacromial impingement syndrome: A systematic review. *J Hand Ther*. 2004;17:152–164.

32. Calis HT, Berberoglu N, Calis M. Are ultrasound, laser and exercise superior to each other in the treatment of subacromial impingement syndrome? A randomized clinical trial. *Eur J Phys Rehabil Med*. 2011;47:375–380.

33. Matti N. Pulsed ultrasound treatment of the painful shoulder a randomized, double-blind, placebo-controlled study. *Scand J Rehab Med*. 1995;27:105–108.

34. Gursel YK, Ulus Y, Bilgic A, et al. Adding ultrasound in the management of soft tissue disorders of the shoulder: a randomized placebo-controlled trial. *Phys Ther*. 2004;(84)4:336–343.

35. Bal A, Eksioglu E, Gurcay E, et al. Low-level laser therapy in subacromial impingement syndrome. *Photomed Laser Surg*. 2009;27(1):31–36.

36. Yeldan I, Cetin E, Ozdincler AR. The effectiveness of low-level laser therapy on shoulder function in subacromial impingement syndrome. *Disabil Rehabil*. 2009;31(11):935–940.

37. Bang M, Deyle G. Comparison of supervised exercise with and without manual physical therapy for patients with impingement syndrome. *J Ortho Sports Phys Ther*. 2000;30:126–137.

38. Conroy DE, Hayes KW. The effect of mobilization as a component of comprehensive treatment for primary shoulder impingement syndrome. *J Ortho Sports Phys Ther*. 1998;28:3–14.

39. Senbursa G, Baltaci G, Atay A. Comparison of conservative treatment with and without manual physical therapy for patients with shoulder impingement syndrome: a prospective, randomized clinical trial. *Knee Surg Sports Traumatol Arthrosc*. 2007;15:915–921.

40. Tate AR, McClure PW, Young IA, Salvatori R, Michener LA. Comprehensive impairment based exercise and manual therapy for patient with subacromial impingement syndrome: a case series. *J Orthop Sports Phys Ther*. 2010;40(8):474–493.

41. Borstad JD, Ludewig PM. Comparison of three stretches for the pectoralis minor muscle. *J Shoulder Elbow Surg*. 2006;15(3):324–330.

42. McClure P, Balaicuis J, Heiland D, Broersma ME, Thorndike CK, Wood A. A randomized controlled comparison of stretching procedures for posterior shoulder tightness. *J Orthop Sports Phys Ther*. 2007;37:108–114.

43. Haahr JP, Ostergaard S, Dalsgaard J, et al. Exercises versus arthroscopic decompression in patients with subacromial impingement: a randomised, controlled study in 90 cases with a one year follow up. *Ann Rheum Dis*. 2005;64:760–764.

44. Ludewig PM, Borstad JD. Effects of a home exercise programme on shoulder pain and functional status in construction workers. *Occup Environ Med.* 2003;60:841–849.

45. Rahme H, Solem-Bertoft E, Westerberg CE, Lundberg E, Sorensen S, Hilding S. The subacromial impingement syndrome. A study of results of treatment with special emphasis on predictive factors and pain generating mechanisms. *Scand J Rehab Med.* 1998;30:253–262.

46. Walther M, Werner A, Stahlschmidt T, Woeffel R, Gohlke F. The subacromial impingement syndrome of the shoulder treated by conventional physiotherapy, self-training, and a shoulder brace: results of a prospective, randomized study. *J Shoulder Elbow Surg.* 2004;13:417–423.

47. Kibler WB, Sciascia AD, Uhl TL, et al. Electromyographic analysis of specific exercises for scapular control in early phases of shoulder rehabilitation. *Am J Sports Med.* 2008;36:1789–1798.

48. Ludewig PM, Hoff MS, Osowski EE, et al. Relative balance of serratus anterior and upper trapezius muscle activity during push-up exercises. *Am J Sports Med.* 2004;32:484–493.

49. Cools AM, Declercq GA, Cambier DC, et al. Trapezius activity and intramuscular balance during isokinetic exercise in overhead athletes with impingement symptoms. *Scand J Med Sci Sports.* 2007;17:25–33.

50. Moraes GF, Faria CD, Teixeira-Salmela LF. Scapular muscle recruitment patterns and isokinetic strength ratios of the shoulder rotator muscles in individuals with and without impingement syndrome. *J Shoulder Elbow Surg.* 2008;17: 48S–53S.

51. Cools AM, Dewitte V, Lanszweert F, et al. Rehabilitation of scapular muscle balance: which exercises to prescribe? *Am J Sports Med.* 2007;35:1744–1751.

52. Townsend H, Jobe FW, Pink M, Perry J. Electromyographic analysis of the glenohumeral muscles during a baseball rehabilitation program. *Am J Sports Med.* 1991;19:264–272.

53. Reinnold MM, Wilk KE, Fleisig GS, et al. Electromyographic analysis of the rotator cuff and deltoid musculature during common shoulder external rotation exercises. *J Ortho Sports Phys Ther.* 2004;34(7):385–394.

54. Ekstrom RA, Donatelli RA, Soderberg GL. Surface electromyographic analysis of exercises for the trapezius and serratus anterior muscles. *J Orthop Sports Phys Ther.* 2003;33:247–258.

55. Kaya E, Zinnuroglu M, Tugcu I. Kinesio taping compared to physical therapy modalities for the treatment of shoulder impingement syndrome. *Clin Rheumatol.* 2011;30(2):201–217.

56. Hsu YH, Chen WY, Lin HC, Wang WT, Shih YF. The effects of taping on scapular performance in baseball players with shoulder impingement. *J Electromyogr Kinesiol.* 2009;19(6):1092–1099.

57. McClure PW, Bialker J, Neff N, Williams G, Karduna A. Shoulder function and 3-dimensional kinematics in people with shoulder impingement syndrome before and after a 6 week exercise program. *Phys Ther.* 2004;84(9):832–848.

58. Rathbun JB, Macnab I. The microvascular pattern of the rotator cuff of the shoulder. *J Bone Joint Surg.* 1970;52B:540.

59. Graichen H, Hinterwimmer S, von Eisenhart-Roth RVR, et al. Effect of abducting and adducting muscle activity on glenohumeral translation, scapular kinematics and subacromial space width in vivo. *J Biomech.* 2005;38:755–760.

60. Brox JI, Gjengedal E, Uppheim G, et al. Arthroscopic surgery versus supervised exercises in patient with rotator cuff disease (stage II impingement syndrome): a prospective, randomised, controlled study in 125 patients with a 2 ½ year follow-up. *J Shoulder Elbow Surg.* 1997;8:102–111.

61. Brox J, Staff P, Ljunggren A, Brevik J. Arthroscopic surgery compared with supervised exercises in patients with rotator cuff disease. *BMJ.* 1993;307:899–903.

62. Hawkins RJ, Schutte JP. The assessment of glenohumeral translation using manual and fluoroscopic techniques. *Orthop Trans.* 1988;12:727–728.

63. Jobe FW, Moynes DR. Delineation of diagnostic criteria and a rehabilitation program for rotator cuff injuries. *Am J Sports Med.* 1982;10:336–339.

64. Leroux JL, Thomas E, Bonnel F, Blotman F. Diagnostic value of clinical tests for shoulder impingement syndrome. *Rev Rhum Engl Ed.* 1995;62:423–428.

Rotator Cuff Tendinopathy

Christopher J. Visco, Gaurav Raj Telhan, and Edward R. Calem

INTRODUCTION

The rotator cuff is composed of the supraspinatus, infraspinatus, teres minor, and subscapularis muscles. These muscles provide both stability and dynamic range of motion (ROM) to the shoulder girdle complex. Rotator cuff tendinopathy (RCT) is the most common cause of shoulder pain in all age groups, accounting for approximately 30% of shoulder-related pain (1). The classification for rehabilitation purposes may be based on the type of injury to the rotator cuff tendons. There is recent research clarifying the pathophysiology and biomechanics, which lead to the development of tendinopathy. The primary proposed cause of tendinopathy is from a blunted inflammatory response to tendonitis, leading to a cycle of degeneration. The repetitive strain subjected to the rotator cuff as it fulfills its role as the primary dynamic stabilizer of the glenohumeral joint also may contribute to recurrent thickening, degeneration, and acute tears (2). The mechanism of injury may be either direct, acutely inflicted trauma, or insidious from accumulated chronic repetitive strains. Microtrauma is usually seen in the younger athlete who participates in overhand sports causing repetitive strain (3). Regardless of the cause of tendinopathy, shoulder rehabilitation is best achieved with a synchronous approach between strengthening, stabilization, ROM, and proprioceptive/neuromuscular reeducation, while avoiding further exacerbation of the underlying injury.

Pathophysiologic etiology may also include muscle ischemia and altered healing or repair processes, and apoptosis of tenocytes. Repeated mechanical stress and recurrent injuries with an absent or blunted inflammatory process may lead to the development of angiofibroblastic hyperplasia (i.e., fibroblasts and vascular granulation tissue) (4–6). Resulting pathologic changes include macrostructural thickening and increased vascularity. Microstructure changes include degeneration and disorganization of collagen fibers, increased cellularity, and

minimal inflammation. The build-up of mucopolysaccharide in fibrous tendon sheath leads to mucoid (myxoid) degeneration. This cycle repeats itself and leads to globular degeneration and the production of matrix metalloproteinases (MMPs), tenocyte apoptosis, chondroid metaplasia of the tendon, and expression of protective factors such as insulin-like growth factor 1 (IGF-1) and nitric oxide synthetase (NOS) causing recurrent and chronic pain (7–11). Overall, whether through acute or chronic repetitive strain, the rotator cuff tendons become swollen and hypercellular, resulting in disruption of the tendon collagen matrix which leads to tendon compromise (7).

Classification of rotator cuff injuries may be based on rotator cuff pathology and classified into five major types: primary impingement, secondary impingement, posterior impingement, repetitive overload, and traumatic events. *Primary impingement* results from compression of the rotator cuff tendons between the humeral head and the overlying acromion, coracoacromial ligament, coracoid, or acromioclavicular joint. *Secondary impingement* is due to an underlying instability of the glenohumeral joint. Laxity in the capsular ligaments from throwing or overhead activities or due to congenital laxity of the patient can lead to anterior instability of the glenohumeral joint. This can lead to impingement of the biceps tendon and rotator cuff (12,13). Labral insufficiency can also lead to instability and impingement. Secondary impingement can cause compressive damage to the tendon or increase the tensile stresses to the rotator cuff tendons. *Posterior impingement* results from placement of the shoulder in a position of 90° abduction and 90° external rotation (e.g., late cocking phase of throwing), causing supraspinatus and infraspinatus tendons to rotate posteriorly. This positions the tendons such that their undersurface rubs on the posterior-superior glenoid rim. *Repetitive overload* is due to heavy repetitive eccentric forces in overhead activities. This can be seen often in overhead sports activities leading to overhead failure of the tendon. *Traumatic events* can lead to partial or full thickness tears of the cuff tendons or associated structures.

Calcific shoulder tendonitis is another example of RCT and it develops through four stages outlined by Uhtoff and Loehr in a manner distinctly different than the repetitive strain mechanism described above. In the formative phase, fibrocartilage ingrowth develops along living tendon tissue, gradually enlarging (14). In the subsequent resting phase, the calcific formations may cause mechanical clicking and ROM changes depending on the size of the calcific deposits. During the resorptive phase, painful inflammation and vascularization develops around the sites of calcification. Macrophages and giant cells with vascular access to the calcifications absorb the deposits and breakdown products can leak into the subacromial bursa causing severe pain. Lastly, in the postcalcific phase, fibroblasts restructure the tendinous collagen pattern (14).

Rupture type injuries from macrotrauma are also possible in contact sports (3). There is a direct correlation between incidence of tears and increasing age, with as many as 34% of asymptomatic patients found to have rotator cuff tears (28% in patients ≤60 years old and 54% in patients >60 years old) (15). Cadaveric studies have demonstrated a 39% incidence of full thickness tears in patients >60 years old (16). The majority of rotator cuff tendinopathies involve the supraspinatus tendon, which is most susceptible to subacromial impingement. Patients with curved or hooked acromions have a higher risk of RCT than those with flat acromions (17).

A thorough history and physical examination are crucial in the evaluation, classification, and treatment of a patient with rotator cuff pathology. *Historical features* of RCT include descriptions of dull, aching, and occasionally sharp pain. Usually, pain is focal, nonradiating, and improves with rest, ice, and nonsteroidal anti-inflammatory drugs (NSAIDs). The pain typically worsens with activity. Important historical points include prior injury of the affected limb, systemic illnesses, and recent use of medications such as fluoroquinolones. Other presentations could include a history of an acute rupture (due to underlying tendinopathy) or complaints of an intermittent or chronic "snapping tendon." Activities performed at less than 90° of abduction tend to be painless, whereas overhead activities may reproduce pain, crepitus, or a catching sensation. RCT can be a source of nocturnal pain, especially when lying on the affected side. Pain may also be referred along the deltoid muscle and chronic tears may lead to muscle atrophy and eventually cuff arthropathy.

Key elements of the physical examination include inspection, palpation, ROM, neurologic, and vascular exams. Palpation may reveal tenderness anywhere from the enthesis to myotendinous junction. Adjacent soft tissues may also be tender, often due to compensatory movement patterns. Postural assessment and biomechanical analysis are important to identify predisposing factors. A detailed shoulder girdle examination with functional assessment, special tests, and provocative maneuvers also help to establish the diagnosis and to develop an individualized exercise prescription.

Neer's impingement sign involves passive shoulder flexion greater than 90° and the examiner may stabilize the scapula to provoke symptoms. Pain with this maneuver implies that subacromial structures, such as the supraspinatus, are being compressed between the acromion and greater tuberosity of the humerus. Hawkin's impingement sign involves passive flexion to 90°, followed by internal rotation of the shoulder; pain with this maneuver also suggests subacromial impingement. The painful arc sign is positive when pain occurs with abduction of the arm between 60 and 120° and is suggestive of rotator cuff irritation beneath the subacromial space. The supraspinatus or "empty can" test is positive when the examiner elicits pain and/or weakness with resisted shoulder elevation at 90°, within the plane of the scapula (also known as scaption) and maximum internal rotation. Resisted external rotation is utilized to assess the function of the infraspinatus and teres minor. Lastly, the drop arm test is positive when the patient is unable to slowly lower the arm to their side after the shoulder has been passively abducted to 90° by the examiner, suggesting a rotator cuff tear. A combination of a positive painful arc sign, drop arm sign, and weakness in external rotation accurately predicts full-thickness rotator cuff tear, while a combination of three negative tests makes the diagnosis unlikely (18).

Radiology is highly utilized for the evaluation of shoulder pain. MRI is the gold standard for evaluation of rotator cuff compromise and is capable of delineating the degree of muscular tear as well as rotator cuff calcification. Large chronic tears are associated with superior migration of the humeral head and fatty atrophy of the supraspinatus and infraspinatus muscle bellies (19). Plain films may be useful in the diagnosis of chronic tears when they demonstrate superior migration of the proximal humerus, flattening of the greater tuberosity, and subacromial sclerosis (20). Musculoskeletal ultrasound is an excellent imaging modality to evaluate for tendinopathy, particularly to compare to the unaffected limb/tendon and evaluate extra-articular soft-tissue pathology. Ultrasound and MRI are both highly accurate for diagnosing full-thickness rotator cuff tears, but less so for partial-thickness tears with an overall accuracy rate for both imaging tests of 87% (21).

Limitations of musculoskeletal ultrasound include clinical availability, examiner experience, and inability of ultrasound to assess deep intra-articular structures, such as the biceps anchor, labrum, and glenohumeral cartilage.

ROTATOR CUFF TENDINOPATHY

■ RCT is among the most prevalent causes of shoulder pain in patients of all age groups

■ It arises from the repetitive strain incurred by the rotator cuff as it fulfills its role as the primary dynamic stabilizer of the glenohumeral joint

■ Clinical features of RCT include: pain, crepitus or catching with overhead activity such as throwing or swimming, pain referred along the deltoid muscle, nocturnal pain, and muscular atrophy

■ Key elements of the physical examination include inspection, palpation, neurovascular examination, and a detailed shoulder girdle examination with ROM and provocative maneuver testing

■ MRI is the gold standard for evaluation of rotator cuff compromise and is capable of delineating the degree of muscular tear as well as rotator cuff calcification. Ultrasound and MRI are both highly accurate for diagnosing full-thickness rotator cuff tears but less accurate for partial thickness rotator cuff tears

THE REHABILITATION PROGRAM

The phases of rehabilitation seen throughout this book should be followed with the following key principles for rehabilitation of patients with RCT:

1. Rehabilitation should be an individualized and evaluation-based program designed to address specific findings from the examination
2. Rehabilitation should be based on addressing the causes of the tendinopathy (e.g., biomechanical causes)
3. Any comprehensive rehabilitation program should emphasize restoration of normal joint arthrokinematics. Ideally, scapular control and glenohumeral joint ROM should be addressed simultaneously

The focus of the acute phase of rehabilitation (phase I) for shoulder tendinopathy is promotion of tissue healing via

reduction of pain and inflammation, avoidance of aggravating maneuvers, and gradual promotion of pain free ROM in conjunction with scapular stabilization. In phase II, ROM should begin in pain-minimized arcs and initially kept below 90° of abduction using pendulum exercises and capsular stretching. Isometric scapular exercises can be followed by closed chain exercises. Once tissue healing has progressed to the point that there is minimal pain with increasing ROM and underlying scapular dyskinesis has begun to be addressed, patients may progress to the recovery phases of rehabilitation (phases III–IV). In the recovery phases a multifaceted approach of stretching, strengthening, and stabilization is aimed at achieving normal active and passive shoulder ROM and normalizing shoulder arthrokinematics in single then multiple planes of motion. Additional scapular control exercises along with progressive upper extremity and isolated rotator cuff exercise may also be employed. Strengthening and proprioceptive exercises can be advanced when full pain free ROM is present. Lastly, in the functional phase (phase V) of rehabilitation, goals include increasing power and endurance in job- and exercise-specific movements and achieving normal muscle firing patterns and movement patterns throughout the entire shoulder ROM. If the patients desire is to return to playing a specific sport, then return to play criteria should be met (Table 9.1).

Therapeutic Modalities

Initial management of RCT aims to decrease aggravating factors and limit inflammation through the application of ice. There is currently limited evidence supporting NSAIDS, therapeutic ultrasound, interferential electrical stimulation, laser, magnetic field therapy, or local massage. Nonetheless, clinical experience and traditional practice patterns have led to the continued use of modalities as a component of comprehensive rotator cuff rehabilitation regimens. While not proven in noncalcific tendonitis to help symptom management and pain control, a study of patients with symptomatic calcific tendonitis of the shoulder found that pulsed therapeutic ultrasound treatment helped more rapidly resolve calcifications that affect the rotator cuff

TABLE 9.1: Return to Play Criteria for RCT

Pain free ROM

Strength is equivalent to at least 80% to 90% of contralateral strength measurements

Provocative impingement signs are negative

tendons and is associated with short-term clinical improvement (22). Likewise, extracorporeal shock wave therapy may help in the short-term for calcific tendinopathy but does not alter the ultimate patient outcome (23,24). Despite a trend toward greater improvement in the treatment group, a study using acetic acid iontophoresis and physiotherapy for the treatment of calcifying tendinitis of the shoulder did not result in better clinical and radiologic effects than those observed in subjects treated by physiotherapy alone (25). The use of transcutaneous nitrous oxide directly over the area of tendinopathy may enhance healing and provide pain relief in the treatment of shoulder tendinopathy (24) although it remains at this time an experimental treatment.

Manual Therapy

Joint mobilization is believed to be an effective treatment for enhancing ROM in patients with rotator cuff impingement (26). One study found that manual therapy applied by experienced physical therapists combined with supervised exercise is better than exercise alone for increasing strength, decreasing pain, and improving function in patients with primary shoulder impingement syndrome. Typical manual therapy treatment in this study included techniques to: enhance glenohumeral caudal (or inferior) glide in positions of flexion or abduction, increase physiological flexion or internal rotation, improve the combined physiological movements of the hand behind back or shoulder, increase upper thoracic extension and side bend, and enhance extension, rotation, or side bend of the cervical spine. Techniques also included soft tissue massage and muscle stretching particularly of the pectoralis minor, infraspinatus, teres minor, upper trapezius, sternocleidomastoid, and scalene musculature (27).

Therapeutic Exercise

ROM, stretching, strengthening, and stabilizing exercises are crucial to the successful rehabilitation of RCT because they help correct glenohumeral instability, muscle weakness, incoordination, soft tissue tightness, and impaired scapulohumeral rhythm. To begin, ROM exercises for RCT should be performed daily and aim to achieve full painless and eventually full glenohumeral ROM through shoulder pendulum exercises, internal/external rotation stretches, adduction/abduction stretches, and biceps/triceps stretches among others (28).

Resistive exercises commence as inflammation and pain levels decrease, ROM improves, and the patient's pain

level guides progression with resistive exercises. Eccentric exercise has been shown to be effective in the rehabilitation of tendinopathy and can be progressed as scapular positioning, control, and stabilization are achieved. Concentric exercises should be commenced with submaximal resistance, usually favoring low levels of resistance and high repetition. Progression should be made to closed chain exercises and eventually plyometrics and specific return to activity interventions. Closed chain exercises can be progressed from standing with hands on wall to prone on elbows to four point stance. Exercise can then be progressed to include the plank or push up position or the use of a physio ball or rollers positioned under the hands or legs to create increased challenge and demand at the glenohumeral and scapulothoracic joints. Plyometric exercises can commence with a simple toss of a one pound medicine ball from hand to hand ensuring scapular stabilization, advanced to transferring the ball behind the back, around the trunk toss and catch in the air, and finally progressed to wall dribbles in various ranges of shoulder flexion and abduction. The exercises described above can help the patient advance from phase II toward phase V of rehabilitation.

Identification and correction of muscular imbalances may play a role in the secondary prevention of RCT. Expert consensus identifies decreased rotator cuff strength or an imbalance between internal and external rotators of the shoulder as predisposing risk factors to the development RCT. Physical therapy (PT) should involve strengthening of the external rotators, which are often weak in comparison to the internal rotators (29). Systematic reviews have emphasized the utility of resistance band therapy focusing on internal rotation with the arm adducted to the side, external rotation with the arm adducted to the side, and scaption (abduction/adduction in the scapular plane) (30). Patients may also begin with isotonic side-lying external rotation (with a towel roll placed between the medial arm and side of the trunk, as described in the "Shoulder Impingement Syndromes" chapter) (Figure 9.1) and prone shoulder extension with an externally rotated (thumb up) position and progress to prone horizontal abduction and prone external rotation exercises with scapular retraction (31). Interestingly, resistance exercise during external rotation should be performed using low-load isometric contractions, which preferentially recruit the infraspinatus muscle (31,32). Previous studies have generally emphasized pain free strengthening of the shoulder depressors (i.e., subscapularis, infraspinatus, and teres minor) (33). Three sets of 15 to 20 repetitions are recommended to create a fatigue response and target the development of local muscular endurance (31,34).

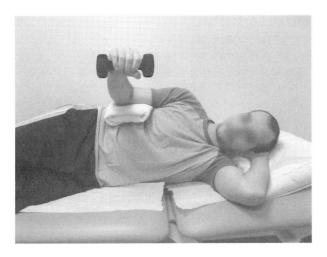

FIGURE 9.1: Isotonic side-lying external rotation.

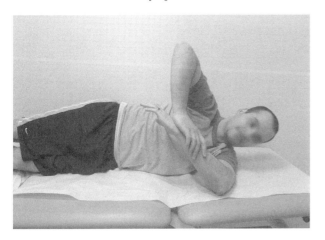

FIGURE 9.2: The sleeper stretch.

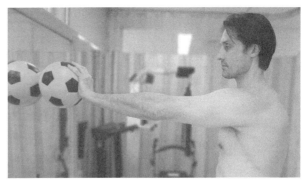

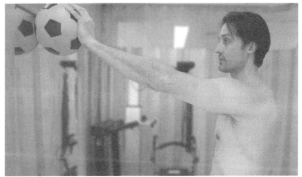

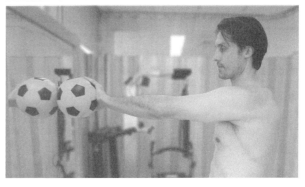

FIGURE 9.3: The scapular clock exercise.

Scapular instability and dyskinesis must be addressed throughout the rehabilitation program with a twofold approach: (a) flexibility addressed through stretching and mobilization techniques and (b) muscle recruitment normalization through conscious muscle retraining (31). Kibler defines scapular dyskinesis as an alteration in the normal position or motion of the scapula during coupled scapulohumeral movements (29). Deficits in scapular stability resulting from lack of soft tissue flexibility may be addressed through stretching of the scapular muscles, especially the pectoralis minor, levator scapulae, rhomboids, and latissimus dorsi; the glenohumeral capsule and posterior cuff should also be addressed, especially the posterior capsule and infraspinatus (31). Specific stretching exercises include: the sleeper stretch (Figure 9.2), the cross arm stretch, the internal rotation stretches and the unilateral corner stretch (31,35,36). Also refer to the shoulder

impingement chapter for a description and reference to a self-stretch for the pectoralis minor. The role of eccentric muscle stretching remains controversial, but preliminary studies have found eccentric stretching of the supraspinatus and deltoid resulted in reduction of pain on the visual analog scale and subjective increase in patient satisfaction with rehabilitation progress (37).

Deficits in scapular stability resulting from suboptimal muscle performance may be addressed through neuromuscular reeducation to achieve balanced use of cocontraction and force couple patterns, as well as through strengthening of the lower trapezius, middle trapezius, and serratus anterior (31). Scapular orientation exercises

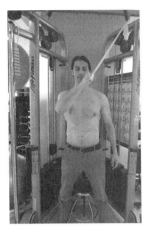
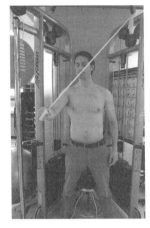
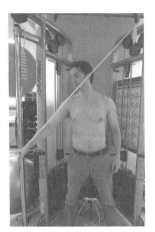

FIGURE 9.4: PNF diagonal with resistance band.

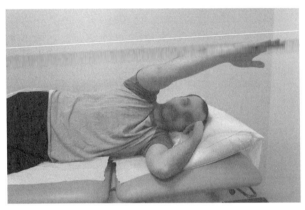

FIGURE 9.5: Side-lying forward flexion.

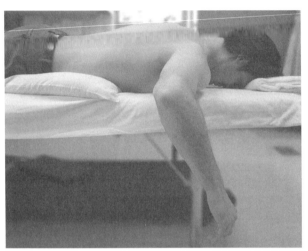

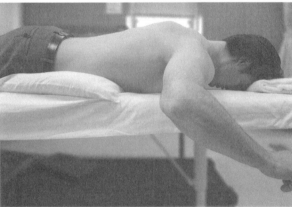

FIGURE 9.6: Prone horizontal abduction with external rotation.

such as the scapular clock (Figure 9.3), reinforcing proprioceptive neuromuscular facilitation (PNF) patterns (Figure 9.4) by postural positioning (in upward/downward rotation, internal/external rotation, and anterior/posterior tilt) to activate the lower trapezius selectively have been described (31,38). Scapular muscle training also involves muscle control to ensure appropriate co-contraction of scapular force couples and muscle strengthening via exercises like the low row, lawnmower, push up progressions, chair presses, and scaption maneuvers (30,31,36). Lastly, exercises with proportionately greater involvement of the serratus anterior and low trapezius muscle groups as compared to the upper trapezius are critical to selectively strengthen typically weaker muscles (31). Cools et al found the following exercises to be the most effective in maximizing proportional activation of the middle and lower trapezius versus the upper trapezius: side-lying external rotation (Figure 9.1), side-lying forward flexion (Figure 9.5), prone horizontal abduction with external rotation (Figure 9.6), and prone extension (39).

Specialized Techniques

Once a patient has progressed to full painless ROM and makes significant strength gains, interval overhead throwing exercises can be used to facilitate return to play and return to play criteria (refer to Table 9.1) can be utilized to guide a safe return to sport for the athlete. Additionally, eccentric muscle strengthening combined with shoulder taping may also be used in conjunction to promote shoulder stabilization. The application of Kinesio tape for shoulder pain is effective for immediate pain relief and increased ROM, but does not have long-term effects (40).

Home Exercise Program

An effective home exercise program (HEP) should be performed in concert with supervised PT from the time of initial evaluation to the completion of an organized PT program. After an initial period of rest, ice, inflammatory control, and tissue healing, ROM, and stretching exercises should be performed daily. Self or assisted stretches may be used to promote ROM and as painless ROM increases, progressive resistive exercises may be initiated. External and internal rotation exercises using resistance bands or weights may be supplemented with chair presses, upright rows, and the push-up plus. Crucial to all flexibility and strength training therapy is a scapular stabilization program (i.e., scapular clock exercises) to reinforce proper PNF patterns, improve control, and counteract forces of scapular instability, which can lead to the recurrence of RCT.

SUMMARY

RCT arises from the repetitive strain incurred by the rotator cuff as it fulfills its role as the primary dynamic stabilizer of the glenohumeral joint and is among the most prevalent causes of shoulder pain in patients of all age groups. After reduction of pain and inflammation in the acute phase (phase I), therapy must be aimed at reestablishing painless ROM (phase II) and laying down the foundation of scapular control. In the recovery phase (phases III–IV), a multifaceted approach of stretching, strengthening, and stabilization must be aimed at achieving normal active and passive shoulder ROM and normalizing shoulder arthrokinematics in single then multiple planes of motion. Lastly, in the functional phase of rehabilitation (phase V), goals include increasing power and endurance in job and exercise specific movements.

SAMPLE CASE

A 30-year-old, right-hand-dominant male with no significant past medical history presents to your office with a chief complaint of right-sided shoulder pain that began 1 month without a specific inciting event. The patient is a recreational athlete whose activities include pitching for his baseball league on the weekends and cycling on a daily basis. Review of systems (ROS) is unremarkable and he denies prior musculoskeletal injury. His examination reveals pain and mild catching with overhead activity. He also has positive impingement signs, a painful arc and tightness of the pectoralis minor on physical examination. Neurovascular examination is unremarkable and plain radiographs do not reveal acute fracture or dislocation. Clinical findings are consistent with a diagnosis of RCT.

 ### SAMPLE THERAPY PRESCRIPTION

Discipline: Physical or occupational therapy.

Diagnosis: Right shoulder RCT.

Problem list: decreased and painful shoulder ROM, tight pectoralis minor.

Precautions: weight bearing as tolerated (WBAT).

Frequency of visits: 2 to 3x/week.

Duration of treatment: 3 to 4 weeks; or an alternative—provide a total of 8 to 12 visits used at the therapist's discretion.

****PT/OT evaluation including analysis of shoulder and upper extremity biomechanics.

Treatment:

1. *Modalities:* Cryotherapy (ice pack, ice massage), moist heat as needed (PRN)

2. *Manual therapy:* glenohumeral joint mobilization/stretching to enhance glenohumeral ROM

3. *Therapeutic exercise:* ROM, stretching and strengthening. Advance from pendulum

exercises to passive and active ROM.
Strengthening progress from isometrics to
pain-free resisted ROM, then to progressive
resistive exercises. Stretching/flexibility also
include pectoralis minor self and assisted
stretching. Scapular stabilization exercises (i.e.,
scapular clock, low rows, push up progressions,
force couple recruitment training), and
neuromuscular reeducation (with PNF
techniques) to promote proper arthrokinematics
and promote return to pain free activity

4. *Specialized treatments:* sports-specific
exercises and Kinesio taping (40)

5. *Patient education:* HEP, proper positioning
during the day and with sleep

Goals: Decrease pain and swelling, restore
shoulder ROM, flexibility, and strength. Then
return to sport if criteria met (refer to Table 9.1)

Reevaluation: in 4 weeks by referring physician.

REFERENCES

1. van der Windt DA, Koes BW, de Jong BA, Bouter LM. Shoulder disorders in general practice: incidence, patient characteristics, and management. *Ann Rheum Dis.* 1995;5412):959.
2. Lyons PM, Orwin, JF. Rotator cuff tendinopathy and subacromial impingement syndrome. *Med Sci Sports Exerc.* 1998;30(Suppl 4):S12–17.
3. Blevins FT. Rotator cuff pathology in athletes. *Sports Med.* 1997;24(3):205–220.
4. Khan KM, Cook JL, Bonar F, Harcourt P, Astrom M. Histopathology of common tendinopathies. Update and implications for clinical management. *Sports Med.* 1999;27:393–408.
5. Ljung BO, Forsgren S, Friden J. Substance P and calcitonin gene-related peptide expression at the extensor carpi radialis brevis muscle origin: implications for the etiology of tennis elbow. *J Orthop Res.* 1999;17:554–559.
6. Soslowsky LJ, Thomopoulos S, Tun S, et al. Overuse activity injures the supraspinatus tendon in an animal model: a histologic and biomechanical study. *J Shoulder Elbow Surg.* 2000;9:79–84.
7. Jones GC, Corps AN, Pennington CJ, et al. Expression profiling of metalloproteinases and tissue inhibitors of metalloproteinases in normal and degenerate human achilles tendon. *Arthritis Rheum.* 2006;54:832–842.
8. Lian O, Scott A, Engebretsen L, Bahr R, Duronio V, Khan K. Excessive apoptosis in patellar tendinopathy in athletes. *Am J Sports Med.* 2007;35:605–611.
9. Scott A, Cook JL, Hart DA, Walker DC, Duronio V, Khan KM. Tenocyte responses to mechanical loading in vivo: a role for local insulin-like growth factor 1 signaling in early tendinosis in rats. *Arthritis Rheum.* 2007;56:871–881.
10. Szomor ZL, Appleyard RC, Murrell GA. Overexpression of nitric oxide synthases in tendon overuse. *J Orthop Res.* 2006;24:80–86.
11. Yuan J, Murrell GA, Wei AQ, Wang MX. Apoptosis in rotator cuff tendonopathy. *J Orthop Res.* 2002;20:1372–1379.
12. Jobe FW, Kvitne RS, Giangarra CE. Shoulder pain in the overhand or throwing athlete. The relationship of anterior instability and rotator cuff impingement. *Orthop Rev.* 1989;18(9):963–975.
13. Wilk KE, Andrews JR, Arrigo CA. The abductor and adductor strength characteristics of professional baseball pitchers. *Am J Sports Med.* 1995;23(6):778.
14. Uhthoff HK, Loehr JW. Calcific tendinopathy of the rotator cuff: pathogenesis, diagnosis, and management. *J Am Acad Orthop Surg.* 1997;5(4):183–191.
15. Sher JS, Uribe JW, Posada A, Murphy BJ, Zlatkin MB. Abnormal findings on magnetic resonance images of asymptomatic shoulders. *J Bone Joint Surg Am.* 1995;77(1):10–15.
16. Bigliani LU, Morrison DS, April EW. The morphology of the acromion and its relationship to rotator cuff tears. *Orthop Trans.* 1986;10:228.
17. Toivonen DA, Tuite MJ, Orwin JF, Acromial structure and tears of the rotator cuff. *J Shoulder Elbow Surg.* 1995;4(5):376–383.
18. Hegedus EJ, Goode A, Campbell S, et al. Physical examination tests of the shoulder: a systematic review with meta-analysis of individual tests. *Br J Sports Med.* 2008;42(2):80–92.
19. Iannotti JP, Zlatkin MB, Esterhai JL, Kressel HY, Dalinka MK, Spindler KP. Magnetic resonance imaging of the shoulder. Sensitivity, specificity, and predictive value. *J Bone Joint Surg Am.* 1991;73(1):17–29.
20. Sanders TG, Jersey SL. Conventional radiography of the shoulder. Elsevier Semin Roentgenol, *Semin Roentgenol.* 2005;40(3):207–222.
21. Teefey SA, Petersen B, Prather H. Shoulder Ultrasound vs MRI or rotator cuff pathology. *PMR.* 2009;1(5):490–495.
22. Ebenbichler GR, Erdogmus CB, Resch KL, et al. Ultrasound therapy for calcific tendinitis of the shoulder. *N Engl J Med.* 1999;340(20):1533–1538.
23. Albert JD, Meadeb J, Guggenbuhl P, et al. High-energy extracorporeal shock-wave therapy for calcifying tendinitis of the rotator cuff: a randomised trial. *J Bone Joint Surg Br.* 2007;89(3):335–341.
24. Andres BM, Murrell GAC. Treatment of tendinopathy: what works, what does not, and what is on the horizon. *Clin Orthop Relat Res.* 2008;466(7):1539–1554.
25. Leduc BE, Caya J, Tremblay S, Bureau NJ, Dumont M. Treatment of calcifying tendinitis of the shoulder by acetic acid iontophoresis: a double-blind randomized controlled trial. *Arch Phys Med Rehabil.* 2003;84(10):1523–1527.
26. Nitz AJ. Physical therapy management of the shoulder. *Phys Ther.* 1986;66(12):1912–1919.
27. Bang MD, Deyle GD. Comparison of supervised exercise with and without manual physical therapy for patients with shoulder impingement syndrome. *J Orthop Sports Phys Ther.* 2000;30(3):126–137.
28. Kibler, BW. Shoulder rehabilitation: principles and practice. *Med Sci Sports Exerc.* 1998;30(Suppl 4):S40–S50.

29. Kibler WB, McMullen J. Scapular dyskinesis and its relation to shoulder pain. *J Am Acad Orthop Surg*. 2003;11(2):142–151.

30. Kuhn JE. Exercise in the treatment of rotator cuff impingement: a systematic review and a synthesized evidence-based rehabilitationprotocol. *J Shoulder Elbow Surg*. 2009;18(1):138–160.

31. Ellenbecker TS, Cools A. Rehabilitation of shoulder impingement syndrome and rotator cuff injuries: an evidence-based review. *Br J Sports Med*. 2010;44(5):319–327.

32. Bitter NL, Clisby EF, Jones MA, Magarey ME, Jaberzadeh S, Sandow MJ. Relative contributions of infraspinatus and deltoid during external rotation in healthy shoulders. *J Shoulder Elbow Surg*. 2007;16(5):563–568

33. Morrison DS, Frogameni AD, Woodworth P. Non-operative treatment of subacromial impingement syndrome. *J Bone Joint Surg Am*. 1997;79(5):732–737.

34. Fleck SJ, Kraemer WJ. *Designing Resistance Training Programs*. Champaign, IL: Human Kinetics; 2004.

35. Borstad JD, Ludewig PM. Comparison of three stretches for the pectoralis minor muscle. *J Shoulder Elbow Surg*. 2006;15(3):324–330.

36. Kennedy DJ, Visco CJ, Press J. Current concepts for shoulder training in the overhead athlete. *Curr Sports Med Rep*. 2009;8(3):154–160.

37. Jonsson P, Wahlström P, Ohberg L, Alfredson H. Eccentric training in chronic painful impingement syndrome of the shoulder: results of a pilot study. *Knee Surg Sports Traumatol Arthrosc*. 2006;14(1):76–81.

38. Mottram SL. Dynamic stability of the scapula. *Man Ther*. 1997;2(3):123–131.

39. Cools AM, Dewitte V, Lanszweert F, et al. Rehabilitation of scapular muscle balance: which exercises to prescribe? *Am J Sports Med*. 2007;35(10):1744–1751.

40. Thelen M, Dauber J, SToneman P. Randomized, double-blinded, clinical trial the clinical efficacy of kinesio tape for shoulder pain: *A J Orthop Sports Phys Ther*. 2008;38(7):389–395.

Glenohumeral Osteoarthritis

Erik S. Brand, Terrence G. McGee, Mark S. Hopkins, and Joanne P. Borg-Stein

INTRODUCTION

Shoulder pain has an estimated prevalence of 4% to 26% and is the third most common musculoskeletal complaint in the primary care setting (1). Referrals for nonoperative community-based musculoskeletal care of shoulder pain are commonly attributed to the rotator cuff (65%), peri-capsular musculature (11%), acromioclavicular joint (10%), neck (5%), glenohumeral osteoarthritis (GHOA) (3%), or adhesive capsulitis (1.5%) (1–4). Primary GHOA is relatively rare due to the nonweight-bearing nature of this joint and is significantly less common than primary osteoarthritis (OA) of the hands, feet, knees, and hips. However, posttraumatic secondary OA of the shoulder is at least as common as that of the hips, knees, feet, and hands and GHOA represents the third most common indication for joint replacement after the knee and hip (5–8). The frequency of GHOA increases with age and it is more common in women (6). Onset can be traumatic or nontraumatic. Predisposing factors for secondary OA include rotator cuff arthropathy, shoulder surgery to correct instability, systemic arthritis, avascular necrosis, congenital malformation, crystalline arthropathy, and other trauma (e.g., dislocation, humeral head or neck fracture) (9–11).

The anatomical structures commonly affected include the articular cartilage, labrum, and humeral head, with development of osteophytes and loose bodies (5,12). Coexisting pathology often includes glenohumeral instability, subacromial inflammation, and adhesive capsulitis (5,13,14). After the development of GHOA, the individual will commonly report gradual onset of anterior shoulder stiffness and pain worsening over months to years, in addition to swelling and possibly night pain. Symptoms are distinct from rheumatoid arthritis (RA) in that they are usually monoarticular. Classically, OA can be distinguished from RA because it is often aggravated by activity and relieved by rest. However, this distinction does not always hold true, as RA shoulder synovitis may also worsen with activity and be relieved by rest.

Initial evaluation includes a detailed history and physical examination. *Key elements of the physical examination* include inspection, palpation, neurovascular examination, and a detailed neck and shoulder examination. Inspection may reveal anterior effusion, increased anteroposterior (AP) diameter, or infraclavicular or generalized effusion compared to the asymptomatic shoulder. Palpation may reveal anterior joint line tenderness that can be elicited under the coracoid process by pressing laterally and slightly cranially (12). Examination of active/passive range of motion (AROM/PROM) in supine may elicit less pain and, therefore, allow a more complete examination of the glenohumeral joint. This benefit may be due to scapular stabilization provided by the supine position which allows the postural stabilizers (e.g., trapezius, rhomboid, and levator scapulae) to rest and/or isolation of the glenohumeral joint stabilizers (e.g., rotator cuff muscles). AROM/PROM will likely reveal pathognomonic end range stiffness. There may be loss of arm abduction and flexion; and external rotation may be less than the normal 90° (with the limb positioned in 90° of both arm abduction and forearm flexion, if possible). While concomitant cervical spine OA may be present, this should not cause limited range of motion (ROM) of the glenohumeral joint. The Apley scratch test may demonstrate asymmetry and limited internal rotation with inability to reach the normal T8-T10 level, consistent with rotator cuff arthropathy, adhesive capsulitis, or GHOA. Anterior crepitation caused by humeral head motion across damaged glenoid cartilage can be palpated or may be audible in advanced cases. This can be elicited by the release of resisted abduction in midrange, or by simple palpation during PROM (8,15).

Plain radiographs help distinguish GHOA from adhesive capsulitis, which may have a very similar physical examination demonstrating capsular restrictions. However, there is often a lack of crepitus if adhesive capsulitis occurs in the absence of OA (10,12). Recommended views include true AP and axillary lateral (10,12,16,17). When clinically indicated, other views may include external rotation and Y-outlet. Narrowing of the inferior articular cartilage may be evident if the joint space is narrowed more than the usual 3 to 4 mm thickness (12). Also witnessed are subchondral sclerosis, cyst formation, and marginal osteophytes on the inferior humeral head (17). Advanced disease may cause flattening of the humeral head. Early GHOA can be detected with CT arthrography, which can demonstrate thinning of inferior glenoid articular cartilage and MRI represents a reasonable alternative (12,18). Once the diagnosis is confirmed, severity of the condition is determined and concomitant conditions (e.g., fracture, dislocation, rotator cuff pathology, cervical or neurovascular injury) are ruled out, a comprehensive rehabilitation program can be planned.

Treatment for the majority of patients with symptomatic GHOA is nonoperative (5). While the lack of conclusive literature precludes strong recommendations, treatment options include physical therapy for the initial and postoperative treatment of GHOA (19,20). Nonoperative treatment includes therapeutic exercise, manual therapy (massage, joint mobilization, or manipulation), acupuncture, hydrotherapy, and/or other physical modalities (e.g., phonophoresis, iontophoresis, ultrasound, laser, and/or electrical stimulation) (19). Limited evidence suggests that pre and post-operative range of external rotation are closely related and that the amount of glenohumeral erosion does not affect the outcome of arthroplasty, should this surgical option become necessary (17).

GLENOHUMERAL OSTEOARTHRITIS

■ This condition has an increasing prevalence with age and female gender

■ Mechanism of injury is usually chronic, following trauma or other predisposing factors such as systemic arthritides, rotator cuff arthropathy, or congenital malformation

■ Key elements of the physical examination include inspection, palpation, neurovascular assessment, and a detailed neck and shoulder examination

■ Symptoms of GHOA may be identical to RA, but monoarticular versus polyarticular involvement are key distinguishing factors

■ Physical examination may also be very similar to adhesive capsulitis. In these situations radiographs are diagnostic and help distinguish between the two

THE REHABILITATION PROGRAM

As noted in previous chapters, a structured and supervised rehabilitation program, following the phases of rehabilitation discussed throughout this book, will facilitate a faster recovery and return to prior level of function. Rehabilitation should occur according to the stage of healing and the degree of irritability that is present. The degree of irritability can be determined through a detailed history, which includes inquiry into the patient's pain behavior, such as aggravating and alleviating factors, as well as the frequency, intensity, and duration of symptoms. Pain at rest is more indicative of a high level of irritability and characteristic of acute inflammation. Localized pain typically indicates less irritable conditions. Chronicity is marked by loss of active and passive ROM, and tends to be less irritable in nature.

Initial management should follow the traditional principles of PRICE (protection, relative rest, ice, compression, elevation) plus MEM (manual therapy, early motion, and medication) (21). Shoulder slings and orthoses are rarely indicated in the treatment of GHOA. However, following the PRICEMEM principles may require immobilization of the upper limb with an orthosis, the most common being the traditional canvas style sling with or without the addition of a swath (Figure 10.1). Generally, the intent is for short-term immobilization or for intermittent use based on the severity of pain and/or instability. For longer term use, fabric shoulder stabilizers are available and are most effective as a kinesthetic reminder, general compression and warmth, and for protection of gross instability (Figure 10.2).

Numerous treatment modalities are available for the management of shoulder pain, including cryotherapy, thermotherapy, therapeutic ultrasound, transcutaneous electrical nerve stimulation (TENS), and therapeutic exercise. Among practitioners, there is discrepancy in treatment approaches, likely related to the uncertainty about the efficacy of these multiple interventions (22). Restoration of scapular kinematics is imperative as there is evidence that alterations in scapular mobility have been associated with shoulder impingement, rotator cuff tendinopathy, rotator cuff tears, glenohumeral instability, adhesive capsulitis, and stiff shoulders. There is also evidence of altered muscle activation in these patient populations (23). Additionally, rehabilitation should take place in the scapular plane rather than straight planes, such as flexion, extension, and abduction, which are less functional. As the rehabilitation program advances, it is important to reproduce those forces and loads that approach the patient's daily functional demands in order to ensure a safe return to prior level of function.

Therapeutic Modalities

The use of thermal agents within any rehabilitation program has been well documented. It is generally agreed that cold should be applied during the first 24 to 48 hours of onset to decrease fluid infiltration into the interstitium, decrease inflammation and pain, and decrease the overall metabolic rate at the site (24). Following cold application, superficial or deep heating modalities may be applied to warm superficial joints, provide patient comfort, cause a deeper heating effect to structures such as muscles, or to heat collagen tissue in order to increase extensibility. Additional modalities such as therapeutic ultrasound and TENS have also been widely investigated in the treatment of shoulder pain. However, there is a lack of evidence supporting their continued application in the daily practice of physical rehabilitation (22). Thus, further investigation into their efficacy is warranted, in particular, in patients with GHOA.

Manual Therapy

The role of passive joint mobilization alone for the treatment of GHOA has not been well documented. There have been some small clinical trials looking at passive joint mobilizations provided to the shoulder joint, but these studies lacked the statistical power to detect the small but clinically significant effects of joint mobilization (25). Systematic reviews have found evidence in support of manual therapy; however, these reviews included studies that investigated joint mobilizations to both the shoulder and vertebral column (15,26,27).

The concept of *regional interdependence* is one that has recently grown in favor within the manual therapy community. It refers to the concept that "seemingly unrelated impairments in a remote anatomical region may contribute to, or be associated with, the patient's primary complaint" (28). This concept further suggests that many musculoskeletal disorders may respond more favorably to a regional treatment regimen in addition to localized treatment. Keeping this concept in mind, there is now mounting evidence in support of manipulative therapy applied to the cervical and thoracic spine to supplement the treatment of shoulder dysfunction and pain. Future studies are necessary to further validate these findings (29).

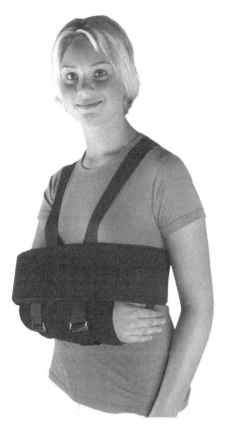

FIGURE 10.1: Traditional-canvas-style sling with swath.

Source: Courtesy of Ossur.

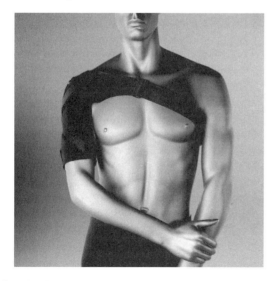

FIGURE 10.2: Fabric shoulder stabilizer.

Source: Courtesy of Ottobock.

Therapeutic Exercise

The use of therapeutic exercise as a sole intervention in the treatment of GHOA has not been adequately studied. As such, no recommendations can be made for therapeutic exercise as a stand-alone modality (22). No published controlled clinical trials have evaluated the efficacy of physical therapy for GHOA (20). Common practice includes early active assisted (AAROM) and PROM exercises performed in all planes of shoulder movement to eliminate symptoms, restore the normal biochemistry of the tissue, and to restore pain-free ROM, if possible. Again, initial AAROM/PROM may elicit less pain in the patient if they are performed in a supine position. Common exercises employed during the acute phase include Codman's or pendulum exercises as well as AAROM utilizing a wand or cane (Figure 10.3). Additionally, in the later acute stage, over the door pulley exercises (Figure 10.4) are also often employed as tolerated. Caution should be advised during ROM exercises, as structural joint remodeling of GHOA may cause a mechanical block (20). Flexibility exercises to stretch both the joint capsule and the shoulder girdle muscles are a vital component of the rehabilitation process as well (21).

Resisted scapular exercises should also be introduced at this time in the form of isometrics in single planes, and progress to movement of the entire scapula to restore its upward rotation required for full and pain-free elevation. Hydrotherapy may be considered for early strengthening, as it provides partial body weight support and resistance that can be titrated according to the rate of

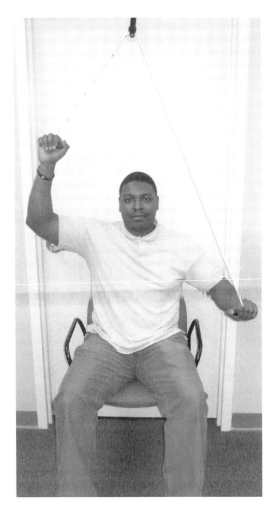

FIGURE 10.4: Shoulder pulley exercises for AAROM with elevation.

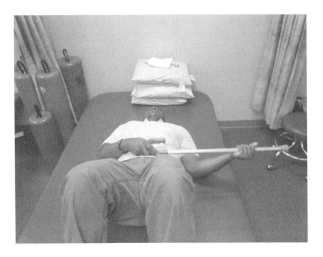

FIGURE 10.3: Wand exercises—AAROM in external rotation (ER) using a cane for the assistance.

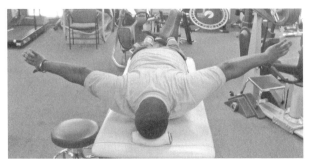

FIGURE 10.5: Scapular stabilization exercises, demonstrated here in the prone T position for strengthening of the middle trapezius and other periscapular muscles.

movement through the water. In addition to scapular stabilization exercises (Figure 10.5), strengthening the rotator cuff muscles is advocated. As the patient progresses out of the acute phase, continued emphasis should be placed on restoration of both glenohumeral and scapulothoracic movement. During the functional phase of recovery, improved neuromuscular control and restoration of the normal force couples should be emphasized. In addition to addressing the shoulder complex, clinicians must address the entire kinetic chain involved in the activity to which the patient is intending to return. This may include rehabilitation of the legs, hips, and core to focus on the production of appropriate activity-specific force and velocity from the lower limbs (21), such as in rehabilitation of the overhead throwing athlete.

Specialized Techniques

Poor posture has been implicated in the identification of potential causes of shoulder pain. As such, a thorough postural examination should be part of the rehabilitation for GHOA. Thoracic posture has been shown to produce alterations in scapular positioning. Additionally, the "forward head with rounded shoulders" posture frequently identified by treating therapists produces alterations in scapular mechanics. Kinesio Taping® is another form of modality that has recently gained favor, especially in the treatment of shoulder pain and instability. It has been found to be more effective than physical therapy alone in decreasing pain in the first week and disability in the second week of treatment (30). However, Kinesio Taping® has not been found to make any change in glenohumeral joint laxity, proprioception, or function (31).

Home Exercise Program

Before prescribing a home exercise program (HEP), the clinician should take into account the time that it will take the patient to perform the prescribed exercises. In addition, the level of tolerance and motivation to exercise varies among individuals, and is based on their diagnosis and stage of healing (21). Each HEP must be individualized to meet the patient's specific needs to help improve adherence and as a result, treatment success. Early monitoring of patient adherence and motivation will further ensure a successful resolution of the patient's symptoms and a return to prior level of function.

SUMMARY

GHOA is a relatively uncommon cause of shoulder pain. Proper diagnosis requires a detailed history, physical examination (including the cervical spine), and radiographs. Conservative treatment of this condition should follow a logical progression through the phases of rehabilitation. Early acute rehabilitation (phase I) should follow the PRICEMEM protocol including immobilization with an upper limb orthoses, if needed. Recommended therapeutic modalities during this phase include cold for the first 24 to 48 hours post injury. Therapeutic exercise in this phase commonly includes AAROM, PROM, and pendulum exercises. Phase II rehabilitation may incorporate superficial heat to aid the recovery of ROM. Other treatment options include ultrasound (deeper heat), TENS, passive joint mobilization, and therapeutic exercise, though none of these have been adequately studied. Phase III of rehabilitation includes gentle strengthening with scapular isometrics, then isotonic scapular stabilization and eventually rotator cuff strengthening. Phases IV and V can emphasize glenohumeral and scapulothoracic proprioception and functional movements for eventual return to prior activities. The functional phase of rehabilitation should emphasize key concepts such as regional interdependence of the kinetic chain including the core muscles, postural improvements, restoration of neuromuscular control and force couples in order to meet functional demands. The HEP should be individualized and include frequent reassessment of the program, the patient's tolerance, and their adherence.

SAMPLE CASE

A 65-year-old female presents with left shoulder pain and stiffness. Her past medical history is remarkable for right rotator cuff arthropathy, which responded well to physical therapy and nonsteroidal anti-inflammatory drugs. On review of systems she denies any prior significant musculoskeletal or sports injuries to the left shoulder. She has morning stiffness (lasting <30 minutes) but reports no other joint pains. The pain is worse in the evening after gardening, but better in the morning. Inspection reveals increased AP diameter of the left shoulder but no overlying ecchymosis. Palpation of the inferior glenohumeral joint line reveals tenderness. Other upper limb joint examinations are unremarkable. AROM/PROM is notable for glenohumeral glenohumeral external rotation of 15°. Neurovascular examination was unremarkable. Left-sided Apley scratch test is restricted and reaches T12, compared to T8 on the right. Single leg stance reveals bilateral Trendelenburg sign. Plain radiographs including true AP and axillary lateral views are negative for fracture but reveal a "club-like deformity" of the humeral head, joint space narrowing, marginal osteophytes and subchondral sclerosis.

 SAMPLE THERAPY PRESCRIPTION

Discipline: Physical or occupational therapy.

Diagnosis: Glenohumeral osteoarthritis.

Precautions: Use caution if encouraging patient to "push through the pain" as structural changes of OA may cause a mechanical block to ROM (20).

Frequency of visits: 2 to 3x/week.

Duration of treatment: Upward to 6 to 8 weeks depending on the severity and chronicity of symptoms.

Treatment:

1. *Modalities:* Cryotherapy progressing to heating agents

2. *Manual therapy:* Grade I–V joint mobilizations for both neurophysiologic effects on pain as well as mechanical effects on joint restrictions. Recommend regional approach with cervico-thoracic assessment as well

3. *Therapeutic exercise:* A/AA/PROM to restore glenohumeral and scapulothoracic motion. Strengthening of the scapular stabilizers first, then the rotator cuff musculature

4. *Specialized treatments:* Thorough postural examination and potentially ergonomic assessment of home/work environment

5. Patient education: Home exercise program

Goals: Decrease pain and swelling, restore ROM/flexibility then restore strength, improve proprioception, safely return to functional activities (e.g., sport, hobbies, work).

Reevaluation: In 4 weeks by referring physician. Additional request for weekly updates to referring physician for tailoring of therapy prescription and for consideration of additional management options (e.g., medications, injections).

REFERENCES

1. Urwin, M, Symmons D, Allison T, et al. Estimating the burden of musculoskeletal disorders in the community: the comparative prevalence of symptoms at different anatomical sites, and the relation to social deprivation. *Ann Rheum Dis.* 1998;57:649 655.
2. Wofford JL, Mansfield RJ, Watkins RS. Patient characteristics and clinical management of patients with shoulder pain in U.S. primary care settings: Secondary data analysis of the National Ambulatory Medical Care Survey. *BMC Musculoskelet Disord.* 2005;6:4.
3. Murphy RJ, Carr AJ. Shoulder pain. *Clin Evid.* (Online). 2010;2010:1107.
4. Vecchio P, Kavanagh R, Hazleman BL, King RH. Shoulder pain in a community-based rheumatology clinic. *Br J Rheumatol.* 1995;34(5):440–442.
5. Weinstein DM, Bucchieri JS, Pollock RG, Flatow EL, Bigliani LU. Arthroscopic debridement of the shoulder for osteoarthritis. *Arthroscopy.* 2000;16(5) 471–476.
6. United States Bone and Joint Initiative. *Burden of Musculoskeletal Diseases in the United States: Prevalence, Societal and Economic Cost.* Rosemont, IL: American Academy of Orthopaedic Surgeons; 2008.
7. Lawrence RC, Hochberg MC, Kelsey JL, et al. Estimates of the prevalence of selected arthritic and musculoskeletal diseases in the United States. *J Rheumatol.* 1989;16(4):427–441.
8. Buckwalter JA, Saltzman MD, Brown T. The impact of osteoarthritis: implications for research. *Clin Orthop Relat Res.* 2004;(Suppl 427):S6–S15. Review.
9. Nakagawa Y, Hyakuna K, Otani S, Hashitani M, Nakamura T. Epidemiologic study of glenohumeral osteoarthritis with plain radiography. *J Shoulder Elbow Surg.* 1999;8(6):580.
10. Anderson BC, Tugwell P, Romain PL. Glenohumeral osteoarthritis. UpToDate. Version 19.1. January 2011. Updated February 17, 2011.
11. Carfagno DG, Ellenbecker TS. Osteoarthritis of the glenohumeral joint: nonsurgical treatment options. *Phys Sportsmed.* 2002;30(4):19–30.

12. Anderson BC. The 67 most common outpatient orthopedic conditions. In: Anderson BC, ed. *Office Orthopedics for Primary Care: Treatment*. Philadelphia, PA: Elsevier; 2006: 44–46.

13. Ellman HA, Harris E, Kay S. Early degenerative joint disease simulating impingement syndrome: Arthroscopic findings. *Arthroscopy*. 1992;8:482–487.

14. Johnson CC. The shoulder joint: An arthroscopic perspective of anatomy and pathology. *Clin Orthop*. 1987;223:113–125.

15. Desmeules F, Cote CH, Fremont P. Therapeutic exercise and orthopedic manual therapy for impingement syndrome: a systematic review. *Clin J Sport Med*. 2003;13:176–182.

16. Green A, Norris TR. Imaging techniques for glenohumeral arthritis and glenohumeral arthroplasty. *Clin Orthop Relat Res*. 1994;(307:7–17.

17. Iannotti JP, Norris TR. Influence of preoperative factors on outcome of shoulder arthroplasty for glenohumeral osteoarthritis. *J Bone Joint Surg Am*. 2003;85-A(2):251–258.

18. Jahnke AH Jr, Petersen SA, Neumann C, Steinbach L, Morgan F. A prospective comparison of computerized arthrotomography and magnetic resonance imaging of the glenohumeral joint. *Am J Sports Med*. 1992;20(6):695–700; discussion 700–701.

19. Izquierdo R, Voloshin I, Edwards S, et al. American Academy of Orthopedic Surgeons. Treatment of glenohumeral osteoarthritis. *J Am Acad Orthop Surg*. 2010;18(6):375–382.

20. Moskowitz RW, Blaine TA. An overview of treatment options for persistent shoulder pain. *Am J Orthop (Belle Mead NJ)*. 2005;34(Suppl 12):10–15.

21. Dutton, M. *Orthopaedic Examination, Evaluation & Intervention*. New York, NY: McGraw-Hill; 2004.

22. Tugwell P, Abright J, Allman R, et al. Philadelphia panel evidence-based clinical practice guidelines on selected rehabilitation interventions for shoulder pain. *Phys Ther*. 2001;81(10):1719–1730.

23. Ludewig PM, Reynolds JF. The association of capular kinematics and glenohumeral joint p. *Phys Ther*. 2009;39(2):90–104.

24. Michlovitz, SL. *Thermal Agents in Rehabilitation*. Philadelphia, PA:F.A. Davis Co; 1990.

25. Yiasemides R, Halaki M, Cathers I, Ginn KA. Does passive mobilization of shoulder region joints provide additional benefit over advice and exercise alone for people who have shoulder pain and minimal movement restriction? A randomized controlled trial. *Physi Ther*. 2011;91(2):178–189.

26. Green S, Buckbinder R, Hetrick S. Physiotherapy interventions for shoulder pain. *Cochrane Database Syt Rev*. 2003;2:CD004258.

27. Michener LA, Walsworth MK, Burnet EN. Effectiveness of rehabilitation for patients with subacromial impingement syndrome: A systematic review. *J Hand Ther*. 2004;17:152–164.

28. Wainner RS, Flynn TW, Whitman JM. *Spinal and Extremity Manipulation: The Basic Skill Set for Physical Therapists*. San Antonio, TX: Manipulations, Inc; 2001.

29. Mintken PE, Cleland JA, Carpenter KJ, Bieniek ML, Keirns M, Whitman JM. Some factors predict successful short-term outcomes in individuals with shoulder pain receiving cervicothoracic manipulation: A single-arm trial. *Phys Ther*. 2010;90(1):26–42.

30. Kaya E, Zinnuroglu M, Tugcu I. Kinesio taping compared to physical therapy modalities for the treatment of shoulder impingement syndrome. *Clin Rheumatol*. 2011;30(2):201–207.

31. Bradley T, Baldwick C, Fischer D, Murrell GAC. Effect of taping on the shoulders of Australian football players. *British J Sports Med*. 2009;43(10):735. Abstract Retrieved May 3, 2011 from ProQuest Direct database.

Glenohumeral Joint Instability

Gerard A. Malanga, Ricardo Vasquez, Ripal Parikh, and Amrish D. Patel

GLENOHUMERAL INSTABILITY

The glenohumeral (GH) joint is the most mobile joint in the body, but the potential cost of mobility is stability. This makes the GH joint potentially the most unstable joint in the body and is often described as "a golf ball on a tee." To maintain mobility and stability of the GH joint requires a fine balance between the action of several muscles and tendons, bones and ligaments. These structures comprise the static and dynamic stabilizers of the shoulder complex that allow for simple activities like combing your hair to complex activities like throwing a football. A breakdown in either a static and/or dynamic stabilizer can lead to GH joint instability (1–4).

The static stabilizers of the shoulder (the noncontractile elements) include the bony articulation and alignment of the glenoid (a small ovoid shaped cavity that by itself does not provide much support) and the humeral head, the clavicle with the acromion process, clavicle to the manubrium of the sternum, and the pseudoarticulation between the scapula and thorax (4–6). The GH joint is further reinforced by the GH ligaments, which are thought to be thickened portions of the joint capsule, and the labrum, a fibrocartilaginous ridge that lines the glenoid deepening the socket and acting like a plunger. There is also the vacuum phenomenon created by the negative pressure within the joint capsule and the synovial fluid that creates some adhesion and cohesion between the joint surfaces (4–6). The static stabilizers then allow for the dynamic stabilizers to create motion at the GH joint while keeping the bones closely approximated.

The dynamic stabilizers (contractile elements) of the shoulder include the rotator cuff muscles, biceps tendon, and scapular stabilizers and other muscles that indirectly stabilize the scapula and act as dynamic stabilizers, such as the latissimus dorsi and pectoralis minor (4,6,7). These structures must work in balance to allow for the greatest mobility without losing stability (2). This requires neuromuscular control and the use of proprioceptive input to allow synchronous muscle activation that keeps the humeral head centrally located and approximated to the glenoid fossa (2,4). Dysfunction of any static and/or dynamic stabilizers can lead to GH instability (1).

GH instability refers to a spectrum of disorders that present with symptoms ranging from a feeling of shoulder "looseness" or just shoulder pain to frank dislocations and subluxations. The history is vital to collecting data and will allow for a clinical classification of the instability. Important aspects of the history include the age of the patient, which is the most important prognostic factor for risk of recurrent instability. The timing of the injury is another factor: Was, it acute or chronic and is it recurrent? Was the cause traumatic, atraumatic, or voluntary? Direction: did it dislocate anteriorly (most common), posteriorly (least common), inferiorly, or is it multidirectional? Did it sublux or fully dislocate? Did it have to be relocated or did it reduce spontaneously? Any associated injuries including loss of blood flow to the arm, associated bony injury, or associated neural injury to the arm with numbness, tingling, or weakness (6)?

The most common dislocation in trauma is an anterior dislocation often of the abducted and externally rotated arm (4). Posterior dislocations are uncommon but can be seen in patients who have seizures or significant posterior force on the shoulder as can be seen with weight lifters or with motor vehicle accidents (4,6). Multidirectional instability (MDI) is another type of instability that is considered to be very rare, although patients may present with varying degrees of instability that contribute to their symptoms. Classically MDI involves diffuse ligamentous laxity that can result from repeated microtraumas or congenital laxity, such as from Ehlers Danlos or Marfan's syndrome. Beighton criteria can be positive for diffuse hypermobility in those with multidirectional atraumatic GH instability (6).

Shoulder dislocations tend to occur in a bimodal distribution occurring in the second and sixth decades of life. Anterior dislocations are the most common accounting for up to 98% of shoulder dislocations and only about 2% with posterior dislocations (4). A large majority of primary dislocations are associated with some form of traumatic dislocation and a major complication of this is recurrent dislocations, which have been reported up to 78% of the time in younger patients within 2 years (8). Recurrent dislocations are far more common in the adolescent population and decreases with increasing age (4,8).

Taking a thorough history and physical examination will allow for the appropriate classification of GH instability. Two broad reasons why instability at the GH joint occurs are: (a) structural deficiency, either from trauma or an underlying structural deficiency that leads to repeated microtraumas, or (b) muscular imbalances and incorrect firing leading to increased translation of the humeral head over the glenoid and the development of secondary injury to static stabilizers. The underlying mechanism of injury initially led to an early classification system for GH instability as either traumatic, unilateral, Bankart lesion surgery (TUBS) or atraumatic, multi-directional, bilateral, rehabilitation, inferior capsular shift surgery (AMBRI). TUBS referred to a traumatic injury, often an anterior dislocation that resulted in unilateral instability often with an associated Bankart lesion, a tear of the labrum off the anterior portion of the glenoid resulting in anterior instability and requiring surgery. A possible associated injury following a traumatic dislocation also includes a Hills-Sachs lesion, which is a compression fracture of the posterolateral aspect of the humeral head. AMBRI referred to an atraumatic or minor injury that may have an associated MDI often with bilateral shoulder laxity found on examination that was treated with rehabilitation and, if surgery was needed, with an inferior capsular shift. Lastly there were voluntary dislocators which were thought to have psychiatrist disorders or secondary gain which should not be treated surgically (4,6).

A more recent system of classification looks at and takes into account the overlap between traumatic and atraumatic dislocations/subluxations. The Stanmore classification has three basic groups: traumatic structural, atraumatic structural, and habitual nonstructural. These groups could then be further subcategorized into acute, persistent, or recurrent and could be applied to anterior and posterior dislocations and subluxations. This system is also thought to allow for the continuum that can occur from one group to the next as GH instability progresses and changes (4,6,9).

Key elements of the physical examination include inspection, palpation, range of motion (ROM), strength,

sensation, reflex testing, and special tests. A key part of the acute examination is to determine if there was a true dislocation. In the subacute or chronic phase, evaluation of deficiency of static or dynamic stabilizers becomes crucial and whether there is multidirectional or unilateral instability should be determined. A Beighton score can often help determine if there is underlying ligamentous laxity (10). Often an acute first time traumatic shoulder dislocation will not relocate on its own, whereas a subluxation might. If a traumatic dislocation occurred, x-rays are recommended to rule out a fracture and confirm position of the humeral head and the type of dislocation (11). Following reduction of the dislocation, post reduction x-rays must be taken to confirm proper reduction, assess appropriate alignment, and to rule out other possible bony pathology (6,11). A critical part of the physical examination initially and at follow up includes a thorough neurovascular examination to rule out injury to the brachial artery or a plexus injury.

In the subacute and chronic phases a thorough examination of scapular stability, mobility, and control is crucial as the scapula is the foundation of proper motion at the GH joint. Evaluation of the rotator cuff and supporting muscles should be performed to look for underlying weakness or pain as described in the earlier chapters on rotator cuff pathology and impingement syndromes. Assessment of ligamentous laxity and subluxation through a series of special tests and assessment of GH joint mobility is the key component of the physical examination.

The Jobs apprehension and relocation tests for anterior instability is one of the key tests for dislocation and subluxation. The apprehension test should be performed in a supine position, although it may be performed in a seated position, with the shoulder at 90° of abduction. Then the GH joint is slowly rotated into external rotation (ER) which will cause fear of dislocation or subluxation if positive. The relocation test is performed immediately after the apprehension test with a posterior force applied to the anterior GH joint followed by attempting further passive ER. A positive relocation test is when the patient tolerates this motion, demonstrating increased ER without signs of apprehension (12).

The Jerk test and sulcus sign are other special tests used to assess for GH instability. The jerk test for posterior instability is performed with the shoulder and elbow in 90° of flexion, full internal rotation of the shoulder while applying a posteriorly directed force. If positive, the patient will jerk the arm away to prevent posterior subluxation/dislocation (12). The sulcus sign for inferior instability is performed with the patient sitting and the arm resting in a neutral position. The examiner pulls the arm inferiorly at the elbow. A positive test is noted if there is gapping or dimpling noted inferior to the acromion (12).

Review of the literature does not support the use of a standard sling for immobilization to prevent recurrent dislocation (13). The resting position of the arm that improved GH contact has been determined to be with the arm adducted and externally rotated. Many studies also looked at recurrence, yet few definitively showed decreased recurrence rates with any period of immobility. However, one larger study did show better results, for patients 30 years or younger, immobilized for a period of 6 to 8 weeks compared to less than 6 weeks (13).

Literature on the role of exercise in the management of nonoperative traumatic anterior dislocations is limited. However, the small number of studies that do exist support the use of a period of immobilization followed by a therapeutic exercise program. The same holds true for the nonoperative management of atraumatic dislocations (13). The principle goals remain to increase the GH surface contact and restore normal scapulothoracic motion and proprioception to the shoulder (13,14). Lifestyle modification is also a key element to the rehabilitation program and may help to prevent recurrent dislocation. Treatment options range from operative to nonoperative management that includes pain control, relative rest with immobilization, and activity restriction and then progression to an active therapy program (10).

THE REHABILITATION PROGRAM

The rehabilitation program for those with both traumatic and atraumatic instability should follow the five phases of rehabilitation that have been utilized throughout this book. In the case of acute traumatic shoulder dislocations, once the shoulder dislocation has been reduced and imaging has ruled out any acute bony pathology (e.g., fractures) the rehabilitation process begins. Once pain and inflammation has been controlled with the PRICE protocol and as needed (PRN) analgesic medications, then the focus of the rehabilitation program is to restore the underlying muscle imbalance and neuromuscular control, especially of the dynamic stabilizers of the scapula and shoulder, and as strength and control is gained ROM may be gradually restored. Soft tissue mobilization promotes ROM and flexibility in the appropriate direction, avoiding positions that will put stress on already weakened static stabilizers;

GLENOHUMERAL JOINT INSTABILITY

- GH instability can be classified into three basic groups: traumatic structural, atraumatic structural and habitual nonstructural (Stanmore classification)

- The most frequent direction of GH joint dislocation is anteriorly

- Immediate management includes reduction of the dislocation, use of pre and post reduction x-rays, along with assessment and monitoring of the neurovascular status

- Classifying the dislocation type, frequency and direction helps guide treatment

- Age and activity level must also be considered, since recurrent dislocation rates are higher for traumatic dislocations especially in younger, active patients

- Nonoperative management is similar for the three types of dislocations and consists of pain control, NSAIDs as needed, joint protection and then a progressive rehabilitation program

proprioception and muscular control retrain the neuromuscular control and stability, strength, and lifestyle modification prevent recurrence (1,4,11,15).

Rehabilitation will likely take months, with the treating physician guiding a multidisciplinary approach to care, including the help of a physical and/ or occupational therapist, athletic trainer, and possibly a psychologist. There is no consensus on rehabilitation of shoulder instability. Much of the literature that exists on rehabilitation for shoulder instability exists for the postoperative management. However, nonoperative management should be approached with the same care and principles as the postoperative management. Some evidence is present to support the use of rehabilitation without surgery (16), although each case must be carefully considered and individualized before deciding on nonoperative versus operative management.

Early management should consist of protecting the soft tissues to allow healing while balancing prevention of stiffness, postural dysfunction, muscle atrophy, loss of proprioception, and aberrant movement patterns. The nontraumatic and habitual dislocations usually do not need periods of immobilization given their gradual onset, however they may have a greater abundance of faulty movement patterns (1,4).

The overall length of recovery for GH instability will vary based on the individual, their activity level, and the type of instability they present with. Traumatic dislocations that have undergone surgery may return to sport on an average of 4 months, atraumatic and habitual instability on average can return to sport around 6 months (4). The latter two subtypes must be educated on the risk of recurrence when taking on new challenges or sports where the neuromuscular system will be put under new and different challenges. Younger individuals who may undergo a growth spurt and therefore have changes in the posture and muscle balance will also be at greater risk for recurrence if they do not maintain postural balance and scapular stability (1,4).

Therapeutic Modalities

Limited literature is available to support the use of therapeutic modalities for GH instability and many choices are based on expert opinion. However, after any acute dislocation or subluxation, cryotherapy can be used to reduce pain, inflammation, and swelling. After the acute phase, thermotherapy may be utilized to improve soft tissue pliability for any stretching that may need to be performed or to improve tolerance to a therapeutic exercise program. If pain continues to be an issue the use of electrical stimulation, specifically a TENS unit, may be considered.

Manual Therapy

Manual therapy techniques that focus on correcting muscle-firing patterns and assisting symmetric movement of the scapula should be incorporated. Manual resistance, such as the utilization of positional neuromuscular facilitation (PNF) techniques (e.g., rhythmic stabilizations) (Figure 11.1), may be used to offer graded increases in resistance at various positions of the GH joint in a controlled manner (1) while directly monitoring for patient apprehension or overexertion. These techniques may allow the patient to gradually restore neuromuscular control, strength, ROM, and confidence. The goal is to restore proximal stability to the shoulder complex, which will allow return to activities that require distal mobility of the upper limb.

Addressing any capsular, soft tissue, or muscular restrictions that may lead to poor biomechanics should

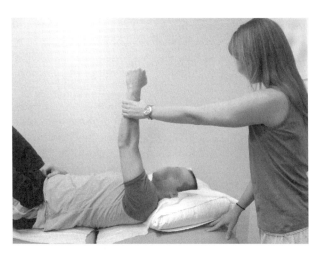

FIGURE 11.1: Manual resistance applied to the shoulder in multiple planes to improve shoulder strength and muscle recruitment (based on PNF technique known as rhythmic stabilization).

also be addressed with the appropriate soft tissue massage, myofascial release, or GH joint mobilizations. Any soft tissue mobilization must be done in areas that are restricted as to not overstretch an area with previous laxity.

The shoulder, cervical, and upper thoracic spine may be addressed as a unit and any soft tissue or joint restrictions of the cervical or thoracic spine should be treated to restore normal motion at the shoulder girdle. Restriction of the ribs should also be addressed since these restrictions may alter muscle-firing patterns and potentially cause increased scapular dyskinesis (4). Pain from the cervical or thoracic spine may also cause muscle inhibition resulting in altered scapular and therefore GH joint kinetics (4).

Therapeutic Exercise

As with many musculoskeletal (MSK) rehabilitation programs, therapeutic exercise is the most crucial aspect of the program. However, for shoulder instability therapeutic exercises will not be advanced in the same stepwise fashion as other MSK conditions discussed throughout this book. The goal of the first phase remains the same and is to reduce pain and swelling but the next phase doesn't focus on fully restoring ROM prior to restoration of joint strength, proprioception, and neuromuscular control (phase II–IV). Instead, these three phases are addressed almost simultaneously. Neuromuscular control and proprioceptive exercises are emphasized along with scapula stabilization and rotator cuff strengthening to avoid recurrent

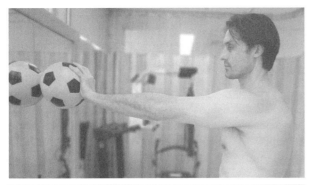

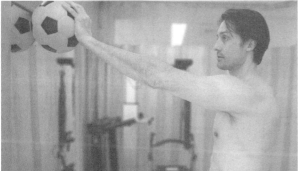

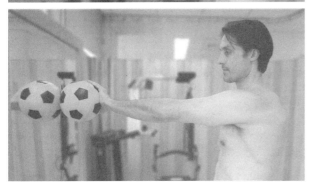

FIGURE 11.2: Closed kinetic chain exercises for the upper limb.

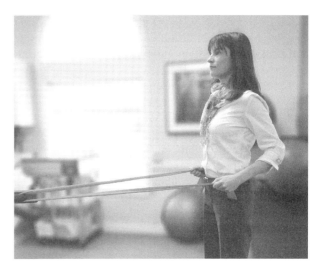

FIGURE 11.3: Using resistance bands for scapular strengthening.

dislocations or subluxations. Only when improved neuromuscular control, proprioception, and strength develop can the functional ROM be safely progressed.

To expand on the initial statements regarding therapeutic exercise for GH joint instability, during the early management of shoulder dislocations, after capsular-ligamentous injury has occurred affecting afferent feedback and therefore altering muscle-firing patterns, a strengthening program that corrects the firing pattern and yet protects the joint is warranted (1,4). Closed kinetic chain exercises can help promote rotator cuff co-contraction promoting increased stability and proprioception (Figure 11.2). This can also encourage scapular stability while not increasing the shear force across

the GH joint. Isometric strengthening of the subscapularis is also encouraged to provide secondary structural support against anterior translation of the humeral head (4). For posterior dislocations, isometric strengthening of the external rotators is encouraged. In atraumatic and habitual dislocators, increasing postural tone may help gain selective rotator cuff recruitment, so performing strengthening exercises while challenging the core and postural muscles may provide benefit (1,17). Activation of postural muscles can help optimize GH joint alignment and promote activation of deep stabilizing muscles. Regardless of the classification of shoulder dislocations-shoulder girdle position, avoiding inappropriate muscle firing patterning and strengthening is important to the early phases of rehabilitation (1,4,18).

Strength training should use lighter weights with higher repetitions to avoid overloading the muscles and prevent abnormal firing patterns, especially seen in the traumatic and atraumatic dislocators. Scapular stability can be addressed with the use of resistance bands for strengthening (Figure 11.3). Rotator cuff strengthening in an adducted position is important for those with secondary impingement; however, for those with inferior instability, deltoid with rotator cuff activation may be desirable (1). This can be achieved by performing internal and external rotator strengthening with the shoulder in slight abduction. In those with habitual instability, biofeedback techniques (see the section of specialized techniques) may be used to help correct abnormal muscle firing. As discussed in the prior paragraph, closed chain exercises are important and can be advanced by performing them on an unstable base. This exercise becomes a proprioceptive training tool, but has not been shown to alter upper limb muscle activation. In the habitual dislocators, using an unstable base under their feet may improve postural control and prevent inappropriate compensatory muscle activation that can occur with an unstable base at the upper limb (1,4).

After obtaining improved strength, postural control, proprioception, and muscle balance, it is important to regain any lost ROM (1). The atraumatic subtype may develop glenohumeral internal rotation deficits, also known as GIRD; this restriction should be addressed in therapy and at home with the "sleeper stretch" (Figure 11.4). Regaining this ROM is a key step in the rehabilitation program, but remember strengthening throughout the newly obtained range should also continue (4).

In the final phases of rehabilitation, therapeutic exercises should focus on full restoration of strength, muscular endurance, and appropriate muscle activation and movement patterns to obtain functional goals. Challenging dynamic stabilization, plyometrics, and use of light weight Swiss balls and medicine balls can all be used to obtain improved speed, strength, and endurance. PNF techniques, including diagonal movement patterns, can be used to gain stability, strength, and control in various movement patterns and even at end ROM (Figure 11.5). An exercise that has been shown to aid in proprioception is the sidelying plank with the affected side elevated toward the ceiling and holding an object in the hand with the eyes closed. Advancement toward sport-based activities is crucial to help with cognitive motor retraining at this point in the rehabilitation program (1).

Specialized Techniques

Biofeedback, postural taping, and the use of mirrors can be employed to facilitate correct muscle activation. Biofeedback for shoulder girdle position and correct posture should be employed early in the rehabilitation program. Facilitation can also be encouraged with manual feedback; some physical therapists utilize surface electromyography (EMG) biofeedback. These methods are often used in those with habitual shoulder instability, likely secondary to their underlying aberrant muscle activation (1).

Home Exercise Program

Education is the key to patient compliance and will help improve strength and stability while preventing recurrent

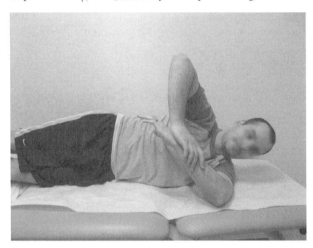

FIGURE 11.4: The sleeper stretch.

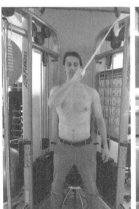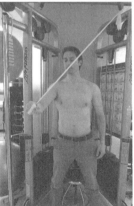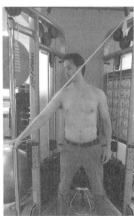

FIGURE 11.5: PNF diagonal techniques can be used to gain stability, strength, and control.

dislocations. Slow progression of a rehabilitation program that will likely continue for several months will start with movements to avoid redislocation. The initial focus of the HEP will include protection from recurrent dislocation and may require behavioral modifications. The HEP should initially focus on isometric exercises, postural correction, scapular stability, and mobility. ROM should initially be guided by your therapist, in order to avoid subluxation or recurrent dislocation. As therapy is advanced and stability improves then strengthening can progress throughout the available ROM. Focus should be on regaining mobility, strength, and neuromuscular control of the scapulothoracic and GH joints. Progression towards sport specific activity will need to be guided by a physical or occupational therapist or certified athletic trainer.

SUMMARY

GH joint instability is a condition that can be traumatic or atraumatic in origin. Traumatic instability occurs from dislocations, especially in the younger population, tends to recur despite aggressive physical therapy (PT). A number of different papers have reported greater than a 75% success rate with PT alone, but these studies have not been reproduced with the same level of success. Furthermore, there is little agreement on a specific therapy protocol post dislocation. Often stratification based on the type of GH instability can help guide the therapeutic program. There is a lack of consensus on the use of immobilization after a dislocation, such as shoulder positioning and duration of immobilization. Despite appropriate rehabilitation for young, active patients, much of the literature suggests that traumatic dislocations with associated soft tissue (labral tears) and bony injury (humeral head or glenoid compression fractures) will eventually require surgery to prevent recurrent dislocation and successful return to sport. The recovery process will take several months and require the guidance of a skilled physical or occupational therapist or athletic trainer and physician to guide the rehabilitation program.

SAMPLE CASE

A 22-year-old male who is s/p right anterior shoulder dislocation two days ago. He has no significant past medical history/past surgical history (PMH/PSH/Meds). He was playing basketball and when he went up to get a rebound he had his right shoulder hyperextended in a flexed position and immediately noted pain and a deformity of his anterior shoulder. He had the shoulder dislocation reduced in the ER and was placed in a sling. Review of systems (ROS) is unremarkable and he denies prior significant MSK or sports injuries. X-rays from the emergency department were negative for fracture. His examination is significant for arm in an internally rotated/adducted position in a sling. +Mild anterior shoulder swelling and tenderness to palpation (TTP) over many portions of anterior shoulder. Active ROM limited in flexion, abduction and ER secondary to pain and guarding. Neurovascular exam unremarkable except for limited AROM of shoulder as noted above. Positive apprehension and relocation tests.

 SAMPLE THERAPY PRESCRIPTION

Discipline: Physical therapy.

Diagnosis: Right anterior shoulder dislocation and traumatic instability.

Precautions: Dislocation precautions (avoid end range shoulder abduction and ER).

Frequency of visits: 2 to 3x/week.

Duration of treatment: 4 weeks.

Treatment:

1. *Modalities:* Cryotherapy (ice pack, ice bath, ice massage) used acutely. Heat modalities after acute phase.

2. *Manual therapy:* Muscle energy to help restore ER mobility, myofascial release, and assisted scapulothoracic motion. Mobilization of cervical and thoracic vertebrae as well as the ribs if restrictions are present and preventing recovery of normal shoulder mechanics

3. *Therapeutic exercise:* Strengthening of shoulder stabilizers such as the rotator cuff muscles and scapular stabilizers, including the trapezius (especially the middle and lower trapezius), rhomboids, and serratus anterior. A/AA/AROM will be advanced slowly and only when the patient demonstrates adequate neuromuscular control to prevent dislocation/subluxation. PNF techniques (diagonal movement patterns, rhythmic stabilizations). Posterior capsular stretch if GIRD is present. Progress to proprioceptive training at full strength, then sports specific activities.

4. *Specialized treatments:* Neuromuscular retraining of shoulder stabilizer muscles

5. *Patient education:* Home exercise program

Reevaluation: In 4 weeks by referring physician

REFERENCES

1. Jaggi A, Lambert S. Rehabilitation for shoulder instability. *Br J Sports Med*. 2010;44(5):333-340.
2. Labriola J, Lee T. Stability and instability of the glenohumeral joint: The role of shoulder muscles. *J Shoulder Elbow Surg*. 2005;14:S32-S38.
3. Myers J, Lephart S. Sensorimotor deficits contributing to glenohumeral instability. *Clin Ortho and Rel Research*. 2002;400:98-104.
4. Hayes K, Callanan M. Shoulder instability: Management and rehabilitation. *J Orthop Sports Phys Ther*. 2002;32:10.
5. Omoumi P, Teixeira P. Glenohumeral joint instability. *J Magn Reson Imaging*. 2011;33:2-16.
6. Itoi E, Newman S. Dynamic anterior stabilizers of the shoulder with the arm in abduction. *British Editorial Society of Bone and Joint Surgery*. 1994;76-/B:834-836.
7. Hoelen M, Burgers A. Prognosis of primary anterior shoulder dislocation in young adults. *Arch Orthop Trauma Surg*. 1994;110:51-54.
8. Burkhead WZ Jr, Rockwood CA Jr. Treatment of instability of the shoulder with an exercise program. *J Bone Joint Surg Am*. 1992;74:890-896.
10. Dodson CC, Cordasco FA. Anterior glenohumeral joint dislocations. *Orthop Clin North Am*. 2008;39(4):507-518, vii. Review.
11. Penzak M, Nho S. Management of acute anterior shoulder instability in adolescents. *Orthop Nurs*. 2010;29(4):237-243.
12. Malanga G, Nadler S. *Musculoskeletal Physical Examination: An Evidence-Based Approach*. Elscvier Health Sciences; 2006:87-101.
13. Smith T. Immobilisation following traumatic anterior glenohumeral joint dislocation a literature review. *Int J Cardiovasc Intervent*. 2006;37:228-237.
14. Itoi E, Hatakeyama Y, Sato T, et al. Immobilization in external rotation after shoulder dislocation reduces the risk of recurrence: a randomized controlled trial. *J Bone Joint Surg*. 2007;89(10):2124-2131.
15. Boileau P, Zumstein M. The unstable painful shoulder (UPS) as a cause of pain from unrecognized anteroinferior instability in the young athlete. *J Shoulder Elbow Surg*. 2011;20(1):98-106.
16. Burgess B, Sennett B. Traumatic shoulder instability, Nonsurgical management versus surgical intervention. *Orthop Nurs*. 2003;22(5): 345-350.
17. Kiss R, Illyes A. Physiotherapy vs. capsular shift and physiotherapy in multidirectional shoulder joint instability. *J Electromyogr Kinesiol*. 2010;20:489-501.
18. Gerber C, Nyffler R. Classification of glenohumeral joint instability. *Clin Orthop Relat Res*. 2002;400:65-76.

Adhesive Capsulitis

Theresa A. Chiaia and Jo A. Hannafin

INTRODUCTION

Adhesive capsulitis is a condition of the shoulder characterized by pain and subsequent gradual loss of shoulder motion. Two types of adhesive capsulitis are described. *Primary adhesive capsulitis, an idiopathic condition of unknown etiology, is the focus of this chapter.* In secondary adhesive capsulitis, or frozen shoulder, there is an underlying or possibly concurrent pathology or inciting injury (1). Adhesive capsulitis occurs in 2% to 5% of the population with an age range of 40 to 60 years (2). It is more common in females and the nondominant extremity. Of significance, 20% to 30% of individuals who develop unilateral adhesive capsulitis will develop it in the opposite shoulder; however, it rarely recurs in the same shoulder (3).

The onset of adhesive capsulitis is insidious, with a progressive worsening of pain ranging from a constant ache at the deltoid insertion, to sharp pain with sudden movements to night pain. *The key element of the physical examination is range of motion (ROM) testing, performed both passively and actively, and initially reveals a subtle loss of external rotation (ER) followed by decreased internal rotation (IR) and abduction.* Neviaser (1) described four stages of adhesive capsulitis by correlating physical exam with the arthroscopic findings: the preadhesive stage, the freezing stage, the frozen or maturation stage, and the thawing stage. Hannafin (4) demonstrated the histopathologic progression of Neviaser stages one through three. These stages represent a continuum rather than distinct well-defined stages (Table 12.1) (5).

Diagnosis and staging of adhesive capsulitis is made by the history and clinical examination. The differential diagnoses to consider when patients present with shoulder pain include cervical radiculopathy, facet syndrome, impingement syndromes, subacromial bursitis, calcific tendinopathy or tendonitis, and osteoarthritis.

Once cervical spine causes have been ruled out, patients with impingement syndromes typically present with shoulder pain with resisted shoulder movements and in isolated impingement typically do not have restricted passive ROM, though they may experience pain. Patients with subacromial bursitis present with similar complaints of pain; but the pattern of pain limited ROM is with elevation, abduction, and IR as opposed to ER, and pain during end range of active motion. Glenohumeral osteoarthritis (OA) typically has increased pain with IR, limited ROM greatest of IR, and associated crepitus. Radiographs can help rule out osteoarthritis, long-standing rotator cuff disease, and calcific tendinopathy.

THE REHABILITATION PROGRAM

Clinical decision making in the rehabilitation of a patient with adhesive capsulitis can be optimized by recognizing the stage of presentation, as well as the irritability of the shoulder joint. Irritability (6) is determined by pain, ROM, and extent of disability and appears to correlate with the stage of adhesive capsulitis.

The goals of rehabilitation are to address the functional impairments and problems that are commonly associated with adhesive capsulitis. They include: pain, loss of function, sleep disturbance, loss of motion due to pain, and/or secondary capsular tightness. The goal is to maximize the function in the presenting stage. This is achieved through decreasing the inflammatory response and pain, increasing ROM, and reestablishing normal shoulder and scapular biomechanics. Treatment includes therapeutic modalities to decrease pain and inflammation, to promote relaxation, and increase tissue extensibility and therapeutic exercise and manual therapy to improve tissue extensibility, ROM, and to reestablish force couples to normalize scapulohumeral rhythm (Table 12.2).

TABLE 12.1: Stages of Adhesive Capsulitis

Stage	I	II	III	IV
Duration	0 to 3 months	3 to 9 months	9 to 15 months	> 15 months
Complaints	Constant ache at deltoid insertion, sharp pain with movement; night pain	Pain persists; Severe night pain; pain in upper trapezius extending to neck; ROM loss	Minimal pain; night pain; Shoulder stiffness	Shoulder stiffness
ROM	A & passive range of motion (PROM) limited by pain	Loss of ROM in capsular pattern	Loss of ROM in capsular pattern	Gradual ROM improvement
Signs	Empty end feel; capsular pain on deep palpation of capsule	Pain at end ROM; hiking of shoulder girdle w/arm elevation	Capsular end feel; resistance before pain; hiking of the shoulder girdle w/arm elevation	Capsular end feel; resistance before pain
Diagnosis	Early loss of ER ROM with intact strength; Intra-articular anesthetic injection restores ROM; evaluation/examination under anesthesia (EUA) reveals normal or minimal ROM loss	ROM improves but is not fully restored with intra-articular injection	No improvement in ROM with EUA or with local anesthetic; exam reveals sense of mechanical block	
Diagnostic tests	X-ray to r/o calcific tendonitis, early OA, longstanding rotator cuff (RC) disease; MRI to r/o RC injury	X-ray to r/o calcific tendonitis, early OA;	X-ray to r/o calcific tendonitis, early OA;	
Arthroscopic findings	Diffuse fibrous synovial inflammatory reaction; NO adhesions or capsular contracture	Insertion of 'scope reveals tight capsule, rubbery dense feel; some loss of axillary fold; Christmas tree appearance, hypervascular synovitis	Thick capsule on insertion of 'scope; loss of capsular volume; remnants of fibrotic synovium; loss of axillary recess	Fully mature adhesions
Biopsy	Hypertrophic, hypervascular synovitis; rare inflammatory cell infiltrates; normal capsule	Hypertrophic, hypervascular synovitis; perivascular and subsynovial scar; fibroplasia and scar in the capsule	Resolving synovitis; dense scar formation in capsule	Data is not available
Irritability	High		Moderate	Low

TABLE 12.2: Rehabilitation Approach Based on the Stage of Adhesive Capsulitis

Stage	Goals	Modalities	Therapeutic Exercise	Manual Therapy
I	Disrupt inflammatory-pain cycle; control pain; educate in support of the upper limb, activity modification; retard progression from synovitis to fibroplasia	To control pain and inflammation; moist heat, cryotherapy, TENS	Pendulums, PROM/AAROM exercises in PoS: elevation in supine with opposite hand, cane ER, IR	Grade I mobilizations
II	Control inflammation/pain, minimize ROM loss, reestablish force couples to maximize S-H rhythm.	To decrease pain and inflammation, and to promote relaxation and increase tissue extensibility.	ROM exercises, pain-free periscapular strengthening, closed chain exercises, hydrotherapy.	Mobilizations: A-P, inferior; soft tissue release; medical massage; PNF techniques.
III	Increase ROM/ flexibility, restore function, avoid painful arcs of active motion, AROM = PROM	To increase tissue extensibility	Frequent ROM/flexibility exercises, pain-free periscapular strengthening, closed chain exercises, hydrotherapy	Mobilizations: A-P, inferior; medical massage; PNF techniques

Patient education is a mainstay of any rehabilitation program. In patients with adhesive capsulitis, education about the diagnosis, the stages of the disease process, and the goals for each stage will encourage patient compliance and minimize patient frustration. The individual is taught self-management of symptoms through positioning, during activities of daily living (ADLs), and a home exercise program. Helping the patient find a position of comfort for the shoulder will afford the patient rest. The patient is instructed to support the arm on a pillow in supine, as the shoulder tends to be more comfortable in the plane of the scapula (PoS) with the elbow at the same height or slightly higher than the shoulder. The pillow should also support the lack of IR; thereby, decreasing the stress on the capsule and helping to relieve pain. Use of the extremity is encouraged through movement in a pain-free arc. Disuse of the arm will result in loss of shoulder mobility and, strength and osteopenia; while continued use of the arm through pain may result in impingement of the subacromial space and altered biomechanics of the shoulder girdle. Education about the importance of early recognition and treatment should symptoms appear in the contralateral shoulder must be discussed. It is the authors' experience that early treatment is associated with shorter duration of disability.

The goal of early treatment of stage I adhesive capsulitis is to retard the progression from synovitis to capsular fibroplasia. Thus, communication with the physician is paramount for successful management. Referral for a glenohumeral corticosteroid injection is indicated to relieve pain, control inflammation, improve motion, and ultimately halt progression through the stages of adhesive capsulitis. Others have suggested use of a suprascapular nerve block to provide pain relief by blocking afferent capsular pain fibers, which may improve ROM.

The goals of treatment for the patient presenting in stage II are pain control, modulation of ROM loss, and reestablishment of force couples. The patient may still benefit from an injection, but requires ROM and joint mobilization to increase capsular extensibility. Recording the improvement in ROM is important as the patient will continue to perceive pain at the end of the ROM and may not recognize the gains. Pain-free active range of motion (AROM) and strengthening are performed in the PoS to optimize scapulohumeral rhythm and discourage deleterious compensatory movements.

In stage III, the patient presents with a stiff, painless shoulder; thus, the goal of rehabilitation is to improve ROM and flexibility, and to restore function.

Since change in capsular extensibility takes time, the goal is to have AROM = PROM. This allows the patient to use the arm during daily activities which will enhance ROM gains and maximize function. Medical massage, active warm-up, joint mobilizations, frequent ROM exercises, and active use of the arm are emphasized. Strengthening of the periscapular musculature in the available ROM will normalize scapulohumeral rhythm as PROM improves.

The phases of rehabilitation will be based on presentation in *stage II adhesive capsulitis*, as this is when the majority of patients present for treatment. The duration of each phase will be determined by the success of initial treatments. Achievement of phase specific goals will determine the advancement to the next phase. The patient's individual goals will determine discharge.

Therapeutic Modalities

Therapeutic modalities are used to reduce pain (transcutaneous electrical nerve stimulation [TENS] (7), and cryotherapy), control inflammation (cryotherapy), and promote relaxation (moist heat) (8). Low power laser therapy was more effective than placebo treatment in reducing pain and disability scores (9), but requires further investigation. Ultrasound, phonophoresis, and iontophoresis reduced the likelihood of improvement (10).

Manual Therapy

Manual therapy techniques are utilized throughout the course of this disease, and will be modified based on the stage and irritability of the shoulder (6). Low grade joint mobilization will be used in stage I and early stage II to modulate pain (11). With decreased capsular volume and a decrease in the axillary recess (12), joint mobilization will focus on tissue extensibility (13). Posterior directed mobilization of the glenohumeral joint has been shown to be more effective than anterior directed mobilization in improving ER ROM (14).

Proprioceptive neuromuscular facilitation (PNF), such as contract-relax techniques to stretch into IR, can be very helpful for improving flexibility of the posterior cuff. Medical massage has been recommended for soft tissue release of the subscapularis (15) and rotator cuff interval (16) and to achieve scapulohumeral dissociation, but further investigation is needed to help define its role.

Therapeutic Exercise

Therapeutic exercise will address soft tissue imbalances created by pain, disuse, and loss of capsular volume and contracture. Pendulum exercises create a distraction at the shoulder joint (Figure 12.1). An active, pain-free warm-up utilizing upper body ergometry provides deep heating of soft tissues and increases blood flow.

ROM exercises (17) are performed to the patient's and their shoulder's tolerance. It is important to get to know their shoulder and its response to treatment. This will guide the dosage frequency, intensity, and duration of ROM exercises. The total end range time (TERT) is determined by manipulating these variables and is based on the irritability of the shoulder (18). ROM exercises

beyond the shoulder's pain threshold may delay progress (19). Pulley exercises are introduced with adequate ROM (~135° elevation) and humeral head control to avoid anterosuperior migration of the humeral head, thus causing subacromial impingement. Advancement to self-stretching of the posterior capsule is initiated when horizontal adduction and "sleeper stretch" can be performed without impingement symptoms or anterior-superior migration of the humeral head (20).

Strengthening will focus on improving scapulohumeral rhythm with emphasis on the periscapular musculature and addressing force couples necessary for arm elevation (serratus anterior, rhomboids, lower trapezius) (21). Resistance exercises should be performed in available ROM with minimal, but tolerable, pain.

Closed chain exercises will help combat osteopenia, and encourage co-contraction of the stabilizing musculature (22). This is an essential and often overlooked part of the rehabilitation program.

Specialized Techniques

Early treatment with intra-articular corticosteroid (23–25) injection may provide a chemical ablation of the synovitis, thus decreasing pain, limiting the development of fibroplasia, and shortening the natural history of the disease (5). Hazelman reported that the success of the treatment with injection is dependent on the duration of symptoms (26); therefore, it is critical to determine the presenting stage. Fluoroscopic or ultrasound guidance is often recommended to ensure accuracy of an intra-articular glenohumeral joint (GHJ) injection.

Hydrotherapy can be utilized for its buoyancy and hydrostatic pressure properties (27). This can often help patients tolerate increased activity and motion when pain and fear of movement are limiting factors to progress.

There is no evidence to support taping for adhesive capsulitis; however, it can be utilized to inhibit or facilitate muscles and provide tactile/postural feedback (28).

Home Exercise Program

A home program should be included in the management of adhesive capsulitis. ROM exercises and flexibility exercises within the shoulder's tolerance are initiated

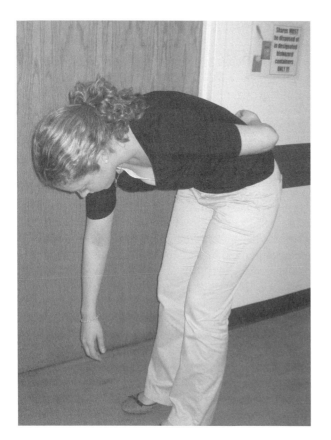

FIGURE 12.1: Pendulum exercises.

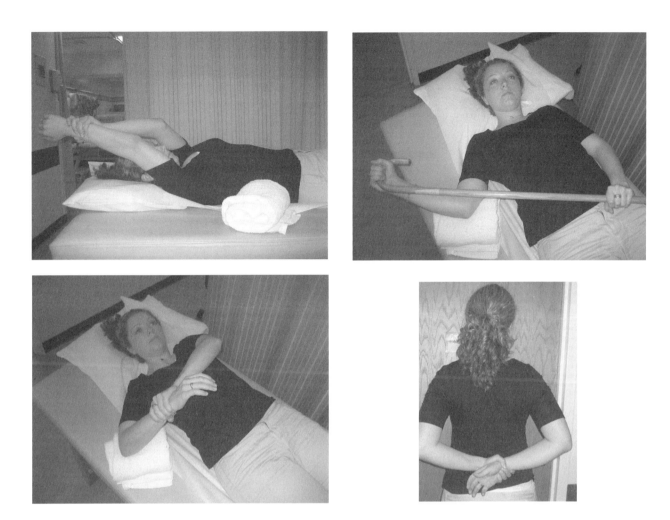

FIGURE 12.2: Adhesive capsulitis home exercise program. A). Active assisted shoulder flexion. B). Active assisted external rotation with cane. C). Active assisted internal rotation. D). Active assisted internal rotation, adduction in standing position.

immediately, and periscapular strengthening exercises are introduced in a pain-free arc of movement. The ROM exercises (Figure 12.2) prescribed as a home exercise program will support the gains made in their supervised physical therapy sessions. It is also important that the individual understands the role of modalities and upper limb positioning, as well as how to use the arm during daily activities to maintain ROM gains and how to modify activity so as not to flare the shoulder.

SUMMARY

Adhesive capsulitis occurs more commonly in females in their fifth and sixth decades of life. It progresses through four stages, from an insidious onset of pain to shoulder stiffness and ultimate resolution within 24 months, if left untreated. Recognition of the stage of adhesive capsulitis at the time of presentation is critical for successful intervention. Early treatment, in the form of an intra-articular steroid injection, has been shown to halt the progression in stage I and to decrease pain in these early stages. ROM exercises in varying dosages will be prescribed in all stages. In the early stages, pain and inflammation will be addressed, whereas in the later stages soft tissue balance will be the focus. Regardless of the stage of presentation, the goal of treatment is to optimize the patient's function.

SAMPLE CASE

A 51-year-old female was referred to physical therapy with the diagnosis of rule out right shoulder adhesive capsulitis. She reported a dull ache in her dominant right shoulder for 2 months. The patient reported pain which she described as an ache at night which disturbed sleep, a sudden sharper pain when reaching into the back seat of her car, and trouble reaching behind her back for dressing and hygiene. Her pain is 3/10 at rest and increases to 6/10 with aforementioned ADLs. Physical examination reveals normal cervical ROM without pain or radicular symptoms. She has tenderness to palpation over the anterior shoulder and long head of the biceps. ROM assessment in the PoS is significant for an empty end feel during PROM 150° elevation; 70° ER; IR 60°, and AROM IR to T10 spine level. She presents with pain and increased scapula elevation in the 80° to 130° arc of elevation. Manual muscle testing reveals 4+/5 strength but mild pain with ER at side and empty can. A positive impingement sign is noted. X-rays are negative.

 ## SAMPLE THERAPY PRESCRIPTION

Discipline: Physical therapy.

Diagnosis: Right shoulder pain and reduced ROM, suspect adhesive capsulitis.

Precautions: Closely monitor ER ROM; avoid painful ROM exercises, painful strengthening. Monitor irritability of the shoulder.

Frequency of visits: 1 to 2x/ week.

Duration of treatment: 6 weeks or 10 to 12 visits to be used over duration of the therapist discretion

Treatment:

1. *Modalities, prn:* moist heat, TENS, cryotherapy

2. *Manual therapy:* ROM exercises, joint mobilizations, soft tissue release, prn

3. *Therapeutic exercise:* AA/PROM exercises for ER, IR, and elevation in the PoS. Strengthening of the periscapular muscles to restore S-H Rhythm

4. *Specialized treatments:* Hydrotherapy, if available

5. *Patient education:* Proper positioning, home exercise program, activity modification, sleep positioning

Goals: Decrease pain to intermittent; able to sleep undisturbed with increased awareness of UE positioning; able to raise arm to shoulder height then overhead with normal scapulohumeral rhythm; improve IR for independent dressing; strength and ROM to meet the demands of ADLs.

Reevaluation: Continue to monitor ROM; F/U with referring physician in 6 weeks.

REFERENCES

1. Neviaser RJ, Neviaser TJ. The frozen shoulder diagnosis and management. *Clin Orthop and Rel Res.* 1987;223:59–64.
2. Wolf JM, Green A. Influence of comorbidity of self-assessment instrument scores of patients with idiopathic adhesive capsulitis. *J Bone Joint Surg Am.* 2002;84:1167–1172.
3. Binder AI, Bulgen DY, Hazleman BL, Roberts S. Frozen shoulder: a long-term prospective study. *Ann Rheum Dis.* 1984;43(3):361–364.

4. Hannafin JA, DiCarlo ED, Wickiewicz TL, et al. Adhesive capsulitis: capsular fibroplasia of the glenohumeral joint. *J Shoulder Elbow Surg.* 1994;3(Suppl 5):435.

5. Neviaser AS, Hannafin JA. Adhesive capsulitis: a review of current treatment. *Am J Sports Med.* 2010;38(11):2346–2356.

6. Kelley MJ, McClure PW, Leggin BG. Frozen shoulder: evidence and a proposed model guiding rehabilitation. *J Orthop and Sports Phys Ther.* 2009;39(2):135–148.

7. Rizk TE, Christopher RP, Pinals RS, et al. Adhesive capsulitis (frozen shoulder): a new approach to its management. *Arch Phys Med Rehabil.* 1983;64(1):29–33.

8. Wadsworth CT. Frozen shoulder. *Phys Ther.* 1986;66:1878–1883.

9. Stergioulas A. Low-power laser treatment in patients with frozen shoulder: preliminary results. *Photomed Laser Surg.* 2008;26(2):99–105.

10. Jewell DV, Riddle DL, Thacker LR. Interventions associated with an increased or decreased likelihood of pain reduction and improved function in patients with adhesive capsulitis: a retrospective cohort study. *Phys Ther.* 2009;89:419–429.

11. Owens-Burkhart H: Management of frozen shoulder. In: Donatelli RA, ed. *Physical Therapy of the Shoulder.* New York, NY: Churchill Livingstone; 1991:91–116.

12. Neviaser JS. Adhesive capsulitis and the stiff and painful shoulder. *Orthop Clinics of North Am.* 1980;11(2):327–331.

13. Nicholson GG. The effects of passive joint mobilization on pain and hypomobility associated with adhesive capsulitis of the shoulder. *J Orthop Sports Phys Ther.* 1985;6(4):238–246.

14. Johnson AJ, Godges JJ, Zimmerman GJ, Ounanian LL. The effect of anterior versus posterior glide joint mobilization on external rotation range of motion in patients with shoulder adhesive capsulitis. *J Orthop Sports Phys Ther.* 2007;37(3):88–99.

15. Simons DG, Travell JG, Simons LS. *Travell and Simons' Myofascial Pain and Dysfunction. The Trigger Point Manual. Volume 1. The Upper Body.* 2nd ed. Lippincott, Williams and Wilkins; 1999:96–612.

16. Ozaki J Nakagawa Y, Sakurai G, Tamai S. Recalcitrant chronic adhesive capsulitis of the shoulder. Role of contracture of the coracohumeral ligament and rotator interval in pathogenesis and treatment. *J Bone Joint Surg Am.* 1989;71:1511–1515.

17. Griggs SM, Ahn A, Green A. Idiopathic adhesive capsulitis. A prospective functional outcome study of nonoperative treatment. *J Bone Joint Surg Am.* 2000;82(10):1398–1407.

18. Flowers KR, LaStayo P. Effect of total end range time on improving passive range of motion. *J Hand Ther.* 1994;7(3):150–157.

19. Diercks RL, Stevens M. Gentle thawing of the frozen shoulder: a prospective study of supervised neglect versus intensive physical therapy in seventy-seven patients with frozen shoulder syndrome followed up for two years. *J Shoulder Elbow Surg.* 2004;13(5):499–502.

20. Harryman DT, Sidles JA, Clark JM, McQuade KJ, Gibb TD, Matsen FA. Translation of the humeral head on the glenoid with passive glenohumeral motion. *J Bone Joint Surg Am.* 1990;72(9):1334–1343.

21. Lin JJ, Wu YT, Wang SF, Chen SY. Trapezius muscle imbalance in individuals suffering from frozen shoulder syndrome. *Clin Rheumatol.* 2005;24:569–575.

22. Kibler BW. Shoulder rehabilitation: Principles and practice. *Med Sci Sports Exer.* 1998;30(Suppl):S40–S50.

23. Carette S, Moffet H, Tardif J, et al. Intraarticular corticosteroids, supervised physiotherapy, or a combination of the two in the treatment of adhesive capsulitis of the shoulder. *Arth Rheum.* 2003;48(3):829–838.

24. Van der windt DAWM, Koes BW, Deville W, et al. Effectiveness of corticosteroid injections versus physiotherapy for treatment of painful stiff shoulder in primary care: randomized trial. *Br Med J.* 1998;317:1292–1296.

25. Ryans I, Montgemery A, Galway R, Kernohan WG, McKane R. A randomized controlled trial of intra-articular triamcinoline and/or physiotherapy in shoulder capsulitis. *Rheumatolgy (Oxford).* 2005;44(4):529–535.

26. Hazelman BD. The painful stiff shoulder. *Rheumatol Phys Med.* 1972;11:413–421.

27. Speer KP, Cavanaugh JT, Warren RF, Day L, Wickiewicz TL. A role for hydrotherapy in shoulder rehabilitation. *Am J Sports Med.* 1993;21:850–853.

28. Page P Andre L. Adhesive capsulitis: use the evidence to integrate your interventions. *North AM J of Sports Phys Ther.* 2010;5(4):267–273.

Lateral Epicondylopathy

Gerard A. Malanga, Steve Matta, and Brian Owens

INTRODUCTION

In 1873, Runge termed the condition of "lawn tennis elbow" based on a group of athletes who shared a common type of pain located at the lateral epicondyle (1). Eventually, lawn tennis elbow was shortened to its now more familiar name, tennis elbow. *Tennis elbow* is commonly known as lateral epicondylitis, although the proper term is epicondylosis as histopathological studies have demonstrated that the injured tendon shows no sign of inflammation, but rather angiofibroblastic dysplasia and neovascularization (2). Therefore, lateral epicondylopathy refers to injury of the wrist extensors originating from the lateral epicondyle of the humerus. The primary muscle affected is the extensor carpi radialis brevis, although other wrist extensors may be involved such as the extensor digitorum communis or the extensor carpi radialis longus (3). It affects about 1% to 3% of the general population (4,5) (Figure 13.1). Normally, there is a history of repetitive wrist extension, such as from the backhand motion in tennis or from occupational use like working on cars, cutting meat, or plumbing. Patients suffering from lateral epicondylosis often report symptoms of pain at the lateral epicondyle with activities related to wrist extension, pronation, and/or grasping objects.

Key elements of the physical examination include inspection, palpation, neurovascular exam, and assessment of pain with range of motion (ROM) and strength testing. This begins with inspection for soft tissue swelling followed by wrist ROM which should be performed with the elbow in full extension and assessment of wrist supination, pronation, flexion, and extension. On palpation of the elbow, there is usually tenderness 1 to 2 cm distal to the lateral epicondyle, near the insertion of the extensor carpi radialis brevis. The presence of pain with resisted wrist extension and resisted third finger extension is suggestive of lateral epicondylosis, although studies have failed to demonstrate the reliability of these tests for diagnosis (6,7). In consideration of other

causes of lateral elbow pain, the clinician should screen the cervical spine for referred pain from the C6-C7 nerve root. Radial capitellar joint arthritis and radial nerve entrapment are also included in the differential diagnosis.

If the diagnosis is unclear or pain is refractory to treatment, imaging may provide useful information, but is unnecessary in the majority of cases. X-rays are often normal, with the exception of occasional calcific changes related to chronic tendinopathy (8). Ultrasonography and MRI are better for soft tissue evaluation and may show edema and tendinopathic changes such as thickening and disruption of the normal tendon architecture (9). Ultrasonography provides the added benefit of dynamic evaluation of soft tissues and sonopalpation.

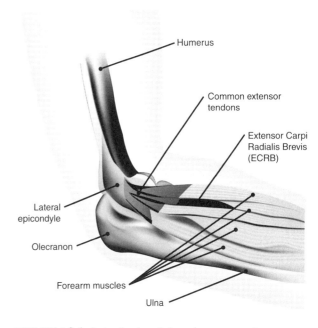

FIGURE 13.1: Lateral epicondyle and common extensor muscles.

LATERAL EPICONDYLOPATHY

- This is a common cause of lateral elbow pain secondary to tendinosis and/or partial tears of the wrist extensors, most often the extensor carpi radialis brevis

- Individuals with a history of overuse of the wrist extensors such as athletes and laborers are at increased risk for lateral epicondylopathy

- Key elements of the physical examination include inspection, palpation, and assessment of ROM. The presence of local tenderness 1 to 2 cm distal to the lateral epicondyle and pain with resisted wrist extension and resisted long finger extension is highly indicative of the lateral epicondylopathy

- Imaging is not necessary in the majority of cases although ultrasonography can be very helpful in delineating the tendinotic region and any associated enthesophytes or tears

THE REHABILITATION PROGRAM

The rehabilitation of lateral epicondylosis can sometimes be a difficult and frustrating process. The key to proper rehabilitation is a step-wise approach beginning with obtaining and performing a proper history and physical examination. When gathering historical information, the provider should inquire about activities which illicit pain whether they are occupational, recreational, or environmental, since the first step in rehabilitation is to avoid any aggravating activities. If the patient is in the acute phase, then ice may be applied to the area for 15 to 20 minutes 3 to 4 times daily. Anti-inflammatory medications have historically been recommended but recent evidence raises concerns regarding their use both in terms of inhibiting tendon healing as well as the potential secondary issues on the gastrointestinal and cardiovascular systems. Recent nutrition reviews have suggested that increased omega-3 consumption via diet or nutritional supplements to increase the ratio of omega-3 to omega-6 may have a natural anti-inflammatory effect (10), without the negative effects on tendon healing, gastrointestinal, or cardiovascular systems. Patients should also be guided in simple

ROM exercises. A counterforce brace, also known as a tennis elbow brace, can also be prescribed and applied to the proximal forearm. This may decrease the tension of the common wrist extensors and decrease pain during daily activities and sports (11). Following this phase, if the patient continues to have pain, they should be directed to a more formal rehabilitation program under the supervision of an allied health care professional (physical or occupational therapist, athletic trainer).

Therapeutic Modalities

The purpose of therapeutic modalities for the treatment of lateral epicondylosis should be for the comfort of the patient as they are undergoing rehabilitation and should not be used as a substitute for a therapeutic exercise program. Ice may be employed in the initial phase of treatment and may also be applied after the completion of workouts. Heat has been used but provides no additional benefit beyond patient comfort. Iontophoresis with the use of cortisone is sometimes used for treatment, but studies have not shown it to be more effective than placebo (12). Phonophoresis and iontophoresis with topical naproxen have also been investigated. They showed similar short-term benefit; however, there was no placebo control making it difficult to draw any conclusions from this study (13).

Extracorporeal shock wave therapy (ESWT), commonly used to treat achilles tendinopathy and other tendinopathies, has been investigated but failed to demonstrate successful outcomes. In fact, research suggests poor outcomes with ESWT and the recommendation is against its use for lateral epicondylopathy (14,15).

Manual Therapy

The role of manual therapy in the management of lateral elbow pain can be useful, but few techniques have been reported in high quality studies. While further research is needed to identify the most appropriate application of several reported techniques, contributing authors have achieved greater success with an eclectic approach versus the utilization of one particular procedure.

Manual therapy may be utilized to target joint structure and mobility, which may also influence response of the muscle tissue surrounding the joint. During the initial stages of rehabilitation, joint mobilization efforts may be useful to address pain and ROM deficits. Mobilization techniques may also improve joint tissue extensibility, joint proprioception, and joint nutrition. Many manual therapy techniques exist and include low and high grade joint mobilization, soft tissue mobilization and massage, muscle energy techniques, and myofascial release.

Thrust mobilization or manipulation of the elbow joint and wrist complex, cervical spine, and ribs has been reported in previous studies (16,17). While several manipulation techniques have been reported for the treatment of tennis elbow, Mill's manipulation has been identified with the greater potential to stretch the affected tendon with the least potential to harm the joint (18). Several low-level studies have found Mulligan's mobilization with movement to result in an immediate increase in pain free grip force (19,20). Postulated mechanisms of pain relief include restoration of bony positional faults at the elbow complex, changes in local neural receptors in surrounding soft tissue, and central control mechanisms (21,22). Additional manual therapy techniques such as soft tissue mobilization and myofascial release may be considered at the elbow complex and surrounding regions in addition to joint mobilization throughout the rehabilitation process. Further high quality studies are needed to identify effective manual therapy techniques to expedite the rehabilitation management of lateral epicondylopathy.

Therapeutic Exercise

A common recommendation in addressing lateral elbow pain following the initial examination includes beginning a home exercise program (HEP) to minimize pain, and muscle atrophy and restore premorbid functional performance. Important initial therapeutic exercises include addressing limitations of elbow, forearm, and wrist ROM. The treating physician should identify gross limitations of ROM and compare ROM of the involved upper limb to the noninvolved upper limb. It is important to restore symmetric flexibility (Figure 13.2) at the involved anatomical site prior to initiating progressive strengthening and functional activities as part of the rehabilitation process. The rehabilitation professional should screen regions proximal and distal to the elbow, such as the cervical and/or thoracic spine, shoulder girdle complex, and wrist. The concept of regional interdependence suggests patient complaints may result from seemingly unrelated impairments at remote anatomical regions

The literature surrounding therapeutic exercise for lateral epicondylopathy supports the implementation of eccentric strengthening as the key part of the program. While previous studies have reported favorable results with eccentric strengthening of various tendinopathies, eccentric training programs have also been implemented in cases of chronic lateral epicondylar tendinopathy (23). Stasinopoulos and colleagues reported supervised and home-based exercise programs consisting of stretching and eccentric exercises were effective in the management of lateral elbow tendinopathy to reduce pain and improve overall level of function (24). Tyler et al investigated eccentric training for chronic lateral epicondylosis in a prospective, randomized trial. They reported significant improvement with the addition of an eccentric wrist extensor exercise program to standard physical therapy for certain dependent variables such as the disabilities of

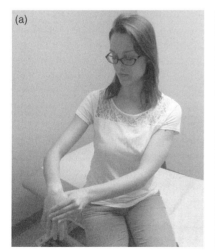 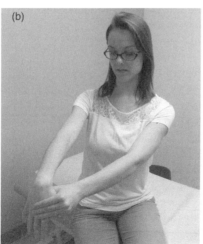

FIGURE 13.2: Forearm extensor mass stretching.

The patient begins with the involved upper limb in front of the body. Instruct the patient to perform wrist flexion at the involved upper limb and provide gentle overpressure with the contralateral hand. Maximum stretch occurs when the wrist is flexed and the elbow extended. The patient should experience mild discomfort, but no pain. Hold stretches for 30 seconds, perform 4 to 6 repetitions and perform them 1 to 2 times daily.

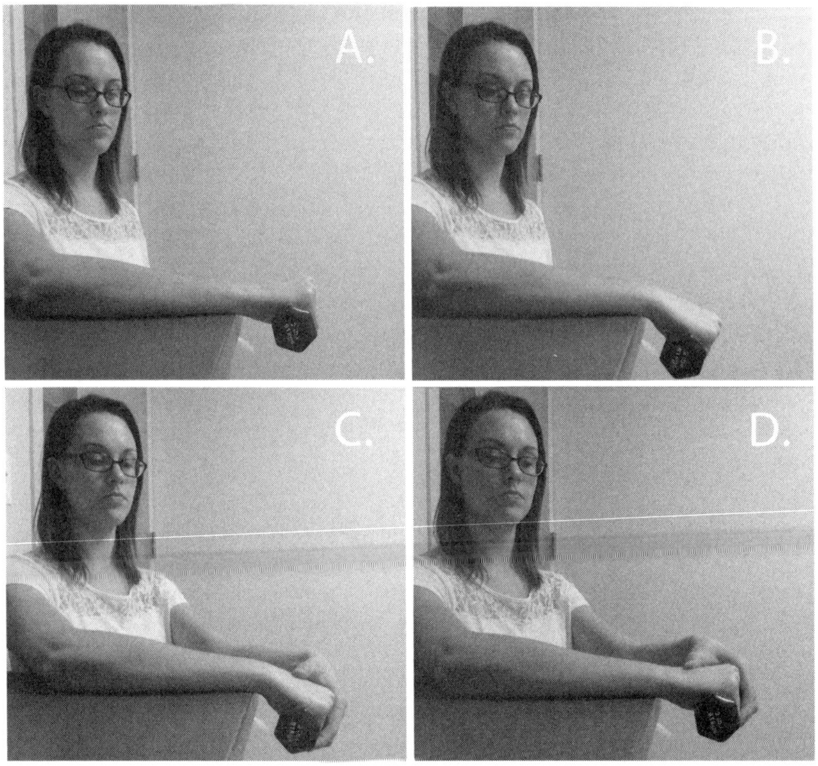

FIGURE 13.3: Wrist extensor eccentric exercise with hand weight.

The patient begins with the arms resting on a table, wrist and hand holding a hand weight off the end of the table. Begin with the elbow and wrist fully extended while holding a hand weight. Instruct the patient to slowly lower the involved wrist into flexion while holding the hand weight. Then use the uninvolved hand to move the hand weight and wrist back into extension (starting position) and repeat by slowly lowering the weight again. Instruct the patient to perform 3 sets of 15 repetitions daily.

arm, shoulder, hand (DASH) Visual Analog Scale (VAS) and for strength; but not a significant difference regarding duration of treatment, duration of symptoms, and number of patient visits (25). The eccentric wrist extensor exercise (Figure 13.3) has been identified as a cost effective supplement to rehabilitation efforts and may be implemented as a valuable component of a HEP (26). From a practical standpoint, many patients are unable to tolerate eccentric training due to pain. As an alternative strengthening exercise, Park and colleagues noted an isometric strengthening program in patients with lateral epicondylosis improved pain and level of function within 4 weeks (27). While prior studies and a recent systematic review reveal that resistance exercise, most commonly eccentric exercise, results in substantial improvement in pain and grip strength for those with lateral epicondylosis, optimal dosing for resistance exercise is still yet to be defined (28) (Figure 13.4).

Initial studies examining eccentric strengthening for tendinopathies advocated performing exercises without pain (23) and others have reported successful eccentric training strategies while training to pain in Achilles tendinopathy (29). However, no known studies to date have investigated strengthening to pain in patients with lateral epicondylopathy. As an explanation to this treatment's effectiveness, authors have noted that eccentric

strengthening, as part of a treatment regimen for Achilles tendinopathy, may produce favorable results secondary to decreased neovascularization and paratendon capillary blood flow (29,30).

In addition to addressing strength and ROM deficits about the elbow, a comprehensive rehabilitation program will include all aspects of the kinetic chain. The initial screen includes evaluation of the entire shoulder girdle complex, scapular motion, cervical and thoracic spine alignment and mobility, and core strength. After dysfunction is identified, the patient should be instructed in the necessary exercises to correct those dysfunctions. After completing their rehabilitation program, the patient should be familiar with exercises involving not only their wrist and forearm, but also their rotator cuff, scapular stabilizers, and core.

Overall, our current recommendation is for the patient to begin with wrist/forearm ROM exercises, gentle isometrics, and eventually pain-free eccentric strengthening exercises to improve patient compliance (Figure 13.5). Initial goals include improving ROM, flexibility and strengthening muscles of the elbow/forearm complex without pain, and then to offer a comprehensive therapeutic program; the kinetic chain should be evaluated and addressed.

Specialized Techniques

The initial conservative management of lateral epicondylosis should consist of decreasing activity that aggravates elbow pain, and ice and analgesics for pain control, with the emphasis of stretching and strengthening of the wrist extensors (e.g., eccentric strengthening exercises), which is the most important aspect of a treatment regimen.

The use of injection techniques, and most commonly corticosteroid injections, for lateral epicondylosis is a common but a controversial practice among clinicians. Historically, it was theorized that tendonitis was an inflammatory condition and that the use of corticosteroids would stop the inflammatory process and aid in the healing of tendon. Nirshl et al studied histologic specimens of tendons from individuals suffering from lateral epicondylopathy and found angiofibroblastic dysplasia rather than inflammatory mediators within the tendon (2). In addition, studies comparing corticosteroids to physical therapy and a "wait and see" approach have shown that, although corticosteroids aid in pain relief for the first 6 weeks following the injection, patients report worse pain at 12 months compared to physical therapy or the "wait and see" approach (31).

Platelet-rich plasma injections have recently been used in refractory lateral tendinopathy with excellent results (32). Ultrasound-guided percutaneous needle tenotomy has also demonstrated very promising results. In this method, tendinotic tissue is first identified by ultrasound followed by ultrasound guided needle fenestration of the tissue and breaking up of any calcifications. In one study, 63.6% of patients suffering from lateral epicondylopathy had excellent outcomes following the procedure, and additional studies have verified its effectiveness (33–35).

Supportive Devices

Patients commonly utilize and healthcare professionals commonly recommend forearm straps, also known as counterforce braces or wrist splints to conservatively manage lateral elbow pain. Wrist splints complement the PRICE protocol and allow the involved tendons, the common extensors, to rest during the initial phases of rehabilitation. A recent prospective, randomized study concluded that wrist extension splints allow a greater degree of pain relief than forearm straps for patients with lateral epicondylitis (36). However, a multicenter, prospective cohort study revealed that workers with epicondylitis treated with wrist splints, many for prolonged periods of time, had more medical visits and required a longer duration of treatment than those managed without splints (37). Therefore, wrist splints may be best utilized as a short-term option for symptomatic management. As another option, counterforce braces or forearm straps are preferred by some patients and therapists. They provide a comfortable alternative to

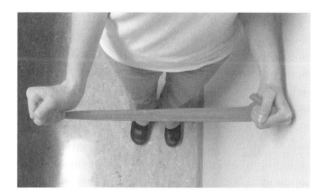

FIGURE 13.4: Wrist extensor eccentric exercise with resistance band.

The patient begins with the involved elbow bent to 90°, wrist fully extended while holding a resistive exercise band. Instruct the patient to pull the opposite end of the resistive band with the noninvolved hand, maintaining wrist position with the involved upper limb. Slowly release the involved wrist into flexion. Remove tension from band and repeat. Instruct the patient to perform 3 sets of 10 to 15 repetitions daily.

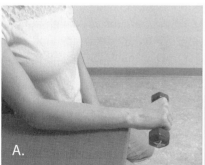 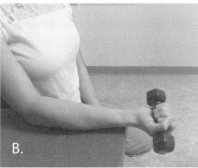

FIGURE 13.5: Wrist supination—resisted ROM.

The patient begins with the involved upper limb supported, wrist in neutral to pronated position while holding a hand weight or dumbbell. Instruct the patient to rotate the palm up or perform forearm supination, without pain and then return to the starting position. Perform 3 sets, 10 to 15 repetitions and perform at least daily.

the wrist splint that doesn't interfere with manual tasks. Prior research supports their use for symptom management and to complement the therapy program, but they should not be used in place of a good therapeutic exercise program (38,39).

Home Exercise Program

A HEP should begin with any initial treatment. The goal of the HEP for lateral epicondylopathy is to educate the patient not only on the right exercises to engage in while treating their condition, but also to encourage them to maintain the necessary strength and ROM to prevent recurrent episodes of pain.

The initial HEP should focus on active range of motion (AROM) and passive range of motion (PROM) exercises while the patient is avoiding aggravating activities. During this phase, the patient should be instructed to avoid exercises or activities that will place additional load on the tendons involved. Passive stretching may be accomplished by instructing the patient to apply pressure to the dorsum of their hand to gently flex their wrist while feeling the stretch at their lateral epicondyle. Initially, this should be done with some elbow flexion progressing toward full extension at completion for the maximum passive stretch on the tissue. Once the patient's pain is improved, they may gradually begin a strengthening program, ultimately utilizing eccentric exercises to restore normal function and decrease or eliminate pain from their daily activities.

SUMMARY

Lateral epicondylopathy is the most common cause of lateral elbow pain as the result of overuse of the wrist extensors. Although it is often referred to as "tennis elbow," the condition is found in other populations which include manual laborers, chefs, and mechanics to name a few. Patients will often complain of pain at the lateral elbow, worsened with increased loading of the wrist and grasping of objects. Physical examination commonly demonstrates tenderness to palpation just distal to the lateral epicondyle, reproduced with resisted wrist and third finger extension. History and physical examination is normally

all that is needed to make a clinical diagnosis although ultrasonography can be helpful in delineating the location and extent of the tendinopathy and to assess for the presence of associated tears and enthesophyte formation. Treatment should begin with relative rest from aggravating activities, ice and analgesics for pain control, and a counterforce brace to help with daily activities. Stretching exercises should begin with initial treatment, followed by an exercise program that includes strengthening of the wrist extensors, as well as addressing other deficits along the entire kinetic chain. Addressing improper technique, grip size, racket, and other sport-specific issues is essential in all patients but especially high level athletes. Patients whose symptoms have not resolved with rest and a HEP should be directed to an allied health professional for a more comprehensive rehabilitation program. If the patient's symptoms are refractory to these treatments, then more invasive treatment options such as injection based treatments (e.g., needle tenotomy or platelet-rich plasma [PRP] injection) may be considered.

SAMPLE CASE

A 45-year-old male presents with left elbow pain which has been present for 3 months. He has no significant past medical history (PMH), past surgical history (PSH) or current medications. He works as a building superintendent and often must use power tools for his work. He now has pain in his elbow not only when working with tools but also turning doorknobs, shaking someone's hand, and even lifting a coffee mug. Physical examination reveals pain at his lateral elbow worse with active and passive wrist flexion (performed with the elbow in full extension), as well as pain with resisted wrist extension and resisted long finger extension and tenderness to palpation at the lateral epicondyle of the humerus. There is no swelling. Neurovascular examination is unremarkable.

SAMPLE THERAPY PRESCRIPTION

Discipline: Physical therapy.

Diagnosis: Left lateral epicondylopathy.

Precautions: No heavy lifting.

Frequency of visits: 2 to 3x/week.

Duration of treatment: 3 to 4 weeks; or an alternative would be to provide a total of 8 to 12 visits used at the therapist's discretion.

Treatment: *Modalities:* cryotherapy (ice pack, ice massage)

1. *Manual therapy:* low and high grade joint mobilization, muscle energy techniques, and myofascial release

2. *Therapeutic exercise:* A/AA/PROM to restore wrist flexion, supination, stretching (self stretching, therapist assisted stretching) including wrist extensor stretching, progressive resistive exercise (PRE) focusing on *eccentric strengthening* and correcting biomechanical deficiencies in the shoulder girdle complex, cervical and/or thoracic spine, and core musculature

3. *Specialized treatments:* none

4. *Patient education:* HEP, activity modification

Goals: Decrease pain; restore wrist ROM and flexibility then restore strength, improve function, safely return to functional activities (e.g., sport, hobbies, work) and prevent recurrent injury.

Reevaluation: In 4 weeks by referring physician.

REFERENCES

1. Cyriax JH. The pathology and treatment of tennis elbow. *J Bone Joint Surg Am*. 1936;18(4):921–940.
2. Kraushaar BS, Nirschl, RP. Current concepts review—tendinosis of the elbow (tennis elbow). Clinical features and findings of histological, immunohistochemical, and electron microscopy studies. *J Bone Joint Surg Am*. 1999;81(2):259–278.
3. Greenbaum B, Itamura J, Vangsness CT, Tibone J, Atkinson R. Extensor carpi radialis brevis: An anatomical analysis of its origin. *J Bone Joint Surg Br*. 1999;81-B(5):926–929.
4. Practice C, Finestone HM. Practice tips tennis elbow no more. *Canadian Family Physician*. 2008;54:1115–1116.
5. Allander E. Prevalence, incidence, and remission rates of some common rheumatic diseases or syndromes. *Scan J Rheumatol*. 1974;3(3):145–153.
6. Cortazzo MH, DeChellis DM. UPMC rehab grand rounds. *Terminology*. 2011;4(10):16.
7. Malanga GA, Nadler S. *Musculoskeletal Physical Examination: An Evidence-Based Approach*. Philadelphia, PA: Hanley & Belfus; 2006.
8. Pomerance J. Radiographic analysis of lateral epicondylitis. *J Shoulder Elbow Surg*. 2002;11(2):156-157.
9. Walz DM, Newman JS, Konin GP, Ross G. Epicondylitis: pathogenesis, imaging, and treatment. *Radiographics*. 2010;30(1):167.
10. Wall R, Ross RP, Fitzgerald GF, Stanton C. Fatty acids from fish: the anti-inflammatory potential of long-chain omega-3 fatty acid. *Nutrition Reviews*. 2010;68(5):280–289.
11. Johnson GW, Cadwallader K, Scheffel SB, Epperly TD. Treatment of lateral epicondylitis. *American Family Physician*. 2007;76(6):843–848.
12. Runeson L, Haker E. Iontophoresis with cortisone in the treatment of lateral epicondylalgia (tennis elbow): a double-blind study. *Scan J Med Sci Sports J*. 2002;12:136–142.
13. Başkurt F, Ozcan A, Algun C. Comparison of effects of phonophoresis and iontophoresis of naproxen in the treatment of lateral epicondylitis. *Clinical Rehab*. 2003;17(1):96–100.
14. Bisset L, Paungmali A, Vicenzino B, Beller E. A systematic review and meta-analysis of clinical trials on physical interventions for lateral epicondylalgia. *BMJ*. 2005;39(7):411–422.
15. Buchbinder R, Green SE, Youd JM, et al. Systematic review of the efficacy and safety of shock wave therapy for lateral elbow pain. *J Rheumatol*. 2006;33(7):1351–1363.
16. Radpasand M. Combination of manipulation, exercise, and physical therapy for the treatment of a 57-year-old woman with lateral epicondylitis. *J Manipulative Physiol Ther*. 2009;32(2):166–172.
17. Vicenzino B, Cleland JA, Bisset L. Joint manipulation in the management of lateral epicondylalgia: a clinical commentary. *The Journal of Manual & Manipulative Therapy*. 2007;15(1):50–56.
18. Kushner S, Reid DC. Manipulation in the treatment of tennis elbow. *J Orthop Sports Phys Ther*. 1986;7(5):264–272.
19. Vicenzino B, Paungmali A, Buratowski S, Wright A. Specific manipulative therapy treatment for chronic lateral epicondylalgia produces uniquely characteristic hypoalgesia. *Manual Therapy*. 2001;6(4):205–212.
20. Abbott JH, Patla CE, Jensen RH. The initial effects of an elbow mobilization with movement technique on grip strength in subjects with lateral epicondylalgia. *Manual Therapy*. 2001;6(3):163–169.
21. Herd CR, Meserve BB. A systematic review of the effectiveness of manipulative therapy in treating lateral epicondylalgia. *The Journal of Manual & Manipulative Therapy*. 2008;16(4):225–237.
22. Paungmali A, O Leary S, Souvlis T, Vicenzino B. Hypoalgesic and sympathoexcitatory effects of mobilization with movement for lateral epicondylalgia. *Physical Therapy*. 2003;83(4):374–383.
23. Croisier J-L, Foidart-Dessalle M, Tinant F, Crielaard J-M, Forthomme B. An isokinetic eccentric programme for the management of chronic lateral epicondylar tendinopathy. *BMJ*. 2007;41(4):269–275.

24. Stasinopoulos D, Stasinopoulos I, Pantelis M, Stasinopoulou K. Comparison of effects of a home exercise programme and a supervised exercise programme for the management of lateral elbow tendinopathy. *BMJ*. 2010;44(8):579–583.

25. Tyler TF, Thomas GC, Nicholas SJ, McHugh MP. Addition of isolated wrist extensor eccentric exercise to standard treatment for chronic lateral epicondylosis: a prospective randomized trial. *J Shoulder Elbow Surg*. 2010;19(6):917–922.

26. Martinez-Silvestrini JA, Newcomer KL, Gay RE, et al. Chronic lateral epicondylitis: comparative effectiveness of a home exercise program including stretching alone versus stretching supplemented with eccentric or concentric strengthening. *J Hand Ther*. 2005;18(4):411–419, quiz 420.

27. Park J-Y, Park H-K, Choi J-H, et al. Prospective evaluation of the effectiveness of a home-based program of isometric strengthening exercises: 12-month follow-up. *Clin Orthop Surg*. 2010;2(3):173–178.

28. Raman J, Joy C, MacDermid JC, Grewal R. Effectiveness of different methods of resistance exercises in lateral epicondylosis—A systematic review. *J Hand Ther*. Available online Nov 2011.

29. Alfredson H. Chronic midportion Achilles tendinopathy: an update on research and treatment. *Clin Sports Med*. 2003;22(4):727–741.

30. Knobloch K, Kraemer R, Jagodzinski M, et al. Eccentric training decreases paratendon capillary blood flow and preserves paratendon oxygen saturation in chronic achilles tendinopathy. *J Orthop Sports Phys Ther*. 2007;37(5):269–276.

31. Smidt N, Windt DAWM van der, Assendelft WJJ, et al. Corticosteroid injections, physiotherapy, or a wait-and-see policy for lateral epicondylitis: a randomised controlled trial. *Lancet*. 2002;359(9307):657–662.

32. Mishra A, Pavelko T. Treatment of chronic elbow tendinosis with buffered platelet-rich plasma. *Am J Sports Med*. 2006;34(11):1774–1778.

33. McShane JM, Nazarian LN, Harwood MI. Sonographically guided percutaneous needle tenotomy for treatment of common extensor tendinosis in the elbow. *J Ultrasound Med*. 2006;25(10):1281–1289.

34. McShane JM, Shah VN, Nazarian LN. Sonographically guided percutaneous needle tenotomy for treatment of common extensor tendinosis in the elbow: is a corticosteroid necessary? *J Ultrasound Med*. 2008;27(8):1137–1144.

35. Housner JA, Jacobson JA, Misko R. Sonographically guided percutaneous needle tenotomy for the treatment of chronic tendinosis. *J Ultrasound Med*. 2009;28(9):1187–1192.

36. Garg R, Adamson GJ, Dawson PA, Shankwiler JA, Pink MM. A prospective randomized study comparing a forearm strap brace versus a wrist splint for the treatment of lateral epicondylitis. *J Shoulder Elbow Surg*. 2010;19(4):508–512.

37. Derebery V, Devenport J, Giang G, Fogarty W. The effects of splinting on outcomes for epicondylitis. *Arch Phys Med Rehabil*. 2005; 86:1081-1088.

38. Solveborn SA. Radial epicondylalgia ('tennis elbow'): treatment with stretching or forearm band: a prospective study with long-term follow-up including range-of-motion measurements. *Scan J Med Sci Sports*. 1997;7:229–237.

39. Clements LG, Chow S. Effectiveness of a custom-made below elbow lateral counterforce splint in the treatment of lateral epicondylitis (tennis elbow). *Can J Occup Ther*. 1993;60:137–144.

Medial Epicondylopathy

Eric Wisotzky, Anna-Christina Bevelaqua, Daniel Tufaro, and Jennifer L. Solomon

INTRODUCTION

Epicondylitis is among the most common disorders affecting the upper limb and can occur both laterally and medially. Medial epicondylitis, often referred to as *golfer's elbow*, is characterized by pathologic changes to the musculotendinous origin of the common flexor tendon and pronator teres at the medial epicondyle (1). The pronator teres and the flexor carpi radialis both attach to the anterior aspect of the medial epicondyle, the supracondylar ridge, and are most commonly involved in medial epicondylitis (Figure 14.1) (2). At one time, epicondylitis was thought to be solely an inflammatory process; however it is now believed to represent a degenerative process caused by repetitive stress and overuse leading to tendinosis (making medial epicondylosis more accurate terminology.) (1,2). Studies have shown that while the initial phase of epicondylitis may display characteristics of generalized inflammation, later stages of injury demonstrate tendon degeneration and microtearing with fibrotic changes and occasionally calcifications (1). These tendon changes may ultimately lead to altered biomechanics at the elbow.

Lateral epicondylitis occurs seven to ten times more frequently than medial epicondylitis (3). Medial epicondylitis typically presents insidiously with pain along the medial elbow, but may also occur with acute trauma. Pain is exacerbated with resisted wrist flexion and forearm pronation (4). Patients may have a history of participating in sports activities as stated above (3). Studies have estimated the prevalence of medial epicondylitis to range between 0.2% and 5.0% (5). It is seen most frequently between the ages of 45 and 54 and occurs equally in men and women (6). It occurs more commonly in the dominant hand (6). Although medial epicondylitis is often called "golfer's elbow," it is often seen in those who participate in a variety of sports including tennis, football, racquetball, bowling, weight lifting, and other throwing sports. It has also been associated with occupations that require repetitive forceful forearm pronation and wrist flexion, such as carpenters (7). One study showed an association between smoking and medial epicondylitis (5). Another study demonstrated an increased prevalence of medial epicondylitis in patients with C6 and C7 radiculopathies (8).

In throwing athletes, studies of biomechanics of the medial elbow have shown that there are intense valgus forces on the medial elbow during the acceleration phase of throwing (1,2). These forces are transmitted to

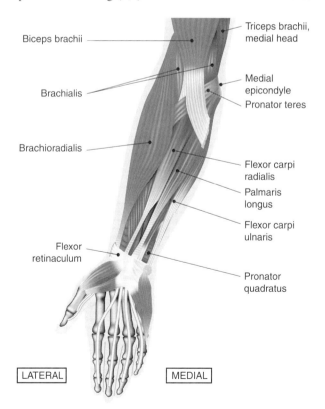

FIGURE 14.1: Medical epicondyle with flexor-pronator muscles.

the flexor-pronator muscle group and then to the deeper medial structures, such as the ulnar collateral ligament (Figure 14.1). When these forces are large, they may exceed the strength of the muscles, tendons, and ligaments of the medial elbow and lead to degenerative changes. This valgus stress can also be seen in the acceleration phase of the tennis serve and in golf when the club is swung from the peak of the backswing downward behind the ball (1–3). One study looking at muscle activity in both professional and amateur golfers found that amateur golfers had more muscle activity in the pronator teres in the *trail arm* in the forward swing phase and the acceleration phase. In contrast, the professional golfers had increased pronator teres muscle activity in the *lead arm* in the acceleration phase and in the early follow through phase (9). It is speculated that the increased activity in the trail arm in amateur golfers may lead to medial epicondylitis.

Key elements of the physical examination include inspection, palpation, range of motion (ROM), manual muscle testing, neurovascular examination, and key special tests. Inspection may demonstrate swelling at the medial epicondyle. Palpation may reveal tenderness 5 to 10 mm anterior and distal to the medial epicondyle, over the pronator teres and flexor carpi radialis (1,3). There is typically normal strength and ROM (10). If a concomitant ulnar neuropathy (also commonly seen in throwing athletes) exists, there may be diminished sensation in an ulnar distribution (2). It is important to also check for medial collateral ligament instability which may occur with medial epicondylitis, especially in throwing athletes secondary to increased valgus forces (1,3). Ulnar collateral ligament instability can be assessed by placing a valgus stress on the elbow (1), usually with the elbow flexed 20 to 30°. Tinel's sign over the ulnar nerve in the region of the retroepicondylar (ulnar) groove should also be checked to rule out the presence of ulnar neuropathy at the elbow. Elbow pain may be reproduced by resisted wrist flexion, sometimes called the "Reversed Cozen's" test.

Initially, imaging is not necessary. Elbow radiographs are most often normal; however, there may be medial collateral ligament calcifications and medial traction spurs seen especially in throwing athletes (2,3,11). In refractory cases or when there is medial instability, MRI imaging may be useful to evaluate the medial collateral ligament. MRI findings in medial epicondylitis include increased signal in the common flexor tendon and soft tissue edema around the common flexor tendon (11). Ultrasonography may also be useful to look for tendinopathy, ligamentous injury, or edema. It also allows for dynamic imaging assessment (12).

MEDIAL EPICONDYLITIS

▪ This condition is much less common than lateral epicondylitis

▪ Mechanism of injury includes repetitive valgus stress on the medial epicondyle

▪ Commonly involves the pronator teres and flexor carpi radialis tendons

▪ Commonly referred to as *golfer's elbow*, although it is often seen in overhead throwing sports, racquet sports, or in occupations requiring repetitive forearm pronation and wrist flexion

▪ Presents with tenderness to palpation over the common flexor tendon mass and pain is reproduced with resisted wrist flexion

▪ Initially a clinical diagnosis is sufficient, but MRI and ultrasound imaging may be useful in refractory cases and to evaluate for concomitant joint, ligamentous, or even nerve injury

THE REHABILITATION PROGRAM

Conservative care of medial epicondylosis begins once the clinical diagnosis is made. The initial phase of rehabilitation requires activity modification, including the avoidance of provocative postures and activities. Therapeutic modalities are often utilized during the initial phase to reduce inflammatory pain. Once pain and swelling, if present, is controlled, gentle ROM and stretching exercises may begin in phase II. The most important phase of rehabilitation in the management of chronic tendinopathies appears to be phase III, and should include eccentric strengthening exercises. The comprehensive rehabilitation program will be discussed in further detail in the remainder of this chapter.

Therapeutic Modalities

In the acute stage, the application of ice to the affected elbow may have local vasoconstrictive and analgesic effects (13). Blood flow studies have shown the application of ice to cause skin vasoconstriction with an increase in skin blood flow following removal of the ice as a physiologic reflex to protect tissue from ice damage (14). Studies have shown that ice should be applied to the skin in increments of 10 to 20 minutes at a time for maximum benefit (14). One study showed that intermittent application of ice for 10 minutes on and 10 minutes off the skin maximized pain relief after acute soft tissue injury (15). Over-icing may lead to a temporary ulnar neurapraxia (16).

Ultrasound has been used to treat a variety of musculoskeletal disorders. It has both thermal and nonthermal mechanical effects on tissue. It is thought to cause an increase in local metabolism, circulation, and tissue regeneration, leading to a decrease in pain and improved functional ROM (17,18). Despite the use of ultrasound clinically, a review of literature shows little evidence to support its effectiveness for soft tissue injuries (19). A study of low intensity ultrasound therapy for lateral epicondylitis showed no significant reduction in pain when compared to placebo (20).

There have been limited studies on the use of iontophoresis with topical dexamethasone to treat epicondylitis. One randomized controlled study showed a mild reduction in pain with the use of iontophoresis with dexamethasone, which was not statistically significant and no long-term benefit was shown (21). A study comparing iontophoresis with naproxen and phonophoresis with naproxen showed no significant difference between the two groups (22). Therefore, cryotherapy provides symptomatic relief of pain and is reasonable to utilize but other traditional modalities (e.g., ultrasound, iontophoresis) show no additional benefit and should not take time away from better supported treatment techniques, such as therapeutic exercise.

Less traditional modalities such as low level laser therapy (LLLT) and extracorporeal shock wave therapy (ESWT) have also been investigated. Low-level laser therapy has also been studied as a treatment modality for medial and lateral epicondylitis. Low-level laser therapy has been used to treat a variety of musculoskeletal conditions, although the exact mechanism of action has not been elucidated. It is believed the treatment may increase the pain threshold, increase levels of serotonin, increase local circulation and lymphatic flow, and decrease inflammatory agents (23). There is limited evidence that LLLT is effective in reducing pain and increasing functional ability in patients with medial epicondylitis (23,24).

ESWT has been used for the treatment of a variety of soft tissue injuries, including plantar fasciitis and tendinopathy. ESWT is thought to provide analgesia by hyperstimulating the area to painful levels, thereby provoking inhibitory pathways descending from the brainstem through the spinal cord to relieve pain. Studies have not shown it to be significantly better than placebo in medial epicondylitis (25–27).

Manual Therapy

The objective of these therapeutic techniques is to relieve pain and to stimulate healing of soft tissues surrounding the medial epicondyle. Transverse or deep friction massage can be used in theory to improve blood flow, prevent the formation of scar tissue, and to stimulate collagen production with proper alignment in the damaged tissue. Deep friction massage is not recommended for patients who are still in the acute phase as it can be poorly tolerated (28). Joint mobilizations or manipulations of the elbow, proximal or distal radio-ulnar joint may be beneficial to address specific motion restrictions. Overall, these manual therapy techniques require additional investigation and currently should be viewed as unproven but potentially beneficial under certain circumstances.

Therapeutic Exercise

Most of the degenerative changes in medial epicondylitis occur in soft tissues of the palmaris longus, flexor carpi radialis, and the pronator teres (28). Although the following exercises can be generalized to other muscles within the forearm, most discussions of medial epicondylitis revolve around these three muscles, commonly referred to as the flexor-pronator mass. Therapeutic intervention for this condition follows the same phases of rehabilitation discussed throughout this book.

Phase I is comprised of pain relief and activity modification. Conservative management of medial epicondylitis typically includes protection, relative rest, ice, and avoiding tasks that provoke discomfort at the elbow. Clinicians also need to modify their patient's daily activities if these tasks provoke symptoms. Patient education on proper body mechanics during everyday tasks and leisure-related activities is imperative. For example, instead of carrying grocery bags with the hand, patients may want to loop the bag around a pronated forearm and carry the bag close to their side. When the forearm is supinated, the pronator teres and the flexor carpi radialis may act as elbow flexors, exacerbating the patient's pain. Thus keeping the forearm pronated will put these muscles on slack and less active. These remedies can be used as an early intervention, especially for less severe injuries, and activity modification is arguably the most important aspect of the initial phase of rehabilitation.

After the pain is well controlled, phase II is initiated and includes stretching the involved musculature and ROM exercises. Stretching of the wrist flexors is performed by gently moving the wrist into extension (Figure 14.2). The elbow should be in a flexed position with the forearm pronated initially to minimize pain. The exercises can then be performed with the elbow extended and the forearm supinated, as tolerated by the patient. The wrist flexors should be gradually stretched in the following sequence of positions, from gentle to full stretch of the flexor-pronator mass:

1. Elbow flexed and forearm pronated

2. Elbow flexed and forearm supinated

3. Elbow extended and forearm pronated

4. Elbow extended and forearm supinated

Each stretch should be held for at least 15 seconds (29). The stretches can first be performed actively by the patient, and then passively by the therapist.

With pain under control and ROM and flexibility improved, the strengthening phase (phase III) can now be initiated. Initially, pain-free, isometric exercises with gentle wrist, forearm, and elbow ROM are performed. Again, the elbow should be flexed during the early stages and progressed toward extension as the patient improves. If discomfort does not occur, the patient can perform progressive resistive exercises (PREs) starting with light-weight concentric contractions, then progressing to eccentric exercises (30).

Continuous observation and monitoring of symptoms during the initial three phases of rehabilitation is important. If pain resumes, regression to the previous phase is recommended until symptoms again dissipate. Farber and colleagues discussed the clinical relevance and importance of exercise in golfers with medial epicondylitis. They emphasize stretching and strengthening of the pronator teres, specifically for athletes, to rehabilitate or prevent recurrences of this condition (9).

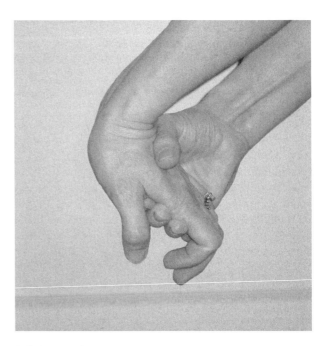

FIGURE 14.2: Wrist flexor stretch.

During the final two phases of rehabilitation, kinetic chain analysis of the upper and lower limbs, specifically joints above and below the elbow (e.g., shoulder girdle, wrist, and hand) should occur to assess for contributing biomechanical deficits. Deficits in ROM or strength in one or more upper limb joints or muscles can lead to improper loads at the elbow, leading to medial epicondylitis, especially if sports participation (e.g., swimming, golf, or overhead sports) was believed to be the inciting event. In throwing sports and golf, evaluation of hip ROM is important to include in the kinetic chain analysis. Strengthening of proximal upper limb muscles, such as the scapular stabilizers or the rotator cuff, can and should occur at this time, as long as this does not exacerbate elbow pain. A therapeutic program should set out to obtain greater than preinjury strength and flexibility, because preinjury conditions were not suitable to prevent tissue damage.

Supportive Devices

During the initiation of conservative management of medial epicondylitis, the most common type of splint provided is a wrist support, or wrist splint. An occupational or physical therapist will usually provide this customized or prefabricated volar splint with the wrist positioned in neutral to 15 degrees of flexion to offer adequate wrist support (29). Although commonly worn at night, this type of splint can also be worn during the day, as it allows the patients to grossly function through active use of their digits. The clinical benefits of these splints remains under review, however they are widely used to allow for rest and healing of the flexor and pronator musculature (28,30). In some more severe cases, a therapist can fabricate a thermoplastic splint to maintain complete immobility at the forearm and elbow. A sugar-tong splint can position the patient's wrist in neutral or a slightly flexed position (Figure 14.3). Each patient requires an individualized approach when prescribing supportive devices or fabricating splints as patient compliance can be poor if factors unique to each individual are not considered (31).

An elbow counterforce brace (or golfer's elbow band) may be applied over the proximal forearm. The brace is placed approximately 10 cm distal to the elbow joint over the muscle bellies of the flexor group on the anterior forearm (30) (Figure 14.4). It acts as a new origin point for the flexor musculature. The counterforce brace may decrease contraction forces of the flexor-pronator muscles on the medial epicondyle (32). Studies using electromyography (EMG) analysis have demonstrated decreased muscle activity while wearing a counterforce brace (33). Snyder-Mackler and colleagues showed that there was significantly less muscle activity at the elbow proximally with placement of a counterforce brace (34). These braces also allow the soft tissue at the medial epicondyle to rest. It should not interfere with the elbow's ability to perform its normal or full active ROM. The braces can be used for therapeutic and preventative purposes. These types of counterforce braces may offer the greatest relief during the first 6 weeks following initial injury (30). One precaution is that with enough pressure from the brace, it is possible to compress the anterior interosseous nerve, which has previously been reported (35).

Specialized Techniques

Elbow taping may also be useful and has been shown to increase pain-free grip strength in lateral epicondylitis (Figure 14.5). It may also be useful in medial epicondylitis (32). A small study comparing taping and counterforce bracing in patients with lateral epicondylitis showed taping to be more effective at relieving pain than

counterforce bracing, but there was no significant difference in grip strength among the two groups (33). The disadvantage of taping is that it must be reapplied by a trained professional.

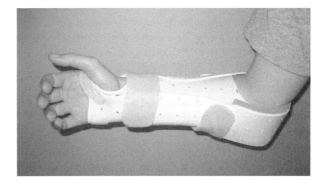

FIGURE 14.3: Sugar-tong splint.

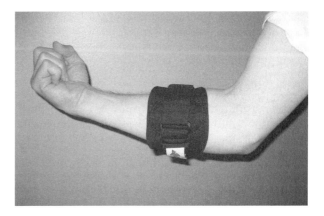

FIGURE 14.4: Counterforce brace or golfer's elbow band.

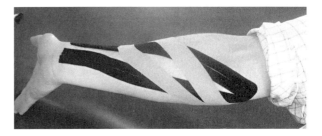

FIGURE 14.5: Kinesiology taping for medial epicondylitis.

Home Exercise Program

Early stages of a home exercise program (HEP) follow the initial phases of the rehabilitation program. Patients are often times instructed to maintain immobility at the elbow while resting the wrist and finger flexors. Splints during functional activities or at rest may be indicated in addition to activity modification. Ice can be used frequently in the acute stage, then only post exercise or during episodes of pain as progress is made. Depending on the patient's initial presentation, early stretches should be performed with the elbow in a flexed and pronated position and progress toward elbow extension with a supinated forearm. When pain has subsided or is under control, strengthening exercises are instituted following the same elbow and forearm positions as above. Initially isometric exercises are performed, followed by concentric and eventually an eccentric strengthening program. It is important for patients to also focus on strengthening other proximal upper limb muscles, such as the deltoids, rotator cuff, and periscapular muscles, which may have been identified as a contributing factor to the development of medial epicondylitis. In order to prevent this condition from recurring, if the mechanism of injury is sports related, patients can be recommended to see a sport specific coach or instructor for evaluation of their body mechanics and technique.

SUMMARY

Medial epicondylitis is significantly less common than lateral epicondylitis, but can be seen in golfers, overhead throwing athletes, and people with specific occupations that require forceful and/or repetitive activities. Rehabilitation should focus on activity modification and relative rest to decrease pain, followed by stretching, and then progressive strengthening exercises. Ice is effective for initial pain control, but evidence is weak for the use of other therapeutic modalities or manual therapy techniques. There is some literature to support the use of counterforce bracing and elbow taping. Counterforce bracing and taping can continue to be used as a preventative measure in patients with recurrent symptoms. Functional restoration and return to sport should be addressed in the final phase of rehabilitation.

SAMPLE CASE

A 55-year-old diabetic, right-hand dominant male reports several months of worsening right medial elbow pain. He recently retired and has begun golfing 2 to 3 times per week. Review of systems is unremarkable and he denies any significant prior musculoskeletal injuries. Physical examination reveals tenderness of the flexor-pronator mass at the medial elbow. Symptoms are reproduced by resisted wrist flexion. X-rays of the elbow are unremarkable.

 ### SAMPLE THERAPY PRESCRIPTION

Discipline: Occupational therapy

Diagnosis: Right medial epicondylitis/wrist flexor tendinopathy

Precautions: Diabetic—use caution with heat/ice

Frequency of visits: 2 to 3x/week

Duration of treatment: 4 to 6 weeks

Treatment:

1. *Modalities*: cryotherapy (ice pack, ice massage)

2. *Manual therapy:* transverse or deep friction massage to flexor-pronator mass, as needed to restore ROM and flexibility

3. *Therapeutic exercise: active, active assisted, and passive range of motion (*A/AA/PROM) of wrist/elbow, stretching wrist flexors—first with elbow flexed/pronated progressing to the elbow extended/supinated. Strengthening wrist flexors and pronators—isometric, concentric, then eccentric. Strengthen other weak areas of upper limb (scapular stabilizers, rotator cuff)

4. *Bracing:* consider cock-up splint, counterforce brace, and/or taping

5. *Patient education:* HEP, activity modification

Goals: Decrease pain, restore wrist/elbow ROM then restore strength, safe and gradual return to golf, prevent recurrent injury

Reevaluation: In 4 to 6 weeks by referring physician

REFERENCES

1. Ciccotti MC, Schwartz MA, Ciccotti MG. Diagnosis and treatment of medial epicondylitis of the elbow. *Clin Sports Med*. 2004;23:693–705.
2. Jobe FW, Ciccotti MG. Lateral and medial epicondylitis of the elbow. *J Am Acad Orthop Surg*. 1994;2:1–8.
3. Walz DM, Newman JS, Konin GP, Ross G. Epicondylitis: pathogenesis, imaging, and treatment. *Radiographics*. 2010; 30:167–184.
4. Wilson JJ, Best TM. Common overuse tendon problems: a review and recommendations for treatment. *Am Fam Physician*. 2005;72(5):811–818.
5. Shiri R, Viikari-Juntura E, Varonen H, Heliovaara M. Prevalence and determinants of lateral and medial epicondylitis: a population study. *Am J Epidemiol*. 2006;164:1065–1075.
6. Hamilton PG. The prevalence of humeral epicondylitis: a survey in general practice. *J R Coll Gen Pract*. 1986;36:464–465.
7. Descatha A, Leclerc A, Chastang JF, Roquelaure Y. Medial epicondylitis in occupational settings: prevalence, incidence and associated risk factors. *J Occup Environ Med*. 2003; 45(9):993–1001.
8. Lee AT, Lee-Robinson AL. The prevalence of medial epicondylitis among patients with C6 and C7 radiculopathy. *Sports Health: A Multidisciplinary Approach*. 2010;2:334–336.
9. Farber AJ, Smith JS, Kvitne RS, Mohr KJ, Shin SS. Electromyographic analysis of forearm muscles in professional and amateur golfers. *Am J Sports Med*. 2009;37(2):396-401.
10. Pienimaki TT, Siira PT, Vanharanta H. Chronic medial and lateral epicondylitis: a comparison of pain, disability and function. *Arch Phys Med Rehabil*. 2002;83:317–321.
11. Kijowski R, de Smet A. Magnetic resonance imaging findings in patients with medial epicondylitis. *Skeletal Radiol*. 2005;34:196–202.
12. Park GY, Lee SM, Lee MY. Diagnostic value of ultrasonography for clinical medial epicondylitis. *Arch Phys med Rehabil*. 2008;89:738–742.
13. Hubbard TJ, Denegar CR. Does cryotherapy improve outcomes with soft tissue injury? *J Athl Train*. 2004;39(3):278–279.
14. MacAuley DC. Ice therapy: How good is the evidence? *Int J Sports Med*. 2001;22:379–384.
15. Bleakley CM, McDonough SM, MacAuley DC. Cryotherapy for acute ankle sprains: a randomized controlled study of two different icing protocols. *Br J Sports Med*. 2006; 40:700–705.
16. Seegenschmiedt MH, Guntrum F, Krahl H. Lateral and medial epicondylitis. Radiotherapy for non-malignant disorders. *Medic Radiol*. 2008;3:281–294.
17. van der Windt D, van der Heijden G, van der Berg S, Riet G, de Winter A, Bouter L. Ultrasound therapy for musculoskeletal disorders: a systemic review. *Pain*. 1999;81:257–262.
18. Sandmeier R. Diagnosis and treatment of chronic tendon disorders in sports. *Scand J Med Sci Sports*. 1997;7:96-106.
19. Robertson VJ, Baker KG. A review of therapeutic ultrasound: effectiveness studies. *Physi Ther*. 2001;81:1339–1350.
20. D'Vaz AP, Ostor AJ, Speed CA, Jenner JR, Bradley M, Prevost AT. Pulsed low-intensity ultrasound for chronic lateral epicondylitis: a randomized controlled trial. *Rheumatology (Oxford)*. 2006;45(5):566–570.
21. Nirschl RP, Rodin DM, Ochiai DH, Maartmann-Moe C. Iontophoretic administration of dexamethasone sodium phosphate for acute epicondylitis. *Am J Sports Med*. 2003;31(2):189–195.
22. Baskurt F, Ozcan A, Algun C. Comparison of effects of phonophoresis and iontophoresis of naproxen in the treatment of lateral epicondylitis. *Clin Rehabil*. 2003;17(1):96–100.
23. Simunovic Z, Trobonjaca T, Trobonjaca Z. Treatment of medial and lateral epicondylitis—tennis and golfer's elbow—with low level laser therapy: a multicenter double blind, placebo controlled clinical study on 324 patients. *J Clin Laser Med Surg*. 1998;16(3):145–151.
24. Bjordal JM, Lopes-Martins RA, Jeoensen J, et al. A systematic review with procedural assessments and meta-analysis of low level laser therapy in lateral elbow tendinopathy (tennis elbow.) *BMC Musculoskelet Disorders*. 2008;9:75.
25. Crowther MA, Bannister GC, Huma H, Rooker GD. A prospective, randomized study to compare extracorpeal shock-wave therapy and injection of steroid for the treatment of tennis elbow. *J Bone Joint Surg Br*. 2002;84(5):678–679.
26. Krischeck O, Hopf C, Nafe B, Rompe JD. Shock-wave therapy for tennis and golfer's elbow- 1 year follow-up. *Arch Orthop Trauma Surg*. 1999;119:62–66.
27. Melikyan EY, Shahin E, Miles J, Bainbridge LC. Extracorporeal shock-wave treatment for tennis elbow: A randomized double blind study. *J Bone Joint Surg (Br)*. 2003;85B:852–855.
28. Fedorczk JM. Elbow tendonopathies: clinical presentation and therapist's management of tennis elbow. In: Skirven TM, Osterman AL, Fedorczk JM, Amadio PC eds. *Rehabilitation of the Hand and Upper Extremity*. 6th ed. Philadelphia, PA: Elsevier; 2011:1098–1108.
29. Cannon NM, Beal BG, Walters KJ. *Diagnosis and Treatment Manual for Physicians and Therapists. Upper Extremity Rehabilitation*. 4th ed. Indianapolis, IN: The Hand Rehabilitation Center of Indiana; 2001.
30. Jayanthi N. UpToDate. Epicondylitis (tennis and golf elbow). http://www.uptodate.com/contents/epicondylitis-tennis-and-golf-elbow. Updated February 9, 2011.
31. Sellards R, Kuebrich C. The elbow: diagnosis and treatment of common injuries. *Prim Care Clin Office Pract*. 2005; 32(1):1-16.
32. Shamsoddini A, Hollisz M, Azad KM. Comparison of initial effect of taping technique and counterforce brace on pain and grip strength of patients with lateral epicondylitis. *J Rehabil*. 2006;7(1(24)):38–42.
33. Vicenzino B, Brooksbank J, Minto J, Offord S, Paungmali A. Initial effects of elbow taping on pain-free grip strength and pressure pain threshold. *J Orthop Sports Phys Ther*. 2003;33(7):400–407.
34. Snyder-Mackler L, Epler M. Effect of standard Aircast tennis elbow bands on integrated electromyography of forearm extensor musculature proximal to the bands. *Am J Sports Med*. 1989;17:278.
35. Ciccotti M, Schwartz M, Ciccotti M. Diagnosis and treatment of medial epicondylitis of the elbow. *Sports Med Arthrosc Rev*. 2003;11(1):57–62.

Other Elbow Disorders

Anjan P. Kaushik, John McMurtry, Jeffrey T. Smith, Daniel C. Herman, and D. Nicole Deal

INTRODUCTION

The elbow presents a wide spectrum of pathophysiology that can include not only the joint itself, but also the stabilizing connective tissues, musculotendinous units, and neurovascular structures surrounding this unique joint. Most patients with elbow disorders, as seen in the previous chapters describing medial and lateral epicondylitis, respond quite well to nonoperative options, and physical and/or occupational therapy techniques play an integral part in the rehabilitation of these patients. Occasionally patients may also require surgery, in which case postoperative rehabilitation requires multidisciplinary collaboration involving surgeons, therapists, and patients themselves during the recovery process. Although a comprehensive account of all elbow disorders is beyond the scope of this text, we present several common pathologies and therapeutic recommendations for these disorders: (a) olecranon bursitis, (b) biceps tendinopathy, (c) ulnar neuropathy, and (d) ulnar collateral ligament injury.

OLECRANON BURSITIS

INTRODUCTION

The olecranon bursa is a synovium-lined pouch positioned just deep to the skin overlying the olecranon process, making it vulnerable to direct or repetitive trauma. The primary function is to decrease pressure and reduce friction on the olecranon process. Trauma is thought to precipitate bursitis through increased vascularity, which in turn leads to excess bursal synovial inflammation (1). Olecranon bursitis is common in activities such as lacrosse, basketball, hockey, swimming, gymnastics, and wrestling.

Olecranon bursitis can present as acute or chronic in nature. Bursitis can also be differentiated into septic and nonseptic, depending on the presence or absence of an infectious process. In septic bursitis, where patients present with acute edema, erythema, and warmth, *Staphylococcus aureus* is isolated as the causative organism in greater than 80% of cases (2). There can also be an inflammatory cause of bursitis, which is frequently seen in patients with arthropathies such as rheumatoid arthritis. Chronic bursitis has an insidious onset with a gradual increase in symptoms not attributable to any single event (3,4).

Key elements of the physical examination include inspection, palpation, and range of motion (ROM). Upon inspection a fluctuant mass that can vary in volume is consistently present over the olecranon process. In chronic bursitis there is bursal thickening that is more subtle, whereas extensive swelling is commonly found in acute bursitis. Patients typically have painless ROM except when the bursa comes under tension (1,4).

A key part of the diagnosis is distinguishing septic versus nonseptic bursitis. The findings of erythema, painful ROM, and warmth can suggest a diagnosis of septic bursitis. In contrast, nonseptic bursitis presents with more subacute, mild pain, with edema and induration (5). Olecranon bursitis is primarily diagnosed on physical exam, with imaging techniques having a secondary diagnostic role. Standard radiographs can demonstrate an olecranon spur in 30% of cases, which is loosely associated with bursitis (1).

Bursal aspiration is essential with suspicion of an inflammatory or septic pathogenesis. In order to minimize formation of a chronic draining sinus, aspiration should be performed via a lateral approach. Septic bursitis contains greater than 1500 white blood cells per field, with a neutrophil predominance (1).

OLECRANON BURSITIS

▨ Injury commonly found in athletes, laborers, and desk workers who place excess pressure on the extensor surface of the elbow

▨ Injury mechanism involves acute or chronic trauma to the olecranon

▨ On examination, the presence or absence of erythema, pain, fluctuance, and warmth indicate a septic or nonseptic process, respectively

▨ When a septic process is suspected, the bursa must be aspirated

TREATMENT AND REHABILITATION

In all suspected cases of olecranon bursitis, the primary treatment is to prevent any further injury to the elbow through modified behavior and elbow protection. Conservative management is the most common treatment modality, which includes prescription of nonsteroidal anti-inflammatory drugs (NSAIDs), compression, and aspiration of the bursal fluid for symptomatic relief (4).

In acute nonseptic bursitis NSAIDs and aspiration are used in addition to protection, rest, ice, compression, and elevation (PRICE). One month after conservative management with bursal aspiration, greater than 70% of patients had resolution of bursal effusions. In that same patient group greater than 90% had complete resolution of symptoms at 6 months (6). For recurrent nonseptic bursitis, intrabursal corticosteroid injection can be utilized. Injection has been shown to hasten recovery and resolution of symptoms, but is not recommended for routine use because there is an increased risk of infection, skin atrophy, tendon rupture, and pain (7). Surgical intervention with olecranon bursectomy is indicated when chronic nonseptic bursitis has failed nonoperative treatment strategies. Surgery is more effective for nonrheumatoid patients (3,4).

For septic olecranon bursitis, a more aggressive treatment approach is necessary. Proper treatment centers on appropriate antibiotic coverage for common causative organisms and adequate bursal fluid drainage. Patients lacking systemic signs of infection can be managed on oral antibiotics geared toward treating *S. aureus* and are appropriately changed according to culture sensitivities. Conversely, patients with severe local or systemic signs of infection should be managed on intravenous antibiotics geared toward

treating *S. aureus*. Antibiotic therapy for 14 days resolves most cases of septic bursitis but can be tailored to symptoms and patient history. Daily aspiration, if needed, commonly provides adequate drainage and should be continued until fluid no longer accumulates or is sterile (2,5).

Therapeutic Modalities

As in any injury that involves inflammation the principles of PRICE provide clear symptomatic benefit. Additional therapies, including ultrasound stimulation, electrical stimulation, and phonophoresis have been suggested for the temporary relief of pain and encouragement of microcirculation. However, there is no compelling clinical data to warrant utilizing these supplemental modalities. Heat therapy is useful when restriction of motion is due to increased muscle tension in the absence of residual swelling. Use of heat modalities in the presence of an active infection is contraindicated (6).

Manual Therapy

Manual techniques such as soft tissue mobilization for edema control and joint mobilization for restoration of ROM are useful approaches for the care of olecranon bursitis. However, there is no compelling clinical data to warrant utilization of a specific manual therapy technique.

Therapeutic Exercises

Many cases of olecranon bursitis do not warrant physical therapy unless significant deficits in ROM or strength are present. In these cases, focused therapeutic activities under the guidance of a therapist or athletic trainer are sometimes necessary. Most important, avoidance of prior injurious activities is paramount to successful therapy.

If a supervised rehabilitation program is necessary, ROM and flexibility exercises are integral to restoring function to the elbow and upper limb. Progression to resistive ROM should begin only after preinjury ROM and flexibility are restored. As in any therapeutic protocol, strengthening begins in a single plane and consists of resistance bands for constant tension and free weights for variable resistance. As uniplanar strength increases, advancement to multiplanar exercises is possible, and exercises can incorporate daily activities and work-related tasks. In athletes, eventual progression to sport-specific exercises should be included before return to play (1,6).

SUMMARY

Olecranon bursitis is a common musculoskeletal injury associated with acute or chronic trauma to the olecranon process. Treatment of nonseptic bursitis is initially conservative with PRICE and NSAIDs, but also involves aspiration of bursal fluid, corticosteroid injection, and lastly surgical modalities if the condition is refractory to conservative management. More urgent therapy is necessary for septic bursitis with antibiotics, and corticosteroids are contraindicated. Physical rehabilitation of these injuries is often unnecessary, but includes early ROM, flexibility, and strengthening to restore deficits. The most important precursor to therapy is educating the patient about which activities will cause recurrence or exacerbation of an already inflamed olecranon bursa.

DISTAL BICEPS TENDINOPATHY

INTRODUCTION

The biceps brachii muscle serves the functions of flexing and supinating the forearm, in addition to contributing to shoulder stability. The long head originates from the supraglenoid tubercle and superior glenoid labrum, and the short head from the coracoid process. The distal insertion is onto the radial tuberosity and bicipital aponeurosis. Tendinopathy and ruptures of the distal biceps tendon commonly occur between the age of 40 and 55. They are more common in males and usually involve the dominant limb. Other risk factors for biceps pathology include occupations with repetitive forearm motion (plumbers, laborers, and athletes), smoking, and chronic steroid use (8,9).

Injuries often occur when an unexpected extension force and eccentric load is placed on the forearm in a partially flexed elbow at 90°. Distal biceps injuries can be either partial or complete. Partial ruptures and tendinopathy warrant referral to a physical therapist to improve or maintain ROM and to avoid progression of the injury. Complete biceps ruptures, which are more common, result in significant weakness during supination (30% loss of strength in flexion, 40%–50% in supination), and permanent weakness can result if the tendon is not surgically repaired. Early referral to an orthopaedic surgeon

is recommended, as chronic biceps rupture repairs have poorer outcomes for postoperative strength and return to work than acute repairs (10,11).

Key elements of the physical examination include inspection, palpation, ROM, manual muscle testing, neurovascular examination, and key special tests. Examination begins with inspection and palpation, followed by assessment of elbow ROM. Patients with distal biceps ruptures describe a distinct "pop" at the elbow and immediate pain, swelling, and ecchymosis in the proximal forearm. Complete ruptures commonly result in "popeye deformity" in the upper arm, and a palpable gap can be noted at the rupture site. A positive Hook test, or inability to palpate the distal biceps tendon by hooking the index finger over the tendon from the lateral side, confirms the diagnosis. Significant weakness is noted in supination and flexion of the elbow, in comparison to the uninjured arm. Loss of supination is normally more functionally debilitating for the patient. Distal biceps tendinosis presents with a thickened tendon with tenderness to palpation and pain often reproduced by passive stretch or resisted contraction. If rupture is suspected, it is also important to rule out vascular injury to the brachial artery and neurologic injury to the median nerve, as well as compartment syndrome (8,10,12).

Plain radiographs are unremarkable and very rarely demonstrate small avulsions of the radial tuberosity or local hypertrophy. Magnetic resonance imaging (MRI) can be used as a confirmative test when differentiating between partial and complete ruptures, and can also depict tendinosis if the tendon is intact.

DISTAL BICEPS TENDINOPATHY

- Injury that occurs from eccentric load onto a partially flexed elbow
- Commonly seen in males 40 to 55, in the dominant arm
- Distinct "pop" noted, with significant swelling and palpable gap in antecubital fossa, often with "popeye deformity" in upper arm
- Partial ruptures and tendinosis can be managed with nonoperative options and physical therapy, but early surgical repair is recommended for complete ruptures, with postoperative physical therapy

TREATMENT AND REHABILITATION

Nonsurgical management of ruptures with NSAIDs and physical therapy for ROM and strengthening is considered for patients with tendinosis and partial ruptures, as well as for patients with complete ruptures who have significant medical comorbidities that preclude surgery or patients who cannot follow an extensive postoperative rehabilitation program. Indications for surgical repair include complete distal biceps ruptures, as well as partial biceps ruptures that fail to respond to nonoperative measures (10,12).

Therapeutic Modalities

Nonoperative management of patients with biceps tendinosis or rupture may include modalities such as cryotherapy, ultrasound, and heat therapy. The initial focus is on resolution of inflammatory pain and edema with cryotherapy and then proceeds toward thermal and nonthermal agents that facilitate healing and restoration of ROM.

Manual Therapy

The role for massage and other manual techniques for conservatively managed distal biceps rupture focuses on resolving localized edema and pain control. There may be a role for massage techniques, such as transverse friction massage in the treatment of tendinosis, but this technique requires further investigation, as do other manual therapy techniques in this setting.

Therapeutic Exercises

Immediately after a partial or complete distal biceps rupture, the patient may be immobilized in a long arm splint or sling to rest injured structures and to prevent further aggravation of local soft tissues. A hinged elbow brace is effective in the first 1 to 6 weeks to protect the elbow and control ROM (8,10).

ROM is limited at first with the hinged elbow brace set to 30° short of full extension, up to 120° flexion, as well as 90° of pronation and supination. The first 3 weeks of rehabilitation emphasizes ROM more than strengthening. Then from week 3 to 6 elbow extension is progressed toward full, forearm ROM is begun by 6 weeks and light

strengthening with elastic bands and 2-pound weights, as well as grip strengthening, may begin after 5 to 6 weeks. Finally, from 6 weeks to 6 months, a gradual strengthening program improves supination and grip strength (13). In the case of tendinosis, prior research on other types of tendinopathy (e.g., Achilles tendinopathy) suggests the need for an eccentric strengthening program before the rehabilitation program is complete, and this may be the case for biceps tendinosis, but further investigation is necessary.

SUMMARY

Rupture of the distal biceps tendon is an injury seen in laborers and athletes who experience an acute eccentric load on a partially flexed elbow. Complete ruptures are most common and result in a "popeye deformity" as well as weakness, pain, edema, and a palpable gap in the antecubital fossa. Early surgical repair is recommended for acute complete ruptures within 2 to 3 weeks to avoid chronic shortening or elbow contracture. Rehabilitation of partial ruptures and tendinosis should follow the phases of rehabilitation, focusing on ROM once pain and swelling have been controlled and later on elbow strengthening for forearm supination and flexion and eventually functional retraining. The role of eccentric training for biceps tendinosis requires further investigation.

ULNAR NEUROPATHY

INTRODUCTION

Compression of the ulnar nerve around the elbow joint, known as cubital tunnel syndrome, can occur at several anatomic sites, including the arcade of Struthers, medial intermuscular septum, medial head of triceps, medial epicondyle, Osborne's ligament in the cubital tunnel, anconeus epitrochlearis, and the flexor carpi ulnaris aponeurosis. Sources of compression include tumors (peri neuromas, hamartomas, vascular lesions), ganglion cysts, osteophytes, and excessive fibrosis of tendons and connective tissues around the elbow. Fractures and dislocations can result in acute ulnar neuropathy, whereas chronic neuropathy is seen more frequently with tumors, osteophytes, and cubitus valgus. Other risk factors include diabetes, thyroid disease, inflammatory arthritides, and vitamin deficiencies (14,15).

Symptoms include numbness and paresthesias to the ring and small fingers, and intrinsic muscle weakness in the hand. Clawing of the ulnar digits can occur late in the course of ulnar neuropathy. Patients may report clumsiness with gripping and fine motor activities, night pain, as well as hand fatigue. Sympathetic nervous system dysfunction can also cause changes in skin color, moisture, and temperature. Symptoms may be exacerbated, for example, by resting the medial elbow on hard surfaces or by keeping the elbow flexed while driving (14–16).

Key elements of the physical examination include palpation, ROM, and most important a detailed neurovascular examination. Extreme flexion of the elbow reproduces the paresthesias of ulnar neuropathy, as well as percussion of the nerve at the posteromedial elbow (Tinel sign). Strength and neurosensory testing (Semmes-Weinstein monofilaments, two-point discrimination) are integral to the examination. Intrinsic hand weakness can be seen when there is compensatory thumb interphalangeal joint flexion when pinching a piece of paper (Froment sign). Wartenberg sign refers to the persistent abduction and extension of the small finger, also secondary to interosseous muscle weakness (15).

Imaging with plain radiographs is usually unremarkable but can occasionally demonstrate large posteromedial osteophytes. MRI may be needed to determine if a tumor or cyst is compressing the nerve. Electrodiagnostic testing can confirm examination findings of cubital tunnel syndrome and rule out other sites of neuropathology, including the cervical spine and Guyon's canal at the wrist (14,15).

ULNAR NEUROPATHY

- ■ Cubital tunnel syndrome is caused by compression of the ulnar nerve around the elbow

- ■ Symptoms include numbness and paresthesias to the ring and small fingers, as well as intrinsic hand muscle weakness

- ■ Neurological examination may reveal weakness of the intrinsic hand muscles and abnormal sensory testing in the ulnar distribution. Extreme flexion or tapping on the medial elbow repeatedly (Tinel sign) may reproduce symptoms

- ■ Avoidance of aggravating factors, NSAIDs, nighttime bracing, and physical therapy are normally effective, but some patients may require surgical ulnar nerve decompression or transposition

TREATMENT AND REHABILITATION

Patient education for avoidance of aggravating activities for at least 3 months is essential for management of early cubital tunnel syndrome. Avoidance of activities involving elbow flexion >45°, use of ergonomic keyboard designs, avoiding pressure of the medial elbow on hard surfaces, and keeping the elbow straight while sleeping with nighttime bracing (Figure 15.1) or a towel around the elbow can all be effective (17).

Nonsurgical treatment with NSAID medications, wrist flexion and extension exercises, and formal physical or occupational therapy to focus on neural glides or nerve mobilization are all recommended prior to considering surgery. Referral to a physical therapy (PT) or

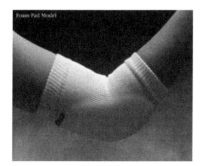
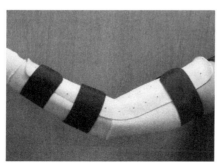

FIGURE 15.1: Elbow padding and nighttime bracing.

Source: Adapted from Sammons Preston Catalog. www.pattersonmedical.com.

occupational therapy (OT) who is a certified hand therapist (CHT) may be advisable. Steroid injections around the nerve are generally avoided to decrease the risk of intraneural injection and nerve damage (15,16).

Surgery is recommended for patients with late findings of ulnar neuropathy (intrinsic muscle wasting), patients with electrodiagnostic evidence of neuropathy who fail >3 months of nonoperative treatment, and those with progressive nerve palsy. Surgical techniques include decompression in situ (without transposition), anterior ulnar nerve transposition (subcutaneous, submuscular, or intramuscular), and, rarely, medial epicondylectomy (14,15).

Therapeutic Modalities

Moist heat therapy can be effective prior to starting an exercise regimen, particularly when the flexor carpi ulnaris is significantly tight and restricted. Ultrasound also shows some promise, based on studies indicating that low intensity pulsed ultrasound can promote earlier nerve regeneration, but evidence is limited and requires further investigation (18). There is limited evidence supporting iontophoresis as a beneficial modality, despite its anecdotal acceptance.

Manual Therapy

The therapist must be careful in the use of manual techniques for ulnar neuropathy, as excessive manipulation can aggravate nerve symptoms. Gentle tension and movements promoting sliding and gliding of the nerve along its path can be effective if done at a subsymptomatic threshold (19).

Therapeutic Exercises

In the acute phase of therapy, strict avoidance of irritating sensitive structures is vital. In severe cases, 24 to 48 hours of strict rest and immobilization in 45° of elbow flexion, with patient education regarding avoidance of aggravating factors, is effective. Palliative effects of pulsed ultrasound and active range of motion (AROM) exercises can then be utilized. After improvements in pain-free ROM are achieved, the use of ulnar nerve gliding, flossing, and tensioning exercises can be done initially with one-on-one formal therapy and later with a self-paced home exercise program (HEP). This often helps patients feel that they are active participants in their rehabilitation, but patients should be advised to stop if they experience further aggravation of symptoms (16,19).

Specialized Techniques

Ergonomic instruction, jobsite adaptation, and postural education are the mainstays of avoidance techniques in the treatment of ulnar neuropathy. In industrial settings, a certified professional ergonomist (CPE) can facilitate productivity without aggravating ulnar nerve symptoms. Patients should be instructed on attention to elbow position, pressure along the nerve, and spinal alignment during occupational and recreational activities (16).

SUMMARY

Cubital tunnel syndrome, or ulnar nerve compression at the elbow, presents with numbness and paresthesias to the ring and small finger, as well as intrinsic hand muscle weakness. Symptoms are aggravated by repetitive contact of the medial elbow against hard surfaces and persistent elbow flexion during occupational activities. Most cases of ulnar neuropathy can be managed nonoperatively with avoidance techniques, nighttime bracing, anti-inflammatory medications, and physical therapy; however, persistent cases and patients with progressive nerve palsy require surgical consultation and may need surgical ulnar nerve decompression or transposition at the elbow.

ULNAR COLLATERAL LIGAMENT INJURY OF THE ELBOW

INTRODUCTION

Injuries to the ulnar collateral ligament (UCL) of the elbow are common in overhead throwing athletes and occur as a result of repetitive, high-velocity valgus stress to the medial aspect of the elbow. These injuries can result in a UCL sprain, which causes attenuation of the ligament, or a complete rupture of the UCL. The UCL consists of three bundles: anterior, posterior, and transverse. It originates from the medial epicondyle and has been classically described to insert on the sublime tubercle of the ulna. A rupture of the anterior bundle, which serves as the strongest structure within the ligament, results in instability of the elbow under varus extension stress. Injuries typically occur in the late cocking and acceleration phases of throwing, when the UCL experiences the highest stresses (20,21).

Patients may present either with an acute UCL injury, where medial elbow pain can be attributed to a single pitch or throw that leads to loss of velocity and control, or chronic repetitive UCL injury, which has a more insidious onset of medial elbow tenderness. Ulnar nerve symptoms are also present in 25% of patients, as valgus load results in stretch of the nerve in the cubital tunnel. Untreated valgus overload can lead to radiocapitellar arthritis in the long term (21).

Key elements of the physical examination include inspection, palpation, ROM, manual muscle testing, neurovascular examination, and key special tests. Palpation of the UCL with the elbow flexed 20° to 30° may elicit tenderness. UCL injury can be diagnosed with the valgus stress test, in which the elbow is flexed, the shoulder abducted, and valgus force applies across the elbow joint. Valgus instability of the elbow is only demonstrable with the valgus stress test in 50% of patients because the elbow instability is dynamic. The O'Driscoll moving valgus stress test, in which the elbow is repeatedly flexed and extended with valgus force, is more sensitive for detecting UCL injury while the elbow is in 70° to 130° of flexion (20,21).

Plain radiographs typically do not show any pathology but may depict an avulsion fracture. Valgus stress radiographs can show increased widening medially with complete UCL ruptures. Magnetic resonance (MR) arthrogram of the elbow is highly sensitive for detection of UCL rupture. Ultrasound is also commonly used clinically to diagnose UCL injury (21).

ULNAR COLLATERAL LIGAMENT INJURY

▪ Pain at the medial elbow as a result of excessive repetitive valgus force to the elbow, commonly seen in overhead throwing athletes

▪ Injury may be a UCL sprain or a complete rupture and may be acute or chronic. Ulnar nerve symptoms can also occur with this injury

▪ Clinical diagnosis of elbow instability with valgus stress test can be confirmed with MR arthrogram. Ultrasound examination with dynamic testing is also gaining acceptance

▪ Nonoperative treatment with bracing, medications, and physical therapy is often successful, but complete ligament ruptures may require surgical UCL reconstruction, particularly in high-functioning athletes

TREATMENT AND REHABILITATION

Nonoperative treatment includes rest, ice, compression, and elevation, as well as nonsteroidal anti-inflammatory medications and physical therapy modalities, which are detailed below. Nighttime splinting or a hinged elbow brace, along with a progressive physical therapy stretching and strengthening program, are usually effective for treatment of UCL sprains. Patients undergo at least 6 weeks of nonoperative treatment prior to reassessment for possible surgical UCL reconstruction, which is considered in patients with persistent medial elbow pain despite extended therapy (21,22).

Therapeutic Modalities

The use of therapeutic modalities such as pulsed ultrasound and electrical stimulation *may* stimulate the inflammatory elements of initial healing and movement of fibroblasts to facilitate collagen synthesis. As the patient's acute symptoms resolve, a gradual staged rehabilitation program of AROM and use of moist heat may be started, as detailed below (23).

Manual Therapy

The literature has minimal discussion of manual therapy techniques in UCL sprain rehabilitation. Manual joint mobilization and muscle energy techniques can be useful adjuncts in cases of postinjury stiffness that may develop in the affected elbow joint. Soft tissue mobilization of edema can be helpful early in the inflammatory process to clear local inflammatory mediators that can cause persistent tissue irritation, but this is strictly theoretical. Light scar massage is integrated into the rehabilitation of the postoperative patient after UCL reconstruction (22,23).

Therapeutic Exercises

The initial goal after UCL injury is to reduce inflammation, pain, and edema, as well as to facilitate collagen synthesis by fibroblasts for healing. The following phases of rehabilitation differ from those used throughout this book, but apply the same principles of rehabilitation and progress from the PRICE protocol to functional or sport-specific training prior to completion.

Phase I, the inflammatory phase over the first 2 weeks, involves immobilization (protection and relative rest) of the affected elbow for the first week in a hinged elbow brace

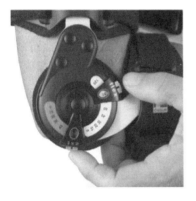 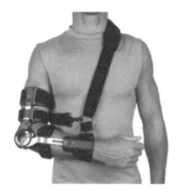

FIGURE 15.2: Hinged elbow brace.

Source: Adapted from Sammons Preston Catalog. www.pattersonmedical.com.

(Figure 15.2) locked at 30° extension. The extension can be gradually increased 10° per week thereafter, with a goal of PROM from 30° to 90°. Active assisted nonpainful ROM is initiated in the second week, with isometric strengthening of wrist and elbow musculature. Shoulder strengthening should avoid internal rotation resistance in order to reduce load on the UCL. As discussed in the modalities section, low-intensity pulsed ultrasound and moist heat packs may be used as adjuncts (22,24).

The second proliferative phase from week 3 to 6 focuses on improvement in AROM toward 0° to 135°, as well as increasing strength and endurance. Isotonic wrist curls, wrist extension, pronation, and supination should be emphasized, along with shoulder external rotation and abduction strengthening. Full, pain-free elbow extension should be achieved by 4 to 6 weeks post injury, but care should be taken to avoid aggravating the healing soft tissues (22).

The third phase from week 6 to 12 focuses on maturation of the healing soft tissues, with improvements in strength, power, and endurance during elbow motion. Emphasis is on increasing neuromuscular control, and high-speed exercise drills are initiated, including the "Thrower's Ten" program and plyometric throwing drills. Other exercises facilitate biceps-triceps co-contraction, supination and pronation, and wrist flexion and extension (22).

The final phase, after week 12, emphasizes fine-tuning of muscle control and throwing technique to allow a patient to return to sports and high-demand activities. This is only possible if the patient has full non-painful ROM, absence of laxity, and satisfactory strength on clinical examination. Recovery of function may take one full year or more during this phase of rehabilitation. A staged return to throwing is detailed by Wilk et al (22) in their hallmark article on UCL rehabilitation.

If symptoms persist at any stage such that pain-free progression is impossible for the patient, the rehabilitation should be regressed to a nonpainful ROM. Failure of the patient to respond to nonoperative treatment with these techniques warrants a referral to the orthopaedic surgeon to consider surgical reconstruction of the UCL (21,23).

Specialized Techniques

Kinesiology taping, aquatic exercise, proprioceptive training, and rhythmic stabilization (a type of proprioceptive neuromuscular facilitation) are occasionally used as alternative methods for UCL rehabilitation, but there is no strong evidence in the literature validating these techniques.

Motion analysis and throwing evaluation is an excellent addition to an athlete's return to sport and should be utilized late in the rehabilitation program to assess readiness for athletic competition (23).

SUMMARY

Elbow UCL sprain or rupture is commonly seen in overhead throwing athletes, and injury generally occurs from valgus overload of the elbow in the late cocking and acceleration phase. Nonoperative management of UCL injuries of the elbow can be a challenging balance of tissue healing, protected ROM, and gradual return to sport. Understanding the frustrations of players, coaches, and parents is vital to keep a young player from becoming a surgical candidate; however, persistent symptoms that prevent pain-free progression in ROM may necessitate surgical UCL reconstruction. Postoperative rehabilitation is also an essential component of the recovery process for this injury.

CONCLUSION

The elbow is a complex joint in which normal functioning depends on the dynamic interactions between stabilizing connective tissues, bony articulations, neurovascular structures, and muscles and tendons surrounding the joint. Pathologic states of the elbow can involve one or more of these components. Physical and occupational therapy modalities and therapeutic exercise play an essential role in the rehabilitation of elbow injuries, and most patients recover well without operative intervention. For the remaining patients who do require surgery, postoperative rehabilitation is also fundamental to recovery. This chapter has illustrated several common disorders of the elbow and serves as an overview to the treatment approaches for these pathologies.

REFERENCES

1. Salzman KL, Lillegard WA, Butcher JD. Upper extremity bursitis. *Am Fam Physician*, 1997;56(7):1797-1806, 1811–1812.
2. Cea-Pereiro JC, Garcia-Meijide J, Mera-Varela A, Gomez-Reino JJ. A comparison between septic bursitis caused by *Staphylococcus aureus* and those caused by other organisms. *Clin Rheumatol,* 2001;20:10–14.
3. Morrey BF. Bursitis. In: Morrey BF, ed. *The Elbow and its Disorders*, 3rd ed. Philadelphia, PA: WB Saunders; 2000:901–908.
4. Bravo CJ. Olecranon bursitis. In: Miller MD, Hart JA, MacKnight JM, eds. *Essential Orthopaedics*. Philadelphia, PA: Saunders Elsevier; 2010:263–265.
5. Zimmerman B, Mikolich DJ, Ho G. Septic bursitis. *Semin Arthritis Rheum*. 1995;24:391.
6. McAfee JH, Smith DL. Olecranon and prepatellar bursitis: Diagnosis and treatment. *West J Med*. 1988;149:607–610.
7. Weinstein PS, Canso JJ, Wohlgethan JR. Long-term follow-up of corticosteroid injection for traumatic olecranon bursitis. *Ann Rheum Dis*. 1984;43:44–46.
8. Golish SR, Bravo CJ. Distal biceps tendon rupture. In: Miller MD, Hart JA, MacKnight JM, eds. *Essential Orthopaedics*. Philadelphia, PA: Saunders Elsevier; 2010:249–252.
9. Safran MR, Graham SM. Distal biceps tendon ruptures: incidence, demographics, and the effect of smoking. *Clin Orthop Relat Res*. 2002;404:275–283.
10. Ramsey ML. Distal biceps tendon injuries: diagnosis and management. *J Am Acad Orthop Surg*. 1999;7(3):199–207.
11. Mazzocca A, Spang J, Arciero R. Distal biceps rupture. *Orthop Clin of North Am*. 2008;39(2):237–249.
12. Miyamoto RG, Elser F, Millett PF. Distal biceps tendon injuries. *J Bone Joint Surg Am*. 2010;92:2128–2138.
13. Hamersly S. Distal biceps repair rehabilitation protocol (pdf). *Methodist Sports Medicine Department of Physical Therapy*. 06/01/2004, Indianapolis, IN. http://www.asset-usa.org/Rehab_Guidelines.html
14. Bravo CJ. Ulnar nerve entrapment. In: Miller MD, Hart JA, MacKnight JM, eds. *Essential Orthopaedics*. Philadelphia, PA: Saunders Elsevier; 2010:266–269.
15. Posner MA. Compressive ulnar neuropathies at the elbow: I. Etiology and diagnosis and II. Treatment. *J Am Acad Orthop Surg*, 1998;6:282–297.
16. Lund A, Amadio P. Treatment of cubital tunnel syndrome: perspectives for the therapist. *J Hand Ther*. 2006;19:170-179.
17. Nakamichi K, Tachibana S, Ida M, Yamamoto S. Patient education for the treatment of ulnar neuropathy at the elbow. *Arch Phys Med Rehabil*. 2009;90:1839–1845.
18. Crisci A, Ferreira A. Low-intensity pulsed ultrasound accelerates the regeneration of the sciatic nerve after neurotomy in rats. *Ultrasound in Med & Biol*. 2002;28(10):1335–1341.
19. Coppieters MW, Butler DS. Do "sliders" slide and "tensioners" tension? An analysis of neurodynamic techniques and considerations regarding their application. *Manual Therapy*. 2008;13(3):213–221.
20. Bravo CJ. Elbow ligament injuries. In: Miller MD, Hart JA, MacKnight JM, eds. *Essential Orthopaedics*. Philadelphia, PA: Saunders Elsevier; 2010:253–257.
21. Chen FS, Rokito AS, Jobe FW. Medial elbow problems in the overhead-throwing athlete. *J Am Acad Orthop Surg*. 2001;9:99–113.
22. Wilk KE, Reinold MM, Andrews JR. Rehabilitation of the thrower's elbow. *Clin Sports Med*. 2004;23(4):765-801.
23. Wilk KE, Marcina L. Rehabilitation for elbow instability: emphasis on the throwing athlete. In: Skirven TM, Osterman AL, Fedorczyk J, Amadio PC, eds. *Rehabilitation of the Hand and Upper Extremity*, 6th ed. Philadelphia, PA: Elsevier; 2011:1143–1150.
24. Schulte-Edelmann J. The effects of plyometric training of the posterior shoulder and elbow. *J Strength Conditioning Res*. 2005;19:129–134.

16

DeQuervain's Tenosynovitis

Christine Pfisterer, Stacia Dyer, and Jeremiah Nieves

INTRODUCTION

DeQuervain's tenosynovitis is a common cause of hand and wrist pain, and is the most common tendonitis of the wrist. References were made to similar entities in the 1983 edition of Grey's anatomy, but the condition was first described by Fritz de Quervain in 1895 (1). In this condition, the tendon sheaths of the abductor pollicis longus (APL) and extensor pollicis brevis (EPB), the tendons of the first dorsal compartment (DC) of the wrist, become compressed at the distal radial styloid (2). Of note, anatomical variations of the first DC exist; occasionally the EPB has its own separate compartment (3). It is felt that repetitive abduction of the thumb and ulnar deviation of the wrist creates tension on the tendons, which when sustained and repeated, can produce friction at the retinacular sheath. Over time, this can lead to swelling or narrowing of the fibro-osseous canal (4).

Patients will often present with complaints of pain in the radial aspect of the wrist, which worsens with abduction of the thumb. Patients usually present in the 5th and 6th decades of life, and women are typically affected more often than men. The condition has also been found to occur in younger women, during pregnancy and lactation, but it typically resolves spontaneously after lactation has stopped (1,2).

Key elements of the physical examination include inspection, palpation, range of motion (ROM), sensorimotor testing, and special test. Patients will often point to the area of pain at the radial side of the wrist. Occasionally swelling or edema may be noted in the area. If chronic or with swelling crepitus may be palpated with ulnar and radial deviation of the wrist. Pain limited thumb abduction and extension may be present on examination and depending on severity some altered sensation may be present over the radial aspect of the wrist and hand. Special test include a positive Finkelstein's test (Figure 16.1), which is performed with the

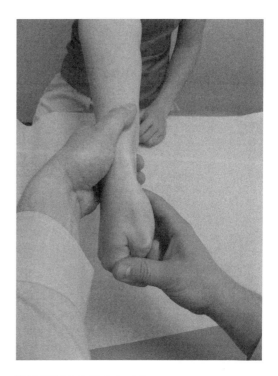

FIGURE 16.1: Finkelstein's test.

patient's thumb clasped in his/her hand followed by passive ulnar deviation of the wrist, which is diagnostic for the condition if it produces concordant pain. Differential diagnoses include, but are not limited to, intersection syndrome, arthritis of the first carpometacarpal or scaphotrapezial-trapezoid joints, or scaphoid fracture. DeQuervain's tenosynovitis is a clinical diagnosis that usually does not require imaging unless other potential causes of pain need to be ruled out. One must rule out cervical radiculopathy or peripheral nerve entrapment that may mimic this pathology. Assessment of shoulder or elbow should be included since pathology at these joints may alter biomechanics of the upper limb, thus alter movement at the wrist leading to overuse conditions.

Treatment will vary, depending on whether the condition is acute or chronic in nature. During the acute phase, relative rest, bracing or splinting, cryotherapy, and anti-inflammatories have been shown to be helpful (2). Physiotherapy, specifically by a an occupational or certified hand therapist (CHT), can be beneficial in the acute or chronic stage, but treatment will vary depending on how long the patient has had symptoms. Steroid injections have also been found to be beneficial; studies have shown 50% to 100% improvement in pain after 1 to 2 injections (1,2). When patients fail to respond to therapy, injections, and activity modification, they can be referred for surgical evaluation and intervention (1,2).

DEQUERVAIN'S TENOSYNOVITIS

▪ DeQuervain's tenosynovitis is a common condition, involving the tendons of the 1st DC of the wrist: APL and EPB

▪ It commonly presents in 40 to 50 year old females

▪ Patients will present with pain and possible swelling at the radial aspect of the wrist

▪ Positive Finkelstein's test is considered to be diagnostic

▪ Conservative treatment includes therapy for teaching of activity modification, dispensement of a splint, and gentle ROM exercises

▪ Anti-inflammatories may be helpful in the acute phase and corticosteroid injections have also been found to be helpful in refractory cases

▪ If the patient fails to respond to these nonoperative measures, they may be referred for surgical evaluation

THE REHABILITATION PROGRAM

All patients can be progressed through the five phases of rehabilitation that are utilized throughout this book. The appropriate referral would be to an occupational or physical therapist who specializes in hand therapy, commonly referred to and credentialed as a CHT. For those who are referred for hand therapy, treatment will be directed based on the duration of the patient's symptoms: Literature on conservative treatment for first DC tenosynovitis is sparse.

Therapeutic Modalities

In the acute phase from 0 to 6 weeks, conservative management can include cryotherapy (e.g., ice massage) given the theory that an inflammatory process is the source of pain. In the subacute phase thermotherapy can potentially be used in an attempt to increase circulation to the region. There is no literature to support these treatments but they can be reasonably and safely trialed. Iontophoresis with dexamethasone may alter the patient's inflammatory response, however; there is no literature supporting the use of these modalities and therefore its efficacy is unknown for this diagnosis.

In the setting of subacute or chronic DeQuervain's tenosynovitis (6 weeks–3 months), cryotherapy is usually not recommended. Also, due to the superficial anatomy and possibility of superficial radial neuritis, further irritability could result from use of ice. Iontophoresis, ultrasound, and phonophoresis are other modalities that are clinically utilized; yet again there is limited to no evidence to support their use. Superficial heat, such as moist hot packs or moist heat (MH), and fluidotherapy are beneficial to prepare tissues for manual treatment, such as soft tissue mobilizations. They also provide comfort and pain relief to the 1st DC (4).

Manual Therapy

This condition's name, "tenosynovitis," (though a misnomer in subacute and chronic phases) indicates that the surrounding myofascial tissue tends to benefit from gentle manual soft tissue mobilization and edema reduction techniques. The goal is to normalize tissue, improve ROM, and encourage healing of the structures (5). There is again no good evidence to support these treatment options. However, assessing more proximal tissues for restrictions and addressing tissue imbalances or even joint restrictions could potentially address biomechanical and kinetic chain disorders.

Therapeutic Exercise

Acutely, once the immobilization period is over with sufficient results, the patient may begin light active ROM (AROM) and isometric exercise to strengthen the wrist and hand with minimal use of splint during heavy activity. Advancing to combined strengthening exercises should only begin when the patient's pain has been reduced

(Figure 16.2 a–d). Strengthening of proximal scapular stabilizers, rotator cuff, and elbow flexors and extensors can add proximal stability and should be initiated earlier in the program. Adding strengthening to antagonistic muscles of the wrist can potentially increase the stability across the wrist. As pain improves, strengthening exercises for the wrist, hand, and forearm may progress.

During this time period, the patient is also educated in passive ROM, and is instructed to remove the splint during light activities only. After a 6-week period, the patient should return to his physician for reassessment. If the patient is significantly better, and there is sufficient relief of symptoms and improved quality of life, he may be able to forgo more invasive treatments like injections or surgical intervention and continue therapy for a strengthening program and functional restoration (6). If the patient has had symptoms for more than 3 to 6 months despite conservative treatment that includes a steroid injection, then surgical intervention may be indicated (5,7,8).

Specialized Techniques

Splinting

In the early phase, conservative treatment is the focus. It is most effective when the symptoms have been present for <3 months (9). Immobilization and patient education are initiated in the first visit. This offers palliative comfort and rests the first DC. It is also used as a form of education for the patient, as it

instructs them in proper body mechanics during aggravating activities (6). The patient may be issued a prefabricated or a custom made splint/orthosis. Over the counter splints must be fitted to the patient to ensure proper fit; however, patient comfort improves with custom made splints to tailor the splint to specific irritable regions (Figure 16.3). It may be called a forearm based static splint, long opponens splint, or a forearm-based thumb spica splint. The IP joint is left free, and the wrist and thumb placed in the following positions:

1. Wrist: 15° of extension

2. Thumb CMC joint: 40° of palmar abduction

3. Thumb MP: 10° of flexion

4. Thumb IP joint: do not immobilize

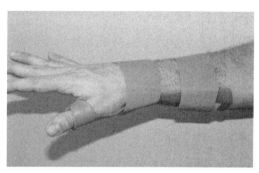

FIGURE 16.3: A long opponens splint.

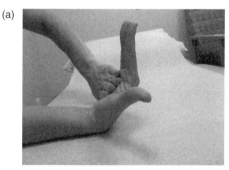
(a)

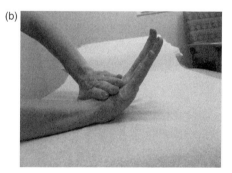
(b)

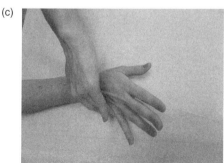
(c)

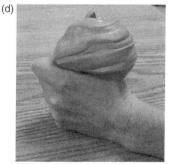
(d)

FIGURE 16.2: Examples of strengthening exercises.

HOME EXERCISE PROGRAM

Gentle passive ROM (PROM) to the affected wrist/digits begins at the first visit, so that patient can maintain joint ROM during the immobilization period. During this period of immobilization, strengthening of more proximal weakness at the shoulder and elbow may provide some benefit to muscle imbalances. As pain subsides, the patient will be instructed in AROM, and then progress to gentle strengthening such as wrist flexion, extension, radial and ulnar deviation, as well as structured grip strengthening. These exercises should also be taught for a home exercise program (HEP). (Figures 16.4-6)

The patient should also be instructed on the following:

1. Use of the "full fist" or power grip position during work or avocation should exclude the thumb during grasping, especially thumb adduction (Figure 16.4)

2. Avoid thumb flexion in combination with wrist ulnar deviation and wrist flexion. Look at patient's tools at work, and have them bring them to therapy if possible. A worksite evaluation may be necessary (Figure 16.5)

3. Promote the use of larger muscle groups to distribute forces when using the hand in a repetitive fashion

4. Keep the forearm and wrist in a neutral position (Figure 16.6)

5. Activity modification. New mothers are especially at risk due to positioning of the infant's head during feedings and lifting the child at the axilla/under armpits to remove from crib

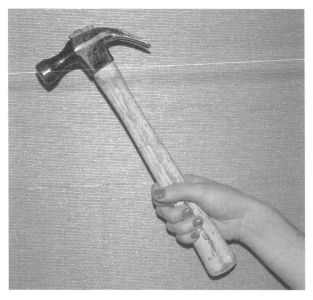

FIGURE 16.5: Improper grip position.

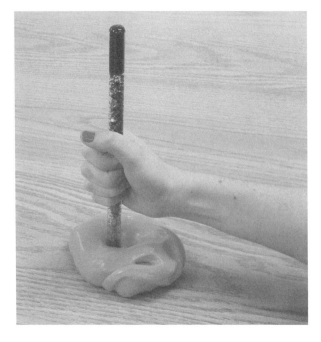

FIGURE 16.4: "Full fist"/power grip position.

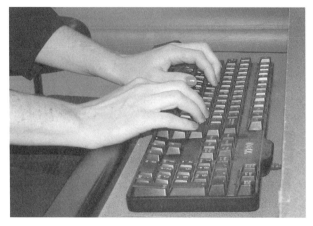

FIGURE 16.6: Proper hand positioning at a computer workstation.

SUMMARY

DeQuervain's tenosynovitis is a common condition, where tendons in the first DC of the wrist, the APL and EPB, become inflamed. Clinical diagnosis is made in the presence of a positive Finkelstein's test. In the acute phase, the patient will likely benefit from referral to a CHT and trial of a thumb splint. Patients may also benefit from corticosteroid injections if they fail to improve with therapy and activity modification alone. When the condition is present for >6 months without alleviation of the symptoms despite comprehensive nonoperative treatment, then patients should be referred to a hand surgeon and consider surgical intervention.

SAMPLE CASE

A 40-year-old female presents to the clinic with a chief complaint of right thumb pain. She states the pain has been present for a few weeks, and denies any specific trauma or other inciting factors. On physical examination, there is minimal swelling at the base of the first digit. She has pain with passive ulnar deviation of the wrist with the thumb held in her fist, demonstrating a positive Finkelstein test. You diagnosis her with DeQuervain's tenosynovitis and refer her to a CHT.

 SAMPLE THERAPY PRESCRIPTION

Discipline: Hand therapy—by CHT, either occupational therapist (OT) or physical therapist (PT).

Diagnosis: DeQuervain's tenosynovitis.

Precautions: Safety, universal.

Frequency of visits: 2 to 3x/week.

Duration of treatment: 4 to 6 weeks.

Treatment:

1. *Modalities:* cryotherapy (ice pack, ice bath, ice massage), superficial heat, and fluidotherapy as tolerated/needed

2. *Manual therapy:* myofascial release and edema management

3. *Therapeutic exercise:* light AROM thumb. Active, passive ROM to the rest of hand and wrist. Isometric exercises to strengthen the wrist and hand as tolerated. Advance to combined strengthening exercises only if patient is pain-free. Shoulder and elbow strengthening program may be included in the acute phase to address proximal muscle imbalances

4. *Specialized treatments:* none

5. *Patient education:* instruct on activity modification, immobilization of thumb, teach HEP

Supportive Devices: Please fabricate and dispense thumb spica splint, position as following: Wrist in 15° of extension, 1st CMC joint in 40° of palmar abduction, thumb MP in 10° of flexion; do not immobilize the thumb IP joint.

Goals: Decrease pain and swelling; restore ROM/flexibility then restore strength, safely return to functional activities (e.g., sport, hobbies, work).

Reevaluation: In 6 weeks by referring physician.

REFERENCES

1. Finnoff JT. Musculoskeletal problems of the upper limb. In: Braddom RL, ed. *Physical Medicine and Rehabilitation*, 3rd ed. Philadelphia, PA: Elsevier; 2007:825–853.
2. Jackson WT, Viegas SF, Coon TM, Stimpson KD, Frogameni AD, Simpson JMJ Anatomical variations in the first extensor compartment of the wrist. A clinical and anatomical study. *Bone Joint Surg Am*. 1986;68(6):923–926.
3. Wolfe S. Other disorders of the upper extremity. Green D, Hotchkiss R, Pederson WC, eds. *Green's Operative Hand Surgery*, 5th ed. Philadelphia, PA: Elsevier; 2005:2150–2154.
4. Piligian G, Herbert R, Hearns M, et al. Evaluation and management of chronic work-related musculoskeletal disorders of the distal upper extremity. *Am J Ind Med*. 2000;37:75–93.
5. Gordon L. Hand and wrist disorders. In: Herrington TN, Morse LH, eds. *Occupational Injuries-Evaluation, Management, Prevention*. St Louis MO, Mosby: 1995:103–124.
6. Ilyas AM. Nonsurgical treatment for DeQuervain's tenosynovitis. *J. Hand Surgery*. 2009;34:928–929.
7. Amadio PC. Dequervain's disease and tenosynovitis. In: Gordon SL, Blair SJ, Fine LJ, eds. *Repetitive Motion Disorders of the Upper Extremity*. Rosemont IL: AAOS; 1995:435–448.
8. Winzeler S, Rosenstein BD. Occupational injury and illness of the thumb. Causes and solutions. *AAOHN J*. 1996;10:487–492.
9. Trumble TE. Tendonitis and epicondylitis. *Principles of Hand Surgery and Therapy*. Philadelphia, PA: Elsevier; 2000:394.

Carpal Tunnel Syndrome

Gautam Malhotra, Lynn A. Ryan, and Shounuck Patel

INTRODUCTION

Carpal tunnel syndrome (CTS) is a very common (1–3/1000/year in the United States) clinical diagnosis, that variably presents as some distressing combination of numbness, paresthesias, pain, and/or weakness involving the hand. Classically patients complain of numbness, paresthesias, and/or pain in the median nerve distribution of the hand, but variability regarding the distribution of symptoms is common. Most patients report their symptoms involve the whole hand. Upon inquiring they may report dropping objects, difficulty with fine motor tasks (e.g., buttoning shirts), waking up due to nocturnal symptoms, and relief by vigorously shaking their hands (aka positive "Flick" sign). There may be a history of repetitive motion activities due to work or hobbies, but not in all cases.

The etiology is intraneural ischemia of the median nerve as it traverses through the carpal tunnel, a palmarly situated space in the distal wrist. Risk factors for this ischemia include anything that can cause increased tunnel pressure such as wrist trauma, diseases associated with neuropathy (e.g., diabetes, hypothyroidism, amyloidosis, alcoholism), inflammatory conditions, fluid retaining conditions (pregnancy, obesity), and synovitis of the flexor tendons traversing the tunnel (1). Due to conflicting reports, at this time it is not entirely clear if a history of repetitive motion or vibration is truly a risk factor.

Key elements of physical examination include inspection, palpation, range of motion (ROM), sensorimotor testing, special test, neural tension testing, and evaluation of the cervical spine and elbow for other possible areas of entrapment. Inspection may reveal atrophy of the thenar eminence, tenderness may be present at the wrist or thenar region, and weakness may be seen when testing thumb abduction and opposition. Sensation testing may reveal decreased sensation in median distribution with or without ring digit involvement. Special tests can reproduce symptoms by increasing the pressure in the carpal tunnel during carpal compression, and include Phalen's or reverse Phalen's maneuvers. Tinel's at the carpal tunnel may reproduce radiation of symptoms into the affected digits. Neural tension testing may also exacerbate symptoms indicating entrapment of the median nerve.

With these presenting symptoms a broad differential diagnosis must be entertained, including but not limited to median mononeuropathy at the wrist, peripheral polyneuropathy, brachial plexopathy, proximal median mononeuropathy, cervical radiculopathy, intracranial pathology, and myofascial pain syndrome. Confirmation of the correct diagnosis is crucial to prevent further loss of function and secure a satisfactory outcome. Although CTS is a clinical syndrome, electrodiagnostic testing with or without ultrasonographic studies should be used to confirm diagnosis, differentiate from other neuromuscular conditions, and quantify severity prior to invasive intervention. Surgical intervention should be sought for significant functional impairments, extensive hand weakness and atrophy, severe trauma, neoplasm, or impending vascular compromise. Otherwise, conservative management should always be pursued first to provide symptomatic relief and prevent development of sequelae due to maladaptive compensatory techniques. It should be noted that, in cases where electrodiagnostically confirmed CTS does not respond to these conservative measures, we believe that referral to a hand surgeon results in more favorable outcomes than a "wait and see" approach.

CARPAL TUNNEL SYNDROME

- History: patients classically complain of numbness, paresthesias, and/or pain in the median nerve distribution of the hand. May report dropping objects, difficulty with fine motor tasks, nocturnal symptoms, "Flick" sign. There may be a history of repetitive motion activities

■ Exam: Sensorimotor and reflex exam of bilateral upper limbs may reveal decreased sensation in the median distribution with or without ring digit involvement and thumb abduction/opposition weakness. Provocative maneuvers include carpal compression, Tinel's at the wrist, Phalen's test, reverse Phalen's test, neural tension testing which may reproduce symptoms

■ Differential to consider: polyneuropathy, brachial plexopathy, proximal median mononeuropathy, cervical radiculopathy, intracranial pathology, myofascial pain syndrome

■ Diagnostic testing: Electrodiagnostic testing to confirm, quantify, and rule out other neurological diagnoses in the differential; lab or imaging testing as appropriate if medical/surgical etiology suspected (e.g., pregnancy, thyroid disease, amyloidosis, malignancy, trauma, etc.)

THE REHABILITATION PROGRAM

Early identification and education about the etiology and prevention of progression are crucial first steps in the management of CTS. Most conservative interventions found in the literature do have some positive effect on short-term reduction of symptoms as compared to no treatment at all. There is no definitive consensus regarding the best practice for conservative interventions. Treatment choice is often determined by cost, convenience, time, severity of symptoms, and the treatment prescriber and provider. Because nerve compression symptoms can be altered by wrist position, external pressures, load applied to structures within the carpal tunnel, and vibration, these principles should guide treatment planning (2). Ideally the prescribing physician should refer to an occupational or physical therapist who has met the requirements to become a certified hand therapist (CHT).

Therapeutic Modalities

Studies on the benefits of therapeutic modalities vary in conclusions, design limitations, and selection bias (3). Those cited include ultrasound, iontophoresis, and low-level laser. There is no conclusive evidence to support any specific frequency or intensity for delivery of ultrasound.

In one study, the use of ultrasound over the carpal tunnel for 15 minutes per session at 1MHz, 1.0 w/cm^2 and a 1:4 duty cycle (20%) for 15 treatments over 3 weeks was found to be effective in decreasing symptoms and increasing pinch strength (4). Iontophoresis with dexamethasone sodium phosphate was found to improve symptoms but was not as effective at 2 and 8 weeks as compared to corticosteroid injections (5). Low-level laser therapy (LLLT) studies present mixed results and some of these studies investigated LLLT in combination with other modalities, for example, splinting (6–9). Another modality that has recently gained some popularity but requires well designed randomized controlled trials to confirm its effectiveness is a carpal ligament traction device that can be used at home (10). Generally, we do not provide modalities unless the patient has not responded to splinting and is not a candidate for surgery; in this situation, we may trial ultrasound and/or low-level laser. Our clinical experience has shown LLLT to benefit some patients when used in combination with patient education and therapeutic exercise.

Manual Therapy

Manual therapy techniques of carpal bone manipulation and flexor retinaculum stretching were found to reduce pain greater than no treatment (3). Massage therapy studies of a number of different techniques including self massage (11) and targeted massage (2,12) are of variable quality. We believe close communication between the prescriber and the therapist is crucial in deciding which manual techniques the therapist is trained for and comfortable providing. In certain situations, these may be included as an adjunct treatment by trained clinicians, although evidence is limited.

Therapeutic Exercises

In addition to pain and sensory changes, the patient may also present with decreased active range of motion (AROM) in the digits, poor flexibility of the long finger flexors as well as thenar muscle atrophy and weakness. Decreased median nerve mobility with CTS has been observed using diagnostic ultrasound (13) possibly due to adherence to the flexor retinaculum, which is not a surprising finding noted by surgeons during open carpal tunnel release. We use median nerve and flexor tendon gliding to improve nerve mobility and tendon excursion

(14,15). Median nerve gliding with forearm supination has been suggested to provide greatest nerve excursion (16) (Figures 17.1 and 17.2). If median nerve symptoms increase with nerve gliding, then the exercise should not be performed to the degree of symptom reproduction; working in a range that does not reproduce symptoms may provide some benefit. Tendon gliding promotes extrinsic flexor tendon excursion at the wrist-palm level (2,8). Note that carpal tunnel incursion by lumbrical muscles during finger flexion (17) and by extrinsic flexor muscles during a combination of finger flexion and wrist extension may contribute to CTS symptoms. One author recommends avoiding AROM and strengthening exercises that promote repetitive flexion (hand balls, grippers, putty) as they increase pressure in the carpal tunnel and suggests instead the use of isometric strengthening of the affected muscles (2). Strengthening should be implemented in some form with monitoring of symptoms, if exacerbated, then modification to exercises should be made to optimize the strengthening program.

Specialized Techniques

Although there are no published studies citing the effectiveness of taping techniques to reduce CTS symptoms, we have noted some benefit using the Kinesio taping® method, which is believed to target receptors in the somatosensory system to reduce pain and decrease inflammation by facilitating lymphatic drainage. It can be used to extend the benefits of manual techniques performed during treatment. Other specialized techniques such as joint protection and ergonomic corrections will be discussed in greater detail.

The importance of joint protection and ergonomics cannot be over emphasized. While splinting plays a passive role, effective symptom relief and/or prevention must include the patient's active participation in optimizing positioning and ergonomics to decrease mechanical stress and symptoms during daily tasks and activities. The prescriber should emphasize the importance of such active participation, and analysis, and even obtain a verbalized commitment from the patient at the time of diagnosis. The occupational therapist's professional training in task/activity analysis, along with activity-based treatment interventions, enables the patient to learn problem solving skills and practice compensatory strategies for daily tasks and activities in areas including activities of daily living (ADL), instrumental activities of daily living (iADL), work, sports, and leisure. Although there is a vast fund of information about CTS available online, there is no substitute for face-to-face assessment and instruction.

The patient should be counseled in general principles of joint protection and ergonomics for CTS including maintenance of a neutral wrist position and avoiding wrist movements that may cause pain and numbness, extreme end ranges (with and without resistance), repetitive gripping or fisting motions, and tasks or tools that expose the nerve to vibration (e.g., power tools).

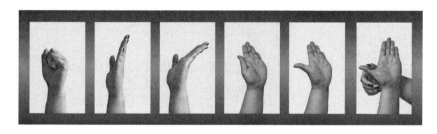

FIGURE 17.1: Median nerve gliding, with positions from left to right numbered 1 through 6.

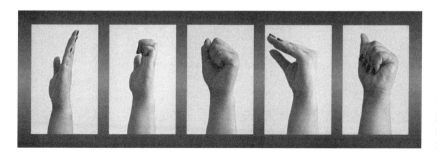

FIGURE 17.2: Tendon gliding, with positions from left to right named straight, hook, fist, table top, and long fist.

Supportive Devices

The literature presents evidence for symptom relief with splinting in a wrist *neutral* position during sleep, during tasks and activities that increase symptoms, and all the time. The recommended position ranges from 2° to 9° of wrist extension and 2° to 6° of ulnar deviation (2). This position decreases the pressure on the median nerve and rests inflamed tendons, the exacerbation of which is contributed to by nocturnal wrist postures. In addition to nightwear, the splint should be worn during tasks and activities (e.g., lawn mowing, driving, grocery shopping) that cause excessive wrist movement, repetitive movements, pain, and numbness in the involved extremity, in order to maintain a wrist neutral position. Splint types are customized thermoplastic or prefabricated: dorsal-based, circumferential, or volar-based.

Dorsal-based splints, usually prefabricated, have the advantage of a neutral wrist position while allowing greater sensory input on the volar surface as well as digit movement. Because only straps cross the volar surface, there is less support allowing some wrist flexion during wear. These splints should be considered when the volar surface is required to be unencumbered during occupational tasks and activities and/or when other volar pathologies are present, for example, scars, skin conditions, hypersensitivity.

Circumferential splints (prefabricated soft fabric wrist cock-up with metal stays of varying forearm length) are the most frequently used splints for CTS (Figure 17.3). They provide some compression and greater support than the dorsal-based splints. It is important that the splint be provided by a clinician who understands the condition and can provide education on relevant splinting concepts. Most prefabricated wrist cock-up splints are manufactured with 20° to 30° of wrist extension. In order to place the wrist in neutral, the stay(s) must be adjusted to attain neutral position. Although there are concerns raised that prefabricated splints do not adequately facilitate a wrist neutral position, compliance will not be achieved unless the patient feels comfortable wearing it. The thought of restricting the hand(s) at night may create

patient anxiety leading to noncompliance. Therefore, the patient's history and activity level may necessitate the use of a shorter forearm-based, lighter weight splint to improve compliance.

In our opinion, volar-based splints, usually thermoplastic with or without metacarpophalangeal (MCP) blocking, provide the most wrist support and reduction in wrist movement (Figure 17.4). The forearm-based thermoplastic splint is heated and molded to the patient's forearm, wrist, and hand, resulting in a custom fit. These splints appear to restrict wrist movement and rest the wrist more effectively than the others. Compared with prefabricated splints, fabrication of thermoplastic splints requires specialized training and increased time for fitting and adjustment. Those who have high activity demands in their daily schedules may not be agreeable to thermoplastic splint wear. The thermoplastic splint should be considered with severe cases of CTS, in patients who are not responding to prefabricated splinting, and/or those who have activity demands that would allow compliance.

Home Exercise Program

The home exercise program (HEP) includes splinting, ROM, and joint protection/ergonomics to reduce stress on the structures within the carpal tunnel. It may also include isometric strengthening of the finger flexors and thenar muscles, and tendon and neural glides.

A prefabricated splint in a wrist neutral position is issued for night wear and during activities that cause stress on the wrist. (If the prefabricated splint does not provide

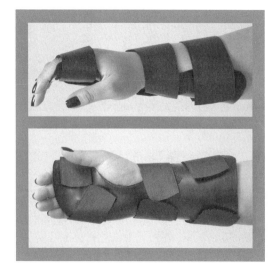

FIGURE 17.4: A custom MCP blocking splint.

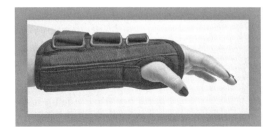

FIGURE 17.3: A prefabricated splint.

relief, a volar-based custom thermoplastic splint with MCP blocking can be trialed). AROM of tendon gliding and median nerve gliding are provided with repetitions and frequency dependent upon severity of ROM deficits. Incorporation of joint protection and ergonomics should be practiced diligently during daily activities. In order to protect from injury, visual cues should be used if a sensory deficit in the median nerve distribution is present.

SUMMARY

After meticulous history, physical examination, and electrodiagnosis has confirmed the clinical diagnosis of CTS, patients should be encouraged to look at how they can optimize their physical habits, ergonomics, and daily activities to avoid compressing the median nerve at the wrist. After such education, management techniques should include splinting in a neutral position and a HEP of tendon and nerve gliding techniques. Therapists may also provide adjunctive treatments with ultrasound, laser, and manual techniques

SAMPLE CASE

A 56-year-old chronically diabetic male presents to an outpatient clinic with bilateral hand numbness, tingling, and pain progressively worsening over the past 3 months. He reports being awakened by the symptoms nightly, dropping his coffee mug occasionally, and difficulty with buttoning his shirt. He has had very minimal but similar symptoms in his feet for many years. He denies neck pain, recent trauma, incontinence, dysarthria, dysphagia, or any constitutional symptoms. He has recently retired and works on home improvement projects. Examination reveals normal neurological examination except for decreased light touch sensation in all of his fingers. Carpal compression reproduces his symptoms in both hands. All other provocative tests are negative. He undergoes electrodiagnostic testing which confirms and quantifies the diagnosis of moderate median neuropathy consistent with the clinical diagnosis of CTS without evidence of a concomitant peripheral polyneuropathy.

 SAMPLE THERAPY PRESCRIPTION

Discipline: Occupational therapy.

Diagnosis: Bilateral CTS.

Precautions: Universal; avoid excessive wrist flexion/ extension and repetitive finger flexion exercises.

Frequency of visits: 1 to 2 visits.

Duration of treatment: 1 to 2 visits.

Treatment:

1. *Modalities:* none

2. *Manual therapy:* trial of carpal bone manipulation and flexor retinaculum stretching

3. *Therapeutic exercise:*
   tendon and nerve gliding techniques
   isometric strengthening of finger flexors/thenar muscles if weakness present
   AVOID strengthening with repetitive flexion (hand balls, grippers, putty)

4. *ADL/iADLs:*
   activity analysis to identify exacerbating factors and teach problem solving skills and compensatory strategies
   identify areas of ADL/iADL impairment
   focus on dressing, home improvement activities
   provide assistive devices as appropriate

5. *Supportive devices:*
   fit and dispense appropriate prefabricated bilateral carpal tunnel splints
   consider custom-molded thermoplastic splint if patient does not tolerate prefabricated splints

6. *Patient education:*
   teach tendon and nerve gliding techniques
   joint protection techniques
   educate in proper ergonomics, maintaining neutral wrist position
   educate and provide handouts for HEP

Goals: Decrease pain/paresthesias, educate effective HEP, provision of appropriate splinting, education to prevent re-exacerbation, optimizing positioning and ergonomics.

Reevaluation: In 4 weeks by referring physician.

REFERENCES

1. Dumitru D. Focal peripheral neuropathies. In: Dumitru D, ed. *Electrodiagnostic Medicine*. Philadelphia, PA: Hanley & Belfus; 1995:1043–1126.

2. Evan R. Therapist's management of carpal tunnel syndrome: a practical approach. In: Osterman AL, Skirven TM, Fedorczyk JM, Amadio PC, eds. *Rehabilitation of the Hand and Upper Extremity*. Philadelphia, PA: Elsevier; 2011:666–677.

3. O'Connor D, Shawn CM, Massy-Westropp N. Non-surgical treatment (other than steroid injection) for carpal tunnel syndrome. *Cochrane Database Syst Rev*. 2003 ;(1):CD003219.

4. Bakhtiary AH, Rashidy-Pour A. Ultrasound and laser therapy in the treatment of carpal tunnel syndrome. *Aust J Physiother*. 2004;50(3):147–151.

5. Gökoğlu F, Fndkoğlu G, Yorgancoğlu ZR, Okumus M, Ceceli E, Kocaoğlu S. Evaluation of iontophoresis and local corticosteroid injection in the treatment of carpal tunnel syndrome. *Am J Phys Med Rehabil*. 2005;84(2):92–96.

6. Branco K, Naeser MA. Carpal tunnel syndrome: clinical outcome after low-level laser acupuncture, microamps transcutaneous electrical nerve stimulation, and other alternative therapies an open protocol study. *J Altern Complement Med*. 1999;5(1):5–26.

7. Irvine J, Chong SL, Amirjani N, Chan KM. Double-blind randomized controlled trial of low-level laser therapy in carpal tunnel syndrome. *Muscle Nerve*. 2004;30(2):182–187.

8. Muller M, Tsui D, Schnurr R, Biddulph-Deisroth L, Hard J, MacDermid JC. Effectiveness of hand therapy interventions in primary management of carpal tunnel syndrome: a systematic review. *J Hand Ther*. 2004;17(2):210–228.

9. Dincer UE, Cakar E, Kiralp MZ, Kilac H, Dursun H. The effectiveness of conservative treatments of carpal tunnel syndrome: splinting, ultrasound, and low-level laser therapies. *Photomed Laser Surg*. 2009;27(1):119–125.

10. Porrata H, Porrata A, Sosner J. New carpal ligament traction device for the treatment of carpal tunnel syndrome unresponsive to conservative therapy. *J Hand Ther*. 2007;20(1):20–7; quiz 28.

11. Madenci E, Altindag O, Koca I, Yilmaz M, Gur A. Reliability and efficacy of the new massage technique on the treatment in the patients with carpal tunnel syndrome. *Rheumatol Int*. 2011 [published online ahead of print].

12. Moraska A, Chandler C, Edmiston-Schaetzel A, Franklin G, Calenda EL, Enebo B. Comparison of a targeted and general massage protocol on strength, function, and symptoms associated with carpal tunnel syndrome: a randomized pilot study. *J Altern Complement Med*. 2008;14(3):259–267.

13. Nakamichi K, Tachibana S. Restricted motion of the median nerve in carpal tunnel syndrome. *J Hand Surg Br*. 1995;20(4):460–464.

14. Wehbe MA, Hunter JM. Flexor tendon gliding in the hand. Part II. Differential gliding. *J Hand Surg Am*. 1985;10(4):575–579.

15. Akalin E, El O, Senocak O, et al. Treatment of carpal tunnel syndrome with nerve and tendon gliding exercises. *Am J Phys Med Rehabil*. 2002;81(2):108–113.

16. Echigo A, Aoki M, Ishiai S, et al. The excursion of the median nerve during nerve gliding exercise: an observation with high-resolution ultrasonography. *J Hand Ther*. 2008;21(3):221–227; quiz 228.

17. Cobb TK, An KN, Cooney WP, Berger RA. Lumbrical muscle incursion into the carpal tunnel during fingerflexion. *J Hand Surg Br*. 1994;19(4):434–438.

Carpometacarpal Osteoarthritis

Neil N. Jasey, Jiaxin Tran, and Stacia Dyer

INTRODUCTION

Carpometacarpal (CMC) joints are articulations between metacarpal and the distal row of carpal bones in the hand. Osteoarthritis in any and all of these five joints is possible, but that of the thumb is most common. The first CMC joint, or thumb joint, is a unique saddle joint that allows for movement in three planes and thus is predisposed to degenerative changes. The thumb CMC is in fact the second most frequently involved arthritic joint in the hand, after distal interphalangeal joints. Prevelance in women is twice that of men and is up to 25% prevelant in postmenopausal females. (1). Repetitive activity, previous injury, and general joint laxity contribute to development of primary osteoarthritis. Secondary causes include: rheumatoid/psoriatic arthritis, gout, collagen vascular diseases, infection, and Lyme disease. Patients usually complain of constant pain localized to the dorsum of the wrist and thumb. Pain is worse with activity and improves with rest, but a dull ache may persist through the night. Some also complain of a grating sensation in the joint with movement. Both pinch and grip strength decrease with time and compromise essential daily activities (e.g., writing, jar opening, and cup holding).

CMC osteoarthritis (OA) is classified into four radiographical stages, which has to correlate with physical examination (2). Stage I reveals joint space widening with mild dorso-radial subluxation of metacarpal base over the trapezium (i.e., "shoulder sign"). Clinical signs are limited to mild effusion and ligament laxity. Stage II is marked by the presence of a small osteophyte (<2 mm) and/or moderate subluxation (at least 1/3 of the metacarpal base). Minimal crepitus can be appreciated on exam. Stage III may include subchondral sclerosis/cyst and large osteophyte (>2 mm) formation, significant subluxation (>1/3 of the metacarpal base), and joint space narrowing. Even so, gross anatomical change is apparent in less than one-third of patients. Finally, stage IV classification includes definitive scaphotrapezial involvement and painless immobilization of the first CMC joint on exam. First web space contracture from thumb adduction and hyperextension deformity of metacarpophalangeal (MCP) joint can be observed at this point. A new stage V has been suggested to categorize pantrapczial arthritis (3).

Key elements of the physical examination include inspection, palpation, range of motion (ROM) and joint stability testing for all joints of both hands. Make note of the patient's grip/pinch strength. Palpate any joint deformities. the dorsolateral and palmar aspects of the thumb base to elicit tenderness. Perform the grind test by grasping the thumb below the MCP joint and applying a gentle axial load during passive rotation. This test is positive if it produces pain; it has a sensitivity of 42% and specificity of 80% (4). Differential diagnoses to evaluate for include: carpal tunnel syndrome, trigger thumb, and tenosynovitis, especially of the first dorsal compartment. Order CMC joint x-ray (Bett's view) as a standard practice to confirm and stage the disease (15), which is then used to plan further management including the comprehensive rehabilitation program.

CARPOMETACARPAL OSTEOARTHRITIS

- Thumb CMC osteoarthritis is a common condition, particularly in postmenopausal women

- It can result in debilitating pain and impaired function due to loss of both pinch and grip strength

- Grind test may reproduce pain, with or without crepitus, and supports the diagnosis of CMC osteoarthritis

- X-ray of CMC joint is a standard order to stage the disease (stage I–IV) and guide rehabilitation program

- Carpal tunnel syndrome and tenosynovitis are commonly associated pathology

THE REHABILITATION PROGRAM

Conservative management of CMC osteoarthritis has been shown to provide long-term relief in the early stages (namely, stages I and II) (5). The main goals of this program include pain management, improved thumb function, activity modification, and restoration of dynamic stability. It is important to not only treat the symptoms but also to empower patients with the knowledge of the disease to minimize impairments. The five phases of rehabilitation seen throughout this book are applied to this condition as well.

Therapeutic Modalities

In the acute phase of this condition, patients generally experience an inflammatory response and cryotherapy options may be considered. In later phases, stiffness and functional deficit are the primary issues. Modalities can always be used for some symptomatic relief. There is additional evidence supporting the use of thermotherapy to improve grip strength and decrease pain (6). Moist hot wraps, paraffin, and fluidotherapy are common superficial heat modalities. The addition of topical analgesic (e.g., capsaicin, menthol, eucalyptus oil, camphor, and methyl salicylate) to paraffin bath can enhance its effect (7). The efficacy of deep heat modalities (e.g., ultrasound) and low level laser therapy have not been established. Ice may have little role in chronic management of CMC osteoarthritis because no study investigated the role of cryotherapy in hand osteoarthritis (8).

Manual Therapy

Immobilization, combined with local inflammation, predisposes the development of contracture. This sequelae is detrimental in the hands because a host of fine motor skills are lost. Careful soft tissues mobilization can help increase ROM by guiding affected collagen fibers to unfold and realign (9). Joint mobilization aims to relieve pain and improve ROM. The latter is accomplished by stretching connective tissues, which are then stimulated to lengthen through remodeling. There is evidence suggesting the benefit of joint mobilization specifically at the MCP (10).

Therapeutic Exercise

It is important to focus on muscle reeducation before strengthening, as the abnormal postures of "overuse" must be unlearned (i.e., "blackberry thumb" causing overused adductor). Focus should begin with closed chain and isometric exercise of the following muscles:

- First dorsal interosseous (can be useful with patients who experience instability)
- Abductor pollicis brevis and longus (Figure 18.1)
- Opponens pollicis (Figure 18.2)
- Flexor pollicis brevis (Figure 18.3)
- Extensor pollicis brevis (Figure 18.4)

A strengthening program is most appropriate in the early stages (11). A markedly unstable or inflamed joint may benefit more initially from rest, splint, and anti-inflammatory medications. Caution should also be taken to avoid isolated strengthening of extensor pollicis longus, which may promote CMC subluxation via its lateral rotation and adduction forces.

Supportive Devices

Prefabricated splints as well as custom-made short opponens splints play a role in pain relief and creating stability to the

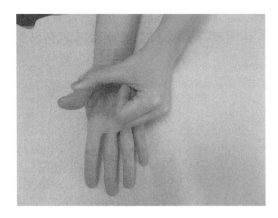

FIGURE 18.1: Abduction of the thumb.

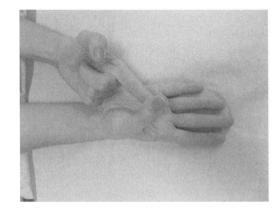

FIGURE 18.2: Opposition of the thumb.

CMC joint. There are various designs that can be purchased or custom-made by a hand therapist. Patient preference, comfort, and lifestyle can contribute to the right choice for the patient. The splint should include the CMC joint in palmar abduction, the metacarpophalangeal joint in 30° of flexion, and interphalangeal joint left free. Moulten showed that 30° of metacarpophalangeal flexion moves the contact area of the trapezium more dorsally, unloading the volar articular surface (12) (see Figures 18.5 and 18.6).

Patient Education

Activity modification is a key element of nonoperative management of CMC osteoarthritis (13). Education in avoidance of aggravating activities allows patients to reflect on their habits and make corrections according to joint protection techniques. The following guidelines can direct the patient:

– Avoid tight pinching, especially the lateral pinch
– Use the following adaptive equipment, in the appropriate patient, to prevent cumulative trauma:
    • Built-up or clip-on handles for various objects (e.g., spoon and pen)—large handle to reduce strain on joints
    • Handle extender or T turning handle—fit over doorknobs and keys for easy grasp and provide leverage
    • Modified jar opener—promote easy grip to jar tops
    • Tab grabber—open twist and pop tops
    • Long loop scissors—self-opening scissors that close with MCP flexion
    • Rocking T knife–semicircular blade that cut with rocking motion
    • Buttonhook—wire loop that guides button through button hole
    • Zipper pull—ring snap onto zipper to extend the pull tab
    • Electronic appliances (e.g., can opener)
– Adhere to a proper splinting schedule to maximize effectiveness and minimize atrophy
– Improve penmanship posture. Encourage metacarpal abduction versus adduction
– Avoid carrying, lifting, and using heavy objects
– Use lightweight utensils and cookware

A prior randomized trial has shown that when the patient is successful at following these recommendations, improved grip strength and pain relief is maintained at one year follow up (14).

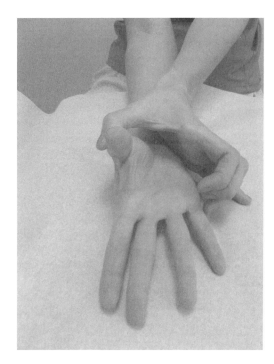

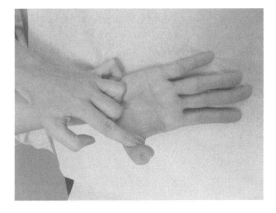

FIGURE 18.3: Flexion of the thumb.

FIGURE 18.4: Extension of the thumb.

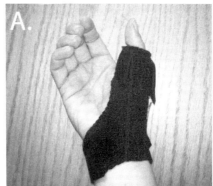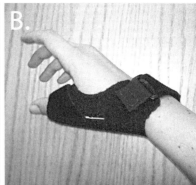

FIGURE 18.5: Custom-made short opponens splint.

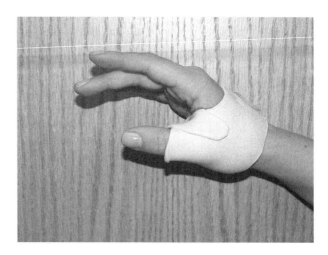

FIGURE 18.6: Prefabricated short opponens splint.

SUMMARY

CMC osteoarthritis is a common site for osteoarthritis and occurs more frequently in females than males. It is often associated with stiffness in the thumb that lasts less than 30 minutes in the early stages. In the later stages, pain occurs with activity and is relieved by rest. Joint swelling, warmth, and deformity can occur as arthritis progresses and difficulty with grip strength can develop. Cryotherapy can help in the acute phase and thermotherapy provides beneficial relief of symptoms as the disease process progresses. X-ray of the CMC joint is the gold standard for staging degeneration of the CMC joint and staging helps to guide further management including the rehabilitation program. Therapy to strengthen around the joint, bracing, and nonsteroidal anti-inflammatory drugs use can often provide symptomatic benefit. Emphases on joint protection and ergonomic changes in patient education are keys to preventing disease progression. Concomitant carpal tunnel syndrome and tenosynovitis may need to be ruled out as possible sources of weakness or alternative diagnoses.

SAMPLE CASE

A 50-year-old right-hand-dominant female has pain at the base of the right thumb. The pain is worse when writing on the blackboard. There is no history of trauma. She is a college professor and enjoys knitting at home. Past medical history (PMH), past surgical history (PSH), and review of systems (ROS) are unremarkable. Visual inspection of the affected hand is notable for mild tenderness and edema at the thenar eminence. The grind test reproduces the patient's pain along with a grating sensation. The rest of the physical examination is unremarkable. X-ray reveals a small trapezium osteophyte suggesting mild osteoarthrosis.

SAMPLE THERAPY PRESCRIPTION

Discipline: Occupational therapy.

Diagnosis: First CMC osteoarthritis of the right hand.

Precautions: Skin, avoid MCP hyperextensions.

Frequency of visits: 2 sessions per week.

Duration of treatment: 4 weeks.

Treatment:

1. *Modalities:* paraffin, fluidotherapy, and cryotherapy

2. *Manual therapy:* soft tissue and joint mobilizations, as needed to improve joint mobility

3. *Therapeutic exercise:* active/active assisted/passive range of motion A/AA/PROM exercise to focus on restoration of muscular balance and gentle strengthening exercises to improve stability of the thumb

4. *Specialized treatments:* assess and dispense thumb splint and adaptive equipment as needed

5. *Patient education:* home exercise program (HEP) and activity modifications

Goals: Decrease pain and swelling; improve strength and ROM, prevent contracture, restore previous functional level.

Reevaluation: in 4 weeks by referring physician.

REFERENCES

1. Armstrong AL, Hunter JB, Davis TR. The prevalence of degenerative arthritis of the base of the thumb in postmenopausal women. *J Hand Surg Br.* 1994;19:340–341.
2. Eaton RG, Glickel SZ. Trapeziometacarpal osteoarthritis. Staging as a rationale for treatment. *Hand Clin.* 1987;3(4):455–471.
3. Tomaino MM, King J, Leit M. Thumb basal joint arthritis. In: Green DP, Hotchkiss RN, Pederson WC, et al. eds. *Green's Operative Hand Surgery*, 5th ed. New York, NY: Churchill Livingstone; 2005:461–485.
4. Merritt MM, Roddey TS, Costello C, Olson S. Diagnostic value of clinical grind test for carpometacarpal osteoarthritis of the thumb. *J Hand Ther.* 2010;23(3):261–267.
5. Day CS, Gelberman R, Patel AA, Vogt MT, Ditsios K, Boyer MI. Basal joint osteoarthritis of the thumb: a prospective trial of steroid injection and splinting. *J Hand Surg Am.* 2004;29:247–251.
6. Valdes K, Marik T. A systematic review of conservative interventions for osteoarthritis of the hand. *J Hand Ther.* 2010;23(4):334-350; quiz 351.
7. Myer JW, Johnson AW, Mitchell UH, Measom GJ, Fellingham GW. Topical analgesic added to paraffin enhances paraffin bath treatment of individuals with hand osteoarthritis. *Disabil Rehabil.* 2011;33(6):467–474.
8. Brosseau L, Yonge KA, Robinson V, et al. Thermotherapy for treatment of osteoarthritis. *Cochrane Database Syst Rev.* 2003;(4):CD004522. Review.
9. Glasgow C, Tooth LR, Fleming J. Mobilizing the stiff hand: combining theory and evidence to improve clinical outcomes. *J Hand Ther.* 2010;23(4):392–400; quiz 401.
10. Ring D, Simmons BP, Hayes M. Continuous passive motion following metacarpalphalangeal joint arthroplasty. *J Hand Surg.* 1998;23A:505–511.
11. Neumann DA, Bielefeld T. The carpometacarpal joint of the thumb: stability, deformity, and therapeutic intervention. *J Orthop Sports Phys Ther.* 2003;33(7):386–399.
12. Moulton MJ, Parentis MA, Kelly MJ, Jacobs C, Naidu SH, Pellegrini VD Jr. Influence of metacarpophalangeal joint position on basal joint-loading in the thumb. *J Bone Joint Surg Am.* 2001;83-A(5):709–716.
13. Yao J, Park MJ. Early treatment of degenerative arthritis of the thumb carpometacarpal joint. *Hand Clin.* 2008;24(3):251–261, v–vi.
14. Hammond A, Freeman K. One-year outcomes of a randomized controlled trial of an educational-behavioural joint protection programme for people with rheumatoid arthritis. *Rheumatology (Oxford).* 2001;40(9):1044–1051.
15. Dela Rosa TL, Vance MC, Stern PJ. Radiographic optimization of the Eaton classification. *J Hand Surg Br.* 2004;29(2):173-177.

Hip Osteoarthritis

Ian Wendel, Todd Stitik, Prathap Jayaram, and Kambiz Nooryani

INTRODUCTION

Osteoarthritis (OA) is a chronic condition that affects synovial joints throughout the body. Primary OA of the hip region is seen predominately in older individuals and is believed to be the result of cumulative biomechanical stresses associated with aging. However, it may occur in younger populations as a result of secondary causes including trauma, osteonecrosis, previous joint infection, femoroacetabular impingement (FAI), and childhood conditions including developmental hip dysplasia, Legg-Calvé-Perthes, and slipped capital femoral epiphysis. In people 55 years or older, the prevalence of radiographic OA changes of the hip ranges from 1% to 25%, with Caucasians having the highest prevalence and Blacks having the lowest prevalence (1).

The hip joint, consisting of the articulation of the pelvic acetabulum with the femoral head, is a major weight bearing joint and thus is particularly prone to OA. Hyaline cartilage produced by chondrocytes lines the femoral head and the acetabulum. Synovial fluid freely flows within the hip joint acting as a lubricant and a shock absorber. The labrum, a fibrocartilaginous structure, rests within the acetabulum to act as a shock absorber and adds stability to the joint by adding depth to the socket. The joint capsule consists of focal thickenings, namely the iliofemoral, pubofemoral, and ischiofemoral ligaments. The aforementioned causes of hip OA degrade hyaline cartilage leading to a lack of joint integrity and the secondary developments of osteophytes. A patient with hip OA classically presents with groin pain. Anterior thigh pain is also commonly reported and may radiate as far down as the knee and typically worsens over time. Various additional or alternative pain patterns from intra-articular hip pathology have also been documented and include referral to the buttocks, distally down the lower limb, and at times all the way to the foot (2), as well as pain to the lateral hip, anterior, posterior, and lateral thigh, and low back (3). Other commonly reported symptoms include limping and morning stiffness that last less than 30 minutes and improve with movement.

Key elements of the physical examination include an assessment of hip range of motion (ROM), provocative maneuvers, and gait analysis. Hip ROM may reveal restricted and painful internal rotation, which is considered to be one of the earliest signs of hip OA. Gait is often antalgic. Provocative maneuvers, including the flexion abduction and external rotation (FAbER) test (Figure 19.1), Stinchfield's test (Figure 19.2), the hip scouring test, the log roll test (Figure 19.3), the anvil test, and the internal rotation over pressure (IROP) test, may be positive in the presence of hip OA. The impingement test for femoral-acetabular impingement (FAI) may also be positive if FAI is present, as well as with other intra-articular pathologies including OA (see Table 19.1).

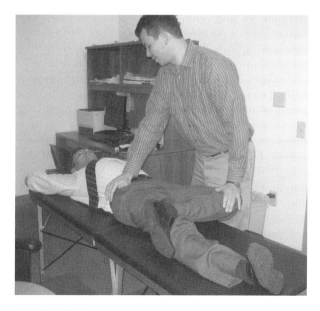

FIGURE 19.1: FAbER physical examination maneuver.

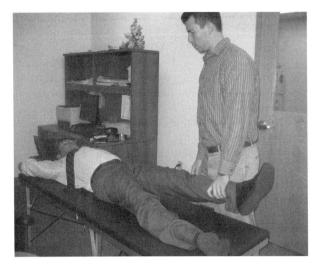

FIGURE 19.2: Stinchfield's physical examination maneuver.

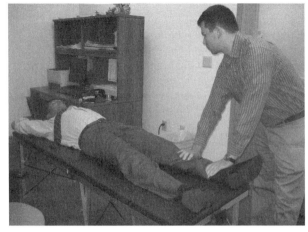

FIGURE 19.3: Log roll test physical examination maneuver.

TABLE 19.1: Physical Exam Maneuvers for Hip OA

Test	Description	Positive Findings
FAbER (Patrick's) (Figure 19.1)	The examiner flexes, abducts, and externally rotates the patient's leg and rests the ipsilateral ankle of the leg on the contralateral, stationary thigh or knee. The examiner then compresses posteriorly on the ipsilateral knee while stabilizing contralateral ASIS	Pain in the groin of the ipsilateral hip joint with posterior compression of the ipsilateral knee is indicative of intra-articular hip pathology and possible OA at the hip, while contralateral buttock pain signifies sacroiliac (SI) joint pathology
Stinchfield's (Figure 19.2)	The patient is in the supine position and flexes a straight leg with the knee extended and the examiner resists hip flexion at 20° to 30°	Ipsilateral pain in the hip region suggests intra-articular hip pathology
Hip scouring test	The patient is in the supine position and the examiner passively flexes the hip and knee of the ipsilateral leg. The examiner then applies a posterior force while internally and externally rotating the leg at multiple angles of flexion	Ipsilateral pain at the hip region suggests intra-articular hip pathology
Log roll test (Figure 19.3)	The patient is in the supine position with the knee extended while the examiner internally and externally rotates the entire leg generally by grasping the ankle	Ipsilateral pain in the hip region suggests intra-articular hip pathology, as well as synovitis. Pain with minimal rotation may be indicative of a septic hip joint or significant trauma
Internal rotation over pressure	The patient is in the supine position with the examiner on the side of the leg being tested. The examiner flexes the ipsilateral hip and knee to 90° and internally rotates this leg (rotating the distal leg more laterally) while applying a gentle lateral pressure to this leg and stabilizing the contralateral ASIS.	Ipsilateral pain in the hip region suggests intra-articular hip pathology
*Impingement test for FAI	The patient is in the supine position with the examiner on the side of the leg being tested. The examiner flexes the ipsilateral hip maximally and ipsilateral knee to 90° and internally rotates this leg (rotating the distal leg more laterally) and adducts the hip joint while stabilizing the contralateral ASIS	Ipsilateral pain at the hip region suggests intra-articular hip pathology. In younger, active individuals, this test may be indicative of FAI

*Variations of the classic hip impingement test have been described.

Maslowski et al conducted a study on the diagnostic validity of the FAbER, Stinchfield's, the scour, and the IROP tests. In their study, they found the IROP and the FAbER maneuvers to be the most sensitive and no one test to be considerably specific (4).

In addition to directly examining the hip, the kinetic chain concept must be kept in mind. Thus an examination of contiguous soft tissue, osseous and articular structures should be conducted to both rule out pathology from these regions as an alternative explanation for the symptoms and for the purposes of detecting biomechanical factors that might be contributing to symptomatic hip OA. For example, the degree of lumbar lordosis and pelvic tilt should be assessed since they can influence the effects of acetabular anteversion or retroversion and lead to altered force production at the hip joints.

The history and physical examination should be utilized to help rule out referred pain from the lumbosacral spine, sacro-iliac joint, knee pathology, entrapment neuropathies (including ilioinguinal, genitofemoral, lateral femoral cutaneous, and obturator neuropathy) as well as gastrointestinal, genital, and dermatologic conditions, which can cause pain similar to that of hip OA. If hip OA remains high within the differential diagnoses, the examiner should order imaging studies, especially a hip radiograph (often anterior posterior [AP] pelvis and frog-leg lateral), which in the presence of hip OA and depending upon its stage, may show one or more of the following: joint space narrowing, osteophytes, subchondral cysts, and subchondral sclerosis. If the diagnosis is still in question, an image-guided intra-articular hip injection can be done, which may be diagnostic and/or therapeutic depending upon if the injectate is only a local anesthetic or includes a corticosteroid preparation as well. When the diagnosis of hip OA is made by a thorough history, physical examination, imaging studies, and possibly a diagnostic injection, a conservative treatment plan should be initiated. This typically consists of pharmacologic interventions, therapeutic exercise, modalities, assistive devices, and adaptive equipment. If pain and/or functional limitations continue, intra-articular joint injections, if not already done, may be performed and surgical interventions (e.g., total joint arthroplasty) can subsequently be considered if needed.

THE REHABILITATION PROGRAM

A comprehensive rehabilitation program for hip OA should focus on flexibility, static and dynamic muscle

HIP OSTEOARTHRITIS

- Usually presents in older individuals as a result of cumulative biomechanical stresses

- Degradation of hyaline cartilage leads to a lack of joint integrity and osteophytes

- Key elements of the physical examination are the location of the pain, hip joint ROM, gait analysis, and provocative maneuvers that stress the hip joint and reproduce pain

- Radiographs can confirm the diagnosis and depending on the stage of OA commonly exhibit signs of radiographic OA, including joint space narrowing, osteophytes, subchondral cysts, and/or subchondral sclerosis

- Image-guided diagnostic intra-articular injections may be needed to confirm the diagnosis

strength, joint protection, pain reduction techniques, and patient education. Interestingly, it was once believed that offloading joints more effectively treated OA. However, Byers has shown that joint movement and loading allows for proper nutrition of cartilage through a process called imbibition (5). The following are a few examples of some studies demonstrating that improved flexibility and muscle strength are efficacious in improving symptoms associated with hip OA.

Simkin showed that continuous passive motion machines used at the hip joint improved visual analog scores, Sickness Impact Profiles, self-selected walking speed, and decreased amount of pain medications required by some patients (6). In another study, Tak et al compared an exercise group and a standard care group. The exercise group incorporated pulleys, a Bowflex™, and walking on a treadmill into an 8-week program that the standard care group did not. They found that the exercise group had less pain at 3 month follow up compared with the standard care group (7).

Establishing a proper home exercise program (HEP) and educating patients on weight loss and joint protection are likely essential to improving outcomes. Increasing total body weight by as little as 10% has been shown to significantly increase the compressive forces at the hip (8). One of the best ways to offload the hip joint besides weight loss is the use of a cane, typically held in the hand opposite the involved hip. Other assistive walking devices (e.g., walker) may be considered, especially if the patient's balance is significantly impaired. Additionally, important adaptive equipment examples include long-handled reachers and elevated toilet seats, which limit extreme hip flexion.

The therapeutic exercise approach should follow the phases of rehabilitation discussed throughout this book, with a few additional caveats. If an inflammatory flare of hip OA is present (e.g., intra-articular hip effusion as seen on ultrasound), then a patient may need to downgrade the activity level. Gentle ROM, stretching, cryotherapy, and isometric strengthening exercises may be utilized during the acute phase, while isotonic strengthening and aerobic exercise involving the lower limbs should be avoided. Serial ultrasound examinations and the possible judicious use of intra-articular corticosteroid injections can be helpful in detecting and treating the presence of inflammation. Once out of the acute phase, the rehabilitation program may progress to restore ROM, strength, balance, and proprioception. Aerobic conditioning exercises are also very important and, as always, transition to an independent HEP for maintenance of functional gains is of utmost importance. In addition to exercises focusing directly on the hip girdle, other body regions may need to be targeted if pathology exists that is negatively impacting hip joint function as per the kinetic chain concept (a detailed discussion of this is beyond the scope of this chapter).

Therapeutic Modalities

Therapeutic modalities used to treat symptoms of hip OA can include thermotherapy, cryotherapy, and electrical stimulation; however, there is a lack of clinical evidence suggesting improved outcomes with the adjunctive use of these modalities. As OA is a chronic condition, thermotherapy can be self-administered on an intermittent, ongoing basis since various forms of hot packs for home use exist. Thermotherapy can help to relieve chronic stiffness and may be used prior to ROM and stretching exercises. Many OA patients find thermotherapy beneficial as it allows for enhanced flexibility with stretching and works as an analgesic (9). The two thermotherapy modalities most used in a formal physical therapy setting include hydrocollator packs and therapeutic ultrasound. Studies examining outcomes of using hydrocollator packs for hip OA are nonexistent; however, there are

limited studies examining therapeutic ultrasound for this treatment. One such study found that in hip and knee OA, the addition of therapeutic ultrasound to exercise did not significantly improve pain over exercise alone (10). However, it is controversial in the current medical literature if benefit with the use of ultrasound at other joints is seen.

If an inflammatory flare is present, cryotherapy is theoretically preferable, although penetration down to the joint may not occur especially in patients with a high body mass index. Cryotherapy causes vasoconstriction, which limits edema and acts as an anti-inflammatory agent by reducing white blood cell counts and collagenase activity (11). The reduction in inflammation and edema can lead to substantial analgesia.

Electrical stimulation, consisting of pulsed electromagnetic field stimulation or transcutaneous electrical nerve stimulation (TENS) as part of a physical therapy program or self-administered, can also be used as a treatment modality. Theoretically, pulsed electrical stimulation should benefit hip OA patients as it is believed to down regulate articular cartilage turnover by maintaining articular cartilage's proteoglycan composition (12). On the contrary, two studies investigating electrical stimulation in OA patients showed that it was no more beneficial than placebo (13,14).

Manual Therapy

Currently, to our knowledge, there are no specific techniques of manual therapy solely used to treat pain or functional deficits associated with hip OA and very few studies that specifically address this issue. However, the results of one study by Hoeksma et al suggest that manual therapy for patients with hip OA is more beneficial with respect to general improvement and function than exercise therapy. In this study, manual therapy consisted of stretching of shortened muscles, traction, and a maneuver described as traction high velocity thrust technique (15). Furthermore, in the ongoing Management of Osteoarthritis (MOA) Trial, a larger scale trial which compared exercise therapy, manual therapy, and both, manual therapy interventions were tailored for individual patients (16). As patients with hip OA may have different dysfunctions (or restrictions, depending on the manual medicine philosophy), patients with hip OA should have the entire kinetic chain evaluated, especially the hip, knee, pelvis, sacrum, and lumbar spine. Gentler techniques, such as muscle energy or myofascial release may be better tolerated than high velocity low amplitude (HVLA) or other thrust techniques by the majority of older patients who suffer from hip OA.

Therapeutic Exercise

As is true of OA in general, most patients' symptoms from hip OA continually worsen over time. With this in mind, it is very important to initiate therapeutic exercise early in the disease course to maintain ROM, strength, and function. ROM exercises should be performed in all planes including hip abduction/adduction, flexion/extension, and circumduction. One example of this type of exercise is having a patient sit with his or her legs abducted and reach for his or her toes, while maintaining their lumbar lordosis, as this stretches both hip adductors and extensors. Just remember that flexibility exercises need to be individualized to patient tolerance and abilities to avoid exacerbating their pain.

With respect to strengthening, there is a relative paucity of literature in support of its benefits for hip OA compared to knee OA. The general concept is to strengthen hip girdle muscles. Strengthening exercises target hip abductors, adductors, flexors, extensors, and external/internal rotators. Hip abductors, for example the gluteus medius, is a particularly important muscle to strengthen (17). The lower gluteus maximus has also been demonstrated to atrophy with hip OA, whereas muscles like the tensor fascia lata (TFL) maintain muscle bulk and symmetry (18). Studies such as these help to tailor the strengthening program for maximum benefit in patients with hip OA. These isotonic exercises usually are performed in the supine, prone, and side lying positions with gravity used as resistance. As patients progress, ankle weights may be added. Isotonic strengthening exercises may also be performed in the standing position with the inclusion of ankle weights. In addition, similar exercises may be performed with resistance bands. Progression to functional, closed kinetic chain exercises will continue to challenge and strengthen targeted muscles with the appropriate exercises.

Before beginning a program of hip abductor muscle strengthening, one must consider muscle imbalances at the hip girdle. A commonly discussed problem is overactivity of the TFL and decreased activity of the glutei muscles, which may lead to abnormal loading of the hip joint (19). Therefore, it is reasonable to attempt neuromuscular reeducation exercises to correct muscular imbalances before proceeding with aggressive hip abductor strengthening.

Individuals with hip OA have demonstrated knee extensor weakness, in addition to hip girdle weakness (20,21). Knee extensor weakness combined with hip girdle weakness, especially of the hip extensors, can lead to significant functional impairments that include difficulty rising from a chair or climbing stairs. Therefore, the prescribed strengthening exercises should also target the quadriceps muscle.

Another functional impairment found in patients with lower limb OA, including hip OA, is decreased balance and a higher incidence of falls (22). Decreased balance may be attributable to proprioceptive deficits and decreased lower limb strength, including knee extensor weakness. Therefore, patients should eventually progress from strength training to phase IV rehabilitation exercises that include balance and proprioceptive training. Then the gains made in balance and proprioception should be incorporated into the final phase of rehabilitation, functional retraining.

It is also important for patients to partake in a low impact aerobic exercise program. This may include a walking, swimming, and/or a cycling program. Cycling may be particularly beneficial as patients are able to simultaneously work on their ROM and strength. Furthermore, it is thought that aerobic exercise promotes a release of endogenous endorphins leading to an analgesic effect (23).

If a patient is enrolled in a formal therapy program it is also important to continue with their therapeutic exercises at home, as in the setting of hip OA, all the gains made may easily be reversed with immobility and deconditioning.

Specialized Techniques

Aquatic therapy may be beneficial to patients suffering from OA, and it has been shown to improve physical activity levels, walk time, and aerobic conditioning (24). Aquatic therapy offloads weight at the hip joint through the properties of buoyancy, allowing for a reduction of pain during ROM, while providing multidirectional resistance to specific movements that leads to hip girdle strengthening.

Other more invasive specialized techniques include corticosteroid and hyaluronic acid injections, as these techniques are used by some physicians to treat pain and loss of ROM from hip OA. There is clinical evidence that supports their use, however this is less convincing for hyaluronic acid injections specific to hip OA (25,26).

Another specialized technique is prolotherapy. In prolotherapy, a sclerosing agent is used to shorten lax tissue, especially ligaments. Currently, there is a lack of literature specifically addressing hip OA; however, its benefit has been seen for knee and hand OA (27). Finally, injections of platelet rich plasma (PRP) and mesenchymal stem cells (MSCs) may become more popular in the future in an attempt to stimulate growth of degraded cartilage from OA. Currently, there are no trials investigating the efficacy of PRP on hip OA, however, a decrease in pain and an improvement in function has been shown with PRP injections for the treatment of knee OA (28–30). Additionally, there are no current trials evaluating the effects of injectable MSCs on hip OA, however, there is one case report of injectable MSCs used to treat knee OA that demonstrated an increase in articular cartilage volume, an increase in ROM, and a decrease in pain (31).

Home Exercise Program

A HEP is essential to long term improvement in function and pain reduction in patients with hip OA. Regardless if a patient partakes in a formal physical therapy program, a HEP should be initiated as soon as possible and be continued indefinitely. Most of the exercises previously discussed can be done at home. Stretching (Figure 19.4) and strengthening of hip girdle muscles usually only requires an exercise mat, ankle weights, and resistance bands. The aerobic component of the program is usually easy to incorporate as long as the patient has access to a place to walk, swim, and/or bicycle.

(a)
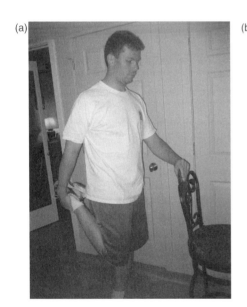

(b)
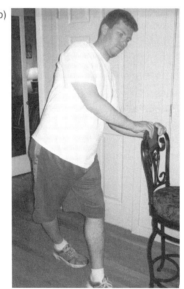

(c)
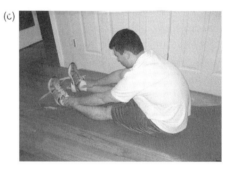

(d)
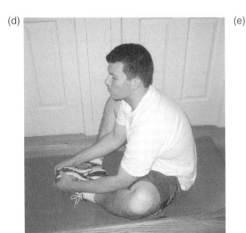

(e)
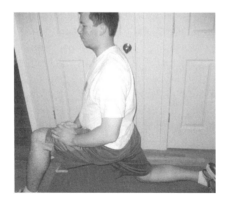

FIGURE 19.4: Self stretches for the lower limbs.

(a) Quadriceps stretch.
(b) Standing Iliotibial band (ITB)/TFL stretch.
(c) Hamstring stretch in long sitting—shown here the lumbar spine is flexed the lumbar spine lordosis can also be maintained with this stretch to isolate the hamstrings and increase the stretch.
(d) Seated short hip adductor stretch.
(e) Hip flexor stretch.

SUMMARY

Once the diagnosis of hip OA is made, treatment should begin with analgesic medications and therapeutic exercise to promote function, decrease pain, and theoretically try to halt the progression of OA. Therapeutic exercise consisting of ROM, strengthening, and aerobic exercises should be initiated as part of a HEP and/or formal physical therapy program depending on the patient's preference, degree of disease, access to facilities, and personal knowledge of exercise. Assistive devices, such as a cane, should be considered to offload the joint. If a comprehensive therapeutic program fails to provide relief, then corticosteroid injections are the current mainstay of injection treatment. Hyaluronic acid injections are available and have some research evidence supporting their use but are not currently covered by insurance for hip OA. Prolotherapy, PRP, and MSC injections are other injection options but remain experimental. Hip arthroplasty remains as an excellent surgical option for refractory cases after conservative treatment options have failed to relieve symptoms and improve function.

SAMPLE CASE

A 67-year-old male with past medical history of hypertension and diabetes who is a retired construction worker presents with a 6-month history of worsening right groin pain that radiates halfway down his antero-medial thigh. He notices the pain when he walks his first couple of blocks but then it subsides with further ambulation. X-rays obtained by his primary medical doctor show right hip joint space narrowing and a moderate sized osteophyte at the right acetabular rim. On examination, he has limited internal rotation, pain limited muscle strength with hip flexion and abduction, and a positive FAbER, IROP, and Stinchfield's on the right. The rest of his physical examination was unremarkable.

 SAMPLE THERAPY PRESCRIPTION

Discipline: Physical therapy.

Diagnosis: Right hip OA.

Precautions: weight bearing as tolerated, cardiac, diabetes

Frequency of visits: 2 to 3x/week (nonconsecutive days).

Duration of treatments: Up to 12 visits.

Treatment:

1. *Modalities:* preheat superficial tissues with moist heat and joint capsule with ultrasound at the beginning of the session. May use ice at the end of the session as needed

2. *Manual Therapy:* may trial gentle joint mobilizations and joint distraction to relieve pain and improve ROM

3. *Therapeutic Exercise:* ROM and lower limb stretching with emphasis on hip girdle muscles after preheating. Lower limb strengthening with focus on hip girdle muscles (e.g., hip abductors) and knee extensors. May need to begin with isometrics and advance to functional, closed kinetic chain exercises as tolerated. Neuro-muscular reeducation of hip abductors if needed. Balance and proprioceptive training. Aerobic conditioning may include low impact exercise such as an exercise bike or elliptical, but only if able to tolerate repetitive hip flexion

4. *Specialized Techniques:* aquatic exercise appropriate initially if available.

5. *Supportive Devices:* train in use of assistive devices (e.g., cane) to be used in the opposite hand

6. *Patient Education:* teach joint protection techniques and HEP

Goals: Decrease pain, improve flexibility, improve gait, and improve activities of daily living.

Reevaluation: By referring physician to coincide with completion of 12 visits.

REFERENCES

1. Felson DT. Epidemiology of hip and knee osteoarthritis. *Epidemiol Rev*. 1988;10:1–28.
2. Lesher JM, Dreyfuss P, Hager N, et al. Hip joint pain referral patterns: a descriptive study. *Pain Med*. 2008;9(1):22–25.
3. Clohisy JC, Knaus ER, Hunt DM, Lesher JM, Harris-Hayes M, Prather H. Clinical presentation of patients with symptomatic anterior hip impingement. *Clin Orthop Relat Res*. 2009;467(3):638–644.
4. Maslowski E, Sullivan W, Harwood JF, Gonzales P. The diagnostic validity of hip provocation maneuvers to detect intra-articular hip pathology. *PMR*. 2010;2:174–181.
5. Kraus BV. Pathogenesis and treatment of osteoarthritis. *Med Clin NA*. 1997;81:85–112.
6. Simkin P, de Lateur BJ, Alquist AD, et al. Continuous passive range of motion for osteoarthritis of the hip: a pilot study. *J Rheumatol*. 1999;26:1987–1991.
7. Tak E, Staats P, van Hespen A, Hopman-Rock M. The effects of an exercise therapy program for older adults with osteoarthritis of the hip. *J Rheumatol*. 2005;32:1106–1112.
8. Neumann D. Biomechanical analysis of selected principles of hip joint protection. *Arthritis Care Res*. 1989,2.146–155.
9. Lehman JF, Masock AJ, Warren CG, et al. Effect of therapeutic temperature on tendon extensibility. *Arch Phys Med Rehabil*. 1970;51:481–487.
10. Puett DW, Griffin MR. Published trials of non-medicinal and non-invasive therapies for hip and knee osteoarthritis. *Ann Intern Med*. 1994;121:133–140.
11. Oostervald FG, Rasker JJ. Effects of local heat and cold treatment on surface and articular temperature of arthritic knees. *Arthrits Rheum*. 1994;37:1578–1582.
12. Liu H, Abbott J, Bee JA. Pulsed electromagnetic fields influence hyaline cartilage extracellular matric comnposition without affecting molecular structure. *Ostearthritis Cartilage*. 1996;4(1):63–76.
13. Oldham JA, Howe TE, Petterson T, et al. Electrotherapeutic rehabilitation of the quadriceps in elderly osteoarthritis patients. A double-blind assessment of patterned neuromuscular stimulation. *Clin Rehab*. 1995;9:10–20.
14. Svarcova J, Trnavsky K, Zvarova J. The influence of ultrasound, galvanic currents and shortwave diathermy on pain intensity in patients with osteoarthritis. *Scan J Rheumatol Suppl*. 1987;67:83–85.
15. Hoeksma HL, Dekker J, Ronday HK, et al. Comparison of manual therapy and exercise therapy in osteoarthritis of the hip: a randomized clinical trial. *Arthritis Rheum*. 2004;51(5):722–729.
16. Abbott JH, Robertson MC, McKenzie JE, et al. Exercise therapy, manual therapy, or both, for osteoarthritis of the hip or knee: a factorial randomized controlled trial protocol. *Trials*. 2009;10:11.
17. Stitik TP, Nadler SF, Foye PM, Smith R. Osteoarthritis of the knee and hip: practical non-drug steps to successful therapy. *Consult Consultation Primary Care*. 1999;39(6):1707–1714.
18. Grimaldi A, Richardson C, Durbridge G, Donnelly W, Darnell R, Hides J. The association between degenerative hip joint pathology and size of the gluteus maximus and tensor fascia lata muscles. *Man Ther*. 2009;14(6):611–617.
19. Kummer B. Is the Pauwels' theory of hip biomechanics still valid: a critical analysis, based on modern methods. *Ann Anat*. 1993;175:203–210.
20. Rasch A, Bystrom AH, Dalen N, Berg HE. Reduced muscle radiological density, cross-sectional area, and strength of major hip and knee muscles in 22 patients with hip osteoarthritis. *Acta Orthop*. 2007;78:505–510.
21. Suetta C, Aagaard P, Magnusson SP, et al. Muscle size, neuromuscular activation, and rapid force characteristics in elderly men and women: effects of unilateral long-term disuse due to hip-osteoarthritis. *J Appl Physiol*. 2007;102:942–948.
22. Sturnieks DL, Tiedemann A, Chapman K, et al. Physiological risk factors for falls in older people with lower limb arthritis. *J Rheumatol*. 2004;31:2272–2279.
23. Schwarz L, Kindermann W. Changes in beta-endorphin levels in response to aerobic and anaerobic exercise. *Sports Med*. 1992;13(1):25–36.
24. Bunning RD, Materson RS. A rational program of exercise for patients with osteoarthritis. *Semin Arthritis Rheum*. 1991;21(suppl. 2):33–43.
25. Lambert RG, Hutchings EJ, Grace MG, et al. Steroid injection for osteoarthritis of the hip: a randomized, double-blind, placebo-controlled trial. *Arthri Rheumati*. 2007;56(7), 2278–2287.
26. van den Bekerom MP, Lamme B, Sermon A, Mulier M. What is the evidence for viscosupplementation in the treatment of patients with hip osteoarthritis? Systematic review of the literature. *Arch Orthop Trauma Surg*. 2008;128(8):815–823.
27. Kim SR, Stitik TP, Foye PM, Greenwald BD, Campagnolo DI. Critical review of prolotherapy for osteoarthritis, low back pain, and other musculoskeletal conditions. *Am J Phys Med Rehabil*. 2004;83:379–389.
28. Kon E, Buda R, Filardo G, et al. Platelet-rich plasma: intra-articular knee injections produced favorable results on degenerative cartilage lesions. *Knee Surg Sports Traumatol Arthrosc*. 2010;18:472–479.
29. Filardo G, Kon E, Buda R, et al. Platelet-rich plasma intra-articular knee injections for the treatment of degenerative cartilage lesions ad osteoarthritis. *Knee Surg Sports Traumatol Arthrosc*. 2011;19(4):528–535.
30. Sampson S, Reed M, Silvers H, Meng M, Mandelbaum B. Injection of platelet-rich plasma in patients with primary and secondary knee osteoarthritis: a pilot study. *Am J Phys Med Rehabil*. 2010;89:961–969.
31. Centeno CJ, Brusse D, Kisiday J, et al. Increased knee cartilage volume in degenerative joint disease using percutaneously implanted, autologous mesenchymal stem cells. *Pain Physician*. 2008;11(3):343–353.

Iliopsoas Tendinopathy and Bursopathy

Annemarie E. Gallagher, Pete Draovitch, Jaime Edelstein, and Peter J. Moley

INTRODUCTION

A common complaint among patients is anterior hip pain, which can be due to iliopsoas tendonitis or bursitis. Injury of the iliopsoas may occur secondary to excessive anteversion of the hip, anterior under-coverage of the acetabulum over the head of the femur and resultant hip joint instability, and osteoarthritis. Iliopsoas injury often presents as a deep, aching groin pain with activity or in certain provocative positions. Occasionally, the patient may also experience an audible snap and corresponding pain in the ipsilateral groin. These issues are mainly seen in young adults, women, and those who have arthritis.

For purposes of *anatomical review*, the psoas muscle originates from the five lumbar vertebrae, and the iliacus muscle originates from the ilium Figure (20.1). These two muscles converge and form the iliopsoas, which inserts anteromedially as the iliopsoas tendon onto the lesser trochanter of the femur. The iliopsoas muscle functions as the primary hip flexor and as an external rotator of the femur. The iliopsoas musculotendinous junction traverses a groove between the iliopectineal eminence (medially) and the anterior inferior iliac spine (laterally) and crosses the pelvic brim and capsule (anteriorly).

The musculotendinous junction of the iliopsoas is separated from surrounding structures by the iliopsoas bursa, which is the largest synovial bursa in the body, extending from the iliac fossa to the lesser trochanter (1). The iliopsoas bursa lies adjacent to the anterior hip. Inflammatory conditions, including osteoarthritis, rheumatoid arthritis, and synovial chondromatosis (2), can affect the joint capsule and the iliopsoas bursa, often causing anterior hip pain. The concurrent pain experienced by patients with a snapping hip is thought to be secondary to repetitive iliopsoas tendon subluxation, most likely at the iliopectineal eminence or the anterior inferior iliac spine, resulting in bursitis, tendonitis, or synovitis (1).

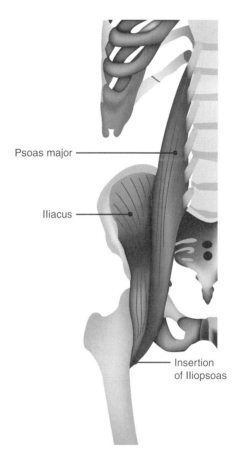

Psoas major

Iliacus

Insertion of Iliopsoas

FIGURE 20.1: Iliopsoas.

For purposes of reviewing *kinesiology*, the psoas muscle connects the lumbar spine to the femur as it inserts onto the lesser trochanter. The psoas functions as the main hip flexor, but has also been shown to serve as a lateral stabilizer of the lumbar spine by activating bilaterally, thereby adding compressive force to the joints of the spine (3,4). The psoas has many functions in controlling the lumbopelvic complex, based on the angle of the hip (4).

Cadaveric studies, both static and dynamic, demonstrated that the psoas has different functions, depending on the degree of hip flexion (5). The psoas major acts as a stabilizer to maintain the erect position of the lumbar spine, and stabilizes the femoral head at 0° to 15° of hip flexion. At 15° to 45°, its primary function is to maintain the lumbar spine in an erect position and it acts less as a hip stabilizer. At 45° to 60°, its main action is to flex the hip (5).

During an active straight leg raise, the iliacus, psoas, rectus femoris, and adductor longus work synergistically and are activated ipsilaterally. The contralateral psoas is also activated, and it is believed that this contralateral recruitment of the psoas aids with lumbar stabilization (6). In the frontal plane, the psoas serves as a lateral stabilizer of the lumbar spine (7). In the sagittal plane, the psoas may also aid in maintaining lumbar lordosis (8).

In asymptomatic hips, frog-leg positioning results in the tendon moving laterally and rotating anteriorly to the iliopsoas muscle. The medial part of the iliacus muscle lies between the iliopsoas tendon and the pubic bone. When in neutral position, the tendon glides and rotates posteromedially, overlying the superior pubic ramus. In the symptomatic hip, as the hip returns from frog-leg position to neutral, the iliopsoas tendon moves in a posteromedial direction, and the muscle is abruptly released laterally, resulting in sudden contact of the iliopsoas tendon against the pubic bone. This typically occurs midway between frog-leg and neutral positions (9).

Iliopsoas bursitis can be associated with Coxa Saltans (snapping hip syndrome), but the patient may develop bursitis with or without snapping. Injury results in inflammation of the tendon and bursa, causing muscle irritation with hip flexion and ultimately pain. The snapping sensation that may be experienced during this inflammatory response is secondary to the subluxation of the iliopsoas tendon over one of the following bony prominences: the anterior inferior iliac spine, the iliopectineal eminence, or the bony ridge of the lesser trochanter (10). Intra-articular causes of internal snapping include labral tears, loose bodies, articular cartilage flaps, transient subluxation of the femoral head, femoral acetabular impingement (FAI), and irregular articular surfaces (11).

A similar but anatomically different snapping can occur at the greater trochanter and is called external snapping. The most common cause is the external, lateral type, where the iliotibial band (ITB) and its connection to the outer border of the gluteus maximus catches the greater trochanter as the hip moves from flexion into extension. This condition is discussed in more detail in the chapter on Greater Trochanteric Pain Syndrome. ITB snapping is generally less audible. The adage is that the clinician can *hear internal* snapping across the room and *see external* snapping across the room.

Patients presenting with anterior hip pain and a snapping hip may have iliopsoas bursitis and/or tendonitis, which may more accurately be described as *iliopsoas syndrome*, involving inflammation of both the tendon and the bursa. Inflammation of one of these structures typically results in an inflammatory response of the other, given their close proximity. These symptoms can be observed in patients who have undergone hip surgery, such as total hip arthroplasty, people with an active or athletic lifestyle, and those with FAI. On the contrary, hypermobile patients may experience *painless* snapping at the hip. Prior hip trauma (in abduction and external rotation) may predispose patients to developing iliopsoas tendon subluxation via a mechanism that damages the retinacular structure that attaches the iliopsoas tendon and the anterior pelvic brim (10).

The three most common causes of iliopsoas bursitis are overuse, trauma, and rheumatoid arthritis. Excessive hip flexion and extension often results in bursitis. It has been hypothesized that with hip flexion, the iliopsoas muscle and anterior bursa move away from the hip, but with hyperextension, the iliopsoas muscle and bursa are stretched, resulting in an inflammatory response at the site of the bursa. It has also been hypothesized that in extension of a flexed, abducted, and externally rotated hip (frog-leg position), the iliopsoas tendon snaps over the femoral head, anterior hip capsule, or the iliopectineal eminence, and pain can ensue (5,12).

Clinical presentation of iliopsoas syndrome includes pain in the anterior inguinal region that radiates down the anterior thigh to the knee (13,14), often aggravated by movement at the hip and alleviated with rest (10,13). Pain is often elicited when the hip is placed in frog-leg position and can be accompanied by a palpable and/or audible snap. Patients can also present with a shortened stride, which intrinsically prevents hip hyperextension. Repetitive snapping of the iliopsoas tendon onto the pubic bone may result in the development of tendinopathy (13). A detailed history and physical examination will help diagnose iliopsoas bursitis from other causes of anterior hip pain.

Key elements of the physical examination include inspection, palpation, range of motion (ROM) testing, neurologic examination, and other specialized tests (e.g., modified FABERs and hip circumduction test). The physical examination should be approached in a systematic and step-wise fashion from inspection to specialized tests. Findings that make iliopsoas bursitis high on the differential include: anterior hip pain worse with activity, tenderness in the femoral triangle (13), weak external rotation when the hip is flexed, and a positive Thomas test. Distal pain in stance phase can also be a clue that iliopsoas bursitis may be present.

Imaging studies can aid with the diagnosis of iliopsoas bursitis. Analyses of plain radiographs have shown that those presenting with iliopsoas bursitis may have

ILIOPSOAS TENDINOPATHY AND BURSOPATHY

- Iliopsoas bursitis results in inflammation of the tendon and bursa, causing muscle irritation with hip flexion and ultimately pain

- The snapping sensation is secondary to the subluxation of the iliopsoas tendon over one of the bony prominences of the hip. Snapping of the iliopsoas is considered internal snapping while snapping over the greater trochanter is external snapping

- Iliopsoas syndrome symptoms include:

  - Pain in the anterior inguinal region, sometimes radiating down the anterior thigh to the knee, aggravated by activity or movement at the hip (e.g., frog-leg position) and alleviated with rest

  - Pain can be accompanied by a palpable and/ or audible snap

  - Shortened stride length

  - Distal pain in stance phase

- Key physical examination findings include tenderness in the femoral triangle, weak external rotation when the hip is flexed, and a positive Thomas test

- Ultrasound, especially dynamic ultrasound, is a useful tool to evaluate the entire course of the iliopsoas tendon and the anatomical cause of snapping

- Conservative management of iliopsoas bursitis includes NSAIDs and a physical therapy program, focusing on stretching in hip extension and hip rotation strengthening exercises

a posteriorly positioned lesser trochanter, affecting the iliopsoas tendon course. MRI has been shown to demonstrate signal changes in the iliopsoas tendon and its surrounding structures. Abnormal iliopsoas tendon motion may also be demonstrated with iliopsoas bursography or tendinography, followed by fluoroscopy (15,16).

Musculoskeletal ultrasound has shown that the most common cause of snapping hip is a sudden "flipping" of the iliopsoas tendon over the iliacus muscle. The audible snap occurs when the tendon makes contact with the pubic bone. Other causes visualized with the ultrasound include bifid tendon heads abruptly moving over each other and the iliopsoas tendon impinging an anterior paralabral cyst. Using ultrasound, dynamic images of the iliopsoas tendon during active hip flexion and extension have shown abrupt movement mediolaterally, resulting in snapping, which can be appreciated in real time (10). Ultrasonography of snapping hips also commonly reveals iliopsoas tendon thickening, indicative of tendonitis, or peritendinous fluid, indicative of iliopsoas bursa distension and a clinical diagnosis of iliopsoas tendonitis and/ or bursitis, respectively.

Conservative management of iliopsoas bursitis should include oral nonsteroidal anti-inflammatories (NSAIDS), as well as stretching in hip extension and rotation strengthening exercises. Ultrasound guidance can be used for diagnostic lidocaine injections placed under the iliopsoas musculotendinous junction (17,15). Furthermore, an ultrasound or fluoroscopically-guided corticosteroid injection into the iliopsoas bursa can provide pain relief, often lasting for more than 3 months (18).

THE REHABILITATION PROGRAM

The iliopsoas muscle is often involved in soft tissue injuries to the groin. A rehabilitation program will focus on stretching and strengthening, while minimizing groin pain or referred pain from the iliopsoas. Rehabilitation of the iliopsoas should focus on correcting muscle imbalances and training errors, and on improving upon core weakness and neuromuscular control (19).

The size and density of the psoas major muscle has been shown to demonstrate gender differences and change with age (20,21). When comparing the psoas muscle versus the quadriceps femoris in women, the psoas muscle showed a steady decrease in cross sectional size from 20 to 60 years of age with dramatic loss after 70 years old. The quadriceps, however, was consistent until into the 40s, with no dramatic decline thereafter

(21). Therefore, an iliopsoas strengthening program is an important component of rehabilitation especially in older female patients. Another important consideration when treating the psoas, regardless of age or gender, is understanding that in most cases, the lumbar plexus is situated within the muscle belly and emerges on the posterior or posterolateral surface of the muscle (22).

Muscle fiber composition of the iliopsoas should be considered when designing a rehabilitation program. The psoas major muscle consists of type I, IIA, and IIX fibers, with type I fibers making up the largest cross sectional area and type IIA fibers showing a predominance. The most clinically relevant component of a study performed by Arbanas et al, which took samples between L1–L4, demonstrated the cranial portion of the psoas to have a postural role, while the caudal portion offered more dynamic characteristics (23). Clinically, this is of significance because often patients diagnosed with hip instability also present with "snapping" hip, whereby the psoas is "snapping" over the iliopectineal eminence or the anterior acetabular rim. If the psoas demonstrates increased tone, releasing this structure, without addressing the inert tissue pathology, could make hip mechanics worse, especially knowing that the caudal portion of the psoas has more dynamic characteristics and less postural stabilization capabilities. Regarding psoas differences between the right and left sides, no changes were demonstrated between young and old males. Although the psoas major does undergo normal aging processes, type IIA fibers became most atrophic, while type I fibers were least affected (24).

Another rehabilitation consideration is the architectural design of the psoas major muscle. In a study of 13 cadavers, it was concluded that the passive biomechanical properties of the psoas resemble erector spinae musculature and become stronger with hip flexion and forward trunk lean (25).

Understanding how the psoas responds to its environment is another factor worth recognizing before designing an exercise or rehabilitation program. Clinicians treating athletes and performing artists, whose sport or activity requires a lot of cutting, change of direction, or a speed component, must take the time to understand the etiology of trunk and hip muscular contributions. It is also important to remember that an essential component of the rehabilitation program will be neuromuscular reeducation of the iliopsoas and surrounding muscles. This can often be achieved with neuromuscular electrical stimulation (e-stim), particularly with isometric hip flexion.

In a study comparing spine and hip motion, motor patterns, and spine load for torso exercises in an erect position, it was found that single plane activities produced the greatest muscle activation, while functional tasks inhibited maximal contraction of the trunk musculature (26). The role of the psoas will vary based on the requirements of the activity to be dynamic versus postural or components of both. Psoas muscle function will also vary if the activity is biased toward the lower body moving on a stable trunk or the trunk moving over a stable lower body.

Overall, the most important factor to consider when designing the rehabilitation program is whether the iliopsoas is truly short and tight or lengthened, overused and weak. The working relationship between the musculoskeletal system and the central nervous system and the muscular response to the sensorimotor system represents the focus of the work of Dr. Vladimir Janda (27). Recognizing imbalance patterns due to inhibition, overstimulation, tightness, or excess length will be the first and most important part of nonoperative management of iliopsoas pathology (28). When treating a truly tight muscle, the treatment of choice is prolonged stretching, active stretching, release techniques, or soft tissue mobilization. Muscles which are inhibited may benefit from techniques, including stretching the antagonist, tactile cueing, facilitation techniques which activate the tissue, or neuromuscular stimulation. Once any contractile tissue achieves a new length, it must be reeducated to ensure the musculature has some working tone in its new end range. When the iliopsoas muscle has become elongated and overworked, the goal should focus on regaining neuromuscular function.

Therapeutic Modalities

As previously mentioned, electrical stimulation (e-stim) may be utilized as part of the neuromuscular training component of the rehabilitation program. Additional modalities to consider using include cryotherapy to help control pain and inflammation during phase I of rehabilitation. Superficial and deep heating modalities (e.g., ultrasound) may be considered as adjunctive treatments to a stretching program, especially if the treatment goal is to improve the length of a shortened iliopsoas. This suggestion is primarily based on expert opinion, since the available literature does not define the role of these treatments and, therefore, may or may not offer benefit over therapeutic exercise alone.

Manual Therapy

Manual therapy techniques are commonly utilized for the iliopsoas and surrounding soft tissue structures to address pain and/or soft tissue restrictions associated with iliopsoas syndrome. Soft tissue mobilization may be considered for the iliopsoas if the desire is to address restrictions and improve the length of a shortened iliopsoas muscle. Our treatment approach also includes the identification and correction of deficits in the kinetic chain, including an assessment of joint mobility and alignment both above and below the pathological tissue (iliopsoas muscle). Therefore, joint mobilization or manipulation techniques may be utilized to address restrictions at the hip, pelvis, or lumbar spine. Although this is a commonly utilized clinical approach, further research is necessary to define the role of specific manual therapy techniques in the setting of iliopsoas syndrome, tendinopathy, or bursopathy.

Therapeutic Exercise Program

Patients with iliopsoas pathology will often present with hip rotation weakness and hip flexor tightness. A sound therapeutic exercise program will, therefore, involve daily strengthening of the hip rotator muscles, using an elastic resistance strap for 2 weeks. A concurrent daily stretching program should involve the hip flexors, quadriceps, and hamstrings. When able to tolerate stretching and strengthening, exercise can then progress to weight-bearing mini-squats on the affected leg (29).

It has also been demonstrated that contraction of the opposite hip flexor causes activation of the inactive side (6). Therefore, opposite limb leg raises may play a role in the treatment of certain conditions requiring psoas activation and stabilization. It is clear that treatment of iliopsoas pathology may be complex. It is also evident that a poorly planned treatment progression for an improperly diagnosed condition can lead to delays in healing and/or unnecessary setbacks.

The success of a rehabilitation program should be based on psoas inhibition, followed by reeducation of the psoas, back extensors, abdominals, and hip musculature that supports the pelvic region (28). Some exercises used for this progression include:

1. Psoas inhibition (Figure 20.2)
   ● Dorsiflex the foot to fire the tibialis anterior
   ● Fire the quadriceps, and keep the hamstrings inhibited

2. Prone multifidus/E-stim with isometric hip flexion (Figure 20.3)
   ● Neuromuscular retraining and education
3. Dynamic bum walk (developed by Erl Pettman, PT) (Figure 20.4)
   ● Based on the multijoint integration during locomotion

The muscular development of the psoas major has also been implicated as a key factor in athletic performance. In a study involving Japanese soccer players, no difference was noted bilaterally when comparing thigh and trunk muscles. The only difference to note was that the cross sectional area of the psoas was greater, even when comparing the whole body-lean tissue mass (30). Regarding sprinting, studies involving both short and long sprints have been conducted. In a group of youth soccer players, times were measured at 10 meters, 20 meters, and the time between 10 and 20 meters. Cross

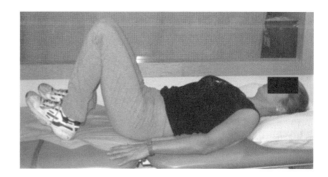

FIGURE 20.2: Psoas inhibition.
Source: Adapted from Ref 31.

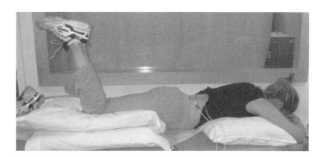

FIGURE 20.3: Neuromuscular reeducation: Electrical stimulation (e-stim) of the multifidus for reeducation of the ipsilateral psoas.
Source: Adapted from Ref 31.

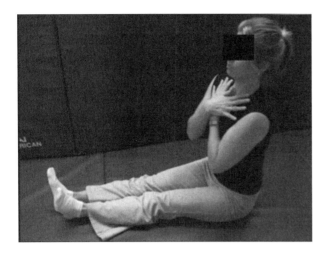

FIGURE 20.4: Psoas bum walk.
Source: Adapted from Ref 31.

sectional areas, measured by MRI, were taken between L1–S1 of the rectus abdominis, obliques, psoas major, quadratus lumborum, and erector spinae. Results demonstrated that erector spinae and quadratus lumborum significantly contributed to performance in sprints less than 20 meters (31). When comparing 100 meter junior sprint times of both genders, it was concluded that better development of the psoas major relative to the quadriceps femoris, as opposed to actual muscle size, was most responsible for achieving improved performance in a race of this length (32).

In a study of elite, subelite, and elite junior wrestlers, increased cross sectional area of trunk flexors was noted to be a significant finding among the elite and elite junior groups, which can be considered a factor for improved performance (33). Although there was no significant difference between the elite and subelite groups regarding trunk musculature, the explanation for their differences in performance level could be traced to factors such as skill, interest level, training methods, coaching, and/or technique.

Home Exercise Program

Once the patient is adequately instructed about how to safely and effectively perform an appropriate exercise regimen, he/she is advised to continue the stretching and strengthening program at home on a daily basis. The home exercises include strengthening the internal and external hip rotators in sitting position and strengthening the hip external rotators and abductors in side-lying. Grade of difficulty can be increased by using an elastic resistance strap. Weight-bearing mini-squats and daily stretching of the surrounding musculature, including the hip flexors, quadriceps, and hamstrings should also be incorporated into the home exercise program (HEP) (29).

SUMMARY

Understanding the iliopsoas as a dynamic muscle of the hip will help aid with the efficacy of a rehabilitation program. Avoidance of pain produced by an internal snapping hip can significantly alter hip mechanics, which can result in more pain, gait instability, and low back pathology. To prevent the sequelae of instability, pain, and ultimate weakness, a rehabilitation program for iliopsoas syndrome must focus on stretching and strengthening not only the iliopsoas, but also the other muscles of the hip joint and core to recreate muscular balance of the hip, pelvis, and lumbar spine. Since this condition is mechanical in nature, compliance with a HEP is of the utmost importance.

SAMPLE CASE

A 24-year-old dancer presents with a history of right anterior groin pain. She reports that her pain has become worse recently, as she has been practicing more for an upcoming show. She has noticed that the pain now radiates down the anterior thigh to the knee. She has also felt a snapping sensation at the right groin, particularly when flexing and abducting the right hip. On physical examination, there is tenderness of the right femoral triangle. There is also right hip external rotation weakness and a positive FABER test on the right. Neurovascular examination is otherwise unremarkable.

SAMPLE THERAPY PRESCRIPTION

Discipline: Physical therapy.

Diagnosis: Iliopsoas bursitis.

Precautions: None.

Frequency of visits: 1 to 2x/week.

Duration of visits: 6 to 12 weeks.

Treatments:

1. *Modalities:* Ice applications prn, e-stim for neuromuscular reeducation

2. *Manual therapy:* Myofascial release of the iliopsoas, soft tissue mobilization of the thigh

3. *Therapeutic exercise*:

    a. Stretching: Daily stretching of the hip flexors, quadriceps, piriformis, and hamstrings

    b. Neuromuscular reeducation of the psoas, back extensors, abdominals, and hip musculature via psoas inhibition and by using e-stim with isometric hip flexion

    c. Strengthening: For 2 weeks, daily strengthening of the internal and external hip rotators while in sitting position using an elastic resistance strap. For 2 additional weeks, daily strengthening of the hip abductors and external hip rotators in side-lying with an elastic resistance strap. When these exercises are tolerated well, progress to weight-bearing mini-squats on the affected leg and opposite limb leg raises

    d. Functional retraining: Walking and light jogging can be pursued initially, and can be advanced to movements associated with the patient's sport or daily functional activities, as tolerated

4. *Specialized treatments:* Biomechanical analysis of the kinetic chain and stride length, review and correct the biomechanics of walking, running, and kicking

5. *Patient education:* Development of progressive, consistent HEP

Goals: Decrease pain with hip flexion and external rotation, restore hip flexion and external rotation strength and ROM, correct imbalances in running mechanics, return to sport, and initiate a HEP to prevent symptom recurrence.

Reevaluation: In 4 to 6 weeks by referring provider.

REFERENCES

1. Vaccaro JP, Sauser DD, Beals RK. Iliopsoas bursa imaging: efficacy in depicting abnormal iliopsoas tendon motion in patients with internal hip syndrome. *Radiology.* 1995;197:853–856.

2. Schaberg JE, Harper MC, Allen WC. The snapping hip syndrome. *Am J Sports Med.* 1984;12:361–365.

3. Gardner-Morse MG, Stokes IA. Physiological axial compressive preloads increase motion segment stiffness, linearity, and hysteresis in all six degrees of freedom from small displacements about the neutral posture. *J Orthop Res.* 2003;21:547–552.

4. Yoshio M, Murakami G, Sato T, Sato S, Niryasu S. The function of the psoas major muscle: passive kinetics and morphological studies using donated cadavers. *J Orthop Sci.* 2002;7:199–207.

5. Yoshio M, Murakami G, Sato T, Sato S, Noriyasu S. The function of the psoas major muscle: passive kinetics and morphological studies using donated cadavers. *J Orthop Sci.* 2001;7:199–207.

6. Hu H, Meijer OG, van Dieen JH, et al. Is the psoas a hip flexor in the active straight leg raise? *Eur Spine J.* 2011;20:759–765.

7. Andersson E, Oddsson L, Grundstrom H, Thorstensson A. The role of the psoas and iliacus muscles for stability and movement of the lumbar spine, pelvis, and hip. *Scand J Med Sci Sports.* 1995;5:10–6.

8. Penning L. Psoas muscle and lumbar spine stability: a concept uniting existing controversies. Critical review and hypothesis. *Eur Spine J.* 2000;9:577–585.

9. Pelsser V, Cardinal E, Hobden R, Aubin B, Lafortune M. Extraarticular snapping hip: sonographic findings. *Am J Radiolog.* 2001;176:67–73.

10. Janzen DL, Partridge E, Logan PM, Connell DG, Duncan CP. The snapping hip: clinical and imaging findings in transient subluxation of the iliopsoas tendon. *Can Assoc Radiolog J.* 1996; 47:202–208.

11. Frich LH, Lauritzen J, Juhl M. Arthroscopy in the treatment of hip disorders. *Orthopedics.* 1989;12:389–392.

12. Johnston CA, Wiley JP, Lindsay DM, Wiseman DA. Iliopsoas bursitis and tendinitis: a review. *Sports Med.* 1998;25:271–283.

13. Deslandes M, Guillin R, Cardinal E, Hibden R, Bureau NJ. The snapping iliopsoas tendon: new mechanisms using dynamic sonography. *Am J Radiolog.* 2008; 90:576–581.

14. Choi YS, Lee SM, Song BY, Paik SH, Yoon YK. Dynamic sonography of external snapping hip syndrome. *J Ultrasound Med.* 2002;21:753–758.

15. Schaberg JE, Harper MC, Allen WC. The snapping hip syndrome. *Am J Sports Med.* 1984;12:361–365.

16. Taylor GR, Clarke NM. Surgical release of the "snapping iliopsoas tendon." *J Bone Joint Surg Br.* 1995;77:881–883.

17. Czerny C, Hofmann S, Neuhold A, et al. Lesions of the acetabular labrum: accuracy of MR imaging and MR arthrography in detection and staging. *Radiology.* 1996;200:225–230.

18. Blankenbaker DG, de Smet AA, Keene JS. Sonography of the iliopsoas tendon and injection of the iliopsoas bursa for diagnosis and management of the painful snapping hip. *Skeletal Radiol.* 2006;35:565–571.

19. Maffey L, Emery C. What are the risk factors for groin strain in sport? A systematic review of the literature. *Sports Medicine.* 2007;37(10):881–894.

20. Imamura K, Ashida H, Ishikawa T, Fujii M. Human major psoas muscle and sacrospinalis muscle in relation to age: a study by computed tomography. *J Gerentol.* 1983;38(6):678–681.

21. Takahashi K, Takahashi HE, Nakadaira H, Yamamoto M. Different changes of quantity due to aging in the psoas major and quadriceps femoris muscles in women. *J Musculskelet Neuronal Interact.* 2006; 6(2):201–205.

22. Kirchmair L, Lirk P, Colvin J, Mitterschiffthaler G, Moriggl B. Lumbar plexus and psoas major muscle: not always as expected. *Reg Anasthe Pain Med.* 2008;33(2):109–114.

23. Arbanas J, Klanas GS, Nikolic M, Jerkovic R, Milanovic I, Malnar D. Fibre type composition of the human psoas major muscle with regard to the level of its origin. *J Anat.* 2009;215(6):636–641.

24. Arbanas J, Klasan GS, Nikolic M, Cvijanovic O, Malnar D. Immunohistochemical analysis of the human psoas major muscle with regards to the body side and aging. *Coll Antropol.* 2010;34(Suppl. 2):169–173.

25. Regev GJ, Kim CW, Tomiya A, et al. Psoas muscle architectural design, in vivo sarcomere length range, and passive tensile properties support its role as a lumbar spine stabilizer. *Spine.* 2011;36(26):E1666–E1674.

26. McGill SM, Karpowicz A, Fenwick CM, Brown SH. Exercises for the torso performed in a standing posture: spine and hip motion and motor patterns and spine load. *J Strength Cond Res.* 2009;23(2):455–464.

27. Page P. The Janda approach to chronic musculoskeletal pain. Retrieved from http://www.jandaapproach.com/the-janda-approach; 2007.

28. Edelstein J. Rehabilitating psoas tendonitis: a case report. *HSS Journal.* 2009;5:78–82.

29. Biundo JJ, Irwin RW, Umpierre E. Sports and other soft tissue injuries, tendinitis, bursitis, and occupation-related syndromes. *Curr Opin Rheumatol.* 2001; 3(2):146–149.

30. Kubo T, Muramatsu M, Hoshikawa Y, Kanehisa H. Profiles of trunk and thigh muscularity in youth and professional soccer players. *J Strength Cond Res.* 2010;24(6):1472–1479.

31. Kubo T, Hoshikawa Y, Muramatsu M, et al. Contribution of trunk muscularity on sprint run. *Int J Sports Med.* 2011;32(3):223–228.

32. Hoshikawa Y, Muramatsu M, Iida T, et al. Influence of the psoas major and thigh muscularity on 100-m times in junior sprinters. *Med Sci Sports Exerc.* 2006;38(12):2138–2143.

33. Kubo J, Ohta A, Takahashi H, Kukidome T, Funato K. The development of trunk muscles in male wrestlers assessed by magnetic resonance imaging. *J Strength Cond Res.* 2007;21(4):1251–1254.

Greater Trochanteric Pain Syndrome

Gerard A. Malanga and Monika Krzyzek

INTRODUCTION

Greater trochanteric pain syndrome (GTPS) is a commonly encountered problem in musculoskeletal medicine. It was originally defined as "tenderness to palpation over the greater trochanter with the patient in the side-lying position," (1–4) but as diagnostic studies, especially magnetic resonance imaging (MRI) and hip arthroscopy techniques, have improved we now have a better understanding of the functional anatomy of the hip (4,5). As a result, this clinical entity has broadened to include a number of associated disorders of the lateral, peritrochanteric hip area including greater trochanteric bursitis (normal variant or calcific), tendinopathy and tears of the gluteus medius and minimus, and external snapping hip (external coxa saltans) (4). It has been called the "Great Mimicker" as it tends to frequently be mistaken for other conditions and often coexists with other conditions (e.g., hip osteoarthritis (OA), lumbar spondylosis with or without radiculopathy). It is commonly, and often incorrectly, referred to as trochanteric bursitis; however, this terminology is generally incorrect as the cardinal signs of inflammation, edema, and rubor are uncommon findings (3,6). In addition, imaging studies such as ultrasound and MRI usually fail to demonstrate any significant bursal effusion.

Patients with GTPS present with lateral hip pain or buttock area pain, with or without radiation down the lateral thigh. It is a common condition, affecting between 10% to 25% of the general population (1,4,6) with a higher incidence in women and runners (4). Incidence is also increased in people with low back pain (LBP), ipsilateral iliotibial band (ITB) tightness/tenderness, ipsilateral or contralateral knee OA, and rheumatoid arthritis (1,7). It can present following trauma after a fall or acute sports injury with direct trauma over the greater trochanter. Other causes include overuse or biomechanical muscular imbalances. It can occur in athletes, nonathletes,

even following hip replacements, as well as in the general population.

Differential diagnosis includes intra-articular hip pathology, other sources of extra-articular hip pathology, and referred symptoms from the lumbar spine and pelvis (4–6,8). Trigger points, tendinopathy, muscle tears, femoral neck stress fracture, femoral head avascular necrosis, bone metastasis, hip OA, hip adductor muscle strain, meralgia paresthetica, ITB syndrome, piriformis syndrome or myofascial pain, pelvic floor dysfunction, sacroilliac joint (SIJ) joint dysfunction, lumbosacral radiculopathy, and degenerative disease of the spine (5,6,9) are some of the specific conditions in this extensive list of possible differential diagnoses.

An understanding of the lateral hip anatomy is necessary for a full appreciation of the multiple clinical entities that compromise GTPS. The greater trochanter is the site of attachment for five muscles: obturator internus, obturator externus, and piriformis medially as well as the gluteus medius and gluteus minimus laterally (4). A breakdown of the insertion sites has been proposed based on five facets (10). The gluteus medius tendon has two distinct insertion sites, inserting onto the lateral facet and supero-posterior facet. The gluteus minimus inserts anteriorly to the gluteus medius tendon at the anterior facet (4–10). Superficially to the gluteus minimus and medius tendons lies the gluteus maximus, tensor fascia lata (TFL) and ITB.

Classily described in anatomy textbooks, the dominant, deep subgluteus maximus bursa is thought of as the "trochanteric bursa" associated with trochanteric bursitis, however multiple bursae of the lateral hip area have been described in literature with evidence of anatomical variation in the number of bursae found and their location, in contrast to the classic anatomy taught in medical school. There is evidence in the literature that at least three bursae are consistently present in the lateral area of the greater trochanter, which function as a cushioning mechanism for the glutei tendons, TFL and ITB. These bursae are known as the subgluteus maximus bursa, the subgluteus medius bursa, and the subgluteus minimus bursa (4,6,11,12). The subgluteus maximus bursa is located laterally to the greater trochanter in between the tendons of the gluteus maximus and gluteus medius. Anatomic variation with as many as four separate bursae (deep, secondary deep, superficial, and gluteofemoral) corresponding anatomically to the area of the subgluteus maximus bursa have been described (6,11). The deep subgluteus maximus bursa is the largest and most consistently found, therefore, this is considered the classic "trochanteric bursa" and is thought to be responsible for classic trochanteric bursitis (4,6). The subgluteus medius bursa is deep to the gluteus medius tendon and is composed of up to three separate bursae. These are the anterior subgluteus bursa (largest and most consistently found), the piriformis bursa, and the secondary piriformis bursa. The subgluteus minimus bursa is located deep to the gluteus minimus tendon at the anterior aspect of the greater trochanter and is composed of either one or two bursa (subgluteus bursa, and secondary subgluteus bursa) (4,11).

Trochanteric bursitis presents with inflammation of the bursa thought to be secondary to repetitive friction between the greater trochanter and ITB with flexion and extension of the hip. It is thought to be associated with overuse trauma, or other conditions that alter normal gait patterns. Patients report symptoms with activity, prolonged standing, sitting with the affected leg crossed, running, and stair climbing and trouble sleeping due to pain while lying on the affected side (6).

Patients with gluteus medius or minimus tears also have lateral hip pain, tenderness to palpation at the gluteal insertion onto the greater trochanter, and weakness of hip abduction (4,5,13). They may have weakness with active resisted abduction in extension, external rotation with the hip flexed at 90°, or pain reproduction with single leg stance lasting 30 seconds or longer (13).

External coxa saltans is a painful snapping at the lateral hip with activities that require repetitive flexion, extension, and abduction secondary to a tight ITB and/or tight gluteus maximus tendon snapping over the greater trochanter (4). The patient will have a painful snapping sensation with activities and a snapping ITB can many times be palpated as the patient flexes his hip or can be visualized with dynamic ultrasound.

Key elements of the physical examination include inspection for ecchymosis and other signs of trauma, palpation for point tenderness over specific sites of the greater trochanter, bilateral lower limb strength testing

with careful attention to the hip extensors and hip abductors along with lower extremity flexibility testing, gait analysis, and Trendelenburg testing. If the patient has paresthesias down the leg, then dural tension tests and complete lower limb neurological examination needs to be included to rule out lumbosacral radiculopathy. Patients may also have pain radiating down the lateral thigh with resisted hip abduction, a positive Patrick/FABER and a positive Ober's on the affected side (4,6,8).

Usually, diagnostic studies are not required. However, in cases of a fall on the side or after a sports injury, plain radiographs may be helpful to rule out a hip region fracture or an avulsion type fracture. Plain radiographs may also reveal enthesopathic changes at the greater trochanter or other underlying pathology, such as degenerative joint disease. MRI or ultrasound can show bursitis, tendinopathy, tears of the gluteus medius and minimus, calcifications, or fatty atrophy within the gluteus muscles (4,14–17). Dynamic ultrasound can be used to evaluate for coxa saltans ("snapping hip"), calcific tendonitis, calcific bursitis, tendinopathy, tears, or other abnormalities (4,5). It should be noted that malignancy and infections have been described in the literature to mimic GTPS and, therefore, if there is

---

GREATER TROCHANTERIC PAIN SYNDROME

▓ Typically presents with lateral hip pain localized to the greater trochanter or occasionally may mimic a radiculopathy with pain and pseudo-paresthesias down the leg

▓ *Pertinent positives of the physical examination*: point tenderness over the greater trochanter and/or gluteus medius or minimus insertions, weakness, and occasionally pain with single leg stance >30 seconds on the affected limb

▓ Can be either traumatic or atraumatic, acute or chronic in presentation

▓ In most patients subtle evidence of muscular imbalances will be found on physical examination especially in the hip abductors and hip extensors

▓ Diagnostic testing usually is not needed to initiate treatment but should be considered in cases not responsive to conservative treatment or in patients with a high index of suspicion for bone lesions or infection

no response to conservative treatment or there is a high index of suspicion, diagnostic testing is of value (18–20). Recalcitrant GTPS needs further evaluation and diagnostic testing, as well as possible surgical consultation (e.g., bursectomy, partial resection of greater trochanteric process)

THE REHABILITATION PROGRAM

A structured rehabilitation program will help to decrease acute or chronic pain, improve hip range of motion (ROM), improve gait mechanics, improve sleep by decreasing pain with side-lying, and restore overall function. The program should focus on pain reduction, stretching, and strengthening to restore proper hip biomechanics and balance to the lower limbs, and should especially improve upon strength and control of the hip abductors, extensors, and overall core strength. Gait training is an important component of the program, since gait abnormalities are common with GTPS.

Along with a rehabilitation program, the patient needs to be instructed on proper activity modification, relative rest, avoiding direct pressure on the area as well as the need for an independent home exercise program (HEP). Activity modification is part of the overall plan and includes avoidance of laying/sleeping on the affected side, and avoidance of sitting with the legs crossed. If the patient is involved in athletic activities and training, their running distance and intensity should be modified, the running surface may need to be modified (e.g., avoiding banked tracks), and weight lifting activities such as squatting should be modified if symptoms are being reproduced. In addition to patient education and therapeutic exercise, modalities and manual therapy techniques are frequently utilized. Transcutaneous electrical neuromuscular stimulation (TENS), cold (or low level) laser therapy, pulsed magnetic field therapy, and cross-frictional massage may also be beneficial but have not been properly evaluated for GTPS. Application of the kinetic chain theory or regional interdependence concept is appropriate. Therefore, joint hypomobility and myofascial restrictions of the lumbar spine, pelvis, hip, knee, and/or ankles may be contributing factors to increased friction on the lateral hip area and should be addressed by the rehabilitation program.

Therapeutic Modalities

Both ice and heat have been recommended for the management of pain associated with GTPS, although these treatments have limited evidence to support their efficacy. During the acute phase, it may be better to use ice. Ice massage is one technique that is fast and efficient for treatment during the acute phase. Ice and heat are not to be used independently, but as part of a therapeutic program and may offer additional benefit over exercise alone. Ice remains an excellent home modality and is recommended as a treatment to the painful area for 20 minutes duration every 2 to 3 hours. Ultrasound (deep heating modality) may also be beneficial especially in chronic cases, but studies have not proven its effectiveness (21).

Low-energy extracorporeal shock wave therapy (ESWT) and high dose pulsed ultrasound modalities have also been described as helpful treatments often in patients who have calcific GTPS (22–24). Low-energy ESWT has demonstrated conflicting efficacy, showing treatment success for GTPS in a case controlled study (23), but when compared to a home training program in a randomized controlled trial (RCT) it failed to demonstrate any significant difference in the short or long term (24). Cold laser, TENS, iontophoresis, and phonophoresis have all been used clinically as adjunctive therapeutic modalities, although they currently lack adequate evidence to support their use.

Manual Therapy

Deep tissue massage, myofascial release techniques, and soft tissue mobilization have been suggested as helpful treatments for the soft tissues of the lateral hip. Transverse friction massage (cross-friction) for the treatment of tendinopathy and bursitis is controversial and has not been proven to be beneficial but further evaluation is needed (25). Soft tissue massage of the ITB can be helpful, especially if combined with a therapeutic program to restore length and flexibility to the ITB and strength to the gluteus medius. Osteopathic manipulative therapy may be of benefit for biomechanical factors contributing to the problem, such as mal-alignment and/or mobility problems of the lumbosacral spine, pelvis, sacrum, and lower limb.

In general, manual therapy can be utilized to treat any soft tissue or joint restrictions at the hip, lumbar spine, pelvis, knee, ankle, or foot joint and this may improve gait, restore normal hip mechanics, and decrease frictional forces on the lateral hip. Despite the widespread use of these techniques by many different healthcare practitioners (e.g., physical therapy [PT], chiropractor, osteopathic physician) and an understanding of functional anatomy that rationalizes this approach, larger scale clinical trials are needed to support manual therapy as an adjunctive treatment of GTPS.

Therapeutic Exercise

Relative rest and therapeutic modalities help patients progress from phase I to II of rehabilitation. Many patients with GTPS experience hip joint stiffness and restricted ROM on the affected side. Restoring normal hip ROM during phase II can be achieved with active, active assisted, and passive range of motion (A/AA/PROM) as well as stretching and manual therapy techniques.

Stretching and strengthening of the bilateral lower limbs will help to restore muscular balance and coordination of the buttock and hip muscles. The focus should be on stretching the tight structures and strengthening the weak muscles on the affected side, while exercising both limbs to help achieve better muscular balance, conditioning, and improved function.

The flexibility program for GTPS usually focuses on stretching of the ITB and TFL. Stretching exercises may be also be necessary to address length deficits of the hamstrings, quadriceps, glutei, and piriformis. Stretching may initially need to be therapist assisted to get the best stretch possible, with self-stretching done at home. One technique to stretch the ITB and TFL is in the supine position with different amounts of hip flexion to stretch all parts/fibers of the ITB and TFL. Another good technique is an assisted stretch in side-lying: with the hip extended, the therapist applies a stabilizing force on the hip and a downward force on the lower limb into hip adduction (Figure 21.1). Standing TFL/ITB stretches can mobilize

the hip into extension and adduction to provide a good self-stretch (Figure 21.2). Some physiotherapists suggest the need for gentle stretching of the ITB, since excessive compression via hip adduction across the greater trochanter can aggravate the condition. In addition, stretching of the TFL/ITB alone, without neuromuscular reeducation and strengthening of the glutei muscles (e.g., gluteus medius), may fail to restore muscular balance and lead to poor outcomes with conservative care (26,28).

Strengthening of the hip abductors (especially the gluteus medius), external rotators, and extensors, as well as the knee extensors and core musculature is essential to help improve gait, hip biomechanics, and pelvic stability or control. Ankle weights or resistance bands can be used to aid progress in the early phases of strengthening with a plan to progress to dynamic strengthening. Strengthening can be either weight bearing or nonweight bearing (26), however, these exercises should progress to functional, sport, and

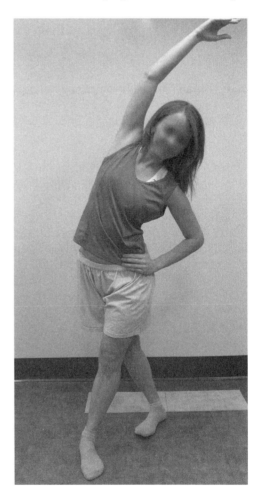

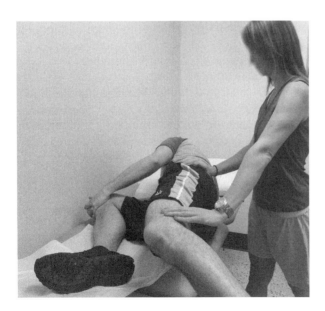

FIGURE 21.1: Therapist-assisted ITB stretch.

FIGURE 21.2: Standing self-stretch of the ITB.

dynamic activity specific strengthening as soon as possible. Recent studies have demonstrated various exercises that have generated the greatest electromyographic (EMG) activity of the hip abductor muscles (29) as well as the hip extensors, such as side-lying hip abduction for the gluteus medius and single-limb squat or single-limb deadlift for the gluteus maximus (26). Neuromuscular and proprioceptive training may help to regain muscle balance and coordination and to prevent further injury and should be included before the final phase of rehabilitation.

In addition, analysis of gait, running, and kinetic chain assessment may identify significant abnormalities that are contributing to the problem. Trendelenberg sign may suggest the need for closed chain hip abductor strengthening; excessive foot pronation may identify the need for stretching/strengthening of the foot and ankle, such as the gastrocnemius, or even the need for orthotics (27). These final steps help to individualize the program and improve the outcome of conservative treatment.

Specialized Techniques

Kinesiology taping has been used for ITB syndrome and Piriformis syndrome. Since ITB tightness tends to accompany GTPS this technique may be of benefit. It has also been used in stroke patients to improve hip extension (30). Thus Kinesio® taping may be beneficial in GTPS also if there are weaknesses of hip extension or ITB tightness but to the best of our knowledge this has not been studied in a patient population with GTPS. One may also consider aquatic therapy to decrease weight bearing forces across the joint, especially at the beginning of a therapeutic exercise program and in patients with co-existing hip OA.

Home Exercise Program

A good HEP will be taught to the patient during their formal therapy sessions and should be reevaluated multiple times to ensure proper exercise technique and patient safety. A HEP should be continued by the patient after completing their therapy program to maintain flexibility, muscle coordination, and strength and to help prevent recurrent GTPS.

Patient education should not only encompass the HEP, but should also teach joint protection strategies, postural training, home modalities for pain management, proper use of assistive device if deemed appropriate, activity modification, and relative rest as well as energy conservation techniques.

SUMMARY

GTPS is a common musculoskeletal condition which tends to respond well to conservative treatment. A comprehensive assessment and individualized rehabilitation program with stretching and strengthening of the appropriate muscle groups as detailed in this chapter is generally successful in decreasing pain and improving function.

SAMPLE CASE

A 25-year-old female has been having left lateral hip pain for 2 weeks. She likes to jog and tends to run on uneven surfaces. She has no significant past medical, surgical, or family history. She has been taking Tylenol for pain with minimal relief. Her pain is worse with activity and when lying on her left side. There are no radicular symptoms, or associated numbness or tingling. Review of systems is unremarkable. She denies ever having an injury to the left lateral hip but notes she had similar pain 1 year ago that went away after she stopped running. On physical examination she is well nourished with normal lower extremity alignment. She has no skin lesions over the lateral hip area and has good muscle bulk at the hip and lower limb. She reports point tenderness to palpation over the left greater trochanter, including the gluteus medius insertion site. There is mild tightness of the left ITB and mild weakness of the left hip abductors and extensors. Otherwise neurological and musculoskeletal exam is unremarkable.

 SAMPLE THERAPY PRESCRIPTION

Discipline: Physical therapy.

Diagnosis: Left GTPS.

Precautions: Full weight bearing. Avoid exercises which worsen pain. Avoid lying on left side for a prolonged time.

Frequency of visits: 2 to 3x/week.

Duration of treatment: 3 to 4 weeks (or a total of 8–12 visits).

Treatment:

1. *Modalities:* Cryotherapy, including home ice massages for acute GTPS; for chronic cases may consider superficial and deep heating modalities

2. *Manual therapy:* Joint and soft tissue mobilization, myofascial release to the lateral hip structures, especially the proximal ITB

3. *Therapeutic exercise:* A/AA/PROM of the hip to address restrictions, therapist assisted stretching of the lower limbs with focus on the left ITB, hamstrings, hip flexors, piriformis, and glutei, Strengthening of the lower limbs with focus on the hip abductors, extensors, and external rotators. Core strengthening (e.g., pelvic floor, multifidus, deep abdominals), balance/proprioceptive training, neuro-muscular reeducation, and aerobic and conditioning exercises as deemed appropriate

4. *Specialized treatments:* Analysis of gait, running, and kinetic chain assessment to identify and address specific biomechanical problems. Kinesio® taping of the ITB and glutei to assist neuromuscular reeducation

5. *Patient education:* HEP to include stretching and strengthening as above, as well as education on proper body biomechanics, proper sleep positioning (to prevent irritation of left hip area), relative rest, and proper running form

Goals: Decrease pain; improve function, restore flexibility and strength, improve balance/proprioception, education and retraining of proper biomechanics (especially while running for the above patient).

Reevaluation: In 4 to 6 weeks by referring physician.

REFERENCES

1. Segal NA, Felson DT, Torner JC, et al. Greater trochanteric pain syndrome: epidemiology and associated factors. *Arch Phys Med Rehabil.* 2007;88(8):988–992.
2. Little H. Trochanteric bursitis: a common cause of pelvic girdle pain. *Can Med Assoc J.* 1979;120(4):456–458.
3. Shbeeb MI. Matteson EL. Trochanteric bursitis (greater trochanter pain syndrome). *Mayo Clin Proc.* 1996;71(6):565–569.
4. Strauss EJ, Nho SJ, Kelly BT. Greater trochanteric pain syndrome. *Sports Med Arthrosc.* 2010;18(2):113–119.
5. Tibor LM, Sekiya JK. Differential diagnosis of pain around the hip joint. *Arthroscopy.* 2008;24(12):1407–1421.
6. Williams BS, Cohen SP. Greater trochanteric pain syndrome: a review of anatomy, diagnosis and treatment. *Anesth Analg.* 2009;108(5):1662–1670.
7. Raman D, Haslock I. Trochanteric bursitis—a frequent cause of "hip" pain in rheumatoid arthritis. *Ann Rheum Dis.* 1982;41(6):602–603.
8. Karpinski MR, Piggott H. Greater trochanteric pain syndrome. A report of 15 cases. *J Bone Joint Surg Br.* 1985;67(5):762–763.
9. Traycoff RB. "Pseudotrochanteric bursitis": the differential diagnosis of lateral hip pain. *J Rheumatol.* 1991;18(12):1810–1812.
10. Robertson WJ, Gardner MJ, Barker JU, Boraiah S, Lorich DG, Kelly BT. Anatomy and dimensions of the gluteus medius tendon insertion. *Arthroscopy.* 2008;24(2):130–136.
11. Woodley SJ, Mercer SR, Nicholson HD. Morphology of the bursae associated with the greater trochanter of the femur. *J Bone Joint Surg Am.* 2008;90(2):284–294.
12. Dunn T, Heller CA, McCarthy SW, et al. Anatomical study of the "trochanteric bursa". *Clin Anat.* 2003;16(3):233–240.
13. Lequesne M, Mathieu P, Vuillemin-Bodaghi V, Bard H, Djian P. Gluteal tendinopathy in refractory greater trochanter pain syndrome: diagnostic value of two clinical tests. *Arthritis Rheum.* 2008;59(2):241–246.
14. Bird PA, Oakley SP, Shnier R, Kirkham BW. Prospective evaluation of magnetic resonance imaging and physical examination findings in patients with greater trochanteric pain syndrome. *Arthritis Rheum.* 2001;44(9):2138–2145.
15. Walsh G, Archibald CG. MRI in greater trochanter pain syndrome. *Australas Radiol.* 2003;47(1):85–7.
16. Kong AA. Van der Vliet, Zadow S. MRI and US of gluteal tendinopathy in greater trochanteric pain syndrome. *Eur Radiol.* 2007;17(7):1772–1783.
17. Kingzett-Taylor A, Tirman PF, Feller J, et al. Tendinosis and tears of gluteus medius and minimus muscles as a cause of hip pain: MR imaging findings. *AJR Am J Roentgenol.* 1999;173(4):1123–1126.
18. Abdelwahab IF, Bianchi S, Martinoli C, Klein M, Hermann G. Atypical extraspinal musculoskeletal tuberculosis in immunocompetent patients: part II, tuberculous myositis, tuberculous bursitis, and tuberculous tenosynovitis. *Can Assoc Radiol J.* 2006;57(5):278–286.
19. Bertoli AM, et al. Soft tissue metastases presenting as greater trochanteric pain syndrome. *J Clin Rheumatol.* 2003;9(6):370–372.
20. Crespo M, Pigrau C, Flores X, et al. Tuberculous trochanteric bursitis: report of 5 cases and literature review. *Scand J Infect Dis.* 2004;36(8):552–558.

21. Butcher JD, Salzman KL, Lillegard WA. Lower extremity bursitis. *Am Fam Physician*. 1996;53(7):2317–2324.

22. Crevenna R, et al. Calcific trochanteric bursitis: resolution of calcifications and clinical remission with non-invasive treatment. A case report. *Wien Klin Wochenschr*. 2002;114(8-9):345–348.

23. Furia JP, Rompe JD Maffulli N. Low-energy extracorporeal shock wave therapy as a treatment for greater trochanteric pain syndrome. *Am J Sports Med*. 2009;37(9):1806–1813.

24. Rompe JD, Segal NA, Cacchio A, et al. Home training, local corticosteroid injection, or radial shock wave therapy for greater trochanter pain syndrome. *Am J Sports Med*. 2009;37(10):1981–1990.

25. Brosseau L, et al. Deep transverse friction massage for treating tendinitis. *Cochrane Database Syst Rev*. 2002(1):CD003528.

26. Distefano LJ, Blackburn JT, Marshall SW, Padua DA. Gluteal muscle activation during common therapeutic exercises. *J Orthop Sports Phys Ther*. 2009;39(7):532–540.

27. Geraci MC, Jr. Brown W. Evidence-based treatment of hip and pelvic injuries in runners. *Phys Med Rehabil Clin N Am*. 2005;16(3):711–747.

28. Bewyer DC, Bewyer KJ. Rationale for treatment of hip abductor pain syndrome. *Iowa Orthop J*. 2003;23:57–60.

29. Bolgla LA, Uhl TL. Electromyographic analysis of hip rehabilitation exercises in a group of healthy subjects. *J Orthop Sports Phys Ther*. 2005;35(8):487–494.

30. Kilbreath SL, Perkins S, Crosbie J, McConnell J. Gluteal taping improves hip extension during stance phase of walking following stroke. *Aust J Physiother*. 2006;52(1):53–56.

Hamstring Strains and Tendinopathy

Annemarie E. Gallagher, Pete Draovitch, and Peter J. Moley

INTRODUCTION

The hamstrings are a collection of three muscles in the posterior thigh: semimembranosus, semitendinosus, and the long and short heads of the biceps femoris. These muscles primarily work as hip extensors and pelvic stabilizers, as well as flexors of the knee. The semimembranosus, semitendinosus, and long head of the biceps femoris originate at the ischial tuberosity. These three muscles cross two joints (the hip and the knee prior to insert onto the proximal tibia and fibula), which makes them prone to injury, particularly during eccentric contraction (Figure 22.1).

Of the hamstrings, the most commonly injured muscle is the biceps femoris. It is hypothesized that this may be due to the dual innervation of the long and short heads of this muscle. The long head of the biceps femoris is innervated by the tibial branch of the sciatic nerve, while the short head is innervated by the peroneal branch of the sciatic nerve. It is thought that the difference in nerve supply leads to asynchronous movements of these parts of the muscle, leading to a propensity for strains and other injuries (1,2). In addition, the sciatic nerve itself passes approximately 1.2cm (on average) lateral to the ischial tuberosity, the origin of the hamstrings, making this nerve susceptible to damage in hamstring injuries as well.

Muscle strains account for approximately 30% of the injuries seen in the practice of Sports Medicine (3) and hamstring strains are the most common. The majority of hamstring injuries occur at the musculotendinous junction of the biceps femoris (4,5). Factors that predispose patients to hamstring injury include a history of a hamstring strain, poor stretching prior to engaging in sport, and limited flexibility (1,6,7). There is also an increased incidence of hamstring injury with increased age, and there is a high recurrence rate of such injury. This may be due to the muscle fiber degeneration that comes with aging.

It is important to review some basic *kinesiology* of the hamstring muscle to further understand hamstring injuries. In the terminal swing phase, the hamstrings are activated and eccentrically contract for the purpose of decelerating the distal leg and controlling knee extension. This is especially important in running. Muscles that cross two joints, as the hamstrings do, work via eccentric contraction. The eccentric contraction of the hamstrings ensures the coordination of hip and knee movement (8). The hamstrings reach their peak length in terminal swing just before foot strike, and this is when the hamstrings are most susceptible to injury (8).

Acute hamstring strains are commonly sustained in a variety of sports (3). Hamstring injuries can be divided into two main categories: injuries of the muscle belly (strains, contusions, and myositis ossificans) and injuries of the tendon origins (tendinopathy, apophysitis, tendon tears, and osseous tears or complete avulsions) (7). In this chapter, we will focus on *hamstring strains and tendinopathy*.

Strains typically occur in extremes of positioning, such as extremes of hip flexion and knee extension with hamstring strains. Hamstring strains can be classified based on how the injury was sustained (i.e., while in eccentric contraction as in sprinting or while in extreme stretch as in dancing). In high speed running, hamstring injury can be consistently localized in the long head of the biceps femoris (9). Meanwhile, in dancers, hamstring injury can be seen after stretching at or beyond joint end range. Strains are often located in the proximal hamstrings, near the insertion site at the ischial tuberosity. Studies have shown that a hamstring strain sustained from stretching often requires increased healing time compared to a hamstring injury from high speed running, and the closer the injury to the ischial tuberosity, the longer the recovery time (9).

Patients typically present with pain in the posterior thigh and tenderness to palpation of the muscle belly.

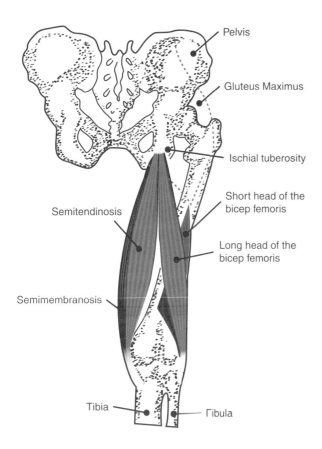

FIGURE 22.1: Anatomy of the hamstring muscles.

Hamstring strains are common in runners, long jumpers, hurdlers, and other sports involving sprinting or kicking. Injuries of the hamstrings often occur despite stretching and strengthening. Patients with proximal hamstring strain or tendinopathy are usually not able to recall a specific inciting event. However, continued stretching of the posterior thigh can exacerbate pain and other symptoms (10).

Hamstring injuries or strains can be graded from I to III. Grade I is a strain, associated with low grade inflammation. Grade II presents as moderate strength loss, and there will often be a concurrent regional hematoma and laminar fluid collection. Grade III is a complete tear, and patients will present with total loss of function (11,12).

Hamstring tendinopathy is a chronic degenerative condition at the origin or insertion of the hamstrings. There may be tenderness over the thickened, chronically inflamed tendon. Tendinopathy of the proximal hamstrings is manifested by lower gluteal discomfort or pain, and can

be exacerbated by strenuous activity or sport, especially sprinting, long distance running, or soccer (13). Prolonged sitting has also been identified as an exacerbating factor with hamstring tendinopathy. Hamstring tendinopathy is caused by mechanical overload and repetitive stretch, resulting in failed healing of an initial injury. This is why initial injury can be caused by such exercises as running (repetitive stretch) and exacerbated by continued exercise (persistent mechanical overload) (14). The repetitive stretching and overloading can cause scarring and adhesions to form around the sciatic nerve, thereby causing additional pain in the posterior thigh (10). Furthermore, the radiating pain that may be felt in swing phase may be secondary to sciatic nerve impingement from a thickened tendon insertion on the lateral ischial tuberosity (10).

Key elements of the physical examination include inspection and palpation of the injured area, passive stretch and resistance testing for the hamstring, and examination of the hip and lumbar spine with a lower limb neurological examination to rule out referred pain. It is important to keep in mind when formulating the differential diagnosis that posterior thigh pain may be referred pain from the lumbar spine and hip. Evaluation of hamstring pain would include range of motion (ROM) testing of the lumbar spine, palpation of the sacroiliac joint, a slump test, and thorough examination of the hip. Positive dural tension signs suggest that the posterior thigh pain is likely referred from above (e.g., nerve root compression). Pain with hip extension can also be a sign of posterior impingement or hip arthritis. Patients often present with reproduction of pain with passive hamstring stretch, prone resisted knee flexion and/or hip extension, and palpation of the posterior thigh.

Severe strains can cause ecchymoses around the injured region and can track into the different compartments of the thigh. Tenderness to palpation, localized to the posterior thigh upon hamstring stretching and resisted contraction, is consistent with hamstring strain or tendinopathy, and the injury may be at the site of attachment, in the tendon, or at the musculotendinous junction. Hamstring strains usually present without significant weakness in knee flexion or hip extension, but pain may be reproduced with resisted contraction. Physical examination and imaging can demonstrate findings consistent with hamstring strain up to 12 months after the initial injury (15). Features suggestive of hamstring strain include an audible "pop" at the time of injury, minor pain in the acute phase of injury, and proximity of the injury to the ischial tuberosity (15).

Patients may present months after the initial injury with persistent pain and posterior thigh cramping, worsened by extreme positioning of the joint in either hip flexion or knee extension, or sitting for an extended period. In chronic injury, patients can experience pain similar to sciatica secondary to scar tissue surrounding the sciatic nerve due to the proximity of this nerve to the ischial tuberosity. Neurolysis may be required to relieve the sciatic symptoms (16). It has been established that injury site, extent of muscle-tendon involvement, and return to play are interrelated. Patients must be reminded, particularly if the injury was sustained months prior to presentation, that this type of injury requires an extensive course of rehabilitation, which prolongs return to play.

Grade I strains are identified on MRI by a small amount of edema and hemorrhage at the injured musculotendinous junction. On T2-weighted images, there is also high intensity signal of the affected muscle (12). With healing, the high intensity signal will return to normal (12). Thinning of the tendons, along with increased amounts of edema and hemorrhage, are consistent with a grade II injury.

On MRI, tendinopathy is seen as increased tendon girth and increased signal heterogeneity at and around the site of origin of the hamstring tendons (2,7,11). The tendons are edematous, and marrow edema of the ischial tuberosity may be seen, as well (11). MRI often demonstrates lateral border semimembranosus tendon thickening with increased signal intensity on T1-weighted and proton density images. The biceps femoris may also show thickening and hyperintensity. Thickening of the tendon insertion lateral to the ischial tuberosity can be visualized as the cause of direct sciatic nerve compression, which also contributes to pain symptoms (11).

MRI can accurately demonstrate the length and extent of the muscle injury, which often correlates with the time required for rehabilitation. With the visualization of edema and fluid signal, consistent with bleeding, the severity of muscle damage and the duration of an anticipated rehabilitation course can be estimated (4). Furthermore, the likelihood of reinjury can be determined based on the length of the muscle damage. Muscle atrophy, fatty infiltration, and scar tissue formation can contribute to reinjury because the mechanics of the muscle is impaired (17). Plain films and electromyography are typically normal. On ultrasound (US) examination, tendinopathy is seen as a thickened, hypoechoic tendon (2). Remember that histological evaluation of tendinopathy reveals round tenocyte nuclei, collagen degeneration, increased vascular proliferation, and increased ground substance (10). Fatty degeneration may also be seen, as evidenced by fat cells present between the collagen bundles. These histological findings provide some insight into how tendinopathy presents on MRI and US imaging studies.

In an acute hamstring injury, pain is mediated by inflammation. Conservative management includes the use of nonsteroidal anti-inflammatory drugs (NSAIDs), which can help to control the resultant inflammatory response, thereby decreasing pain. Conservative management of hamstring tendinopathy includes rest from sport, NSAIDs, corticosteroids, hamstring stretching, and physical therapy, focusing on eccentric strengthening. The early use of NSAIDs after muscle or tendon injuries has recently been debated due to possible impaired healing, with increased fibrosis and decreased tensile strength, secondary to a stunted inflammatory response (18). This is a controversial topic, but should be considered in the acute treatment of muscle and tendon injuries.

HAMSTRING STRAINS AND TENDINOPATHY

- Hamstring strains and tendinopathy are common overuse injuries secondary to repetitive stretch (such as in running) and are exacerbated by persistent mechanical overload from continued exercise

- Hamstring strains are graded as follows:

  1. Grade I: Low grade inflammatory response; no loss of strength or function

  2. Grade II: Tissue damage with resultant decreased strength at the musculotendinous junction

  3. Grade III: Complete tear; significant loss of function

- Key physical examination findings include pain with passive hamstring stretch, resistance testing of knee flexion or hip extension, and palpation of the posterior thigh

- Signs of hamstring strain include tenderness to palpation of the posterior thigh +/- ecchymosis; without significant knee flexion or hip extension weakness, unless a grade III injury has occurred

▨ MRI is a useful tool to analyze the extent of tendon injury and to monitor musculotendinous remodeling.

▨ Conservative management of hamstring tendinopathy includes rest from sport, analgesics or NSAIDs, corticosteroids, hamstring stretching, and physical therapy, focusing on eccentric strengthening by the end of the program to prevent recurrent injury

THE REHABILITATION PROGRAM

Rehabilitation of an injured hamstring can range from managing acute strains to chronic tendinopathies to complete avulsions. Acute strains will follow guidelines for acute insult to contractile tissue, while tendinopathy may respond best to treatment associated with chronic fibrotic-type tissue. Regardless of the type of hamstring injury incurred, the rehabilitation process needs to be progressive in nature (19–21) and should follow the phases of rehabilitation. Recognizing the workload threshold during the process is not always the easiest thing to predict or manage. The location of the injury, combined with the time frame for treatment commencement certainly plays a role in rehabilitation management. In addition, existing structural and environmental variables, such as femoral acetabular impingement (FAI), poor trunk stability, coexisting low back pain (LBP), time of season, prescribed radiologic interventions, previous hamstring history, and even decreased ankle dorsiflexion (22) need to be considered for program development and recovery.

Specific to rehabilitation, evidence is beginning to support the use of eccentric exercise for both tendinopathies and muscle strains (19). Agre recommends that the best treatment is prevention, but after an injury has occurred, a sound rehabilitation program should include work-out variables of strength, flexibility, endurance, coordination, and agility (20). Hamstring injury mechanisms, such as maximum sprinting, kicking, acceleration, and change of direction must be incorporated to ensure a complete functional recovery and neuromuscular adaptation (23–25). Altered neuromuscular control of injured hamstrings has been demonstrated when the leg is preparing for single leg stance (24), therefore, neuromuscular reeducation and proprioceptive training is a key component of rehabilitation and injury prevention.

Therapeutic Modalities

Expert opinion supports the use of cryotherapy during phase I of rehabilitation, as part of the PRICE protocol to control the pain and swelling associated with acute hamstring injuries. Superficial and deep heating modalities combined with stretching have been recommended as treatments to improve soft tissue flexibility and decrease pain. However, these modalities have not been adequately studied in the setting of hamstring injuries and, therefore, have not been demonstrated to be better than stretching alone.

Increased interest in therapeutic shock wave therapy for the nonoperative treatment of tendinopathy has led to many recent studies, including an randomized control trial on shock wave therapy compared to traditional conservative treatment for chronic proximal hamstring tendinopathy in professional athletes. In this study, Cacchio et al found shockwave therapy to be an effective treatment for tendinopathy, as far out as 3 months post treatment. The shockwave group had an 85% success rate. There was at least a 50% reduction in pain versus the traditional treatment group that only had a 10% success rate (26). Additional research is necessary to confirm the results of this study, but shockwave therapy appears to be a promising therapeutic modality for proximal hamstring tendinopathy.

Manual Therapy

Soft tissue techniques, such as massage, myofascial release, transverse friction massage, and soft tissue mobilization are commonly utilized to treat hamstring strains and tendinopathy. Mobilization techniques that include a transversely-directed force have been shown to greatly influence the passive biomechanical properties of the muscle-tendon unit. These techniques combined with longitudinal loading through the hamstring muscle-tendon unit can improve the flexibility of the hamstrings (27).

When applying the principles of regional interdependence, manual therapy techniques such as joint mobilizations or even muscle energy techniques may be utilized for the lumbar spine and pelvis, especially if motion restrictions or poor postural alignment is identified. Pelvic asymmetry and excessive anterior tilt can result in increased tension at the origin of the biceps femoris, leading to increased functional demands on the hamstrings (28). In addition, manual manipulation of the sacroiliac joint has been shown to alter the peak torque of the hamstrings, even more so than moist heat followed by passive stretching alone (29).

Although current research does not definitively support the use of therapeutic exercise combined with modalities and manual therapy over therapeutic exercise alone for the management of hamstring strains or tendinopathy, this type of comprehensive approach is supported by expert opinion. Hopefully future research efforts will clarify the role of these adjunctive treatments on the management of acute and chronic hamstring injuries.

Therapeutic Exercise for Acute Hamstring Strain

According to Khan and Scott (30), 30% to 50% of injuries in sport are tendon injuries. The mechanical variability of the acute hamstring strain can occur in the dancer from slow movement stretching or in the sprinter who pulls up holding the back of their leg. The sprinter's injury may appear more obvious and may present with more of a functional deficit, but research has shown that the recovery may be shorter when comparing these two groups (15). Late swing phase is when the demands placed on the hamstring seem most consistent and is why eccentrics should play a major role in the program (31). Biceps femoris strains accounted for 80% of the 170 hamstring injuries which occurred in athletes in the study by Koulouris and Connell (32). Thelen et al concluded that because the biceps femoris has greatest lengthening and electrical activity during the late swing phase of running, it may be more at risk

for insult than its medial hamstring counterparts (33). The rate of reinjury ranged from 12% to 31% (34,35) and was most likely to occur within the first 2 weeks of return to sport (17).

When reviewing the different rehabilitation programs in the literature, most programs offer no more evidence than expert opinion (36). However, Sherry and Best, compared two different rehabilitation programs, a progressive agility and trunk stabilization (PATS) program and a traditional stretching and strengthening (STST) program. The PATS program focused on frontal and transverse plane training before initiating sagittal plane movement and demonstrated a superior reinjury rate of 0% and 8% at 2 weeks and 1 year, respectively. In comparison, the STST program demonstrated a reinjury rate of 55% at 2 weeks and 70% at 1 year (34).

The initial goal of therapy is to control pain and inflammation and to protect the injured structure. The patient may start safely with mid-range pain-free movement exercises. It is important to begin with trunk stabilization and simple agility drills. As the patient progresses to pain-free walking and light jogging, strengthening should focus on supine bent knee bridge walk outs, supine single leg chair bridge, and single leg balance windmill touches. Fast jogging and sprinting should not be implemented until there is equal bilateral strength at 90°, 45°, and 15° of knee flexion.

Strengthening the strained hamstrings should emphasize eccentric exercises and should include both static and dynamic stretching (see Figure 22.2a and 22.2b) (37). Eccentric prone throw downs are also encouraged

(a)

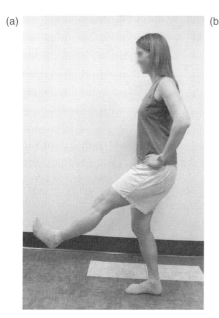

(b)

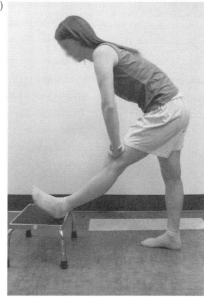

FIGURE 22.2: (a) Dynamic hamstring stretching. (b) Static hamstring stretching.
Source: Adapted from Ref (37).

(see Figure 22.3) (37). Frontal and transverse plane motion should be the focus before progressing to sagittal plane strengthening. Wooden dowel tug of war pulls will also engage the hamstrings in a closed kinetic chain position. The ultimate goal of therapeutic exercise is painless end range swing position for walking and running. In addition, studies suggest that eccentric training is effective, not only for rehabilitation of hamstring strains, but also for primary and secondary prevention (37).

Therapeutic Exercise for Hamstring Tendinopathy

Proximal hamstring tendinopathy presents with a different set of problems than an acute hamstring strain. Whether the mechanism is due to overuse in activities requiring

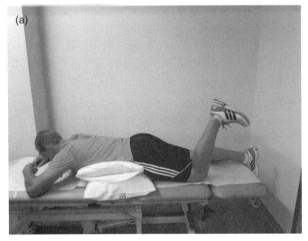

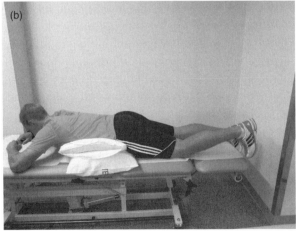

FIGURE 22.3: Eccentric prone throw downs.
Source: Adapted From Ref (42).

long distance running or sprinting, repetitive cutting in soccer, or an offensive lineman being asked to control an opposing force, the athlete will most likely complain of proximal hamstring or buttock pain. Eccentric training may work well for tendinopathy-type problems (36,38,39).

Alfredson was one of the first people to clinically study diseased tendon (39). His work on the Achilles tendon consisted of twice daily eccentric workloads 7 days per week for a period of 12 weeks. The results demonstrated return to pre-injury activity levels, accompanied by significantly decreased pain and increased strength. Physiologically, this makes sense based on the work of Williams in the 1980s. Williams found that during eccentric training, oxygen consumption is 7.5 times lower for tendons and ligaments when compared to skeletal muscle. Lower metabolic rates are required to create loads and tension over long periods of time (38).

Proximal attachment tendinopathy responds best to eccentric exercise. Ideally, the initial treatment of choice is 2 weeks of rest and pain-free activities of daily living (ADLs). Following this rest period, easy stationary cycling and eccentric exercises should commence. Eccentrics include Romanian dead lifts (RDLs) and prone leg lowering 4 days/week for another 2 to 4 weeks. Between the 4th and 6th week, concentric exercises should be the focus in frontal and transverse planes. Sagittal plane exercises commence shortly afterward. Eccentric exercises can include single leg RDLs, windmills, step-downs, hip hikes, Swedish hamstrings, steamboat extensions, stability ball bridges, and single leg bridge lowering (refer to Table 22.1 for exercise descriptions). If accessible, Alter-G or suspension system for initiating jogging/running may provide a more controlled environment.

Dynamic warm-ups may include a wall push running drill, Mach A/B, claws, standing leg swings, and prone throw downs (refer to Table 22.1 for exercise descriptions). Leg press, leg curl, and four-way hip extensions can then be initiated, but caution must be used to ensure that the patient goes up on two legs and down on one leg. Often a spotter is required to aid with the concentric portion of the exercise. Explosive lifting should be initiated with the resistance bands, such as the commercially available Flex Band, performing super 4s (push press, military, overhead squat) and sidestep snatches. This typically helps ensure a safe, neuromuscular progression regarding return to the weight room, if desired.

TABLE 22.1: Advanced Hamstring Exercises With Descriptions

Exercise	Description of the Exercise
Swedish hamstrings	The athlete or patient assumes an upright kneeling position. A half foam roller is then placed underneath the dorsum of the foot for comfort. The therapist or coach then secures the back of the athlete's ankles to hold the body in place. The athlete then falls forward toward the mat while maintaining the upright posture, being sure to catch themselves with their hands before falling into the mat. The athlete then uses their hands to push themselves back up into the starting position. The end position of the fall would be the same as a push up being performed on the knees. 1 to 2 sets of 6 reps are enough of a workload to begin this exercise
Steamboat extensions	The athlete or patient stands on their affected leg and places a looped piece of tubing around the opposite ankle which is attached to a stationary object. The athlete then steps in a backward direction until there is some tension in the tubing. While standing on the affected side, the athlete then moves the opposite leg into an extended position, while the foot is off the ground. The amount of motion on the elastic tubing side should be cued by saying toes to heel and heel to toes in relationship to the foot that remains on the ground. It is important to maintain a stable trunk during the exercise in order not to compensate. It is recommended you perform 2 to 3 sets of 10 to 15 reps beginning with the affected leg being the stance leg for the first sets
Mach A & B & C Drills	These are running drills used by track coaches that attempt to teach good running form. The A drills are used to promote a thigh lifting action while the B drills are used to promote leg reach or pawing action. The C drills are implemented to promote push off or extension. Regarding the hamstring, any reaching, pawing, or push promotes hamstring strengthening whereas any lifting drill promotes recovery. These drills can be found in any track and field sprint book or by searching for technique on the Internet
Claws	This drill is usually done after the A skip drills and attempts to promote proper running form during both the recovery and push off phases of running. It is done in a stationary position with the starting position being the hip, knee, and ankle at 90°. The athlete then throws the leg toward the ground as if they were running, being sure to have the foot hit the ground at a point as close to directly below the hip as possible. The recovery phase is then initiated by pulling the heel toward the buttocks and driving the thigh up toward the original starting position

Both Mach drills and Fast Claw drills are late phase rehabilitation activities and are important things to consider as part of a rehab program for anyone whose sport or activity requires sprinting.

In a study performed by Andersen et al, the highest level of neuromuscular activation (67%–79%) was seen with open kinetic chain resistance exercises, which included isolated knee extension and hamstring curls. These results suggest that neuromuscular activation may be optimized through heavy resistance training, and if incorporated into a rehabilitation program, muscle growth and strength may be significantly stimulated (40).

In addition to eccentric exercise, dynamic warm-ups, and open kinetic chain resistance exercises, a recent Cochrane Review suggested that improved lumbar stability and pelvic motor control could aid in rehabilitation and even decrease the recurrence rate of hamstring injuries. Therefore, therapy for the injured hamstrings should also emphasize lumbar stabilization, sacroiliac and pelvic alignment, and improved posture mechanics (41).

Home Exercise Program

A well-designed home exercise program (HEP) will reinforce the exercises learned during the prescribed and supervised physical therapy sessions. The purpose of these exercises is to regain full function, return to sport, and prevent recurrent injury to the hamstrings. As a result, it is essential that the HEP become part of the patient's daily routine.

After resting for 2 weeks, a formal physical therapy program with home exercises should commence. The HEP should include daily dynamic warm-ups and eccentric stretching, as well as core strengthening and lumbo-pelvic stabilization exercises. As pain improves, open kinetic chain resistance exercises should be incorporated into the rehabilitation program. Fast jogging and sprinting should not be implemented until there is equal bilateral strength at 90°, 45°, and 15° of knee flexion. The ultimate goal of the therapeutic exercise regimen is to return to sport pain-free and to promote hamstring injury prevention.

SUMMARY

About 25 years ago, the hamstring injury mechanism was thought to be due to a combination of poor flexibility, decreased muscle strength and endurance, awkward running style, and early return to sport (20). Due to improved understanding of the biomechanics of sport and movement, in conjunction with more evidence based studies, we are moving in a direction that allows us to design effective rehabilitation and injury prevention programs. Rehabilitation programs need to be designed to mirror the demands of the patient's desired sport or activity and incorporate an eccentric and neuromuscular training regimen. This philosophy best offers us the chance at effective long-term results for managing hamstring pathology.

SAMPLE CASE

A 22-year-old sprinter presents with a 1 month history of right posterior thigh pain that developed following a race about 4 weeks ago. Onset of symptoms was gradual, and the pain is now constant and markedly worse with running and sitting for extended periods of time. Pain is moderately responsive to intermittent NSAID use. On physical examination, palpation of the posterior right thigh reproduces pain. Upon hamstring stretching and resisted contraction, pain is localized to the proximal posterior thigh, near the ischial tuberosity. There is no significant weakness in knee flexion or hip extension. Neurovascular examination is otherwise unremarkable.

SAMPLE THERAPY PRESCRIPTION

Discipline: Physical therapy.

Diagnosis: Right hamstring tendinopathy.

Precautions: None.

Frequency of visits: 1 to 2x/week.

Duration of visits: 6 to 12 weeks.

Treatments:

1. *Modalities:* Ice as needed, therapeutic shockwave therapy if available may be considered

2. *Manual therapy:* Myofascial release to the hamstrings, including soft tissue mobilization with transversely-directed force

3. *Therapeutic exercise:* should commence after 2 weeks of rest and painless ADLs

   a. Stretching: During week 2, eccentric strengthening of the hamstrings should begin. Between week 4 and week 6, concentric exercises should be the focus in frontal and transverse planes. Sagittal plane exercises should commence shortly afterward

   b. Strengthening: Pain-free isometric exercises for the hamstrings and glutei, as well as lumbo-pelvic strengthening. Progress to eccentric strengthening as tolerated

   c. Neuromuscular reeducation with open kinetic chain resistance exercises

   d. Functional retraining: Walking and light jogging can be pursued initially, and can be advanced to fast jogging and ultimately sprinting when knee flexion strength is equal bilaterally at 90°, 45°, and 15°

4. *Specialized Treatments:* Biomechanical analysis of the kinetic chain, review and correction of biomechanics of walking, running, and kicking

5. *Patient education:* Development of progressive, consistent HEP

Goals: Decrease pain with knee flexion and hip extension, restore hamstring ROM and strength, correct imbalances in running mechanics, return to sport, and initiate a maintenance HEP to prevent symptom recurrence.

Reevaluation: In 4 to 6 weeks by referring provider.

REFERENCES

1. Clanton TO, Coupe KJ. Hamstring strains in athletes: diagnosis and treatment. *J Am Acad Orthop Surg.* 1998;6:237-248.
2. Koulouris G, Connell D. Hamstring muscle complex: an imaging review. *Radiographics.* 2005;25:571-586.
3. Brooks JHM, Fuller CW, Kemp SPT, Reddin DB. Incidence, risk, and prevention of hamstring muscle injuries in professional rugby union. *Am J Sports Med.* 2006;34:1297-1306.
4. Connell DA, Schnieder-Kolsky ME, Hoving JL, et al. Longitudinal study comparing sonographic and MRI assessments of acute and healing hamstring injuries. *AJR.* 2004;183:975-984.
5. De Smet AA, Best TM. MR imaging of the distribution and location of acute hamstring injuries in athletes. *AJR.* 2000;174:393-399.
6. Brockett CL, Morgan DL, Proske U. Predicting hamstring strain injury in elite athletes. *Med Sci Sports Exerc.* 2004;36:379-387.
7. Davis KW. Imaging of the hamstrings. *Seminars Musculosk Radiol.* 2008;12:28-41.
8. Petersen J, Holmich P. Evidence based prevention of hamstring injuries in sport *Br J Sports Med.* 2005;39:319-326.
9. Askling CM, Tengvar M, Saartok T, Thorstensson A. Acute first time hamstring strains during high speed running: a longitudinal study including clinical and MRI findings. *Am J Sports Med.* 2007;35:197-206.
10. Lempainen L, Sarimo J, Mattila K, Vaittinen S, Orava S. Proximal hamstring tendinopathy: results of surgical management and histopathologic findings. *Am J Sports Med.* 2009;37:727-734.
11. Bencardino JT, Mellado JM. Hamstring injuries of the hip. *Magn Reson Imaging Clin N Am.* 2005;13:677-690.
12. Palmer WE, Kuong SJ, Elmadbouh HM. MR imaging of myotendinous strain. *AJR* 1999;173:703-9.
13. Fredericson M, Moore W, Guillet M, Beaulieu C. High hamstring tendinopathy in runners: meeting the challenges of diagnosis, treatment, and rehabilitation. *Phys Sports Med.* 2005;33:32-43.
14. Warden SJ. Animal models for the study of tendinopathy. *Br J Sports Med.* 2007;41:232-240.
15. Askling CM, Tengvar M, Saartok T, Thorstensson A. Proximal hamstring strains of stretching type in different sports: Injury situations, clinical and magnetic resonance imaging characteristics, and return to sport. *Am J Sports Med.* 2009;36:1799-1804.
16. Sarimo J, Lempainen L, Mattila K, Orava S. Complete proximal hamstring avulsions: a series of 41 patients with operative treatment. *Am J Sports Med.* 2008;36:1110-1115.
17. Orchard J, Best TM. The management of muscle strain injuries: an early return versus the risk of recurrence. *Clin J Sports Med.* 2002;12:3-5.
18. Shen W, Li Y, Ying Tang Y, Cummins J, Huard J. NS-398, a cyclooxygenase-2-specific inhibitor, delays skeletal muscle healing by decreasing regeneration and promoting fibrosis. *Am J Pathol.* 2005;167(4):1105-1117.
19. Lorenz D, Reiman M. The role and implementation of eccentric training in athletic rehabilitation: tendinopathy, hamstring strains and ACL reconstruction. *Int J Sports Phys Ther.* 2011;6(1):27-44.
20. Agre JC. Hamstring injuries. Proposed aetiological factors, prevention and treatment. *Sports Med.* 1985;2(1):21-33.
21. Mendiguchia J, Brughelli M. A return to sport algorithm for acute hamstring injuries. *Phys Ther Sports.* 2011;12(1):2-14.
22. Gabbe BJ, Bennell KL, Finch CF, Wajswelner H, Orchard JW. Predictors of the hamstring injury at the elite level of Australian football. *Scan J Med Sci Sports.* 2006;16(1):7-13.
23. Brughelli M, Cronin J. Preventing hamstring injuries in sport. *Strength Cond J.* 2008;30:55-64.
24. Sole G, Milosavljevic S, Nicholson H, Sullivan SJ. Altered muscle activation following hamstring injuries. *Br J Sports Med.* 2012;46:118–123.
25. Heidersheit BC, Sherry MA, Silder A, Chumanov ES, Thelen DG. Hamstring strain injuries: recommendations for diagnosis, rehabilitation and injury prevention. *J Ortho Sports Phys Ther.* 2010;40(2):67-81.
26. Cacchio A, Rompe JD, Furia JP, Susi P, Santilli V, DePaulis F. Shockwave therapy for the treatment of chronic proximal hamstring tendinopathy in professional athletes. *Am J Sports Med.* 2011;39(1):146-153.
27. Rushton A, Spencer S. The effect of soft tissue mobilization techniques on flexibility and passive resistance in the hamstring muscle-tendon unit: a pilot investigation. *Man Ther.* 2011;16(2):161-166.
28. Panavi S. The need for lumbar-pelvic assessment in the resolution of chronic hamstring strain. *J Bodyw Mov Ther.* 2010;14(3):294-298.
29. Cibulka MT, Rose SJ, Delitto A, Sinacore DR. Hamstring muscle strain treated by mobilizing the sacroiliac joint. *Phys Ther.* 1986;66(8):1220-1223.
30. Khan KM, Scott A. Mechanotherapy: how physical therapists prescription of exercise promotes tissue repair. *Br J Sports Med.* 2009;43:247-251.
31. Chumanov E, Heiderscheit BC, Thelen DG. Hamstring musculotendon dynamics during stance and swing phases of high speed running. *Med Sci Sports Exerc.* 2011;43(3):525-532.
32. Koulouris G, Connell D. Evaluation of the hamstring muscle complex following acute injury. *Skeletal Radiol.* 2003;32:582-589.
33. Thelen D, Chumanov D, Hoerth M. Hamstring muscle kinematics during treadmill sprinting. *Med Sci Sports Exerc.* 2005;38:108-115.
34. Sherry MA, Best TM. A comparison of 2 rehabilitation programs in the treatment of acute hamstring strains. *J Ortho Sports Phy Ther.* 2004;34:116-125.

35. Peterson J, Holmich P. Evidence based prevention of hamstring injuries in sport. *Br J Sports Med.* 2005;39:319-325.
36. Copland ST, Tipton JS, Fields KB. Evidence based treatment of hamstring tears. *Curr Sports Med Rep.* 2009;8(6):308-314.
37. O'Sullivan K, Murray E, Sainsbury D. The effect of warm-up stretching and dynamic stretching on hamstring flexibility in previously injured subjects. *BMC Musculoskelet Disord.* 2009;16:10:37.
38. Williams JG. Achilles tendon lesions in sport. *Sports Med.* 1986;3:114-135.
39. Alfredson H, Pietila T, Jonsson P, Lorentzon R. Heavy-load eccentric calf muscle training for treatment of chronic Achilles tendinosis. *Am J Sports Med.* 1998;26:360-366.
40. Andersen LL, Magnusson SP, Nielsen M, Haleem J, Poulsen K, Aagaard P. Neuromuscular activation in conventional therapeutic exercises and heavy resistance exercises: implications for rehabilitation. *Phys Ther.* 2006;86(5):683-697.
41. Mason DL, Dickens V, Vail A. Rehabilitation for hamstring injuries. *Cochrane Database Syst Rev.* 2007;24(1):CD004575.
42. Hibbert O, Cheong K, Grant A, Beers A, Moizumi T. A systematic review of the effectiveness of eccentric strength training in prevention of hamstring muscle strains in otherwise healthy individuals. *N Am J Sports Phys Ther.* 2008;3(2):67-81.

Other Hip Disorders

Michael R. Nicoletti, Robert DePorto, and Robert DeStefano

ADDUCTOR STRAIN

INTRODUCTION

The adductor muscle group contains six different muscles: pectineus, gracilis, obturator externus, adductor brevis, adductor longus, and adductor magnus. All are innervated by the obturator nerve, with the exception of the pectineus, which receives innervation from the femoral nerve. The primary function of this muscle group is adduction of the thigh in open chain motions and stabilization of the lower limb and pelvis in closed chain motions. Violent, usually eccentric contractions of these muscles can lead to adductor strain. Despite being a single-joint muscle, the adductor longus is the most commonly injured of the six. It has the least mechanical advantage on adduction of the hip, therefore making it most susceptible to strain (1,2).

Adductor strains are the most common groin injuries in athletes, specifically with kicking sports or sports requiring sudden changes in direction, such as soccer and hockey. The eccentric contraction occurs with the hip in external rotation, and abduction is thought to be the cause of the strain. Inflexibility, previous injury, and strength imbalance between adductors and abductors are common risk factors for adductor strains. The highest risk factor for adductor strain is an adductor-to-abductor strength ratio of 80% or less; decreased adductor strength is a risk factor for recurrent strains (1).

The presentation could range from minor pain with activity to weakness and significant pain limiting or precluding training. The patient usually complains of medial thigh or groin pain, which is accentuated with hip abduction. The involved area is usually slightly swollen and tender with or without an area of ecchymosis. The area most commonly affected is the musculotendinous junction of the adductor longus. Therefore, palpation from the proximal insertion of the muscle belly on the pubic rami distally usually elicits the site of maximal tenderness. Palpable defect may or may not be present. Resisted adduction can provoke symptoms and strains are graded based on strength evaluation. Mild (grade I) strains result in pain with minimal strength loss, moderate (grade II) strains result in strength loss and pain, and severe (grade III) strains result in complete functional and motor loss (1–3).

Adductor strains must be differentiated from other sources of groin pain. History should also include aggravating or alleviating factors to help differentiate from other causes of groin pain. Tenderness to palpation at the pubis may result from osteitis pubis, athletic pubalgia, or muscular origin avulsion injury. Osteitis pubis is marked by tenderness over the pubic tubercle or inguinal ring and can often be differentiated because the symptoms are exacerbated by sit-ups. Athletic pubalgia may have tenderness over the pubic tubercle or conjoined tendon or at a dilated superficial inguinal ring. This pain can also be reproduced with sit-ups, resisted leg adduction or Valsalva maneuver. Inspection for an inguinal hernia should also be performed (1).

Diagnostic imaging is not needed for evaluation or management of most muscle strains because these are treated conservatively. Plain radiographs are often used to evaluate for other causes, such as muscular origin avulsions, osteitis pubis, and stress fractures. Magnetic resonance imaging (MRI) is the imaging method of choice when examining chronic groin pain of unknown etiology, grading strains, and evaluating suspected grade III strains. The cost of the MRI eliminates it as routine testing for evaluation of adductor strains. In athletes, with persistent and suspected athletic pubalgia, MRI with athletic pubalgia protocol can help determine if a conjoined tendon tear is present.

THE REHABILITATION PROGRAM

After the diagnosis is made, a rehabilitation program is initiated and the phases of rehabilitation are followed. This regimen requires intermittent monitoring of range of motion (ROM), pain, and muscle testing. As with other muscle strains, the initial phase of rehabilitation begins with PRICE (protection, rest, ice, compression, and elevation) and possibly nonsteroidal anti-inflammatory drugs (NSAIDs) and/or analgesics to help decrease swelling and inflammation, control pain, as well as protect and prevent further injury. After 24 to 48 hours, passive range of motion (PROM) and submaximal isometric contractions (Figures 23.1A and B) are initiated to limit atrophy and restore ROM. This prevents the adverse effects of immobilization on joint cartilage, tendon, and musculature (1). Therapeutic modalities such as ultrasound and electrical stimulation may be beneficial, although they are not proven adjunctive treatments. During this initial phase, trunk and upper limb weight-training and conditioning may continue to prevent significant deconditioning.

Once ROM has improved and the patient can adduct against gravity without pain, the patient may progress from phase II toward phase III (restoration of strength). During this phase, the patient is allowed to start bicycling and swimming for conditioning as well as isotonic adduction (1). Emphasis is now placed on regaining strength, flexibility, and endurance. The patient is encouraged to gently stretch the short and long hip adductors (Figures 23.2A and B), and start single-leg squats to develop muscular control.

When the adduction-to-abduction strength ratio is equal to 75%, the patient is allowed to progress toward phase IV (proprioceptive training) and eventually phase V (functional/sport specific training). This phase allows increased resistance, speed, and volume of resisted training. The patient is then allowed to start sport-specific training to improve adductor strength and modification of sport specific techniques. When the adduction-to-abduction strength ratio is at least 90% to 100% and the adduction strength is symmetrical, hip ROM is restored and pain is resolved, then resumption of sports training and competition is allowed (1).

Although most patients return in 2 to 3 weeks, severe cases may take 8 to 12 weeks. On return to competition, the patient should continue the adductor rehabilitation program and wear a compressive thigh sleeve. Before training or competition, a warm-up program consisting of cycling and stretching should be performed. An adduction strain prevention program focusing on strengthening of adductor musculature should be initiated during the off-season and maintained throughout the season. This should be reinforced with sport-specific exercises and proper technique (2).

Therapeutic Modalities

The most important therapeutic modality in the treatment of groin strains is the initial PRICE protocol and the application of ice during the first 24 to 72 hours. Ice helps reduce internal bleeding from injured blood vessels by causing vasoconstriction. The more blood that collects, the longer the healing time will be. Ice may be applied for 15 to 20 minutes every hour during the first 24 hours after the injury. Ice may also be applied in the form of an ice massage. After 48 to 72 hours the icing regimen may be stopped. Superficial or deep heat, from either hot packs or ultrasound, may be useful in warming muscles prior to

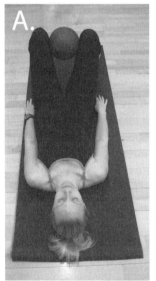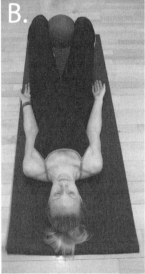

FIGURE 23.1A AND 23.1B: Isometric adduction exercises. Photo courtesy of Marissa Reda, CPT, RYT.

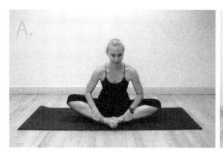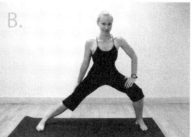

FIGURE 23.2A: Seated short adductor stretch. **B**: Straight leg long adductor stretch. Photo courtesy of Marissa Reda, CPT, RYT.

performing exercises and stretching during the beginning phases of rehabilitation, although it hasn't been proven to be more effective than therapeutic exercise alone.

Manual Therapy

The use of manual therapy in the treatment of adductor strains is not well supported by the currently available literature. Although further research is necessary, expert opinion and several recent studies suggest that manual therapy might be a promising treatment in terms of success rate, recovery time, as well as frequency and duration of treatment (4). The Van den Akker manual therapy method consists of prewarming the muscle group, then positioning the athlete semisupine. Once the patient is relaxed, using the contralateral hand to control the tension in the adductor muscles, the physician uses the ipsilateral hand to move the hip from neutral position into abduction and external rotation, with the knee in full extension (5). Muscle tension is controlled subjectively. This flowing, circular motion is used to apply the maximum tolerable stretch to the adductor muscle group. After performing the movement, the adductor muscle compartment is compressed using one hand while the other hand moves the hip into adduction and slight flexion. This circular movement followed by compression lasts approximately 25 seconds, and is repeated three times in one treatment session (4,5).

Sports massage is sometimes used to release tension in the muscle and to stimulate blood flow and healing. Techniques include effleurage, petrissage, stripping, which involves sustained pressure along the muscle to iron out any lumps, bumps, and knots; and circular friction, which involves deep circular motions to work out any taut and/or tender spots. Always remember, massage must not be performed during the acute stage of injury.

Specialized Techniques

Hydrotherapy, such as aqua jogging or walking and water resistance exercises, utilizes the principle of buoyancy and temperature regulation to allow for more exercise than is permitted on land. Exercises may also be progressed by increasing speed or surface area when moving through the water. Therapies such as compression wrapping, bracing, and kinesiology taping have been used to provide support in the prevention of groin strains as well as to aid in the healing process. While some patients may find relief with these techniques, results are widely inconsistent. They may be employed as supplemental treatment modalities, but should not be used in lieu of a structured rehabilitation program.

Patient Education

After a groin injury, it is important to start the recovery and rehabilitation process as soon as possible. While return to normal activity level should take place gradually to avoid reinjury, therapeutic exercises performed at home are just as important as those done with a medical professional. The PRICE protocol may be initiated immediately in the home setting. Once pain and swelling have improved the patient may begin stretching, isometric, and ROM exercises. As pain-free strength and flexibility improve the patient may begin adduction exercises against gravity (Figures 23.3a and 23.3b), and then progress to light weights for added resistance, such as ankle weights.

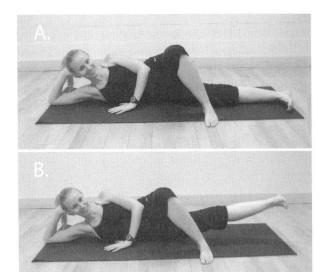

FIGURE 23.3A AND 23.3B: Side lying hip adduction against gravity. Photo courtesy of Marissa Reda, CPT, RYT.

SUMMARY

Adductor strains usually occur with rapid change in direction or kicking. The adductor longus is the most commonly strained muscle of the adductor group. Adductor-to-abductor strength ratio of 80% or less has been identified as the greatest risk factor for adductor strains. History and physical examination should be used to rule out other causes of groin pain including osteitis pubis, athletic pubalgia, hernias, and stress fractures. Treatment should include a short PRICE period, followed by progression through the phases of rehabilitation. Groin strain prevention includes adequate warm-up and strengthening should continue once the rehabilitation program is completed.

SPORTS HERNIA

INTRODUCTION

Sports hernia, also termed Gilmore's groin or *athletic pubalgia*, is a relatively new diagnosis, and the most unique and misunderstood cause of groin pain. Prior to establishing the diagnosis of sports hernia, athletes were diagnosed and treated for chronic groin strains, often resulting in career-ending chronic pain and disability. The pathology of the sports hernia is a broad spectrum of injuries involving the inguinal ligament, conjoined tendon, transversalis fascia, internal oblique muscle, external oblique muscle, and rectus abdominis insertion (1). Sports hernias are believed to develop from a muscle imbalance between the adductor muscle group of the lower limb and the abdominal musculature (1). When strength of the adductors overpowers core strength it leads to weakening and potential tearing of the structures of the pelvic floor.

Athletic pubalgia is seen more frequently in males than in females. Patients often complain of exertional pain in the pubic area, which may radiate into the adductor or genital region and can be aggravated by specific activities. The history may reveal an aggravating injury. Similar to that of adductor strains, the mechanism of injury is described as a hyperextension injury pivoting around the pubic symphysis, seen frequently in hockey and soccer players. Clinical presentation includes an insidious onset of deep groin pain that is exacerbated by prolonged standing, athletic activities that require pivoting and cutting, or coughing or sneezing and is relieved with rest.

Physical examination findings for athletic pubalgia are subtle. Patients may have tenderness along the conjoined tendon or inguinal ring, the pubic tubercle or symphysis, insertion sites of the rectus abdominis, and origin of the adductors. Although uncommon, a small defect may be palpable within the abdominal musculature near the insertion on the pubis. Patients may also have tight hamstrings or limited ROM at the hip, therefore, conditions such as femoroacetabular impingement (FAI) may be contributing factors. Provocative testing includes pain with resisted sit-ups and with resisted adduction of the lower limb with the hip externally rotated (1).

THE REHABILITATION PROGRAM

The first course of intervention in the treatment of athletic pubalgia should be a period of rest followed by 4 to 6 weeks of rehabilitation. Whether the patient is pre-, post-, or mid-season should be taken into account, as well as whether it is a first-time or recurrent episode. For the acute presentation of a first-time episode during pre- or mid-season, treatment should constitute a 2-week period of rest and analgesics and/or anti-inflammatories (1). After this 2-week period, a rehabilitation program should be instituted. Rehabilitation focuses on stretching the abdominal and lower limb muscles and tendons.

In addition, strengthening of the core muscles are emphasized, particularly the transversus abdominis, multifidus, and pelvic floor. During the initial 2 weeks of therapy avoid trunk hyperextension, aggressive hip extension ROM, and contractions of rectus abdominis, as would occur with crunches (6). Core exercises should emphasize neutral spine alignment. Lower body strengthening exercises should always begin with double leg (bilateral) and progress to single leg (unilateral) activities as strength and stability increase. The athlete can return to play when he or she has full lumbar and hip ROM, full and symmetrical strength of the hips, abdominal muscles, and lumbar multifidus, and finally when they can perform activities of daily living (ADLs) and sport-specific activities without pain (6). Recurrent episodes in the pre- or mid-season need to be treated with rest for at least 4 weeks. If pain-free return to play cannot be achieved with physical therapy (PT) and rehabilitation, then proliferative therapy (prolotherapy) injections or surgical consultation should be considered.

Manual Therapy

The effectiveness of hip and lumbar mobilizations/manipulations to address hip dysfunction and lumbar region pain has been well documented. However, utilization of these techniques to address groin pain associated with a sports hernia is still controversial. Techniques including soft tissue mobilization to the lumbar and hip regions, joint mobilization and manipulation to the pelvis, sacroiliac joint (SIJ) and/or hips, neuromuscular reeducation, and manual stretching have all been utilized as part of the rehabilitation protocol (7). Soft tissue mobilization has been used to address muscular tightness in the pelvic musculature and fascia, as well as myofascial restrictions of the lumbar spine and pelvis. SIJ and hip mobilization/manipulation are proposed to have hypoalgesic effects as well as mechanical effects, including connective tissue elongation. The sacroiliac regional thrust manipulation technique has been shown to be effective at decreasing pain associated with hip, lumbar, and SIJ dysfunction. Soft tissue manipulation, or sports massages, such as effleurage and petrissage, have been used in athletic pubalgia to address muscular tightness and to theoretically break up of scar tissue. Neuromuscular reeducation and manual stretching techniques assist in maintaining capsular mobility (7), and together the manual therapy techniques complement the therapeutic exercise program, but the role of manual therapy in the treatment

of sports hernia requires further research for better definition.

Therapeutic Exercise

Progression through the phases of rehabilitation includes PRICE protocol, followed by gentle ROM and stretching, and low impact aerobics which may be initiated in the pool. Core strengthening is arguably the most important part of the therapeutic exercise program and should progress from static to dynamic core training, including exercises designed to challenge the athlete's proprioception and balance. It is very important to retrain these muscles through neuromuscular reeducation exercises before progressing to more advanced dynamic core training. Once the athlete is pain-free, ROM, strength, balance, and proprioception are restored, then the program progresses to the final phase of rehabilitation, sport specific training prior to returning to play.

Specialized Techniques

Hydrotherapy, such as aqua jogging or walking, utilizes the principle of buoyancy and provides temperature regulation to allow for more exercise than is permitted on land. Patients are usually started off with this mode of exercise when they are not ready to work against the full force of gravity. Exercises may be progressed by increasing speed or surface area when moving through the water.

Patient Education

Rest is the key factor during the initial stages of rehabilitation after establishing a diagnosis of sports hernia. Avoiding any activities that aggravate the injury is essential to the length of recovery. Once the recommended period of rest, ice, analgesics, and/or anti-inflammatories is completed, the patient can progress to the functional rehabilitation program. Home exercise should go hand in hand with the supervised program, and should include a combination of flexibility, strength, and stability training. Isometric exercises for abdominal strengthening, such as front and side planks (Figures 23.4 and 23.5), and quadruped position (Figures 23.6a and 23.6b), as well as stretching of the adductors can be performed at home and will aid in recovery. As the patient progresses, exercises can increase in intensity and difficulty.

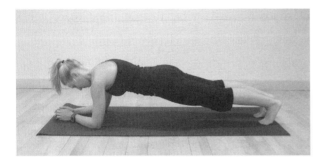

FIGURE 23.4: Isometric front plank. Photo courtesy of Marissa Reda, CPT, RYT.

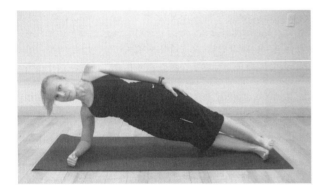

FIGURE 23.5: Isometric side plank. Photo courtesy of Marissa Reda, CPT, RYT.

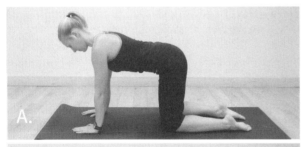
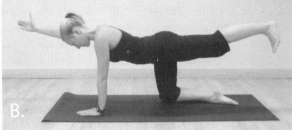

FIGURE 23.6A AND 23.6B: Quadruped starting position, then bird dog exercise for core strengthening. Photo courtesy of Marissa Reda, CPT, RYT.

SUMMARY

Sports hernia usually present insidiously with groin pain that is exacerbated by activity, coughing, or sneezing, and relieved with rest. The mechanism of injury may be an imbalance between the adductors of the lower limb and the abdominal musculature, or related to altered hip biomechanics. Patients diagnosed with a sports hernia should complete a period of rest followed by 4 to 6 weeks of PT. Therapy includes stretching abdominal and lower limb muscles along with neuromuscular retraining and strengthening of the core muscles. If pain-free return to play cannot be achieved with appropriate rehabilitation program, ultrasound-guided prolotherapy injections, although experimental, or sports hernia surgery should be considered and may even be required for return to sport.

HIP LABRAL TEARS

INTRODUCTION

The acetabular labrum is a ring of fibrocartilage that lines the border of the acetabulum and is continuous with the transverse acetabular ligament. Blood vessels supply only the peripheral one-third of the labrum, leaving the remaining two-thirds avascular. This makes the healing potential poor and very much dependent on location of the tear. Labral tears have been reported as the most common form of intra-articular pathology in the hip. There are five recognized causes of labral tears: FAI, hip dysplasia, trauma, capsular laxity, and joint degeneration. Patients with dysplastic hips often have large and floppy labrums making it more susceptible to tearing, particularly with the increased translational motion found with dysplastic hips. Similarly, capsular laxity and hip hypermobility, as seen in Ehlers-Danlos syndrome, also have increased translational forces across the hip joint (1). Patients with joint degeneration are likely to tear the labrum due to repetitive deranged motion of the hip with acetabular edge loading. Finally, traumatic injuries, such as dislocation or subluxation, and loose bodies can be directly responsible for labral tears.

Classic presentation includes groin pain with certain movements, which can be exacerbated by sudden twisting or pivoting motion. There may be a clicking or catching sensation, known as intra-articular snapping hip (1). Examination of the affected hip may reveal decreased and painful ROM.

Labral tears can occur in various locations. In the presence of an anterior labral tear, ranging the hip from a fully flexed, externally rotated, and abducted position to a position of extension, internal rotation, and adduction may elicit pain. Posterior tears may be painful if the hip is brought from a flexed, adducted, and internally rotated position to one of abduction, external rotation, and extension (1).

When there is suspicion of a labral tear, imaging modalities are essential to the diagnosis. Plain radiographs do not demonstrate signs of labral tears but will diagnose underlying pathology, such as acetabular dysplasia, trauma, joint degeneration, and FAI. Computed tomography (CT) scanning is also helpful in determining an underlying cause, but again does not confirm the presence of a labral tear. Magnetic resonance (MR) arthrogram is the diagnostic test of choice. Furthermore, intra-articular injection of lidocaine alone or with steroid, along with the contrast dye, at the time of arthrography can be diagnostic and therapeutic (1).

THE REHABILITATION PROGRAM

Initially an attempt may be made at conservative management, but due to the mechanical nature of the injury and poor healing quality of the labrum, long-term results are inconsistent and require further study to clarify the role of nonoperative management of labral tears. Relative rest and avoidance of provocative positions or activities are initial interventions (PRICE protocol). Intervention should also focus on optimizing the alignment of the hip joint and the precision of joint motion (8). This is accomplished by avoiding excessive force to the anterior hip joint, correcting movement patterns during exercises and gait, and minimizing pivoting motions.

Therapeutic exercise generally targets hip flexion, abduction, external rotation, and extension to restore ROM and strength in these planes. One of the most important interventions is to correct any faulty gait patterns, particularly knee hyperextension, which causes hip hyperextension during stance. When walking on a treadmill, patients must be careful not to let the moving tread contribute to excessive hip hyperextension (8). Functional lifestyle modifications include avoiding sitting in excessive hip flexion (e.g., low chairs), sitting cross-legged, sitting with the hip rotated (neutral position is encouraged), or sitting on the edge of a seat with hip flexors contracted. When getting up from a chair that is behind a desk or out of a car, patients should avoid pushing or rotating the pelvis on a loaded femur. The patient should also avoid

weight training of quadriceps and hamstrings, as well as any exercises causing hip hyperextension (8).

Cycling is a good activity, but recumbent bikes should be avoided because of the excessive hip flexion and the tendency to use the hip flexor muscles to maintain the foot on the pedal. The patient should be trained not to rotate the acetabulum on the femur. Most importantly, therapeutic exercises and functional activities should not cause pain. NSAIDs may be beneficial in the management of pain and signs of inflammation. PT may allow for temporary resolution of symptoms, but the symptoms usually return after the patient returns to full activity. Long-term outcome may be best with surgery in certain subsets of patients, therefore, if the patient is responding poorly to conservative management then consider referral to an orthopedic surgeon experienced in hip arthroscopy.

SUMMARY

Labral tears are the most common source of intra-articular hip pathology. Vasculature supplies only the outer third of the labrum resulting in poor healing potential to injuries in the avascular regions, similar to the meniscus of the knee. Causes of labral tears include FAI, acetabular dysplasia, trauma, capsular laxity, and joint degeneration. Clinical presentation includes groin pain, often worse with athletic activity and exacerbated by sudden twisting or pivoting motion. A clicking or catching sensation may be present and is known as intra-articular snapping hip. Conservative management is recommended initially and includes PRICE protocol +/- NSAIDs, and PT. Therapy focuses on optimizing the alignment of the hip joint, correcting movement patterns during exercise and gait, and patient education on the avoidance of pivoting motions and excessive forces into the anterior hip joint. Conservative treatment may initially relieve symptoms, but surgical management may be required for a successful outcome, especially for return to sport in younger athletes. Many research questions must still be addressed to better clarify the role of nonoperative and operative management of labral tears and their respective long term outcomes.

FEMOROACETABULAR IMPINGEMENT

INTRODUCTION

FAI is another potential cause of hip pain in athletes. Abnormal dynamic contact between the proximal femur and acetabulum results in damage to femoral neck, acetabular rim, hip labrum, and articular cartilage (1). The impingement is classified into three types: Cam impingement, Pincer impingement, and a combination of the two (Figure 23.7). *Cam impingement* is a femur-based pathology. It can occur when there is insufficient offset at the head and neck junction or when the head is "out of round," essentially making the head too large for the acetabulum at the extremes of motion. Standard hip motion then causes abnormal loading of the anterior acetabular cartilage and labrum and increased stress at the acetabular edge. Conversely, *pincer impingement* is an acetabulum-based pathology. The acetabulum may be found to have poor anteversion or may be too deep, essentially enveloping the femoral head and limiting hip motion. The femoral neck continuously loads the anterior acetabular rim, with consequent damage to the cartilage and labrum. The combination of both cam and pincer mechanics can also be seen and can accelerate the occurrence of hip pathology caused by abnormal joint motion (1). Causes include Legg-Calve-Perthes disease, slipped capital femoral epiphysis, trauma, and idiopathic causes.

Patients often complain of groin pain with activities that involve hip flexion. With minimal symptoms, patients complain of hip stiffness or start-up pain and limited ROM. Some patients may present with the clinical finding of a labral tear. Older patients may present with severe secondary osteoarthritis. Patients may have pain with weight-bearing activities. Physical examination reveals limited flexion that can be less than 90°. Patients generally have more passive external rotation than internal rotation. An anterior impingement test is positive if a patient has pain with passive flexion, adduction, and internal rotation (FADIR) (1).

Imaging is essential in the diagnosis. Plain radiographs are arguably the most important study to obtain. They should include an antero-posterior (AP) pelvis and lateral x-rays (e.g., frog leg lateral) with the hip in 15° of internal rotation. Inadequate femoral head and neck offset can be diagnosed on the lateral x-ray and a CAM lesion may be seen on either view. The AP pelvis is also used to rule out the presence of acetabular

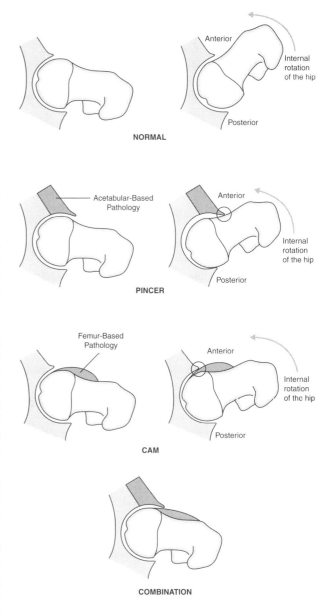

FIGURE 23.7: Hip anatomy: normal, pincer and CAM lesions, and combination type FAI.

dysplasia, over-coverage, or acetabular version. Three-dimensional CT scans can show asphericity within the femoral head and inadequate femoral head-neck offset and is very important for surgical planning. MRI is ideal for assessing the articular cartilage and labrum, besides elaborating on the type and extent of impingement (e.g., cam or pincer).

THE REHABILITATION PROGRAM

Conservative management of FAI is possible; however, it involves significant changes in lifestyle regarding activity levels, modification of certain activities, and a commitment to maintaining hip strength (9). Impingement is a mechanical problem; therefore, nonsurgical management will not change the underlying abnormal hip biomechanics and may contribute to further hip degeneration (1). A good PT program focusing on hip strengthening, specifically hip extensors, external rotators and abductors, and neuromuscular control of the hip and pelvis may be more beneficial than a stretching program, although significant soft tissue restrictions or muscle imbalances should be corrected. Unlike other pathologies, here aggressive stretching can make the symptoms worse. Activity modification should involve avoiding activities that take the hip through extreme ROM. Anti-inflammatory medications can also be utilized in the treatment regimen. Intra-articular steroid-analgesic injection can be both diagnostic as well as therapeutic. In achieving pain relief, the injection then also confirms the origin of the pain to be the intra-articular hip and not another source. Patients with persistently symptomatic FAI that doesn't respond to conservative care should be referred for orthopedic surgical consultation. The role of surgery for long-term hip preservation in the setting FAI is currently being investigated.

SUMMARY

FAI is classified into three types: Cam, Pincer, or a combination of both Cam/Pincer pathologies. Clinical presentation includes groin pain that is typically worse with activities involving hip flexion and rotation. Imaging studies, especially plain radiographs, are essential to the diagnosis of FAI. Nonoperative management involves a commitment to lifestyle change toward lower impact activities, or at least a modification of activities that require end ROM (e.g., yoga). PT should focus on hip and core strengthening, correcting muscular imbalances, and on improving the neuromuscular control of the hip and pelvis, where as aggressive stretching should be avoided since it may worsen symptoms. Patients with persistently symptomatic FAI that hasn't responded to conservative care should be referred for orthopedic surgical consultation.

SAMPLE CASE

A 31-year-old male patient presents with pain in the left groin for the past 6 days. Otherwise healthy, he has no significant past medical history (PMHx), past surgical history (PSHx) notable for right knee arthroscopy 2 years ago for a meniscal tear. He is not currently taking any medications other than a daily multivitamin. The pain began after a recreational rugby match over the weekend. He states that he took some Ibuprofen and felt better a few days later. However, when he attempted to go for a run 2 days ago the pain returned and he was unable to do so. He describes the pain as deep and aching. Review of systems (ROS) is unremarkable other than arthroscopy scars noted around the right knee. On physical examination there is tenderness to palpation (TTP) over the inguinal ring without any palpable mass or defect. Full ROM and strength 5/5 throughout the lower limbs bilaterally, however resisted flexion of the left hip with the knee bent at 90° reproduces pain. Pain was also reproducible with resisted sit-ups. Hip scouring was negative bilaterally. Neurologically intact with normal reflexes bilaterally.

 ### SAMPLE THERAPY PRESCRIPTION

Discipline: Physical therapy.

Diagnosis: Sports hernia/athletic pubalgia.

Precautions: Follow PRICE protocol the first 2 weeks. Avoid trunk/hip hyperextension, rectus abdominis contraction (crunching)—during this time period.

Frequency of Visits: 2 to 3x/week.

Duration of Treatment: 4 to 6 weeks, begins after initial 2 weeks of rest.

Treatment:

1. *Modalities (optional):* Heat or ultrasound preexercise as a mode of muscle warming. Cryotherapy/ice post exercise to minimize any inflammation

2. *Manual therapy (optional):* Mobilization of hip, pelvis, SIJ. Soft tissue manipulation/sports massage—effleurage/petrissage, as needed

3. *Therapeutic exercise:* ROM and stretching of hamstrings, adductors, quads, iliopsoas. Core engagement and strengthening, transversus abdominis and multifidus—static training progressed to dynamic. Lower limb functional strengthening—bilateral activities progressing to unilateral activities. Dynamic single leg and pelvic stability training. Neuromuscular reeducation. Cycling/swimming to maintain cardiopulmonary fitness

4. *Specialized techniques:* Aqua walking/jogging until land program can be tolerated

5. *Patient education:* Home exercise program (HEP).

Goals: Decrease pain. Promote core recruitment
and proper posture. Increase core strength and lower limb flexibility. Gradual and safe return to full preinjury activity level; consider injury prevention program.

Reevaluation: After 4 weeks for either continued treatment or return to sport.

REFERENCES

1. Jesse C, Drez D Jr, Miller MD. *DeLee and Drez's Orthopaedic Sports Medicine.* Philadelphia, PA: Saunders; 2010.
2. Timothy FT, Holly JS, Michael BG, et al. Groin injuries in sports medicine. *Sports Health.* 2010;2:231–236.
3. Tyler TF, Slattery AA. Rehabilitation of the hip following sports injury. *Clin Sports Med.* 2010;29(1):107–126.
4. Weir A, Veger AS, Van de Sande HBA, et al. A manual therapy technique for chronic adductor-related groin pain in athletes: a case series. *Scand J Med Sci Spor.* 2009;19:616–620.
5. Weir A, Jansen JACG, van de Port IGL, et al. Manual or exercise therapy for long-standing adductor-related groin pain: a randomized controlled clinical trial. *Manual Therapy.* 2011;16(2):148–154.
6. Jeffrey SH. Sports hernia repair protocol. *Sports Hernia South.* 2010. Retrieved from http://www.sportsherniasouth.com/Sports-Hernia-Treatment.html
7. Kachingwe AF, Grech S. Proposed algorithm for the management of athletes with athletic pubalgia (sports hernia): a case series. *J Orthop Sports Phys Ther.* 2008;38(12):768–781.
8. Cara LL, Shirley SA. Acetabular labral tears. *Physical Therapy.* 2006;86(1):110–121.
9. Aaron L. Femoral acetabular impingement: an overview of cause, repair, and rehabilitation. *National Strength and Conditioning Association.* 3 September, 2010. Retrieved from http://www.nsca-lift.org/AllNews.asp?news=1478
10. Fred F. *Ferri's Netter Patient Advisor 2010–2011.* Philadelphia, PA: Saunders; 2010.
11. Houglum PA. *Therapeutic Exercise for Musculoskeletal Injuries,* 3rd ed. Champaign, IL: Human Kinetics; 2010.
12. Miller MD. *Review of Orthopedics* 4th ed. Philadelphia, PA: Saunders, 2008.
13. Morelli V, Smith V. Groin injuries in athletes. *American Family Physician.* 2001;64:1405–1414.
14. Nicholas SJ, Tyler TF. Adductor muscle strains in sport. *Am J Sports Med.* 2002;32:339–344.

Knee Osteoarthritis

Eduardo J. Cruz-Colón, Todd Stitik, Kambiz Nooryani, and Prathap Jayaram

INTRODUCTION

Osteoarthritis (OA) affects 27 million people in the United States and the knee is one of the most common joints affected. Knee OA is the leading cause of disability and its prevalence is growing among the general population. Seventy percent of the population over the age of 65 will demonstrate radiographic evidence of knee OA and 12.1% will have clinical symptoms (1,2). An adequate understanding of the nonsurgical options and early diagnosis and management is essential to optimally treating knee OA patients. Knee OA is a degenerative disorder that involves cartilage breakdown, subchondral bony sclerosis, osteophyte formation, abnormal synovial fluid hyaluronate, and an increase concentration of inflammatory mediators (2). Risk factors include obesity, female gender, genetic predisposition, African American race, and weak quadriceps. Obesity is the most important modifiable risk factor for the development of knee OA (3,4).

When evaluating the history, physical examination and radiologic findings, the American College of Rheumatology includes the following criteria for knee OA: pain in the knee, and either morning stiffness less than 30 minutes, age greater than 50 or crepitus on active range of motion (ROM), and x-ray evidence of osteophytes (5). The Kellgren-Lawrence scale can be used to grade radiologic findings of knee OA. Grading is based on osteophytes, deformity of bone contour and joint space narrowing. X-rays done are usually weight-bearing anterior-posterior radiographs of the knee in full extension. It has also been suggested that x-rays may be done in 40° of flexion, as this view demonstrates different weight bearing areas of the femur and tibia and may be more sensitive in identifying arthritic changes (6,7). Other x-ray views include the tunnel view, also called the intercondylar notch view, which helps identify osteochondral loose bodies and the sunrise or merchant view, useful in identifying arthritis at the patellofemoral compartment (6,23).

Key elements of the physical examination include inspection, palpation, evaluation of range of motion, neuromuscular examination, and knee-specific examination including medial joint line tenderness, crepitus with passive ROM, suprapatellar effusion, painful knee flexion, and possibly quad weakness. Ligamentous laxity and concomitant meniscal pathology should also be assessed. Differential diagnoses of patients with suprapatellar effusions should also include infection and inflammatory conditions. If there is a high clinical suspicion for these, further workup such as blood tests and knee aspiration with synovial fluid analysis should be performed (9). Once the diagnosis has been made, treatment should include educating the patients on

KNEE OSTEOARTHRITIS

- Knee OA is the leading cause of disability and its prevalence is growing

- It involves cartilage breakdown, subchondral bony sclerosis, osteophyte formation, abnormal synovial fluid hyaluronate, and an increase concentration of inflammatory mediators

- Risk factors include obesity, female gender, genetic predisposition, weak quadriceps

- Current American College of Rheumatology diagnostic criteria include: knee pain and at least one of the following: age ≥ 50, crepitus, morning stiffness < half an hour, osteophytes on x-ray

- Typical physical examination findings include medial joint line tenderness, crepitus, painful knee flexion, varus deformity, and possibly a suprapatellar effusion depending upon the stage of the OA

risk factors such as obesity and the importance of compliance with a home exercise program (HEP), a comprehensive rehabilitation program with emphasis on quad strengthening, and identification of other components that may help them improve their quality of life including: activities of daily living (ADL) evaluation, assistive devices, and bracing.

THE REHABILITATION PROGRAM

A comprehensive rehabilitation program should include the five phases of rehabilitation with controlling pain and inflammation using the PRICE principal, restoration of ROM, strengthening, proprioceptive training, and functional recovery including aerobic conditioning. Modalities, HEP, weight loss, and bracing also play an important role and should be considered for integration into the rehabilitation program. The main treatment goals include pain reduction, improved ROM, and identifying and then correcting modifiable risk factors. Each patient should have an individualized rehabilitation program to target their respective rehabilitation needs. All exercises should be done without aggravating the signs and symptoms of the underlying OA (4). Although previously controversial, it is now clear that joint loading and movement are essential for cartilage nutrition (1,10). A multidisciplinary approach should also include evaluation of assistive devices, in-office trial of a knee unloader brace, and consideration for lateral wedged insoles for genu varum knee deformities. Education and incorporation of a proper HEP is essential. Having the patient demonstrate the exercises at the follow up physician visits is important in helping to assess compliance with the HEP and to help correct any errors in exercise performance. These treatment guidelines for knee OA are summarized in Table 24.1.

TABLE 24.1: Treatment Guidelines for Knee OA

- Patient education: compliance with HEP, weight loss (if overweight)

- Physical therapy: PRICE, ROM, stretching and quadriceps strengthening, balance and functional recovery

- Occupational therapy: assistive devices, ADLs, joint protection techniques

- Aerobic exercises

- Orthoses and bracing

- Home exercise program

Therapeutic Modalities

Either ice or heat may be used for treatment of knee OA pain depending on the particular treatment goal. An understanding of the physiologic effects of each is essential to using them as effectively as possible. Physiologic effects of cryotherapy include analgesia, edema reduction, decreased tissue elasticity, and localized vasoconstriction. Ice modalities should work best in patients with inflammation and pain, but should be avoided before exercise. Cold will promote increased stiffness of collagen, which leads to decreased flexibility and can predispose to injury (1). Heat also promotes analgesia, but has opposite effects on collagen stiffness and arterial blood flow. Heat modalities may be most effective before exercise to help facilitate stretching and ROM. For example, the application of ultrasound to a contracted knee capsule could promote better ROM if stretching is performed immediately after the ultrasound application.

Although either therapeutic cold or heat can be used, it is unclear which is the most effective in treating knee OA pain. A Cochrane database review evaluated three randomized controlled clinical trials involving 179 patients with clinical and radiographic evidence of knee OA. The studies evaluated the effectiveness of heat and cold versus placebo. The conclusions of the review include the following: ice massage compared to control had a statistically beneficial effect on ROM, function, quad strength, and swelling. However, ice packs did not have significant effects on pain when compared to control. Hot packs had no beneficial effect on edema (12). Studies have also shown that when compared to placebo, transcutaneous electrical stimulation (TENS) has significant benefit for knee pain and knee stiffness (13).

Manual Therapy

Although most physical therapy programs involve aggressive quad strengthening and lower limb stretching, manual therapy does have its role when treating knee OA. Of all manual therapies, joint mobilization is one of the most widely used and can have an important role in some patients with knee OA. Specifically, joint mobilization can be used in patients with limited patellofemoral motion and/or capsular restriction. These interventions include patellar mobilization either by inferior, medial, lateral, or superior patellar glides. Good patellar mobility is needed for full knee flexion/extension and tibial rotation. Distraction of the knee joint, via a distraction force acting on the tibia and femur at the knee joint, can be used in combination with joint mobilization to further stretch the capsule (14). Soft tissue restriction that limits ROM and flexibility usually responds to stretching with or without heat modalities, but under certain circumstances soft tissue mobilizations or myofascial release may be utilized with success to help restore flexibility.

Therapeutic Exercise

Strengthening, ROM, and aerobic exercises are the main components of a comprehensive rehabilitation program. Factors such as pain and edema are important to identify, as multiple studies have shown that they will both cause reflex inhibition of quadriceps muscle activity (14). Both can be present in patients with knee OA, hence these patients will usually present with significant quadriceps atrophy. A major goal of physical therapy is to strengthen the lower limb muscles with emphasis on the quadriceps. Quadricep strengthening has been shown to decrease pain associated with knee OA (1). Furthermore, studies have shown that quadricep weakness correlates with pain severity (15).

The patient should perform exercises without pain and without aggravating the underlying arthritis. Closed kinetic chain exercises are usually preferred as they place less shear forces on the joints, provide increased joint stability, are capable of generating large forces with relatively low velocities of movement, and are generally considered to be safer early in the therapeutic program (4,14). Open chain exercises such as leg extensions may cause exercise induced arthralgia in patients with knee OA (16). If the patient cannot tolerate wall slides or leg presses, which are both very good closed kinetic chain exercises for quadricep strengthening, the patient may begin with an isometric exercise such as quad sets. Although an open kinetic chain exercise, straight leg raise without ankle weights is also a low impact exercise that may be used early in the rehabilitation process. Although the ideal exercise frequency is unknown, the "dosage" of exercise should be individualized to the patient. Hence, depending on the patient, strengthening exercises can be done every third day so that the muscle tissue has adequate time to recover and develop between bouts of exercise. This will also minimize the potential for overuse of the knee joint.

It is desirable to treat poor flexibility aggressively. Functional knee flexion is needed for proper sit-to stand transfers, walking on level surface, ADLs, climbing stairs, etc. (1); neutral knee extension is needed for all of these activities as well (2). Flexion will usually be limited more than extension as this is the typical pattern of capsular restriction (14). Knee flexion contractures will cause increased compressive forces at both the tibiofemoral and patellofemoral articulations (17). Stretching should involve lower limb muscle groups with a special focus on knee extensors and flexors. Evaluation of flexibility deficits involving the hip flexors, iliotibial band, and heel cords should also be addressed. Examples of stretching exercises include a standing quadriceps stretch, a supine hamstring stretch, and heel slides. Flexibility exercises should be tailored to each patient's needs and tolerance level. Heat will decrease collagen stiffness and is recommended before commencing the stretching exercise; a low impact aerobic warm up may be an alternative to heat. For optimal results, stretching should be done daily and be slightly uncomfortable, but not painful. Although the ideal stretching time is not known, the literature supports stretching time to be from 30 seconds to 2 minutes (18–20).

Aerobic conditioning should be incorporated into the rehabilitation program as its advantages include: improved walking speed, better aerobic capacity, reduced painful symptoms due to arthritic joints, improved coordination, and an analgesic effect produced by release of endogenous opioids (1,21). The type of aerobic activity should be according to patient preference and tolerance; some options include treadmill, walking, exercise bike, (usually high seated cycling to avoid excessive knee flexion), upper body ergonometer, or elliptical machine. Aerobic activity ideally should be for 30 minutes a day, no more than 5 times a week, and accompanied by a 5 minute warm up and cool down (22).

Specialized Techniques

Occupational therapy for evaluation of ADLs, assistive devices, and education in joint protection techniques will contribute to optimizing a patient's quality of life and to reducing pain symptoms. Assistive devices may include long handled shoe horns, sock aides, and raised toilets seats, all of which should help decrease activity-related deep knee flexion. Education on joint protection techniques, which is sometimes a mystery to many health specialists, include the following: avoidance of overuse and extreme knee flexion, not maintaining the same position for prolonged periods of time, unloading the joint when it becomes painful, and using correct patterns of motion (16).

Aquatic therapy offers the advantage of decreasing compressive exercise-related forces on lower limb joints and is a very good option for patients with severe pain and disability. The buoyancy of water counteracts the force of gravity and reduces body weight in water to 1/8th that on land. This will result in better tolerance of exercise activity, and unloading of weight bearing joints, providing for ease of movement and having an analgesic effect if the water is maintained at 86° to 96° Fahrenheit (21). Patellar taping should also be trialed in patients with knee OA, particularly in patients with pain from the patellofemoral joint. It should also be kept in mind that procedures such as corticosteroid injections, viscosupplementation, and possibly prolotherapy should be considered in patients with persistent pain despite therapy or may be used as an adjuvant to the therapy program.

Home Exercise Program

The long-term success of a comprehensive rehabilitation program relies strongly on compliance with the HEP. Education in a HEP should include a good understanding of joint protection techniques and the importance of weight loss. Simple weight loss recommendations include eating small portions and frequent meals, usually five to six a day, and a balanced diet of carbohydrates, protein, and fats. The intake of carbohydrates should be minimal after 7 p.m. and aerobic exercises should be done five times a week as noted above. Other weight loss techniques include logging caloric intake, weight loss programs, or consultation with a dietician or nutritionist.

The literature supports quadricep strengthening as a very important component of the HEP. These exercises include the wall slide, quad sets and straight leg raises, particularly since these do not require gym equipment. The patients should start with quad sets, and/or straight leg raises if they have poor quad strength. For the wall slide (Figure 24.1), the back should either be straight against the wall or the trunk flexes with the sacrum making contact with the wall and the knees should not extend past the toes; the patient may hold light weights at their sides to make the exercise more challenging. The patient should avoid deep knee flexion. The width that the feet are placed apart and the relative position of the feet in neutral, externally rotated,

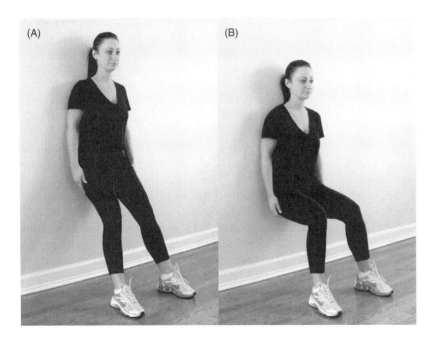

FIGURE 24.1: Wall slide.
Stand with your back against the wall; feet shoulder-width apart. (A) Slide down the wall slowly until you are almost in a chair position but not beyond this. The front of the knees should not extend out past the front of the feet. (B) Hold this position momentarily (for 3-5 seconds) and then slide back to the start position. (A) Positioning the feet inward or outward are variations to target the vastus medialis and vastus lateralis quadriceps muscles respectively. The relative width that the feet are placed apart may also be varied as can the distance that the feet are placed away from the wall.

or internally rotated should be adjusted as needed so that the exercise can be performed without causing knee pain. The patient should be counseled to distinguish quadricep muscle discomfort (desirable effect) from knee joint pain (undesirable effect). Since stretching may be considered boring by some patients, it can be suggested to patients that they do these exercises during the commercials of their favorite TV show. Specific stretching exercises include the standing quadriceps stretch and supine hamstring stretch with a towel. Various other stretching positions are available for the quadriceps and hamstrings. Each patient should be evaluated for the position that they are most capable of performing. The one legged stance is a good balance and proprioceptive exercise that will help patients with knee instability. The stance position should be held for 30 seconds to 2 minutes and then the patient switches sides. Tailoring a program to the individual can help increase compliance if it is easier for the patient to perform.

SUMMARY

Knee OA is one of the leading causes of disability and its risk factors include obesity, female gender, genetic predisposition, and weak quadriceps. A comprehensive rehabilitation program should consist of education on use of ice or heat for pain and inflammation control, lower limb strengthening and stretching with special attention to quad strengthening. Evaluation of assistive devices and ADLs is also strongly recommended in this patient population. For optimal results, the patient should demonstrate adequate understanding of their HEP, and joint protection techniques and should demonstrate to their physician, therapist, or trainer that they can perform the exercises correctly and pain free. Knee unloader braces and lateral wedge insoles are options that can be trialed in a way to reduce stress on this weight bearing joint and provide better tolerance for patients during activity. In some cases, a cane can be used to help unload the affected or more affected knee. Choice of hand (i.e., ipsilateral or contralateral) that the cane is held in is less clear for knee OA than it is for hip OA (24), although we recommend following common practice initially and trialing it on the contralateral side.

SAMPLE CASE

A 63-year-old male with history of hypertension and hyperlipidemia presents with bilateral aching knee pain and stiffness. He denies previous trauma, falls, or any other mechanism of injury; review of systems is negative. He is a retired police officer and wishes to return to his normal daily activities without having so much knee pain. His pain is worse with activity, especially going up and down stairs, and partially relieved with rest. Physical examination reveals bilateral medial joint line tenderness, mild warmth to palpation, painful and limited knee flexion with associated crepitus, and small suprapatellar effusions as confirmed on ultrasound examination. His gait is slightly antalgic and manual muscle testing of the quadriceps was 4+-5. Standing anteroposterior and lateral radiographs revealed medial joint space narrowing, marginal osteophytes, and subchondral sclerosis.

 SAMPLE THERAPY PRESCRIPTION

Discipline: Physical therapy.

Diagnosis: Bilateral knee OA, abnormality of gait, limited knee flexion.

Precautions: Weight-bearing as tolerated (WBAT), cardiac.

Frequency of visits: 2 to 3x/week (nonconsecutive days).

Duration of treatment: Approximately 4 weeks, then physician reevaluation is needed for additional physical therapy. Typical maximum treatment is 3 months.

Treatment:

1. *Modalities:* heat prior to exercise to facilitate ROM (ultrasound and or hydrocollator pack), ice after exercise for pain and inflammation

2. *Manual therapy:* Joint mobilizations as needed for pain relief and to restore ROM

3. *Therapeutic exercise:*

- *Aerobic Conditioning:* 20 to 30 minutes of aerobic conditioning, especially high seated cycling

- *Stretching* lower limb stretching globally (specifically focusing on quadriceps, hamstrings, gastrocnemius/soleus complex)

- *Strengthening* of the lower extremity especially quads with emphasis on wall slides and quad sets, would avoid leg extension, step ups, and lunges

- *Occupational therapy* may also be considered for the assessment of ADL's and need for adaptive equipment.

4. *Patient education:* HEP, joint protection techniques

Goals: Decrease pain; improve knee ROM/flexibility and strength.

Reevaluation: After the initial 12 physical therapy visits by referring physician.

REFERENCES

1. Wrightson JD, Malanga GA. Strengthening and other therapeutic exercises in the treatment of osteoarthritits. Physical medicine and rehabilitation: state of the art reviews. 2001;15(1):43–56.
2. Stitik T, Kim JH, Stiskal D, et al. Osteoarthritis. In: Delisa J, Frontera W. eds. *DeLisa's Physical Medicine and rehabilitation: Principles and Practice,* 5th ed. Philadelphia, PA: Lippincott Williams & Wilkins; 2010:781–810.
3. Stitik T, Hochberg M. Baseline program. In: Moskowitz RW, Altman RD. eds. *Osteoarthritis: Diagnosis and Medical/Surgical Management,* 4th ed. Philadelphia, PA. Lippincott Willaims & Wilkins; 2007:257–263.
4. Stitik T, Ciolino I, Foye P. Rehabilitation for osteoarthritis. *Emedicine.* 2011.
5. Kellgren JH, Lawrence JS. Radiological assessment of osteoarthrosis. *Ann Rheum Dis.* 1957;16:494–502.
6. Sarwark MD. Arthritis of the knee. In: Sarwark JF, ed. *Essentials of Musculoskeletal Care,* 4th ed. Rosemont, IL: American Academy of Orthopedic Surgeons; 2010:650–656.
7. Niinimaki TR. Ojala R. The standing fixed flexion view detects narrowing of the joint space better than the standing extended view in patients with moderate osteoarthritis of the knee. *Acta Orthopaedica.* 2010;81(3):344–346.
8. Hooper M, Holderbaum D, Moskowitz RW. Clinical and laboratory findings in osteoarthritis. In: Koopman WJ. ed. *Arthritis and Allied Conditions: A Textbook of Rheumatology,* 15th ed. Philadelphia, PA. Lippincott Williams & Wilkins; 2005:2228–2231.
9. Stitik TP, Kaplan RJ, Kamen L, et al. Rehabilitation of orthopedic and rheumatologic disorders. 2. Osteoarthritis assessment, treatment, and rehabilitation. *Archives of Physical Medicine and Rehabilitation,* 2005;86(3 Suppl 1):S48–S55.
10. Kraus VB. Pathogenesis and treatment of osteoarthritis. *The Medical Clinics of North America.* 1997;81(1):85–112.
11. Stitik TP, Nadler SF. Sports injuries part 1: When and how to use cold most effectively. *Consultant.* 1998;38(12): 2881–2890.
12. Brosseau L, Yonge KA, Robinson V, et al. Thermotherapy for treatment of osteoarthritis. *Cochrane Database of Systema Rev.* 2003;(4):CD004522.
13. Osiri M, Welch V, Brosseau L, et al. Transcutaneous electrical nerve stimulation for knee osteoarthritis. *Cochrane Database of Systema Rev.* 2000;(4):CD002823.
14. Houglum PA. Therapeutic exercise for musculoskeletal injuries: athletic training education series. *Human Kinetics,* 2010;176-179,855,867–870.
15. Slemenda C, Brandt KD, Heilman DK, et al. Quadriceps weakness and osteoarthritis of the knee. *Annals of Internal Medicine.* 1997;127(2):97–104.
16. Stitik TP, Yonclas P, Foye PM, Schoenherr L. Nonpharmacologic management of knee and hip osteoarthritis. *J Musculoskel Med.* 2005;22:61–67.
17. Bashaw RT, Tingstad EM. Rehabilitation of the osteoarthritic patient: focus on the knee. *Clinics in Sports Medicine.* 2005;24(1):101–131.
18. Bandy WD, Irion JM. The effect of time on static stretch on the flexibility of the hamstring muscles. *Physical Therapy.* 1994;74(9):845-850; discussion 850–842.
19. Feland JB, Myrer JW. The effect of duration of stretching of the hamstring muscle group for increasing range of motion in people aged 65 years or older. *Physical Therapy.* 2001;81(5): 1110–1117.
20. Sainz de Baranda, Ayala F. Chronic flexibility improvement after 12 week of stretching program utilizing the ACSM recommendations: hamstring flexibility. *Int J Sports Med.* 2010;31(6):389–396.
21. Stitik TP, Nadler SF, Foye PM, Smith R: Osteoarthritis of the knee and hip: practical nondrug steps to successful therapy. *Consultant.* 1999;39(6):1707–1714.
22. Haskell WL, Lee IM. Physical activity and public health: updated recommendation for adults from the American College of Sports Medicine and the American Heart Association. *Med Sci Sports Exerc.* 2007;39(8):1423-1434.
23. McKinnis L. *Fundamentals of Musculoskeletal Imaging,* 2nd ed. Philadelphia, PA: F.A. Davis Company; 2005. Retrieved from http://www.R2Library.com/marc_frame.aspx? Resource ID=149
24. Mendelson S, Milgrom C, Finestone A, et al. Effect of cane use on tibial strain and strain rates. *Am J PM&R.* 1998;77(4):333–338.

Patellofemoral Syndrome

Trasey D. Falcone and Gary P. Chimes

INTRODUCTION

Patellofemoral pain syndrome (PFPS) is a description of symptoms and a diagnosis of exclusion that is a common endpoint to the differential diagnosis of anterior knee pain (1). Among patients presenting to sports medicine centers, it is thought to encompass as much as 25% of those with knee complaints. Women and active individuals have been found to be affected at higher rates (2).

There are six anatomic areas thought to contribute to pain within the patellofemoral joint. These include subchondral bone, synovium, retinaculum, skin, nerve, and muscle. Although the etiology of PFPS is essentially multifactorial, a commonly referred to source is joint overload. Activities that can overload the patellofemoral joint include squatting, kneeling, prolonged knee flexion, and ascending or descending stairs. The patellofemoral joint is one of the highest loaded musculoskeletal components in the body (3).

Equally important sources of PFPS include malalignment and trauma. Direct trauma to the patella, trochlea, and surrounding structures can result in patellar dislocation or subluxation, as well as reticular strain or damage to articular cartilage. Malalignment involves abnormality in static patellar position and dynamic tracking problems within the femoral trochlea. Patella alta or baja can influence compressive forces at the patella femoral joint with knee flexion. Patellar tracking abnormalities may arise from reduced patellar mobility, leg length discrepancy, abnormal foot morphology, hamstrings and hip musculature tightness, angular and rotational deformities of the lower limbs, increased quadriceps (Q) angle, and muscle weakness or imbalance (4). Other structural causes may incur from a shallow trochlea, also known as trochlear dysplasia, allowing for increased lateral displacement of the patella.

The diagnosis of PFPS is predominantly clinical; therefore, a detailed physical examination is imperative.

Key elements of the physical examination include inspection, palpation, neurovascular examination as well as a detailed knee joint examination. Proper inspection of the knee should be performed with the patient weight-bearing. Observe body habitus, muscle bulk, looking for atrophy, angular or rotational deformity of the lower limbs, patella height, and signs of inflammation. Note abnormalities in dynamic patellar tracking with squatting and be aware of excessive pronation of the foot when standing or walking. Palpate around the knee joint and note areas that elicit pain, then slide the patella medial and lateral to expose and palpate the patellar facets. Look for discrepancies between the symptomatic and asymptomatic knee. Test flexibility of the quadriceps, hamstrings, gastroc-soleus, iliotibial band (ITB), hip flexors, extensors, and rotators. Assess the patient's gait for signs of quadriceps avoidance and hip abductor weakness. Passively move the knee through full range of motion (ROM) and feel for crepitus. Make note to perform full hip and lumbar spine examination as both are potential sources of referred pain (5).

Special tests performed during the physical examination to assess for PFPS include patellofemoral compression, apprehension test for patellar dislocation, patellar glide, and Q-angle, plus ligamentous and meniscal testing to rule out alternative or concomitant pathology. A positive patellofemoral compression test elicits pain when the patella is directly compressed into the trochlear groove while the leg is extended. The apprehension test for patellar dislocation or instability is performed with the knee flexed to 30° and pressure is applied to the medial patella pushing the patella laterally. The test is considered positive if the patient demonstrates signs of apprehension such as anxiety or reactive knee extension when the patella reaches maximal patellar displacement (6). Patellar hypermobility and retinacular tightness are assessed with the patellar glide test. With the patella passively displaced medially and laterally the extent of patellar translation is assessed. If the translation is limited to less than 1/4 of the patella's width, the retinaculum is tight. If the patella translates 3/4 of patellar width then the test is suggestive of patellar hypermobility. The Q angle is a measurement used to estimate the valgus moment acting on the patellofemoral joint. This measurement is taken from the anterior superior iliac spine to the mid-patella, and then to the tibial tubercle. A Q angle of 20° has been suggested as the upper normative value (5,7). Tests for ligamentous instability include anterior drawer, Lachman, posterior drawer, varus stress, and valgus stress. Meniscal tests include palpation for joint line tenderness, McMurray test, and Apley grind test (6).

Biomechanical analysis of step ups and step downs on the involved and uninvolved limb can be a helpful office based test. While having the patient perform a single leg squat, observe for excessive contralateral pelvic drop and/or hip adduction with internal rotation that can lead to increased valgus stress at the knee. If pain is elicited during a single leg squat, biomechanical modifications can be made to address potential sources of altered tracking such as excessive foot pronation or hip abductor weakness. An arch support can be added, cues can be provided to activate the gluteal muscles, and even patellar taping can be utilized to assess for improvement in symptoms with repeated leg single squats. These tests could be performed in the physician's office or at the physical therapy evaluation.

Initially, radiographic imaging is usually of limited diagnostic value because PFPS is considered a clinical diagnosis. Imaging can, however, be pursued if the patient's symptoms are refractory to initial therapy. X-rays of the knee with weight-bearing posterior-anterior, lateral, and patellofemoral (e.g., Merchant or Sunrise) views can be used to rule out bipartite patella, osteoarthritis, loose bodies, or occult fracture. Additionally, the patellofemoral views can identify lateral displacement, tilting, or rotation of the patella.

MRI can be helpful for detection of chondromalacia patella, articular cartilage injuries, osteochondritis dissecans, or injuries to the patellar retinaculum and medial patellofemoral ligament. Patellar malalignment and subchondral sclerosis can be detected with serial flexion views on CT. Ultrasound can provide insight into patellar tendinopathy. Increased bone activity secondary to subchondral stress can be perceived via bone scan (7,8).

PATELLOFEMORAL PAIN SYNDROME

- Symptoms include pain localized to the anterior knee, typically with insidious onset. The pain can be made worse with activities such as ascending and descending stairs, squatting, and prolonged sitting due to the compressive forces on the joint

- Mechanism of injury is often related to overuse and/or training errors

- Key elements of the physical examination include inspection, palpation, and detailed knee examination including ligamentous testing

- Provocative tests: Patellofemoral compression, apprehension test for patellar dislocation

- Functional tests including single leg squat can be very revealing and may be repeated and symptoms reassessed after correction of biomechanical problems (e.g., excessive foot pronation, patella instability or maltracking, and gluteal muscle inhibition)

- PFPS is a clinical diagnosis; however, radiographic imaging may be useful to rule out other sources of knee pain if the condition remains refractory to treatment

THE REHABILITATION PROGRAM

Development of a rehabilitation program targeted at improving symptoms of PFPS should take into consideration the presumed etiology of pain. Most current research has targeted kinetic chain deficiency involving muscle imbalance, tight soft tissue structures, abnormal patellar mobility, and structural malalignment of the lower limb. Fredericson describes a three-phase treatment algorithm incorporating pain control, correction of malalignment and strength deficits, and long-term functional adaptations for sustained symptom management. Initial management utilizes pain control with activity modification, patellar taping and bracing, and anti-inflammatory medications and modalities (9). The five phases of rehabilitation discussed throughout this book may also be applied, as long as an assessment for and the correction of biomechanical errors, training errors, faulty movement patterns, and muscular imbalances are included.

Dye proposed that primary tissue pathology best accounts for the etiology of PFPS in most patients. Primary tissue pathology describes the responses of musculoskeletal tissues to differential loading homeostasis, loss of homeostasis caused by disuse or overuse, and structural failure. With this idea, the suggested treatment of PFPS exists via staying within this realm of painlessness with loading activity. Any perceived pain within the patellofemoral joint that is activity-induced is an indication of supra physiologic loading event that will subvert any normal healing mechanisms. Potential sources for nociceptive output can come from any patellofemoral structure that possesses a sensory nerve supply (3). A nerve block directed at the infrapatellar branch of the saphenous nerve is a newly proposed intervention for pain management, although no current published study is supportive of this intervention.

Therapeutic Modalities

Modalities proposed to benefit patients with PFPS have included cryotherapy, therapeutic heat, phonophoresis, iontophoresis, monophasic pulsed stimulation, transcutaneous electrical nerve stimulation (TENS), neuromuscular electrical stimulation (NMES), and electromyography (EMG) biofeedback. Lake et al performed a systematic review to examine evidence for the basis of recommendations for or against these modalities, and they revealed no scientific justification for the treatment of PFPS with therapeutic modalities alone. One study reported subjective improvement with the use of ultrasound and ice massage, ice bags, phonophoresis, and iontophoresis, however, this was a low quality study (10,11). However, the use of many other transdermal modalities such as ultrasound therapy, electrical stimulation, iontophoresis, magnet therapy, and topical medications are lacking literary evidence (10).

Complementary therapies for PFPS have also been investigated. Naslund et al conducted a randomized control trial to determine if acupuncture treatment of patients with PFPS was beneficial. At the conclusion of this study, patients had positive outcomes with both electro-acupuncture treatment and subcutaneous needling (12).

Manual Therapy

Physical therapists typically assess the mobility of the patellofemoral and proximal tibio-fibular joints. Hypomobility will be addressed via joint mobilization techniques, whereas hypermobility requires strengthening of the supportive structures (e.g., quadriceps). Patellar mobilization with stretching of tight peri-patellar structures may be useful for controlling symptoms of PFPS when combined with exercise, orthoses, and activity modification (13).

Other manual therapies that have been used for relief of PFPS symptoms include sacroiliac (SI) joint manipulation and chiropractic patellar joint manipulation. There is currently insufficient evidence to suggest that these interventions are effective (14). It is postulated that mechanical dysfunction of the ipsilateral SI joint may be responsible for persistent muscle inhibition of quadriceps muscles that can be observed in PFPS. SI joint manipulation uses a high-velocity low-amplitude thrust to the SI joint ipsilateral to the affected knee. Studies have shown improvements in quadriceps muscle strength and may be beneficial for anterior knee pain associated with SI joint dysfunction (13,15,16), although well designed, randomized controlled studies are required to confirm these results.

Therapeutic Exercise

The mainstay of treatments for PFPS is physiotherapy and has been proven effective for the relief of patellofemoral joint pain (17). Treatment programs should be individualized and styles may vary depending upon physician and therapist preferences. General recommendations include pain control with activity modification, correction of patellar malalignment (if applicable), and stretching and strengthening exercises for the affected lower limb (14). In general tight structures should be mobilized and the kinetic chain should be balanced (1).

Quadriceps muscle imbalances are thought to contribute to maltracking of the patella on the distal femur. Specifically, vastus medialis oblique (VMO) muscle weakness or imbalance relative to the vastus lateralis (VL) causing abnormal lateral tracking and increased patellofemoral contact pressure has been frequently suggested and addressed in the literature as a possible cause of PFPS. There is evidence to suggest that therapy directed at correcting quadriceps muscle imbalance is an effective treatment strategy for PFPS (2). Exercises targeted at retraining VMO and correcting muscle imbalance include isometric VMO contractions and small range weight-bearing squats to 30° of flexion. According to Australian physiotherapist Jenny McConnell small range squats can begin with the feet parallel and then progress to walk stance positioning to simulate the motion of the knee during the stance phase of walking (18). EMG biofeedback during physiotherapy sessions may be utilized to assist in muscle isolation (18). Recent review articles suggest that the VMO may not be activated in isolation; instead it may only be activated along with the rest of the quadriceps. The benefits of VMO specific exercises may be attributable to generalized quadriceps strengthening and improved control of the patellofemoral joint, which has been proven to be effective (19).

More recent studies have focused on hip strength and hip and knee kinematics for PFPS treatments (20). Balanced strengthening of the affected lower limb should include quadriceps, hip flexors, hip abductors, hip extensors, and external rotators. In fact, studies looking at strengthening hip abductors and external rotators have demonstrated moderate pain reduction, whereas the addition of hip extensor and hip flexor strengthening had greater improvement in pain (19). Exercises involving these muscle groups include single leg raises in supine, seated knee extension, seated leg presses, squats, isometric hip abduction, hip abduction with weights, and step up/step down exercises. An effective hip exercise is the four-way straight leg raise. This is performed in supine, prone, and lateral decubitus positions to target the hip flexors, extensors, abductors, and adductors. Elastic bands can be utilized for resistance with standing hip abduction, sitting hip external rotation, and side stepping exercises (21). Both open and closed kinetic chain exercises have been proven effective treatment strategies for PFPS (2). Closed kinetic chain exercises are often preferable as they simulate daily functional mobility and if performed correctly can limit stress or forces across the knee joint.

In addition to muscle strengthening exercises, the comprehensive therapy program should include stretching of tight lower limb soft tissue structures. The focus should be on hamstring, plantarflexor, quadricep, and ITB stretches (21). A "figure of four" position can be used to stretch tight anterior thigh structures (18), but aggressive stretching in this position can cause anterior hip pain and must be avoided (Figure 25.1). The quadriceps can be stretched in the prone or standing position by pulling the ankle toward the buttocks. The ITB can be stretched in the standing position or seated position (Figure 25.3). A supine hamstring stretch is performed by supporting the leg with both hands and slowly straightening the leg (Figure 25.2). The plantarflexors can be stretched by taking a lunge step toward a wall with hands placed on the wall for support. The posterior leg should be straight with the heel of the foot pressing toward the floor (22). Flexibility programs need to address deficits in the individual patient and tailored to what they are able to tolerate.

The home exercise program (HEP) should be a simplified version of treatment prescription that can be performed daily for approximately 5 minutes. It is preferable to provide three to four exercises that do not require use of equipment. Exercises should include hip abduction and external rotation exercises specifically targeting gluteal musculature, small squats, and anterior hip stretches (18).

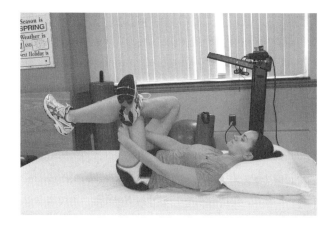

FIGURE 25.1: "Figure of four" stretch.

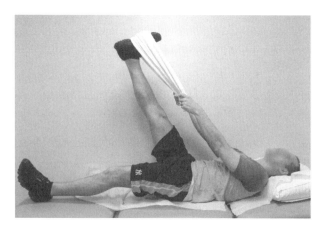

FIGURE 25.2: Supine hamstring stretch.

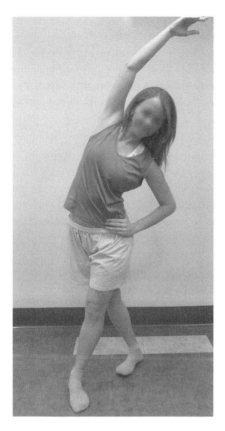

FIGURE 25.3: Standing ITB stretch.

Specialized Techniques

Patellar taping is a widely utilized component of PFPS physiotherapy. This technique has been shown to subjectively relieve pain associated with PFPS (23). The proposed advantage of this is by pulling the patella medially the VMO activity will be increased, thus providing increased patellar stability. Taping may not only increase activity of VMO, but also alter timing of onset of VMO activity (24). However, taping has minimal effect on long term symptoms associated with PFPS. Therefore it should be used in the short term to improve patient tolerance for strengthening exercises (25). Patellofemoral braces have been developed to similarly correct malalignment; however, no current studies have proven their efficacy (26). While the mechanism for taping and bracing remain uncertain, they are still regarded as good adjunctive treatments for PFPS, especially if pain is reduced and the strengthening program is more effective. Foot orthoses may be beneficial for control of foot over-pronation or supination if applicable (14). Prospective studies have demonstrated that PFPS can increase with navicular drop or supination. But, studies still are needed to demonstrate if supporting the arch or absorption of shock provides any long term benefit (19).

Home Exercise Program

The HEP should be able to be performed on a daily basis within a small time allotment, with minimal to no equipment requirements. Optimally this would include three to four strengthening and stretching exercises. It should be noted that an essential component of PFPS treatment is activity modification and pain relief; therefore, the HEP should not reproduce the patient's symptoms. The four-way single leg raise, small squats, and anterior hip stretches can be easily incorporated into a daily regimen for treatment and prevention of PFPS (18).

SUMMARY

PFPS is a descriptive term for anterior knee pain that is generally exacerbated with loading activities such as squatting, kneeling, prolonged sitting, and ascending/descending stairs. This is a clinical diagnosis and treatment should be directed toward pain alleviation and restoration of proper biomechanics. Physical therapy is a proven treatment for the relief of patellofemoral pain. Therapy must be individualized to the patient to address biomechanical factors contributing to their pain, such as weakness of the quadriceps, hip abductors, and external rotators. Patellar taping is a proven short-term adjunctive treatment option; manual therapy may be beneficial when combined with therapeutic exercises, whereas therapeutic modalities lack sufficient evidence to support their use beyond initial symptomatic management. An independent HEP that is performed on a daily basis is important for continued patient progress, maintenance of functional improvements, and prevention of recurrent PFPS.

SAMPLE CASE

A 24-year-old female presents with a 1 month history of right anterior knee pain exacerbated with stair descent, squatting, and prolonged sitting. She denies any recent or previous trauma to the knee joint. She did note that she had recently started a running program to train for an upcoming 10K race. Review of systems is unremarkable. A complete physical examination was performed to assess neuromuscular function. The right knee exhibited significant peri-patellar tenderness, with mild tenderness over the lateral patellar facets on the articular surface, and more diffusely along the lateral and inferior pole of the patella with some extension into the patellar tendon. The right knee was without effusion. ROM was tested by bringing the knee into full flexion and extension. Significant pain and muscle guarding were produced when the right knee was within five to ten degrees of full extension and she had some lateral tracking of the patella. Tests for ligamentous instability of the right knee with anterior drawer, Lachman, posterior drawer, varus stress, and valgus stress were negative. The patient was asked to perform a right single-leg squat that was very limited going from neutral to the first five degrees of flexion. Her two-legged squat produced only marginal pain after ten repetitions, which was made worse with medial arch support. Examination of the left knee was unremarkable. The patient has no previous radiographic studies of her lower extremities.

 SAMPLE THERAPY PRESCRIPTION

Discipline: Physical therapy.

Diagnosis: Patellofemoral pain syndrome.

Precautions: weight bearing as tolerated (WBAT)"

Frequency of visits: 2 to 3x/week.

Duration of treatment: 4 to 6 weeks.

Treatment:

1. *Modalities:* cryotherapy prn

2. *Manual therapy:* assessment of patellar mobility, patellar mobilization as needed

3. *Therapeutic exercise:* stretching exercises focusing on the quadriceps, ITB, hamstrings, and plantarflexors. Strengthening exercises focusing on the quadriceps, gluteus maximus and medius, including but not limited to: seated leg press, small squats, step up/step down exercises, four-way straight leg raise, single leg knee extension

4. *Specialized treatment:* Patellar taping, bracing, foot orthoses, if these treatments improve the patient's ability to comply with the strengthening program

5. *Patient Education:* HEP

6. *Follow up:* Physician follow up after 4 weeks of treatment

REFERENCES

1. Fulkerson J. Diagnosis and treatment of patients with patellofemoral pain. *The Am J Sports Med.* 2002;30(3):447–456.

2. Fagan V, Delahunt D. Patellofemoral pain syndrome: a review on the associated neuromuscular deficits and current treatment options. *Br J Sports Med.* 2008;42:789–795.

3. Dye SF. The pathophysiology of patellofemoral pain: a tissue homeostasis perspective. *Clin Orthop Relat Res.* 2005;436:100–110.

4. Bolgla L, Malone T, Umberger B, et al. Hip strength and hip and knee kinematics during stair descent in females with and without patellofemoral pain syndrome. *J Orthop Sports Phys Ther.* 2008;38(1):12–18.

5. Post W. Clinical evaluation of patients with patellofemoral disorders. *Arthroscopy.* 1999;15(9):841–851.

6. Malanga GA, Andrus S, Nadler SF, et al. Physical examination of the knee: a review of the original test description and scientific validity of common orthopedic tests. *Arch Phys Med Rehabil.* 2003;84:592–603.

7. Haim A, Yaniv M, Dekel S, et al. Patellofemoral pain syndrome validity of clinical and radiological features. *Clin Orthop Relat Res.* 2006;451:223–228.

8. DeLisa JA, Frontera WR, Gans BM, et al. In: Imaging techniques relative to rehabilitation. *DeLisa's Physical Medicine and Rehabilitation Principles and Practice,* 5th ed. Philadelphia, PA: Lippincott Williams & Wilkins; 2010:139–160.

9. Fredericson M, Powers C. Practical management of patellofemoral pain. *Clin J Sport Med.* 2002;12:36–38.

10. Bolin DJ, Transdermal approached to pain in sports injury management. *Curr Sports Med Rep.* 2003;2:303–309.

11. Lake DA, Wofford NH. Effect of therapeutic modalities on patients with patellofemoral pain syndrome: A systematic review. *Sports Health: A Multidisciplinary Approach*, 2011;3:182–189.

12. Naslund J, Naslund UP, Odenbring S, et al. Sensory stimulation (acupuncture) for the treatment of idiopathic anterior knee pain. *J Rehabil Med.* 2002;34(5):231–238.

13. Brantingham JW, Globe G, Pollard H, et al. Manipulative therapy for lower extremity conditions: expansion of literature review. *J Manipulative Physiol Ther.* 2009;32(1):53–71.

14. Crossley K, Bennell K, Green S, et al. A systematic review of physical interventions for patellofemoral pain syndrome. *Clin J Sport Med.* 2001;11:103–110.

15. Sutter E, McMorland G, Herzog W, et al. Decrease in quadriceps inhibition after sacroiliac joint manipulation in patients with anterior knee pain. *J Manipulative Physiol Ther.* 1999;22(3):149–153.

16. Hillermann B, Gomes AN, Korporaal C, et al. A pilot study comparing the effects of spinal manipulative therapy with those of extra-spinal manipulative therapy on quadriceps muscle strength. *J Manipulative Physiol Ther.* 2006;29(2):145–149.

17. Crossley K, Bennell K, Green S, et al. Physical therapy for patellofemoral pain: A randomized, double-blinded, placebo-controlled trial. *Am J Sports Med.* 2002;30:857–865.

18. McConnell J. Rehabilitation and nonoperative treatment of patellar instability. *Sports Med Arthrosc Rev.* 2007;15(2):95–104.

19. Bolgla LA, Boling MC. An update for the conservative management of patellofemoral pain syndrome: a systematic review of the literature from 2000 to 2010. *Inter J of Sports Phys Ther.* 2011;6(2):112–125.

20. Souza R, Powers C. Differences in hip kinematics, muscle strength, and muscle activation between subjects with and without patellofemoral pain. *J Orthop Sports Phys Ther.* 2009;39(1):12–19.

21. Fukuda TY, Rossetto FM, Magalhaes E, et al. Short-term effects of hip abductors and lateral rotators strengthening in females with patellofemoral pain syndrome: A randomized controlled clinical trial. *J Orthop Sports Phys Ther.* 2010;40(11):736–742.

22. Coppack RJ, Etherington J, Wills AK. The effects of exercise for the prevention of overuse anterior knee pain. *Am J Sports Med.* 2011;39(5):940–948.

23. Ng G, Cheng J. The effects of patellar taping on pain and neuromuscular performance in subjects with patellofemoral pain syndrome. *Clin Rehab.* 2003;16:821–827.

24. Christou E. Patellar taping increases vastus medialis oblique activity in the presence of patellofemoral pain. *J Electromyogr Kines.* 2003;14:495–504.

25. Clark DI, Downing N, Mitchell J, et al. Physiotherapy for anterior knee pain: a randomised controlled trial. *Ann Rheum Dis.* 2000;59(9):700–704.

26. McCrory J, Quick N, Shapiro R, et al. The effect of a single treatment of the Protinics system on femoris and gluteus medius activation during gait and the lateral step up exercise. *Gait Posture.* 2004;19:148–153.

Patellar and Quadriceps Tendinopathy

Kim Middleton, Mark A. Harrast, and Lori Sabado

INTRODUCTION

Patellar tendinopathy (PT), frequently termed "jumpers knee," and quadriceps tendinopathy (QT) are conditions of chronic tendon overuse and overload of the knee extensor mechanism, associated with activities involving repeated running, jumping, and kicking. The histology of each condition is consistent with a non-inflammatory disruption of the tendon's extracellular matrix and vascular structures, most commonly localized to the superior patellar pole in QT and to the inferior patellar pole in PT.

The true pain generator is not well established; potential sources are from peripheral peritendinous pain receptors or related to the process of neovascularization that occurs after injury (1,2). Both PT and QT are common conditions, with prevalence estimated in nonelite athletes of 8.5% (PT), highest among volleyball players (14.4%) (3). Identified risk factors include poor hamstring and quadriceps flexibility (4), poor knee joint coordination, reduced ankle dorsiflexion, and increased pronation velocity of the foot (5). By contrast, acute patellar and quadriceps tendon ruptures are quite rare, occurring at any point within the tendon substance, often associated with high force generation in young athletes, steroid or fluoroquinolone antibiotic use, or systemic diseases such as rheumatoid arthritis and diabetes mellitus (6).

Diagnosis of patellar and QT is made clinically based on symptoms and physical exam findings. Patients describe anterior knee pain, insidious in onset, often associated with an increase in training intensity or frequency. Pain may first be present upon initiating activity and then improve after a warm up. Patients may report stiffness with inactivity and sharp pain with initiation of activity. Crepitus may be felt by the patient while walking or moving their knee. Over time, symptoms may become painful throughout sport and commonly with any provocative maneuvers such as kicking or squatting.

Key elements of the physical examination include inspection, palpation, neurovascular examination, passive and active range of motion (ROM) of the knee, quadriceps and hamstring flexibility and strength testing, and testing for ligamentous and meniscal integrity. Examination of the hip and low back should be performed to rule out associated pathology that may present as anterior knee pain. Tenderness is most common at the anterior superior or inferior pole of the patella in QT and PT respectively, with symptoms exacerbated by resisted knee extension and decline squats. Functional testing includes single leg stance, squat and decline squats, single leg hopping, and the dip test (1). Including a kinetic chain assessment with a detailed examination of the hip and ankle, as well as an evaluation of foot alignment and shoewear, is imperative.

Imaging is generally not necessary to make these clinical diagnoses but can be confirmatory in equivocal cases. Ultrasound imaging can reveal evidence of ill-defined hypoechoic zones with thickening of the tendon, and/or MRI by increased signal intensity on T2 images (7). Ultrasound may also provide the added benefit of sonopalpation to further localize the area of pain generation. Since these imaging findings, as well as histologic changes consistent with tendinosis, are also observed in asymptomatic individuals, imaging currently has a limited role in guiding rehabilitative treatments or judging prognosis and may be more appropriate to rule out other pathology such as calcific tendinopathy or tendon rupture.

PATELLAR AND QUADRICEPS TENDINOPATHY

- PT and QT are common overuse injuries in sports involving significant jumping and kicking

- Known risk factors include poor quadriceps/hamstring inflexibility, reduced ankle dorsiflexion, and foot malalignment

- Symptoms include pain to the anterior knee, evolving insidiously and worsening with initiation of activity, improved during exercise and progressively worsening with continued use

- Key physical examination findings include: Pain over inferior or superior patellar poles, aggravated by resisted knee extension and squats, with weakness and/or discomfort provoked by squatting

THE REHABILITATION PROGRAM

Tendon loading stimulates collagen remodeling and repair (8); correspondingly, the cornerstone of treatment for both PT and QT involves a comprehensive rehabilitative program. This program entails managing pain, strengthening the affected muscle-tendon unit with progressive loading, correcting biomechanical deficits that may be contributing factors to the initial injury, as well as improving flexibility, proprioception, and motor coordination in everyday activities and sport-specific training. Manual therapy and modalities help to relieve initial symptoms and complement the rehabilitative exercises to promote tendon recovery and eventual return to sports-specific activities. The five phases of rehabilitation followed throughout this book should be applied to the rehabilitation program.

Therapeutic Modalities

While passive application of ice has little role in these chronic, noninflammatory conditions, specialized strategies such as ice friction massage may help to stimulate a healing response in chronic tendinopathy. Animal studies involving laser and electrical stimulation to postsurgical tendons demonstrated improvements in tendon healing and tensile strength (9,10) but to date there is limited evidence to support these as conservative treatment approaches in nonsurgical PT or QT.

Therapeutic ultrasound is an appropriate complementary treatment for PT and QT, with animal and in-vitro studies demonstrating the benefit of ultrasound to facilitate tendon healing, though compelling evidence remains to be demonstrated (11). Extracorporal shock wave therapy (ESWT) involves transmission of sonic energy pulses to tissues with the goals of providing pain relief and stimulating tissue recovery (2). While there is limited evidence that ESWT provides symptomatic pain relief and improved knee function in PT (12), there is no clear optimal treatment protocol and its utilization is further limited by cost and patient discomfort.

Manual Therapy

Manual techniques are used commonly in treatment of chronic tendinopathy although evidence within literature is sparse. Myofascial tissue treatments such as deep or transverse friction massage, augmented soft tissue mobilization (ASTM)®, and Graston technique® are believed by some to promote tendon recovery, potentially by stimulating fibroblast activity as seen in an animal model (13). Myofascial quadriceps work has been shown to improve pain scores in PT (14). For self-management, patients can be taught friction massage, or ice friction massage, to potentially stimulate the same process as part of a home treatment program. Joint mobilization of the hip, knee, ankle, or foot may be helpful in patients with restricted motion to improve kinetic chain function.

Therapeutic Exercise

As focal discomfort improves, it is appropriate to transition to the next phase of the rehabilitation process to promote flexibility, strength, and endurance, as well as optimize balance and proprioception, with the goal of returning to sport-specific activities.

Stretching across all phases of recovery should include both passive and active techniques for the quadriceps and hamstrings as well as for hip and ankle flexibility. Active strategies, which mirror the eccentric strengthening approach discussed in this chapter (Figure 26.1), include movements such as straight leg marching (hamstrings), eccentric dorsiflexion stretches (gastrocnemius), and active quadricep stretching. Manual therapy, including joint mobilization and myofascial work, can also facilitate soft tissue extensibility in this rehabilitation phase.

After PT and QT injuries, the normal knee extensor muscle activation pattern may potentially be altered with quadriceps muscle inhibition, as seen in patients after

(a)
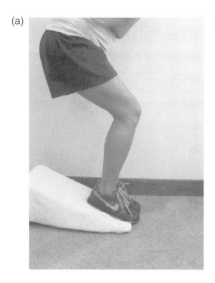
(b)
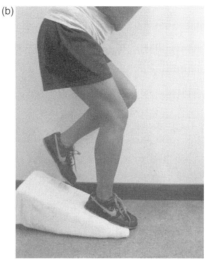
(c)
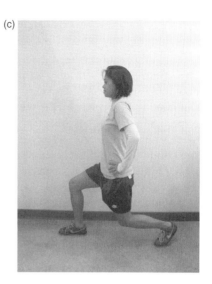

FIGURE 26.1: Eccentric quadriceps strengthening.

(a)
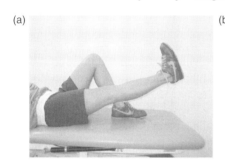
(b)
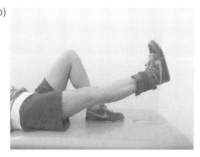

FIGURE 26.2: Isometric quad strengthening.

patellar contusion, ACL tear and repair, and knee replacement (15–17). In affected patients, neuromuscular reeducation strategies can be trialed to correct the muscle firing patterns prior to initiating strengthening efforts and dynamic exercise regimens. This can function to allow for appropriate balanced muscle forces during the strengthening program.

Strengthening regimens for tendinotic conditions traditionally emphasize eccentric exercises (for the quadriceps these include, but are not limited to, deep and decline squats and lunges) which have been shown to help normalize tendon structure and thickness and reduce neovascularization (18,19) (Figure 26.1). However, very early quadriceps strengthening should also include isometric exercises which generally cause less initial discomfort (Figure 26.2). As pain improves, progressing from short arc ROM to full arc sets is a reasonable strategy to increase tendon load and healing. Moreover, rehabilitative efforts should target associated hip and ankle musculature, to build strength as well as proprioception and balance to optimize the forces and mechanics affecting the knee joint (Figure 26.3). As the patient advances further, sports-specific drills and aerobic exercise incorporating lumbo-pelvic movements should be added.

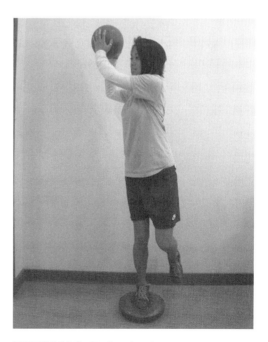

FIGURE 26.3: Challenging single leg balance activities.

These can include cutting, jumping, hopping, and jogging (Figure 26.4).

An evaluation of gait and jumping technique is important as abnormal jumping mechanics can predispose to this condition and reinjury (20,21) (Figure 26.4). Observed malalignments of the foot or ankle may require corrective shoewear or orthotics; similarly, avoidance of concrete in favor of softer surfaces such as tracks and treadmills may also be helpful during the recovery phase. Athletes should be counseled to adjust their training intensity and frequency for symptomatic relief and to accommodate their rehabilitative program.

Specialized Techniques

Athletic taping or bracing, such as a patellar tendon strap or neoprene sleeve with patella buttress, may provide symptomatic relief to the practicing athlete but there is little evidence to support their use (1).

Home Exercise Program

The home exercise program (HEP) reinforces the functional skills and exercises learned during formal physical therapy sessions and should be continued even after return to sport to retain the benefits of treatment and prevent recurrence of symptoms.

Thus, the early HEP should include daily stretching and begin with core strengthening, targeting nonpainful associated hip and ankle joint dysfunction. As symptoms improve, the patient can progress with guidance from their rehabilitation specialist to incorporate eccentric exercises of the quadriceps, hamstrings, and gluteals, and ultimately a graded progression to more dynamic activities including plyometrics, cutting, kicking, and running. In some athletes, teaching taping techniques and ice friction massage for self-management throughout recovery may be useful.

SUMMARY

PT and QT are common chronic overuse conditions causing anterior knee pain. The diagnosis is made clinically and radiographic imaging does not offer further insight unless bony fracture or trauma are suspected. Ultrasound examination may provide the benefit of sonopalpation to localize the site of pathology. The mainstay of recovery involves a graded comprehensive rehabilitative program, focused on stretching, eccentric exercises of hamstrings and quadriceps to build strength and endurance in conjunction with drills to promote coordination, proprioception, and flexibility at the hip, knee, and ankle. Myofascial treatments, therapeutic ultrasound, and ESWT may further help with pain and tendon remodeling. Patellar tendon straps and taping may provide athletes with some symptomatic relief and support during sport. A HEP should reinforce the stretching and strengthening strategies learned in physical therapy, progressing from simple to more dynamic movements and then sport-specific activities in order to facilitate recovery and return to play.

(a) 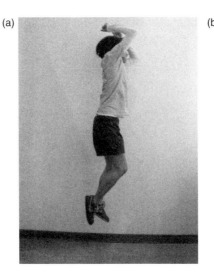 (b)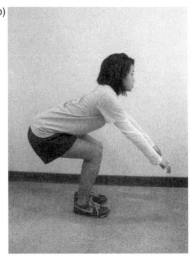

FIGURE 26.4: Proprioceptive and sports-specific training.

SAMPLE CASE

A 25-year-old volleyball player presents with a 4 month history of insidious onset, progressive right anterior knee pain at the inferior pole of the patella. Symptoms were gradual in onset, initially occurring only at the beginning of some practices but now are present throughout every game, and occasionally with simple knee flexion outside of sport. Symptoms have not been responsive to anti-inflammatory medications. On physical examination, he has pes planus foot alignment, reduced ankle dorsiflexion range, and tight hamstrings and quadriceps muscles. Palpation over the inferior pole of the right patella and resisted knee extension reproduce pain. Functional testing reveals single leg squats to be more difficult and painful on the right. Neurovascular examination is unremarkable.

 SAMPLE THERAPY PRESCRIPTION

Discipline: Physical therapy.

Diagnosis: Right PT with poor hamstring/quad flexibility, pes planus.

Precautions: None.

Frequency of visits: 1 to 2X/week.

Duration of treatment: 6 to 12 weeks.

Treatments:

1. *Modalities:* Ice as needed, ice friction massage, therapeutic ultrasound

2. *Manual therapy:* myofascial release to the quads, iliotibial band (ITB), and hamstrings if restricted. Transverse friction massage/soft tissue mobilizations to the patellar tendon

3. *Therapeutic exercise:*

   a. Stretching of the gastroc/soleus complex, hamstrings, quadriceps, ITB, and hip flexors

   b. Neuromuscular reeducation for abnormal muscle-firing patterns (if indicated)

   c. Strengthening: pain-free isometric exercises for quadriceps, hamstrings, and gluteals and progress to eccentric strengthening (decline squats with increasing resistance, lunges, hamstring and calf exercises). Add pain-free proprioceptive training, and lumbo-pelvic stabilization

   d. Functional retraining, stabilization, and strengthening: that is, lateral squats, jumps, hops, running, and cutting drills as tolerated

5. *Specialized treatments:* Biomechanical analysis of gait and the kinetic chain, evaluation of shoes, review and correction of biomechanics of walking/running/jumping/ kicking, and trial of patellar taping/bracing if continuing with sport during rehabilitative course

6. *Patient education:* development of progressive HEP

Goals: Decrease pain with knee flexion, improve leg extension strength, restore hamstring/quad ROM, improve balance/ proprioception, correct any imbalances in running/jumping mechanics, return to sport, and initiation of maintenance exercise program to prevent return of symptoms

Re-evaluation: In 4 to 6 weeks by referring provider if symptoms persist and are not improving so that further management can be discussed

REFERENCES

1. Kountouris A, Cook J. Rehabilitation of Achilles and patellar tendinopathies. *Best Pract Res Clin Rheumatol.* 2007;21(2):295–316.
2. Peers, K.H. and R.J. Lysens, Patellar tendinopathy in athletes: current diagnostic and therapeutic recommendations. *Sports Med.* 2005;35(1):71–87.
3. Zwerver J, Bredeweg S, van den Akker-Scheek I. Prevalence of jumper's knee among non-elite athletes from different sports; a cross-sectional survey. *Br J Sports Med.* 2011; 45(4):324.
4. Witvrouw E, Bellemans J, Lysens R, Danneels L, Cambier D. Intrinsic risk factors for the development of patellar tendinitis

8sm.

in an athletic population. A two-year prospective study. *Am J Sports Med*, 2001;29(2):190–195.

5. Grau S, Maiwald C, Krauss I, Axmann D, Janssen P, Horstmann T. What are causes and treatment strategies for patellar-tendinopathy in female runners? *J Biomech*. 2008;41(9):2042–2046.

6. Kim JR, Park H, Roh SG, Shin SJ. Concurrent bilateral patellar tendon rupture in a preadolescent athlete: a case report and review of the literature. *J Pediatr Orthop B*. 2010;19(6):511–514.

7. Tuong B, White J, Louis L, et al. Get a kick out of this: the spectrum of knee extensor mechanism injuries. *Br J Sports Med*. 2011;45(2):140–146.

8. Morelli V, Rowe RH. Patellar tendonitis and patellar dislocations. *Prim Care*, 2004;31(4):909–924, viii-ix.

9. Reddy GK, Gum S, Stehno-Bittel L, Enwemeka CS. Biochemistry and biomechanics of healing tendon: Part II. Effects of combined laser therapy and electrical stimulation. *Med Sci Sports Exerc*. 1998;30(6):794–800.

10. Gum SL, Reddy GK, Stehno-Bittel L, Enwemeka CS. Combined ultrasound, electrical stimulation, and laser promote collagen synthesis with moderate changes in tendon biomechanics. *Am J Phys Med Rehabil*. 1997;76(4):288–296.

11. Tsai WC, Liang FC. Effect of therapeutic ultrasound on tendons. *Am J Phys Med Rehabil*. 2011. Epub ahead of print.

12. van Leeuwen MT, Zwerver J, van den Akker-Scheek I. Extracorporeal shockwave therapy for patellar tendinopathy: a review of the literature. *Br J Sports Med*. 2009;43(3):163–168.

13. Davidson CJ, Ganion LR, Gehlsen GM, Verhoestra B, Roepke JE, Sevier TL. Rat tendon morphologic and functional changes resulting from soft tissue mobilization. *Med Sci Sports Exerc*. 1997;29(3):313–319.

14. Pedrelli A, Stecco C, Day JA. Treating patellar tendinopathy with Fascial Manipulation. *J Bodyw Mov Ther*. 2009; 13(1):73–80.

15. Williams GN, Buchanan TS, Barrance PJ, Axe MJ, Snyder-Mackler L. Quadriceps weakness, atrophy, and activation failure in predicted noncopers after anterior cruciate ligament injury. *Am J Sports Med*. 2005;33(3):402–407.

16. Mizner RL, Petterson SC, Stevens JE, Vandenborne K, Snyder-Mackler L. Early quadriceps strength loss after total knee arthroplasty. The contributions of muscle atrophy and failure of voluntary muscle activation. *J Bone Joint Surg Am*. 2005;87(5):1047–1053.

17. Manal TJ, Snyder-Mackler L. Failure of voluntary activation of the quadriceps femoris muscle after patellar contusion. *J Orthop Sports Phys Ther*. 2000;30(11):655–660; discussion 661–663.

18. Ohberg L, Lorentzon R, Alfredson H. Eccentric training in patients with chronic Achilles tendinosis: normalised tendon structure and decreased thickness at follow up. *Br J Sports Med*. 2004;38(1):8–11; discussion 11.

19. Ohberg L, Alfredson H. Effects on neovascularisation behind the good results with eccentric training in chronic mid-portion Achilles tendinosis? *Knee Surg Sports Traumatol Arthrosc*. 2004;12(5):465-470.

20. Richards DP, Ajemian SV, Wiley JP, Brunet JA, Zernicke RF. Relation between ankle joint dynamics and patellar tendinopathy in elite volleyball players. *Clin J Sport Med*. 2002;12(5):266–272.

21. Richards DP, Ajemian SV, Wiley JP, Zernicke RF. Knee joint dynamics predict patellar tendinitis in elite volleyball players. *Am J Sports Med*. 1996;24(5):676–683.

Knee Ligament Sprains

Curtis W. Bazemore, Meredith B. Brazell, Stephanie L. Griggs,
Gary A. Levengood, and Harris A. Patel

INTRODUCTION

Ligamentous injuries to the knee account for 20 to 40 percent of sports injuries sustained to the knee. The medial collateral ligament (MCL) is most commonly injured, followed by the anterior cruciate ligament (ACL) (1). Ligamentous injuries are often not isolated events, and multiple structures of the knee are also compromised during a contact or noncontact injury. The ACL and posterior cruciate ligament (PCL) provide rotational stability while the lateral collateral ligament (LCL) and MCL provide lateral stability; when one is injured, all other knee structures become compromised, including but not limited to the previously mentioned ligaments, the menisci, and articular cartilage. The mechanism of ligamentous injury is generally traumatic and involves a forced rotation or direct blow, or both (Table 27.1). There is generally a pop, followed by swelling and instability with weight bearing on the involved limb (if weight bearing is possible at all).

Initial management always requires a detailed history and physical examination. *The key elements of the physical examination* include inspection, palpation, range of motion (ROM) assessment, strength assessment, neurovascular assessment, and special testing for the menisci and ligamentous integrity. Inspection for alignment, patella position, muscle bulk, and effusion should be assessed. An effusion can indicate an intra-articular process. Tenderness to palpation at the joint line may indicate meniscal pathology or collateral ligament injury. Special tests to assess the integrity of the ACL include Lachman's, Anterior Drawer, and Pivot Shift test however, muscle guarding and pain can affect your findings. PCL integrity can be tested using the Posterior Drawer, Posterior Sag, and Godfrey 90/90 test. MCL and LCL integrity is tested using the Valgus and Varus Stress tests, respectively. The patellofemoral ligaments (PFLs) can be assessed with patellar glides, patella dislocation with the Patella Apprehension test (2), patella femoral syndrome with the patella grind test, and an effusion can be tested for with the Ballotable Patella test (2). Sprains to any of these ligaments can vary in degree from grade I to grade III. If significant trauma has occurred then x-rays are recommended to assess whether an avulsion fracture is associated with the injury and/or any arthritic changes that may be present. An MRI can be ordered to determine the degree of the sprain as well as the location and fibers involved in the injury. If the patient has a painful effusion then needle aspiration with or without corticosteroid injection may be considered. Findings from the patient's history, physical examination, and diagnostic studies will allow the treatment team (treating physician, physical therapist, athletic trainer) to determine an appropriate program for the individual's needs and goals for returning to preinjury function The remainder of this chapter will focus on nonoperative ligamentous injuries to the knee, including grade I to II sprains of the LCL, PCL, ACL, and MCL. The approach described below could also be applied to grade III MCL tears as well, in the superior or mid substance of the MCL, since outcomes are usually good with nonoperative management.

THE REHABILITATION PROGRAM

As with other injuries it is important to progress through the phases of rehabilitation discussed throughout this book, and initiate the elements of protection, rest, ice, compression, and elevation (PRICE) as soon as possible after an acute injury. Protection of the injured ligament is essential for prevention of further injury and can be obtained with appropriate bracing and offloading the joint during ambulation

TABLE 27.1: Ligament Injuries of the Knee

	SIGNS/SYMPTOMS	PHYSICAL EXAMINATION	DIAGNOSTICS
ACL	-Audible pop or patient felt pop in the knee -Immediate joint swelling that decreases after several days -Inability to flex or extend the knee fully -Feeling of instability	-Mild/moderate joint effusion -Anterior point tenderness - + Lachman's - + Pivot-Shift - + Anterior Drawer -Occasionally an extensor lag	x-ray: generally normal radiographs; possibly will have associated Segond's fracture U/S: + joint effusion MRI: reveals fibers torn and location of tear
PCL	-Audible or patient felt pop in the knee -Subsequent joint swelling that continues to increase -Feeling of instability -Limitation of motion	-Mild/moderate joint effusion -Diffuse anterior point tenderness - + Posterior Drawer - + Posterior Sag - + Godfrey's 90°/90° - + Reverse Pivot Shift (Jakob Test)	x-ray: generally normal radiographs U/S: + joint effusion MRI: reveals fibers torn and location of tear
MCL	-Mild to moderate swelling in the joint; localized to the medial aspect -Feeling of instability -Limit of motion -Catching/locking sensation	-Mild/moderate medial effusion -Medial joint tenderness/tenderness over origin and attachment of MCL + Valgus Stress Test at 0° and/or 30°	x-ray: possible avulsion of MCL from origin/attachment U/S: can visualize effusion and any discontinuation of MCL MRI: reveals fibers torn and location of tear
LCL	-Mild/moderate swelling in the joint; localized to lateral aspect -Feeling of instability -Limit of motion -Catching/locking sensation	-Mild/moderate lateral effusion -Lateral joint tenderness/tenderness over origin and attachment of LCL + Varus Stress Test at 0° and/or 30°	x-ray: Possible avulsion of LCL from origin/attachment U/S: can visualize effusion and any discontinuation of LCL MRI: reveals fibers torn and location of tear
PFL (medial/lateral)	-Mild to moderate joint/suprapatellar swelling -Patient will have felt like their knee was "out" and came back in -Often presents like an ACL injury -Limit of motion	-Mild to moderate joint effusion -Floating patella -Diffuse tenderness - + Ballotable patella - + Patellar apprehension	x-ray: patella will be displaced and out of trochlear notch; possible avulsion fracture from attachment sites U/S: + joint effusion; can visualized discontinuation/trauma to PFL MRI: reveals fibers torn and location of tear

with an appropriate assistive device if warranted. Strengthening and mobility should be initiated to prevent muscular atrophy and joint stiffness and possible contracture. Progression of activity should be guided by the level of ligamentous injury and pain. Most of post injury rehabilitation is focused on ACL tears and nonoperative and postoperative therapy. The rehabilitation program should be individualized to the patient and progression of therapy is in our expert opinion also individualized to the patient. There is some evidence that progressive exercise does improve knee function especially after ACL tear (3).

Therapeutic Modalities

Early in the acute phase it is important to control and reduce pain and swelling in the knee joint while protecting the other structures from further injury. Along with the patient following the PRICE guidelines, the clinician may use a variety of modalities to assist in pain and edema control, including cryotherapy. There are many methods of decreasing pain and inflammation: cryotherapy, transcutaneous electrical nerve stimulation (TENS) (4), iontophoresis though evidence in literature is lacking, and nonsteroidal anti-inflammatories (NSAIDS). Applying neuromuscular electrical stimulation (using HI Volt/Russian stimulation or combo therapy) while doing quad sets, short arc quad sets (SAQs), and straight leg raise (SLR) have shown benefits in reducing muscle wasting (5).

Manual Therapy

Joint mobilization or deep tissue mobilization, such as Active Release Techniques® (ART®) can be useful in gaining full ROM of the knee as is seen in pilot studies (6) and is also theorized to help maintain the health of the articular surfaces of the knee joint.

Therapeutic Exercise

During the early phase of rehabilitation, while controlling and resolving the pain and swelling, the patient will perform basic strength exercises, such as quad sets (Figure 27.1), SLRs (Figure 27.2), SAQs, side leg raise (Figure 27.3), and hip lifts among others. If the ROM of the knee is not restored, it is useful to teach the patient a program of end range stretching (Figures 27.4 and Figure 27.5). In the author's opinion instructing them to perform these stretches at least 60 or more times and hold for 1 minute at end range will help improve ROM. They are instructed to stretch to the point of discomfort, but not into pain.

As ROM is being restored, the patient is guided through a series of closed chain, weight bearing exercises (as pain allows). The program can begin with simple, standing, multidirectional weight shifts. As the patients gain control of the knee and the pain decreases. They can be advanced to marching in place on varying surfaces to reduce impact to the knee (i.e., mini trampoline). Lower impact squat movements can be performed on units like the Total Gym® (at 30%–40% body weight), or leg press machines, using lower weights and higher repetitions. Patients can use these units as a "warm-up" for their knees by performing 60 to 100 repetitions at a reduced weight using concentric and eccentric loading. When they have gained sufficient ROM (at least 100° of knee flexion), then the stationary bike program is incorporated, using light resistance, along with other forms of cardiovascular training. Next, the patient can be allowed to return to light jogging if stability is good and there is no return of swelling with graded activities

KNEE LIGAMENT SPRAINS

▪ Ligamentous injuries to the knee account for 20 to 40 percent of sports injuries sustained to the knee

▪ The MCL is most commonly injured, followed by the ACL

▪ The mechanism of ligamentous injury is generally traumatic and involves a forced rotation or direct blow, or both

▪ *The key elements of the physical examination* include inspection, palpation, ROM assessment, strength assessment, and special testing for the menisci and ligamentous integrity

▪ If significant trauma has occurred then x-rays are recommended to assess whether an avulsion fracture is associated with the injury and/or any arthritic changes that may be present

▪ An MRI can be ordered to determine the degree of the sprain or to rule out ligament rupture, as well as the location and fibers involved in the injury

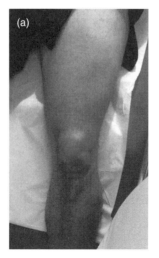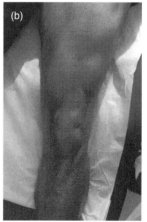

FIGURE 27.1: (a) Quad set start. (b) Quad set finish.

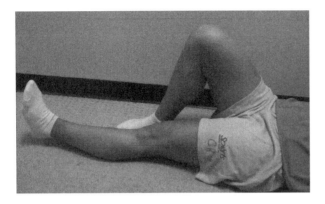

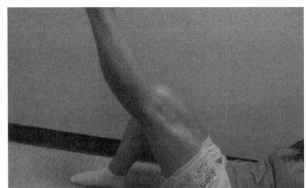

FIGURE 27.2: SLR start/finish.

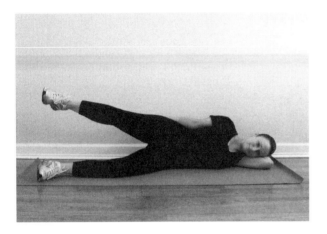

FIGURE 27.3: Hip lifts.

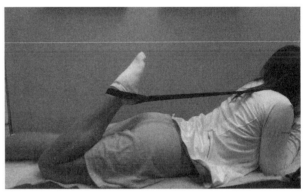

FIGURE 27.5: Prolonged assisted flexion.

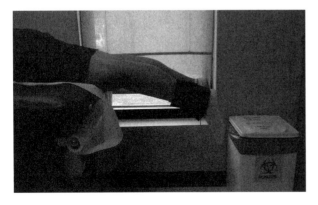

FIGURE 27.4: Prolonged hangs.

In the early phases, care is taken to avoid rotational torque producing drills and to avoid stress on the secondary restraints of the knee. As the patient gains more control and confidence in the knee, they gradually perform more advanced closed chain drills such as wall squats, step-ups, cross over, lateral steps (using resistance bands around ankles), and single leg balance drills on various surfaces (balance discs, foam half-rolls, BOSU® balls, etc.). Then, add resistance to march outs and low hurdle steps, both forward and sideways. With an athlete, the whole body is addressed in the rehabilitation program by including abdominal drills, as well as upper back and other core muscle groups. Further into the progression, plyometric drills with low box jumps, double leg jump ropes, and ski hex jumps (double leg hops to and from a center point in six different directions) among others will be added for more sport-specific goals.

Specialized Techniques

Aquatic therapy, including aquatic treadmills, can be used to begin lighter joint loading while patients perform various exercises including sports simulated activities. Devices such as the anti-gravity treadmill (AlterG®) are also useful in allowing a patient to begin reduced weight bearing walking or running, earlier in their rehabilitation program.

There are other specialized techniques in which fibroblastic proliferation is elicited and the production of new collagen occurs. Some examples of these include Kinesio Taping®, Graston Technique®, and dry needling. (Refer to the Chapter 28 for more techniques that also pertain to ligamentous injury rehabilitation.)

Kinesio Taping® has been shown to potentially reduce edema in patients (7). Kinesio Taping®, although unproven, has clinically been shown to help control pain and increase patient confidence as they resume activities.

Graston Technique® is an instrument-assisted soft tissue mobilization method which reignites the inflammatory process by bringing a controlled amount of microtrauma to the area (8). When done after an acute injury, this technique can accelerate overall tissue healing (9).

It has been demonstrated that dry needling once or twice during the phases of the rehabilitation process decreases pain and improves overall function (10).

Injury prevention in our opinion is the best method of treatment. After injury and once the patient obtains the ability to return to sport, an injury prevention program should be initiated. There is some evidence to show that prevention programs provide benefit from ligamentous knee injuries (11).

Supportive Devices

A variety of knee braces can be used to support an unstable knee and could potentially prevent further injury at low loads but at normal loads seen in sport this has not been validated in the literature. Knee braces can be made of magnesium to fiberglass and come in all different types, from neoprene sleeves for proprioception and biofeedback to custom fit functional braces. For ligament sprains, short, bilateral hinged knee braces have proven to be effective knee braces. Wearing a functional knee brace increases quadriceps activity by as much as 40%, and can increase joint stability (12).

Orthotics, custom or store bought, can also play an effective role in good knee function, in order to prevent further harm to the knee (13). Enhancing the biomechanics of the foot alignment could decrease pain, unload the knee, and improve neuromuscular control and overall function in patients.

SUMMARY

Ligamentous injuries of the knee can range from mild to severe and atraumatic to traumatic causes in any population. Studies show that nonoperative ligament injuries (in our opinions grade I or II MCL sprains, LCL sprains, PCL tears) respond best to a rehabilitation program that includes early ROM and weight bearing exercises, as well as lower extremity strength and conditioning exercises (1). Paired with protective bracing techniques, specialized treatments, and a structured home exercise program (HEP), the goal of returning to normal function will generally be reached.

SAMPLE CASE

A 16-year-old female, who is status post right knee ACL sprain 6 days ago presents. She has no significant past medical history/past surgical history and only takes ibuprofen 800 mg as needed. She is a starting midfielder on her high school soccer team, as well as her club soccer team. Her review of systems is unremarkable and she denies any prior injury to the right knee. X-rays are negative for any fracture/avulsion. Her examination is significant for a slight antalgic gait, moderate suprapatellar effusion, and no ecchymosis. She is tender to palpation at the anterior aspect of the knee and medial/lateral joint lines. She has a positive Lachman's and anterior drawer test, in her case indicating mild laxity of the ACL, however there is a firm endpoint. The remainder of the examination revealed quadricep weakness (4/5 manual muscle test) and slight extensor lag (-10°). Neurovascular examination was unremarkable.

 SAMPLE THERAPY PRESCRIPTION

Discipline: Physical therapy.

Diagnosis: Right knee grade II ACL sprain, antalgic gait, decreased quadriceps/vastus medialis oblique (VMO) strength and decreased knee extension.

Precautions: No pivoting or rotational movements x 4 weeks.

Frequency of visits: 3 x week.

Duration of treatment: 4 weeks; duration of at least 12 to 15 visits at therapist's discretion.

Treatment:

1. *Modalities:* Cryotherapy (ice bath/pack/massage) 3 to 4x/day and after activity; Game Ready® will be used after every therapy session; E-stim (TENS) treatment if needed for pain control: Premod/HiVolt/Russian for pain management and muscle stimulation/reeducation

2. *Manual therapy:* Patellar joint mobilization to restore flexibility; proprioceptive neuromuscular facilitation stretching techniques; massage therapy to increase vascularity and restore ROM/flexibility

3. *Therapeutic exercise:* active/active assisted/passive range of motion (A/AA/APROM) to restore knee flexion/extension, lower extremity stretching to promote flexibility to include hamstrings, gastrocnemius/soleus, quadriceps, hip flexors/extensors, and lower back stretches; open/closed kinetic chain exercises; strengthening/progressive resistive exercises (PREs) including core/abdominal strengthening, quad/hamstring strengthening (particularly VMO), ankle and calf strengthening, balancing/proprioception training, neuromuscular reeducation, aerobic fitness, plyometrics, and sport-specific training

4. *Specialized treatments:* sport-specific training for soccer movements; assess core stability and abdominal strength; assess Q-angle and biomechanical analysis of gait and jumping/landing techniques; bracing options for joint protection

5. *Patient education:* Pain/swelling management (cryotherapy techniques), HEP (open and closed kinetic chain movements), and ACL injury prevention program

Goals: Decrease pain and swelling; Restore full ROM and flexibility of lower extremities; restore strength to bilateral comparison; improve balance and proprioception; improve sport-specific activities (landing/jumping); safely return athlete to functional movements and activities and prevent future knee injury.

Reevaluation: 4 weeks by referring physician.

REFERENCES

1. Miyamoto RG, Bosco JA, Sherman OH. Treatment of medial collateral ligament injuries. *Journal of the American Academy of Orthopaedic Surgeons,* 2009;17:152–161.
2. Konin JG, Wiksten DL, Isear JA Jr, et al. *Special Tests for Orthopedic Examination*, 2nd ed. Thorofare, NJ: SLACK Incorporated; 2002: 219–290.
3. Eitzen I, Moksnes H, Snyder-Mackler L, Risberg MA. A progressive 5-week exercise therapy program leads to significant improvement in knee function early after anterior cruciate ligament injury. *J Orthop Sports Phys Ther.* 2010;40(11):705–721.
4. Kara B, Baskurt F, Acar S, et al. The effect of TENS on pain, function, depression, and analgesic consumption in the early postoperative period with spinal surgery patients. *Turk Neurosurg.* 2011;21(4):618–624.
5. Wright RW, Preston E, Fleming BC, et al. A systematic review of anterior cruciate ligament reconstruction rehabilitation. *The Journal of Knee Surgery,* 2008;21:225–234.
6. George JW, Tunstall AC, Tepe RE, Skaggs CD. The effects of active release technique on hamstring flexibility: a pilot study. *J Manipulative Physiol Ther.* 2006;29(3):224–227.
7. Bialoszewski D, Wozniak W, Zarek S. Clinical efficacy of kinesiology taping in reducing edema of the lower limbs in patients treated with Ilizarov method-preliminary report. *Ortopedia Traumatologia Rehabilitacja,* 2009;11(1):46–54.
8. Hammer WI. The effect of mechanical load on degenerated soft tissue. *Journal of Bodywork and Movement Therapies,* 2008;12:246–256.
9. Loghmani MT, Warden SJ. Instrument-assisted cross-fiber massage accelerates knee ligament healing. *Journal of Orthopaedic & Sports Physical Therapy,* 2009;39(7):506–514.
10. James SLJ, Ali K, Pocock C, et al. Ultrasound guided dry needling and autologous blood injection for patella tendinosis. *Br J Sports Med,* 2007;41:518–522.
11. Sadoghi P, von Keudell A, Vavken P. Effectiveness of anterior cruciate ligament injury prevention training programs. *J Bone Joint Surg Am.* 2012. [Epub ahead of print].
12. Ramsey DK, Wretenberg PF, Lamontagne M, et al. Electromyographic and biomechanic analysis of anterior cruciate ligament deficiency and functional knee bracing. *Clin Biochem.* 2003;18:28–34.
13. Bar-Ziv Y, Beer Y, Ran Y, et al. A treatment applying a biomechanical device to the feet of patients with knee osteoarthritis results in reduced pain and improved function: A prospective controlled study. *BMC Musculoskeletal Disorders.* 2010;11:179.

Meniscal Tears

Curtis W. Bazemore, Meredith B. Brazell, Stephanie L. Griggs, Gary A. Levengood, and Harris A. Patel

INTRODUCTION

The menisci are crescent shaped fibrocartilage structures that provide structural integrity to the knee. They have many functions for the knee which include load bearing, shock absorption, joint lubrication, joint stability, and providing proprioceptive feedback. While the knee is in extension, the meniscus is able to transmit up to 50% of the total load placed on the knee and about 90% of the load while the knee is in flexion. Only a small percentage of the menisci are vascular, and therefore tears located in the vascular region can respond well to surgical repair or heal with nonoperative management. The remainder of the menisci may not heal with conservative measures and may require surgical resection but depends on the severity and type of tear. Any degree of damage to the menisci can result in knee instability, loss of articular cartilage, and eventually lead to degenerative arthritis or further injury. Meniscal tears can be traumatic or degenerative depending on the mechanism of injury, age, and activity level of the patient (refer to Table 28.1). Catching and pain with twisting are among the most common complaints of meniscal pathologies (refer to Table 28.2).

Key elements of the physical examination include inspection, palpation, range of motion (ROM) assessment, strength testing neurovascular examination, and a detailed knee examination with cartilaginous special tests. Inspection may reveal atrophy of the muscle bulk of the leg, joint effusion suggestive of intra-articular pathology, and alignment abnormalities. Palpation may reveal medial or lateral joint line which has shown to be a very sensitive, but not specific diagnostic test for detecting meniscal tears, possibly more sensitive and specific for the detection of lateral than medial meniscal tears (2).The most common special test used during the physical examination is arguably the McMurray's test, which can be used to assess both the medial and lateral meniscus. Apley Grind test, bounce home test, and Thessaly's test are other special tests that can be performed to further assess for intra-articular pathology, specifically for meniscal pathology. Thessaly's test, performed in single leg stance in 20° of knee flexion has been shown to have the highest diagnostic accuracy rate (3).

TABLE 28.1: Features of Degenerative Versus Traumatic Meniscal Tears

	Population	General Complaints	Test Results
Degenerative Meniscal Tears	- Older population/elderly (50+)	- Pain with deep flexion and rotational activities	X-ray: normal; r/o arthritis that may present as meniscal pathology
	- usually have no recollection of injury or no particular mechanism	- Feel a pop or click in the knee with motion or normal ADLs	U/S: trained technicians can visualize a tear; joint effusion will be visualized
			MRI: will reveal size and location of tear
Traumatic Meniscal Tears	- Younger in age	- Pain with deep flexion and rotational activities	X-ray: normal; r/o arthritis that may present as meniscal pathology
	- usually sports related	- Feel a pop or click in the knee with motion or normal ADLs	U/S: trained technicians can visualize a tear; joint effusion will be visualized
	- patient can usually recall a specific twisting event		MRI: will reveal size and location of tear

TABLE 28.2: Features of Lateral Versus Medial Meniscal Tears

	Signs/Symptoms	Physical Exam	Test Results
MMT	- Pop felt in the knee with injury/activity - Gradual onset of swelling/stiffness (2–3 days) - Catching/locking of the knee - Knee buckles or gives way - Limit of motion	- Mild/moderate joint effusion - decreased ROM due to "locked" knee/pain + McMurray Medially + Medial Joint line pain + Apley's Compression Test	X-ray: normal; should r/o arthritis or other associated injury U/S: trained technicians can visualize a tear; joint effusion will be visualized MRI: will reveal size and location of tear
LMT	- Pop felt in the knee with injury/activity - Gradual onset of swelling/stiffness (2–3 days) - Catching/locking of the knee - Knee buckles or gives way - Limit of motion	- Mild/moderate joint effusion - decreased ROM due to "locked" knee/pain + McMurray laterally + Lateral Joint line pain + Apley's Compression Test	X-ray: normal; should r/o arthritis or other associated injury U/S: trained technicians can visualize a tear; joint effusion will be visualized MRI: will reveal size and location of tear

Findings from the patient's history, physical examination, and diagnostic studies will allow the rehabilitation team (treating physician, physical therapist, athletic trainer) to determine an appropriate program for the individual's needs and goals for returning to preinjury function.

For further diagnostic workup, plain radiographs may be necessary to rule out fracture or dislocation in the setting of trauma. X-rays should also be taken to rule out degenerative joint disease (DJD), as the symptoms of DJD are similar to those of a meniscus tear. MRI has become the test of choice for confirming intra-articular pathology and to determine the type and location of meniscal tear, but diagnostic arthroscopy remains the gold standard for confirming the presence of meniscal tears.

THE REHABILITATION PROGRAM

As with other injuries, while progressing through the phases of rehabilitation, it is important to initiate the PRICE protocol as soon as possible after an acute injury. Protection of the injured limb is essential for prevention of further injury and can be obtained with appropriate bracing and offloading the joint during ambulation with an appropriate assistive device if warranted. Strengthening and mobility should be initiated early to prevent muscular atrophy, joint stiffness, or even joint contracture.

Therapeutic Modalities

In the early stage of treating meniscal injuries, swelling and pain need to be controlled first by the PRICE protocol. The

MENISCAL TEARS

▦ The menisci are crescent shaped fibrocartilage structures that provide shock absorption, joint lubrication, joint stability, and proprioceptive feedback to the knee

▦ Meniscal tears can be traumatic or degenerative depending on the mechanism of injury, age, and activity level of the patient

▦ Catching and pain with twisting are among the most common complaints of meniscal pathologies

▦ Key physical examination findings include palpation for joint line tenderness, assessment for effusion, ROM, and special tests (e.g., McMurray, Thessaly)

▦ Plain radiographs, MRI, and diagnostic arthroscopy are tests commonly utilized in the setting of meniscal tears

use of electrical stimulation with an interferential current is helpful in pain management (although this treatment has not been validated with clinical research). Vasopneumatic devices, such as a Game Ready® or Aircast Cryo Cuff®), can be used to reduce inflammation and pain (4). Application of ketoprofen or dexamethasone solutions via iontophoresis may be effective in reducing both pain and swelling in acute injuries (5), but additional high quality research is required to confirm its role in the setting of acute knee injuries.

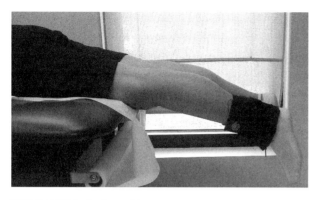

FIGURE 28.1: Prolonged hangs.

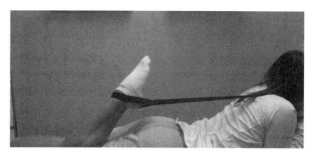

FIGURE 28.2: Assisted flexion.

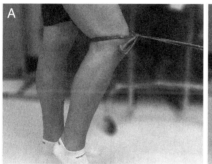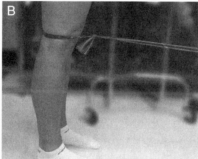

FIGURE 28.3: (A) Terminal knee extensions (TKE)—start. (B) TKE—finish.

Manual Therapy

Meniscal injuries can greatly benefit from deep tissue and soft tissue mobilization of surrounding structures. Joint effusions can lead to quadriceps inhibition leading to altered patella kinematics (6). In our experience mobilization of the patellofemoral joint maintains the biomechanics of the joint along with enhancing ROM. At the beginning of the rehabilitation session, anterior/ posterior and medial/lateral glides are performed for anywhere from 20 to 50 repetitions. If the knee has been immobilized for some period of time, patella mobilization can help maintain the integrity of the articular surfaces.

Therapeutic Exercise

While pain and swelling is being controlled, passive and active ROM exercises begin. In our opinion, if ROM is compromised, the patient should start a program of prolonged end-range stretching (Figures 28.1 and 28.2). If decreased ROM is not present, a basic program of muscle facilitation begins, including quad sets, terminal knee extensions (0–30 degrees) (Figure 28.3), straight leg raises, side leg raises, and hip lifts. Gradually progress the patient to standing, multidirectional weight shifts, marching in place, and single leg balancing (Figure 28.6). Patients can start an "unloaded" full squat using equipment like the Total Gym® or leg press, using light weight and high repetitions (40–50 lbs for 60–100 repetitions).

Closed chain exercises are proven to be safer and more effective than open chain exercises during knee rehabilitation (7), but most therapists would agree that a combination of open and closed chain exercises should be utilized for the best functional outcome. This progression, such as lateral dips, step ups (Figure 28.4), single leg partial squats, wall squats, or chair squats (Figure 28.5) and cross over steps begins as the patient shows increased control of their lower limb. Attempt

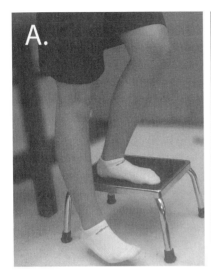
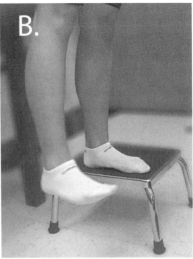

FIGURE 28.4: Lateral dips.

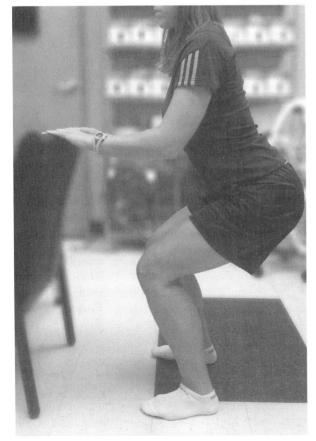

FIGURE 28.5: Chair squats.

to progress patients to more advanced functional drills, such as resisted marching, lunges, hurdle steps, and chop rotation drills. In the early phases, avoid rotational drills that put additional torque stress on the injured knee. Proprioception can be challenged with balance drills such as balance disc squats, BOSU® ball drills, etc (Figure 28.6). Depending on the age and activity level of the patient, they may be progressed to basic plyometric and functional drills including eight inch box jumps, depth jumps, and single hops, among others.

From the start, cardiovascular training should be initiated to maintain the endurance of the cardiopulmonary and muscular system. Stationary biking, elliptical running, treadmill fast walking, or even aquatic swimming or aquatic exercises can be started and progressed as tolerated.

As the patient returns to running, a thorough gait analysis should be performed to verify that they have not developed any poor or altered biomechanics. Functional testing can be performed, comparing things such as vertical leap (single and double leg jumping), long jump, 10 yard sprint, and 5-10-5 shuttle run to established normative data or more practically just to compare to the opposite, uninjured leg; many functional performance tests are still being researched to determine their validity for determining safe return to sport.

Specialized Techniques

Fibroblastic proliferation has been shown in smaller studies to be elicited along with the production of new

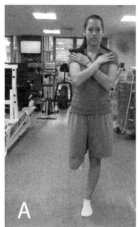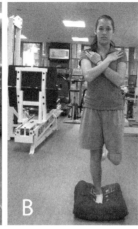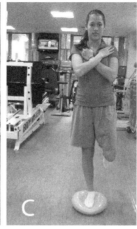

FIGURE 28.6: Balance progression.

collagen with cyclic mechanical stretching (8). Some of the techniques that can be used to obtain this type of stretching include massage therapy, Active Release Technique (ART®), and proprioceptive neuromuscular facilitation (PNF) stretching. (Refer to the prior chapter for more specialized techniques that also pertain to meniscal injury rehabilitation.) Massage therapy has a long history and has been shown to have positive effects on musculoskeletal or chronic pain (9). Patients who use massage therapy demonstrated a significant decrease in knee joint pain and stiffness and an increase in physical function (10).

However, while massage therapy may reduce pain and improve function, deep tissue massage has demonstrated to increase the local blood circulation to the joint (11). ART®, a type of deep tissue massage, improves joint flexibility (12) and the tone of musculature, reduces pain (13), and in our opinion improves function. Studies show, as compared to static, passive, or ballistic stretching, PNF has greater success in regaining compromised range of motion (11). Low impact weight bearing exercises such as aquatic therapy or the anti-gravity treadmill (AlterG®) are used to allow patients to begin walking or running.

Supportive Devices

Various knee braces can be utilized to protect the knee from further injury and to provide external support. Knee braces can be made from magnesium to fiberglass,

neoprene sleeves for proprioception and biofeedback (i.e., Bauerfeind®), or custom-fit functional knee braces. Functional knee bracing increases quadriceps activity by as much as 40% (14).

It has been shown that the use of orthotics is effective in keeping the knee in a neutral position, helping to prevent injury or further harm to the knee (15). Enhancing the biomechanics of the foot through appropriate footwear or orthotics improves neuromuscular control and unloading, decreases pain, and improves overall function in patients.

SUMMARY

Meniscal tears are the most common type of injury to the knee. Rehabilitation should include a gradual and systematic progression through the five phases of rehabilitation discussed throughout this book. Phase I to control pain and inflammation, then the following phases to restore ROM, strengthen, improve proprioception, and eventually advanced neuromuscular re-education exercises and progression to sport-specific activities. The use of protective braces or taping techniques for normal function, as well as a specialized rehabilitation program and HEP can prove important in not only protecting the injured meniscus, but also protecting further structural injury.

SAMPLE CASE

A 50-year-old male presents who developed left medial knee pain after playing soccer three days ago. He denies any trauma or feeling a pop in his knee while playing. He has no significant past medical history/past surgical history and takes Ibuprofen as needed. He is the coach and director of a club soccer association and is regularly active. His review of systems is unremarkable and he denies any previous injury to the left knee. X-rays are negative for fracture/avulsion, but reveal some mild degenerative changes. His examination shows a normal gait, mild anterior swelling and joint effusion, no ecchymosis or deformity. He has medial joint line tenderness, a positive McMurray's test medially, suggesting a tear in the medial meniscus; all other special tests normal. The remainder of the exam showed normal ROM, but mild decrease in quadriceps strength when compared to the contralateral leg. Neurovascular exam was unremarkable.

 SAMPLE THERAPY PRESCRIPTION

Discipline: Physical therapy.

Diagnosis: Right knee medial meniscus tear; decreased quadriceps strength.

Precautions: No shearing/torque movements or forces x 4 weeks.

Frequency of visits: 2 to 3 x week.

Duration of treatment: 4 weeks; duration of at least 8 to 10 visits at therapist's discretion.

Treatment:

1. *Modalities:* Cryotherapy (ice bath/pack/massage) 3 to 4x/day and after activity; Game Ready® will be used after every therapy session; E-stim (TENS®) treatment: Premod/HiVolt/Russian for pain management and muscle stimulation/reeducation

2. *Manual therapy:* Patellar joint mobilization to restore flexibility; PNF stretching techniques; massage therapy to assist in restoring ROM/flexibility

3. *Therapeutic exercise:* AROM to maintain knee flexion/extension, lower limb stretching to promote flexibility (self and therapist assisted) to include hamstrings, gastroc/soleus, quadriceps, hip flexors/extensors/abductors/adductors, and lower back stretches; open/closed kinetic chain exercises; strengthening/progressive resistive exercises (PREs) including core/abdominal strengthening, quad/hamstring strengthening, ankle and calf strengthening, balancing/proprioception training, aerobic fitness, and sport specific training

4. *Specialized treatments:* Kinetic chain analysis/sport-specific training for soccer movements; assess core stability and abdominal strength; biomechanical analysis of gait and jumping/landing techniques; bracing options for joint protection

5. *Patient education:* Pain/swelling management (cryotherapy techniques) and home exercise program (HEP) (closed kinetic chain movements)

Goals: Decrease pain and swelling; maintain full ROM and flexibility of the lower limbs; restore strength; improve balance and proprioception; improve sport-specific activities (landing/jumping); safely return patient to functional movements and activities and prevent future knee injury.

Re-evaluation: 4 weeks by referring physician.

REFERENCES

1. Browner BD, Levine AM, Jupiter JB, et al. *Skeletal Trauma: Basic Science, Management and Reconstruction*, 4th ed. Saunders Elsevier 2009:2167–2200.
2. Eren OT. The accuracy of joint line tenderness by physical examination in the diagnosis of meniscal tears. *Arthroscopy.* 2003;19(8):850–854.
3. Karachalios T, Zibis AH, Zachos V, Karantanas AH, Malizos KN. Diagnostic accuracy of a new clinical test (the Thessaly test) for early detection of meniscal tears. *J Bone Joint Surg Am.* 2005;87(5):955–962.

4. Michlovitz SL, Smith W, Watkins. Mice and high voltage pulsed stimulation in treatment of acute lateral ankle sprains. *Orthop Sports Phys Ther.* 1988;9(9):301–304.

5. Gurney B, Wascher D, Eaton L, et al. The effect of skin thickness and time in the absorption of dexamethasone in human tendons using iontophoresis. *Journal of Orthopaedic and Sports Physical Therapy.* 2008;38:238–245.

6. Hopkins JT. Knee joint effusion and cryotherapy alter lower chain kinetics and muscle activity. *J Athl Train.* 2006;41(2):177–184.

7. Wright RW, Preston E, Fleming BC, et al. A systematic review of anterior cruciate ligament reconstruction rehabilitation. *The Journal of Knee Surgery.* 2008;21:225–234.

8. Skutek, M. Cyclic mechanical stretching modulates secretion pattern of growth factors in human tendon fibroblasts. *European Journal of Applied Physiology.* 2011;86(1):48–52.

9. Perlman AI, Sabina A, Williams AL, et al. Massage therapy for osteoarthritis of the knee. A randomized controlledt. *Archives of Internal Medicine,* 2006;166:2533–2538.

10. Yip YB, Tam ACY. An experimental study on the effectiveness of massage with aromatic ginger and orange essential oil for moderate-to-severe knee pain among the elderly in Hong Kong. *Complementary Therapies in Medicine.* 2008;16:131–138.

11. Spenoga SG, Uhl TL, Arnold BL, et al. Duration of maintained hamstring flexibility after a one-time, modified Hold-Relax Stretching protocol. *Journal of Athletic Training.* 2001;36(1):44–48.

12. George JW, Tunstall AC, Tepe RE, Skaggs CD. The effects of active release technique on hamstring flexibility: a pilot study. *J Manipulative Physiol Ther.* 2006;29(3):224–227.

13. Robb A, Pajaczkowski J. Immediate effect on pain thresholds using active release technique on adductor strains: pilot study. *J Bodyw Mov Ther.* 2011;15(1):57–62.

14. Ramsey DK, Wretenberg PF, Lamontagne M, et al. Electromyographic and biomechanic analysis of anterior cruciate ligament deficiency and functional knee bracing. *Clinical Biomechanics,* 2003;18:28–34.

15. Bar-Ziv Y, Beer Y, Ran Y, et al. A treatment applying a biomechanical device to the feet of patients with knee osteoarthritis results in reduced pain and improved function: a prospective controlled study. *BMC Musculoskeletal Disorder,* 2010;11:179.

16. Konin JG, Wiksten DL, Isear JA Jr, et al. *Special Tests for Orthopedic Examination,* 2nd ed. Thorofare, NJ: SLACK Incorporated; 2002:283–285.

Iliotibial Band Friction Syndrome

Christine Roque-Dang and Peter P. Yonclas

INTRODUCTION

Iliotibial band friction syndrome (ITBFS) is a common cause of lateral knee pain, which has been associated with overuse injuries in endurance athletes (e.g., cyclists and military personnel) (1–6). In runners, ITBFS has been cited as the most common cause of lateral knee pain (4,7,8). Depending on the studied population, the incidence of ITBFS ranges from 1.6% to 52% (2,6,9–11).

The iliotibial band (ITB) originates at the ileum and the anterior superior iliac spine (ASIS). The ITB is formed proximally by the fascial confluence of the tensor fascia lata (TFL), gluteus maximus, and gluteus minimus muscles (1, 2, 12–15). The distal insertions of the ITB include the lateral border of the patella, the lateral retinaculum, and Gerdy's tubercle of the tibia (1,3,14). ITBFS is caused by repetitive and excessive friction at the distal ITB as it slides over the lateral femoral condyle with knee flexion and extension (16–19). Increased tension or friction at the ITB may result in inflammation and irritation. Several studies have reported that ITBFS occurs with approximately 30° of knee flexion (16,20) and an impingement zone mechanism (19) has been previously proposed. However, there is some controversy whether the ITB is a discrete structure versus a thickened zone of the TFL (4,21,22). If the latter anatomical theory is true, some authors argue that anterior-posterior glide at the ITB would be impossible and that ITBFS is actually a misnomer for this overuse condition (4,21,22). Of note, a true bursa has not been associated with ITBFS pathology (15,23).

Various etiologic factors have been suggested for the development of ITBFS. These factors include abnormal foot mechanics including excessive pronation (14,23–26), tight ITB (23,24,26), leg length discrepancies (25,26), genu varum (23–25,27), hill training (12,23–25,27), running on uneven surfaces, presence of a prominent lateral femoral condyle (23,24,26,27), hip abductor weakness (28–31), knee flexor and extensor weakness (14), excessive internal tibial rotation (1,29,30), training errors (14,19,32), mechanical ITB strain rate (29,30), and excessive mileage (14,15,23–25,27).

Primarily, ITBFS is clinically diagnosed with a thorough history and physical examination. Laboratory testing is typically not indicated and radiographic imaging is seldom warranted. Magnetic resonance imaging (MRI) may be helpful in detecting the extent of ITB inflammation (2,33–35). Oftentimes, the patient will complain of intermittently recurring or persistent lateral knee pain, which may radiate to the lateral thigh (12,23,27). Symptoms are usually exacerbated with rigorous physical activities that involve repetitive knee flexion and extension (e.g., running, stair negotiation). However, patients may be symptomatic at rest.

Key elements of the physical examination include inspection, palpation, range of motion (ROM), neuromuscular examination, a detailed knee, hip, foot, and ankle examination, provocative testing maneuvers (i.e., Noble compression test, Ober's test, etc.) and lower limb flexibility testing, and gait analysis. Results of the knee examination may be unremarkable except for localized tenderness at the distal ITB, which is usually located 2 to 3 cm proximal to the lateral knee joint line (3,17). The Noble compression (23) and creak tests (12) are provocative testing maneuvers for ITBFS. A positive test will elicit pain at the distal ITB with approximately 30° of knee flexion (12,23). Ober's test can also be performed to determine whether the patient has ITB tightness. Ober's test is considered positive if the thigh remains suspended despite placing the ITB in a shortened position (36). A Trendelenburg sign may be useful in detecting gluteus medius weakness. The sign is positive if the contralateral pelvis drops during single leg stance (36). Special attention should be placed on differentiating ITBFS pain from intra-articular knee pathology. Differential diagnoses include fracture, osteoarthritis, meniscal pathologies, ligamentous injuries, tendonitis, patellofemoral syndrome, and tumor. If there is a high clinical suspicion for ITBFS and other differential diagnoses, such as fractures, tumor, or intra-articular knee pathology, are excluded, a comprehensive rehabilitation program may be planned.

THE REHABILITATION PROGRAM

Now that a clinical diagnosis has been established, the rehabilitation program may be individualized to the patient and gradually advanced through the phases of rehabilitation (Table 29.1). Therapeutic modalities,

ILIOTIBIAL BAND FRICTION SYNDROME

- ITBFS is a common cause of lateral knee pain and is associated with overuse injuries in active individuals and endurance athletes (e.g., runners, cyclists, skiers)

- ITBFS is the most common cause of lateral knee pain in runners

- The mechanism of injury usually involves repeated friction and microtrauma to the distal ITB as it slides over the lateral femoral condyle with knee flexion and extension

- The diagnosis of ITBFS is often achieved clinically

- Key elements of the physical examination include inspection, palpation, a detailed knee, hip, foot, and ankle examination, provocative testing maneuvers for ITBFS and lower limb flexibility testing, neurological examination, and gait testing

- If there is a high clinical suspicion for ITBFS and other differential diagnoses are excluded, a comprehensive rehabilitation program may be planned

TABLE 29.1: Phases of Rehabilitation

Phase I: Decrease pain and swelling, includes PRICE protocol

Phase II: Restore ROM

Phase III: Strength training

Phase IV: Proprioceptive/balance training

Phase V: Functional/sport specific training

rest, and activity modification are very helpful during phase I. Stretching exercises help to restore ROM and flexibility, but without adequate hip and knee strengthening and correction of faulty movement patterns, the ITB will remain tight and painful. These topics will be discussed in further detail in the remainder of this chapter.

Therapeutic Modalities

The immediate treatment goal is to reduce local inflammation at the ITB. For acute treatment of ITBFS, the early application of ice to the distal ITB is highly recommended. Ice can be applied for 15 to 20 minute intervals and repeated at an hourly frequency for up to 72 hours. An alternative form of cryotherapy is an ice massage applied to the distal ITB (refer to Chapter 3 on Therapeutic Modalities for further details). In conjunction with oral nonsteroidal anti-inflammatory drugs (NSAIDs) and activity modification, the application of ice has been found to be very effective treatment for acute ITBFS (7,16,17). In the acute rehabilitative process, ionophoresis with corticosteroids may be considered, but it is unclear whether this treatment hastens recovery (4,6).

In the restorative rehabilitation phases, modalities should be used to maximize the benefit of each physical therapy session. Prior to each session, moist heat may be applied to the ITB and other affected areas for 5 to 10 minutes. Moist heat application increases blood flow to the area and prepares the tissues for stretching. Similarly, prior to stretching or manual therapy, therapeutic ultrasound at 1.5 to 2 cm² may be employed to the ITB for 5 to 7 minutes though literature on effectiveness of ultrasound is limited. If ultrasound is utilized, therapist assisted stretching should immediately follow the ultrasound application to take advantage of this therapeutic window of improved soft tissue elasticity. After each physical therapy session, ice may be applied to the area for 10 to 15 minutes to decrease inflammation and post exercise soreness.

Manual Therapy

The role of manual therapy in ITBFS remains controversial and there is limited published data on the efficacy of these treatments. However, with resolution of the acute inflammatory phase, manual therapies to restricted muscle groups and the adjacent soft tissues may be considered. Elimination of restrictions may complement physiotherapy and prepare the patient for the strengthening and endurance training phase (3,37). Previously, myofascial release (3,28), strain-counterstrain (38), soft tissue mobilization (37,39), and effleurage massage (39) techniques have been described as potentially beneficial treatments. Consistent clinical benefit has not been found with the use of deep transverse friction massage (DTFM), which is a massage technique that is utilized in subacute and chronic inflammatory conditions (10,16).

Therapeutic Exercise

Usually, the acute inflammatory phase is successfully treated with a combination of activity modification, oral nonsteroidal anti-inflammatory drug (NSAID) use, and adherence to the protection, rest, ice, compression, and elevation (PRICE) protocol. The restorative phases of rehabilitation are essential to regain ROM, strength, flexibility, and to facilitate the safe return to athletic activities. The long-term benefits of a supervised exercise program include prevention of chronic pain and recurrent ITBFS.

Once the acute inflammation resolves, ROM restoration and stretching exercises should be initiated. ROM restoration should include passive range of motion (PROM), active range of motion (AROM), and active assisted range of motion (AAROM) exercises. Self and assisted ITB and TFL stretching exercises are essential to the physiotherapy program. In particular, the literature supports the incorporation of an overhead arm extension to ITB stretches to achieve the increased ITB flexibility (Figure 29.1) (3,7,37,40). Additionally, the quadriceps, hamstrings, gastrocnemius, and soleus muscle groups should be stretched (3,40).

Several studies have demonstrated an association between weak hip abductors with the development of ITBFS (28–31) and the performance of hip abductor

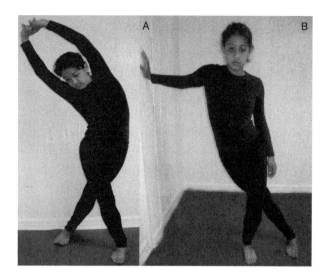

FIGURE 29.1: Iliotibial band stretches.

strengthening exercises to yield symptomatic improvement (3,13,28). Hamstring and quadriceps weakness has been associated with the development of ITBFS (13,14,19,28). Hence, strengthening of the hip abductors and extensors and knee flexors along with the extensors is central to the rehabilitative process.

Once flexibility and ROM are restored, strength and endurance training may commence. Strengthening exercises should begin with open kinetic chain exercises such as side lying leg lifts for hip abductor strengthening (37) (Figure 29.2) and prone leg extensions for hip extensor strengthening (39) (Figure 29.3). With tolerance and mastery of the open kinetic chain exercises, the patient may progress to closed kinetic chain exercises such as pelvic drops and frontal plane lunges for hip abductor strengthening (37) (Figures 29.4 and 29.6A) and wall slides for hip extensors and abductors strengthening (39) (Figure 29.5). In this phase, resistive ROM exercises may be performed with the use of light dumbbells, levers, cables, or resistive exercise bands/ tubing to gradually increase strength. Resisted ROM hip abduction exercises in the standing, seated, and side lying positions should be completed. Short-arc quadriceps extensions, hamstring curls, and prone straight leg raises may be done to strengthen the hip extensors, and knee flexors and extensors (39). Strengthening should commence in the single plane with advancement to exercises focusing on multiplanar strengthening, integrated movement patterns, and eccentric muscle contractions (37). As previously described by Fredericson

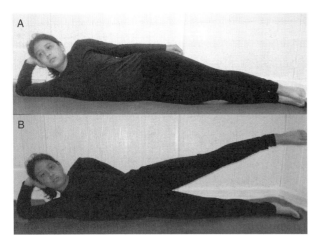

FIGURE 29.2: Side lying leg lifts.

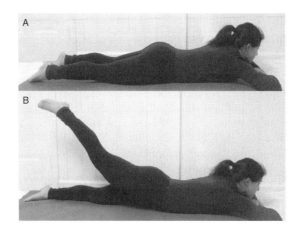

FIGURE 29.3: Prone leg lifts.

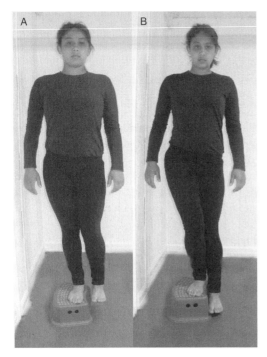

FIGURE 29.4: Pelvic drops.

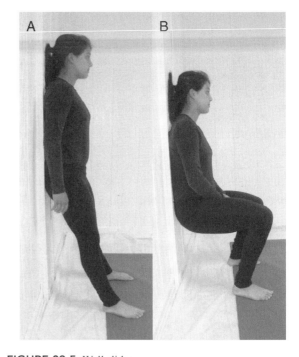

FIGURE 29.5: Wall slides.

et al these neuromuscular education exercises include frontal lunges with medial and lateral reaches (Figures 29.6B, 29.6C), wall bangers, and the modified matrix (3). To further challenge pelvic stability and once the patient is ready for proprioceptive/balance training, single leg balance exercises may be performed on variable surfaces (e.g., flat elevated surface, slant board, wobble board) (39).

Initially, the patient should aim to correctly perform 5 to 8 repetitions of each exercise. As the patient masters the assigned exercises, the goal may be increased to 2 to 3 sets of 15 repetitions. To ensure muscular strengthening, it is strongly recommended that the exercises be completed in the bilateral lower limbs (3).

To maintain or enhance muscular endurance and prevent deconditioning, aerobic exercises need to be incorporated into the program. In the early rehabilitative phases, activities that require repeated knee flexion and extension (e.g., running and cycling) or the activities that reproduce the patient's pain should be avoided. In the initial rehabilitative course, swimming exercises would be ideal (3,13). However, substituted activities such as walking on level surfaces or on

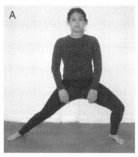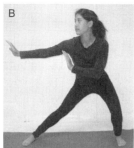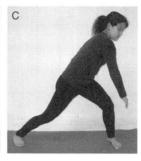

FIGURE 29.6: Lunges.

a treadmill, utilizing elliptical machines with a neutral incline and high seated stationary bicycling are all considered low impact aerobic activities and may be tolerated well.

In preparation for functional and sport-specific training, gait and, likely, running analyses should be completed. Addressing underlying biomechanical dysfunctions and training errors is an absolutely critical aspect of the rehabilitation process (7). If left uncorrected, biomechanical dysfunctions and training errors can lead to recurrent overuse injuries and muscular imbalances.

After the patient is able to properly perform all of the strengthening exercises without pain, he or she may gradually return to sport-specific activities (3,13,37). The return to athletic activities is dependent on multiple factors including the injury severity, compliance with the rehabilitation program and home exercise program (HEP), premorbid functional status, and, if applicable, the patient's co-morbid medical conditions. Initially, patients should participate in these activities at a reduced intensity, pace, frequency, and, if applicable, distance (3,37). For instance, for the first week of return to running, runners may complete short and relatively easy sprints on even surfaces every other day. Biomechanical studies have demonstrated that, due to the knee being flexed beyond 30° at foot strike, fast paced running is less likely to exacerbate ITBFS (19,37). As another example, military personnel may be given training activity restrictions for allowable carried gear weight and distance for running exercises. As tolerated, intensity, pace, frequency, and distance (if applicable) of activities may be gradually increased.

Specialized Techniques and Supportive Devices

For the athlete or active individual, footwear and/or equipment evaluation is certainly warranted. In patients with excessive foot pronation, orthotics and/or corrective footwear may be useful. For patients with worn footwear from issues such as excessive mileage, a new pair of sneakers may be necessary. For cyclists, a change in seat height, cycling position, or pedal/cleat system should be considered (17). In a reported case, neuromuscular electrical stimulation (NMES) as part of a neuromuscular education protocol was successfully utilized in the treatment of ITBFS (39). This approach could be used to train an inhibited and poorly functioning gluteus medius to restore muscular balance between the TFL and gluteus medius.

Home Exercise Program

Patients should perform the HEP starting on the first day of rehabilitation. The early HEP should consists of activity modification, adherence to the PRICE protocol, and performance of PROM and AROM exercises such as ITB stretches. Once flexibility and ROM are restored, open kinetic chain exercises such as side lying leg lifts and, eventually, resisted ROM exercises may be added to the HEP.

As the patient progresses to closed chain kinetic exercises, that is, pelvic drops, these exercises may be incorporated into the HEP. After mastering closed chain kinetic exercises, multidimensional and integrated movement pattern exercises should be added. Also, neuromuscular reeducation, balance, and proprioceptive exercises, including single stance leg activities on varied surfaces, may be employed. Patients should be encouraged to incorporate these activities into a daily routine or while engaging in leisure activities, such as performing wall slides or side-lying leg lifts while watching television.

Return to sports-specific activities should be guided by a physician, therapist, and/or athletic trainer and the patient should be strongly urged to comply with the gradual and steady guidelines set for return to these activities. If an acute exacerbation occurs, the patient should be advised to follow the PRICE protocol, modify his or her activities, and alert the physician, therapist, and/or athletic trainer. To prevent injury recurrence, the patient should continue to perform the HEP after the rehabilitative course has been completed.

SUMMARY

Especially in active populations, ITBFS is a commonly encountered cause of lateral knee pain (1–4,7–11). Participation in a supervised rehabilitation program has been shown to be pivotal in successful conservative treatment and injury prevention (3,16,28,37,39,40). The rehabilitative program should encompass early inflammation and pain control, behavior modification, ROM restoration, stretching, strengthening, endurance training, and gradual return to functional and sport-specific activities.

SAMPLE CASE

A 39-year-old female marathon runner presents to your office with right lateral knee pain, which is described as burning, sharp, intermittent, and is noticeable after her normal running routine. She states that she runs on an asphalt-paved road. When questioned further, she reports that she runs at the edge of the road, which is a banked and uneven surface. She has no significant past medical history/past surgical history (PMH/PSH). Knee x-rays, which were ordered by her primary care physician (PCP) were negative for fracture and other bony pathology. Her examination is significant for tenderness to palpation (TTP) 2 cm proximal to the right lateral femoral condyle, positive right Noble compression test, positive right Ober's test, and a slightly positive right Trendelenburg's sign. The remainder of the knee, hip, foot, and ankle exams were unremarkable. Neurovascular examination was unremarkable. Gait was normal.

 SAMPLE THERAPY PRESCRIPTION

Discipline: Physical therapy.

Diagnosis: ITBFS.

Problem list: Weak right hip abductors.

Precautions: Weight bearing as tolerated (WBAT), avoid excessive knee flexion, avoid running, inclined aerobic exercises, and low-seated cycling exercises.

Frequency of visits: 2 to 3x/week.

Duration of treatment: 8 to 12 sessions.

Treatment:

1. *Modalities:* moist heat to affected areas for 5 to 10 minutes prior to session, cryotherapy (ice pack or ice massage) to affected areas for 10 to 15 minutes following the session

2. *Manual therapy:* myofascial release and soft tissue mobilization techniques to the right ITB/tensor fascia lata (TFL)

3. *Therapeutic exercise:* A/AA/PROM to restore hip abduction, flexion, and extension, stretching (self stretching, therapist assisted stretching) including ITB/TFL, glutes, quadriceps, hamstrings, and ankle plantar flexor stretching. Strengthening/progressive resistive exercise (PRE) for the gluteal muscles (especially gluteus medius), quadriceps, and hamstrings, neuromuscular education (especially for the gluteus medius), aerobic and conditioning exercises

4. *Specialized treatments:* biomechanical analysis of gait, running, and the kinetic chain

5. *Patient education:* HEP.

Goals: Decrease pain and inflammation; restore knee and hip ROM, improve lower limb flexibility, restore strength, safely return to functional activities (e.g., sport, hobbies, work), and prevent recurrent ITBFS.

Reevaluation: In 4 weeks by referring physician.

REFERENCES

1. Powers CM, The influence of abnormal hip mechanics on knee injury: a biomechanical perspective. *J Orthop Sports Phys Ther.* 2010;40(2):42–51.
2. Kirk KL, Kuklo T, Klemme W. Iliotibial band friction syndrome. *Orthopedics.* 2000;23(11):1209–1214; discussion 1214–1215; quiz 1216–1217.
3. Fredericson M, Wolf, C. Iliotibial band syndrome in runners: innovations in treatment. *Sports Med.* 2005;35(5):451–459.
4. Lavine R. Iliotibial band friction syndrome. *Curr Rev Musculoskelet Med.* 2010;3(1–4):18–22.
5. Falvey EC, Clark RA, Franklyn-Miller A, Bryant AL, Briggs C, McCrory, PR. Iliotibial band syndrome: an examination of

the evidence behind a number of treatment options. *Scand J Med Sci Sports.* 2010;20(4):580–587.

6. Ellis R, Hing W, Reid D. Iliotibial band friction syndrome—a systematic review. *Man Ther.* 2007;12(3):200–208.

7. Paluska SA. An overview of hip injuries in running. *Sports Med.* 2005;35(11):991–1014.

8. Taunton JE, Ryan MB, Clement DB, McKenzie DC, Lloyd-Smith DR, Zumbo BD. A retrospective case-control analysis of 2002 running injuries. *Br J Sports Med.* 2002;36(2):95–101.

9. Pinshaw R, Atlas V, Noakes TD. The nature and response to therapy of 196 consecutive injuries seen at a runners' clinic. *S Afr Med J.* 1984;65(8):291–298.

10. Brosseau L, Casimiro L, Milne S, et al. Deep transverse friction massage for treating tendinitis. *Cochrane Database Syst Rev.* 2002(4):CD003528.

11. Jordaan G, Schwellnus, MP. The incidence of overuse injuries in military recruits during basic military training. *Mil Med.* 1994;159(6):421–426.

12. Renne JW. The iliotibial band friction syndrome. *J Bone Joint Surg Am.* 1975;57(8):1110–1111.

13. Khaund R, Flynn SH. Iliotibial band syndrome: a common source of knee pain. *Am Fam Physician.* 2005;71(8):1545–1550.

14. Messier SP, Edwards DG, Martin DF, et al. Etiology of iliotibial band friction syndrome in distance runners. *Med Sci Sports Exerc.* 1995;27(7):951–960.

15. Orava S. Iliotibial tract friction syndrome in athletes—an uncommon exertion syndrome on the lateral side of the knee. *Br J Sports Med.* 1978;12(2):69–73.

16. Schwellnus MP, Theunissen L, Noakes TD, Reinach SG. Anti-inflammatory and combined anti-inflammatory/analgesic medication in the early management of iliotibial band friction syndrome. A clinical trial. *S Afr Med J,* 1991;79(10):602–606.

17. Cosca DD, Navazio F. Common problems in endurance athletes. *Am Fam Physician.* 2007;76(2):237–244.

18. Evans P. The postural function of the iliotibial tract. *Ann R Coll Surg Engl.* 1979;61(4):271–280.

19. Orchard JW, Fricker PA, Abud AT, Mason BR. Biomechanics of iliotibial band friction syndrome in runners. *Am J Sports Med.* 1996;24(3):375–379.

20. Noble CA. The treatment of iliotibial band friction syndrome. *Br J Sports Med.* 1979;13(2):51–54.

21. Fairclough J, Hayashi K, Toumi H, et al. The functional anatomy of the iliotibial band during flexion and extension of the knee: implications for understanding iliotibial band syndrome. *J Anat.* 2006;208(3):309–316.

22. Fairclough J, Hayashi K, Toumi H, et al. Is iliotibial band syndrome really a friction syndrome? *J Sci Med Sport.* 2007;10(2):74–76; discussion 77–78.

23. Noble CA. Iliotibial band friction syndrome in runners. *Am J Sports Med.* 1980;8(4):232–234.

24. Jones DC, James SL. Overuse injuries of the lower extremity: shin splints, iliotibial band friction syndrome, and exertional compartment syndromes. *Clin Sports Med.* 1987;6(2):273–290.

25. Holmes JC, Pruitt AL, Whalen NJ. Iliotibial band syndrome in cyclists. *Am J Sports Med.* 1993;21(3):419–424.

26. Krivickas LS, Anatomical factors associated with overuse sports injuries. *Sports Med.* 1997;24(2):132–146.

27. Sutker AN, Barber FA, Jackson DW, Pagliano JW. Iliotibial band syndrome in distance runners. *Sports Med.* 1985;2(6):447–451.

28. Fredericson M, Cookingham CL, Chaudhari AM, Dowdell BC, Oestreicher N, Sahrmann, SA. Hip abductor weakness in distance runners with iliotibial band syndrome. *Clin J Sport Med.* 2000;10(3):169–175.

29. Ferber R, Noehren B, Hamill J, Davis IS. Competitive female runners with a history of iliotibial band syndrome demonstrate atypical hip and knee kinematics. *J Orthop Sports Phys Ther.* 2010;40(2):52–58.

30. Noehren B, Davis I, Hamill J. ASB clinical biomechanics award winner 2006 prospective study of the biomechanical factors associated with iliotibial band syndrome. *Clin Biomech (Bristol, Avon).* 2007;22(9):951–956.

31. Hamill J, Miller R, Noehren B, Davis I. A prospective study of iliotibial band strain in runners. *Clin Biomech (Bristol, Avon).* 2008;23(8):1018–1025.

32. Messier SP, Pittala KA. Etiologic factors associated with selected running injuries. *Med Sci Sports Exerc.* 1988;20(5):501–505.

33. Nemeth WC, Sanders BL. The lateral synovial recess of the knee: anatomy and role in chronic Iliotibial band friction syndrome. *Arthroscopy.* 1996;12(5):574–580.

34. Ekman EF, Pope T, Martin DF, Curl WW. Magnetic resonance imaging of iliotibial band syndrome. *Am J Sports Med,* 1994;22(6):851–854.

35. Murphy BJ, Hechtman KS, Uribe JW, Selesnick H, Smith RL, Zlatkin MB. Iliotibial band friction syndrome: MR imaging findings. *Radiology.* 1992;185(2):569–571.

36. Magee D. Hip. In: *Orthopedic Physical Assessment.* 2008; Saunders: St. Louis, MO.

37. Fredericson M, Weir A. Practical management of iliotibial band friction syndrome in runners. *Clin J Sport Med.* 2006;16(3):261–268.

38. Pedowitz RN. Use of osteopathic manipulative treatment for iliotibial band friction syndrome. *J Am Osteopath Assoc,* 2005;105(12):563–567.

39. Pettitt R, Dolski A. Corrective neuromuscular approach to the treatment of iliotibial band friction syndrome: a case report. *J Athl Train.* 2000;35(1):96–99.

40. Fredericson M, White JJ, Macmahon JM, Andriacchi TP. Quantitative analysis of the relative effectiveness of 3 iliotibial band stretches. *Arch Phys Med Rehabil.* 2002;83(5):589–592.

41. Gunter P, Schwellnus MP. Local corticosteroid injection in iliotibial band friction syndrome in runners: a randomised controlled trial. *Br J Sports Med.* 2004;38(3):269–272; discussion 272.

42. Drogset JO, Rossvoll I, Grontvedt T. Surgical treatment of iliotibial band friction syndrome. A retrospective study of 45 patients. *Scand J Med Sci Sports.* 1999;9(5):296–298.

43. Hariri S, Savidge ET, Reinold MM, Zachazewski J, Gill TJ. Treatment of recalcitrant iliotibial band friction syndrome with open iliotibial band bursectomy: indications, technique, and clinical outcomes. *Am J Sports Med.* 2009;37(7):1417–1424.

Other Knee Disorders

Daniel C. Herman and James F. Wyss

BURSITIS

INTRODUCTION

Bursae are closed, fluid-filled sacs that serve as gliding surfaces to reduce friction between tissues of the body, such as where connective tissue and muscle rub against bone. Due to the very nature of their function involving repetitive friction, bursae can become chronically inflamed, thickened, and painful. Injury also commonly occurs via direct trauma, particularly at superficial locations without significant intervening tissue, such as the knee. Bursitis is an important condition to consider when developing a differential diagnosis, as it can mimic other conditions such as tendonitis, confusing, maybe it should be a new sentence and read "Also conisder osteoarthritis, rheumatologic conditions and infection in your differential diagnosis." The knee contains 12 or more bursae in total; however, the discussion in this chapter will be confined to those most commonly seen with clinical pathology: the prepatellar, infrapatellar, suprapatellar, and anserine bursae.

Prepatellar

Prepatellar bursitis is often encountered in sports that feature significant amounts of repetitive friction or trauma against external surfaces, such as in wrestling or football. It is also commonly found in occupational settings which require significant amounts of kneeling, such as with carpet and floor laying. Such occupations have been found to have prevalence ratios of up to 11.9 compared to non-kneeling work, and may be much higher when including asymptomatic cases (1). Systemic inflammatory diseases, connective tissue disorders, gout, chronic renal failure, diabetes mellitus, chronic obstructive pulmonary disease, and alcohol abuse may also be causative/contributive factors (2).

Patients will present with complaints of swelling over the patella with or without anterior knee pain. Eliciting an appropriate history will often yield a likely causative exposure as discussed previously. Physical examination findings include prepatellar fluid at the inferior pole of the patella with or without corresponding tenderness to palpation, and may demonstrate crepitus and knee flexion end range of motion (ROM) discomfort and limitation. More chronic cases may have less swelling with higher grade bursal thickening (as demonstrated on ultrasonography) (3). Cases stemming from a single acute traumatic shearing event or chronic cases with poor response to treatment may require ultrasound imaging or magnetic resonance imaging (MRI) to rule out a closed degloving injury (Morel-Lavalle lesion) which may occur in the area of the prepatellar bursa (4).

A septic process must be considered, and the presence or absence of fluctuance, warmth, erythema, and ascending lymphangitis or lymphadenopathy should be noted. The presence of systemic disease as noted above, prior history of bursitis, and occurrence during the summer months are also risk factors for septic prepatellar bursitis (2,5). Aspiration for obtaining a gram stain and culture should be considered in high-risk patients even in the absence of symptoms: 50% of patients in a case series of septic prepatellar bursitis in wrestlers were asymptomatic (6). Aspiration should be completed using a lateral approach to reduce the risk of sinus tract formation. Septic bursitis contains greater than 1000 white blood cells per microliter, with approximately 80% of cases caused by *Staphylococcus aureus* (5).

PREPATELLAR BURSITIS

- Commonly found in occupations (e.g., floor and carpet laying) and sports (e.g., wrestling and football) featuring repetitive external friction or trauma

- Systemic diseases, connective tissue disorders, and alcohol use may be risk factors

- Presentation may include swelling over the patella with or without pain, crepitus, and knee flexion end ROM limitation and discomfort

- Fluctuance, warmth, erythema, and ascending lymphangitis or lymphadenopathy should raise a concern for a septic process, but cannot be ruled out in asymptomatic cases

Infrapatellar

The infrapatellar bursae (superficial and deep) serve to protect the patellar tendon; correspondingly, pain and inflammation may occur in individuals in jumping sports and those with abnormal knee biomechanics. The superficial infrapatellar bursa is also often injured in occupational settings featuring significant amounts of kneeling causing direct repetitive trauma as with prepatellar bursitis discussed above. Although they are typically anatomically distinct, the superficial infrapatellar and prepatellar bursae is often referred to collectively as the prepatellar bursa.

Patients will present with complaints of swelling inferior to the patella in the area of the patellar tendon, with or without anterior knee pain. As with prepatellar bursitis, a likely causative exposure or other risk factor may be found with a thorough history. Physical examination findings include swelling and tenderness to palpation inferior to the patella and superficial to the tendon, or with thickening and tenderness medial, lateral, and posterior to the patellar tendon without swelling anterior to the patellar tendon in cases of isolated deep infrapatellar bursitis (7). Reduced ROM, firmness, and crepitus are often noted, particularly in chronic cases. Such cases may

demonstrate aggregated calcific masses on radiographs; however, it should be noted that synovial sarcomas and chondromas may have similar clinical presentations and appearance on radiographs, so such findings may warrant biopsy and further imaging (7,8). Considerations for septic bursitis are similar to those discussed previously for prepatellar bursitis.

INFRAPATELLAR BURSITIS

- The superficial bursa may be injured in environments similar to prepatellar bursitis, whereas the deep bursa can be injured in jumping athletes with abnormal knee biomechanics

- Presentation may include swelling and tenderness superficial to the patellar tendon if the superficial bursa is involved, or with thickening and tenderness medial, lateral, and posterior to the patellar tendon without anterior swelling if the deep bursa is involved

- Considerations for a septic process are similar as for prepatellar bursitis

Suprapatellar

The suprapatellar bursa is an extension of the synovium of the knee joint proximal to the trochlea. It primarily serves to reduce the friction of the quadriceps tendon. It lies deep to the tendon, and extends to approximately 4 cm proximal to the superior aspect of the patella. It is usually not anatomically distinct and communicates with the knee joint, and is sometimes referred to as the suprapatellar pouch. Bursitis is generally the result of direct trauma at the location of the bursa in high contact sports, and can also occur with rheumatologic diseases and as a result of internal derangement of the knee (9).

Patients will present similarly as previously described, with complaints of swelling in the location of the suprapatellar bursa, with or without anterior knee pain. Physical examination findings include swelling and tenderness to palpation superior to the patella and medial, lateral, and posterior to the quadriceps tendon without significant swelling anterior to the tendon. Pain and tenderness will often manifest in the distal quadriceps musculature as well. Pain will be exacerbated with resisted knee extension, and crepitus is often noted.

Chronic cases or cases with underlying rheumatologic etiology may have significant extensions proximally into the quadriceps musculature, as the synovium or existing suprapatellar plica may thicken and calcify producing a membrane between the bursae and joint proper, forming one-way valves similar to a Baker's cyst (10). Such cases may result in rupture at the apex of the bursa, with secondary inflammation, muscle breakdown, and granulation tissue formation. These cases may present in a fashion similar to a deep vein thrombosis, with thigh pain, swelling, warmth, and erythema (11). Chronic cases that are refractory to conservative therapy may warrant advanced imaging to rule out significant internal derangement. Chronic cases may also have a neoplastic etiology, most commonly secondary to benign entities such as lipoma arborescens and pigmented villonodular synovitis. These cases may present with a greater extent of ROM limitation and intermittent pain and swelling which may mimic the signs and symptoms of an internal derangement.

Considerations for septic bursitis are similar to those discussed previously for prepatellar and infrapatellar bursitis, with one major exception: a low threshold for consideration of joint aspiration, gram stain, and culture should be maintained as, unlike the prepatellar and infrapatellar bursae, the suprapatellar bursa communicates directly with the knee joint.

SUPRAPATELLAR BURSITIS

- Can be the result of direct local trauma in high contact sports, rheumatologic diseases, and internal derangement of the knee

- Presentation includes swelling superior to the patella and medial, lateral, and posterior to the quadriceps tendon with or without anterior knee and distal quadriceps pain that is exacerbated with resisted knee extension

- There should be a low threshold for consideration of a septic process as the suprapatellar bursa communicates with the knee joint

Anserine

The anserine bursa is located at the distal medial aspect of the knee, below the medial joint line and deep to the confluence of the semitendinosus, gracilis, and sartorius tendons, otherwise known as the pes anserine. The bursa serves to reduce the friction of these tendons when pulling along the tibia. Due to its biomechanical function, inflammation and pain may commonly develop in runners, athletes in sports with a high degree of lateral movement requirements, and individuals with a higher degree of frontal plane malalignment such as those with osteoarthritis (12). It is also relatively prevalent in individuals with diabetes mellitus, rheumatoid arthritis, or direct trauma. Although commonly referred to as anserine bursitis, debate exists regarding the exact pathology involved (bursitis, tendonitis, panniculitis, fasciitis, or some combination), and as such is often referred to as "pes anserine syndrome" rather than true bursitis. In spite of a general lack of epidemiologic data, this entity is generally regarded as the second most common knee bursitis behind prepatellar bursitis, and is commonly overlooked, particularly in older patients with osteoarthritis (13).

Patients will have variable presentations. Most commonly, patients present with classic symptoms of proximal tibial swelling and pain along proximal medial tibia in the area of the pes anserine; however, patients may also demonstrate pain that is located along the medial or even posteromedial joint line with an absence of swelling, thus mimicking a medial meniscus tear (14). Saphenous nerve entrapment due to the inflamed bursa has also been reported, further complicating the presentation with tibial pain and paresthesias which may mimic the symptoms of a tibial stress fracture (15). Despite these variations, patients will commonly report pain with ascending and/or descending stairs, when rising from a seat, and at night and in the morning (16). Imaging with ultrasound and MRI has not been demonstrated to be consistently useful in helping establish the diagnosis due the variability of the presence of swelling and the prevalence of asymptomatic cases, which further contributes to the debate regarding the true pathology involved (12). An injection of a local anesthetic may aid diagnosis (12). Although septic anserine bursitis is not commonly reported, the clinician should keep in mind that the anserine bursa does occasionally communicate with the knee joint, particularly in those with a prior history of surgery.

ANSERINE BURSITIS

- Commonly found in runners, athletes in sports with a high degree of lateral movement requirements, and individuals with a higher degree of frontal plane malalignment (e.g., osteoarthritic knees)

- Female gender and history of diabetes mellitus, obesity, and arthritis are also risk factors. It is commonly overlooked in those with knee arthritis

- Presentation is variable, with proximal tibial swelling and pain along proximal medial tibia in the area of the pes anserine considered as classic, with exacerbations with ascending and/or descending stairs, rising from a seat, and with night/early morning times of the day

- Septic anserine bursitis is uncommon, but the bursa may communicate with the joint, particularly in those with a surgical history at the symptomatic knee

TREATMENT AND REHABILITATION

Initial management of bursitis typically begins with use of prescription of nonsteroidal anti-inflammatory drugs (NSAIDs), oftentimes preceded by fluid aspiration for highly symptomatic cases and in cases where there is a suspicion for a septic process, particularly when involving the suprapatellar bursa. As with other inflammatory conditions, use of protection, rest, ice, compression, and elevation (PRICE) treatment is employed. Protection is a particularly important component with prepatellar and infrapatellar bursitis so as to minimize further environmental exposure to friction or repetitive trauma as recurrence is common. Addressing contributing co-morbidities should also be part of a comprehensive treatment plan. Diabetes, rheumatologic, and other systemic diseases should be optimally controlled. Obese patients should be placed on an appropriate nutrition and exercise-based weight-reduction plan, and screening for alcohol use should be considered.

Use of a local steroid injection is generally reserved for cases with a disabling level of pain after a septic etiology has been ruled out, although more dramatic effects have been generally reported for anserine bursitis and thus may warrant earlier consideration in these cases. Guidelines for treatment of septic bursitis have been previously detailed in the chapter Other Elbow Disorders, with antibiotic coverage targeted towards *S. aureus* until the causative organism can be confirmed. Surgical referral for bursectomy may be considered in those who have not responded to conservative treatment and have had bothersome symptoms for greater than a year, and after other conditions have been ruled out.

Therapeutic Modalities

In addition to PRICE treatment, there is some limited evidence that ultrasound therapy may be helpful in the treatment of anserine bursitis (17); however, no significant evidence exists regarding the use of other modalities such as electrical stimulation and iontophoresis. Home treatments with ice massage (refer to the Therapeutic Modalities chapter for further details) can be an important modality for symptom management of pes anserine bursitis, which is based on the authors' prior clinical experience.

Manual Therapy

As detailed in the chapter concerning olecranon bursitis, soft tissue mobilization and joint mobilization are useful for edema control and maintenance/restoration of ROM, with no compelling evidence favoring a particular technique.

Therapeutic Exercises

The efficacy of physical therapy is dependent on the type of bursitis found. Prepatellar and superficial infrapatellar are most often caused by repetitive trauma and friction, and thus warrant protection and environmental modification with physical therapy reserved for cases that include ROM deficits. However, deep infrapatellar, suprapatellar, and anserine bursitis often have biomechanical etiologies and may benefit from a course of physical therapy. Deep infrapatellar and suprapatellar bursitis are often associated with disorders of the knee extensor mechanism, whereas anserine bursitis is often associated with increased forces in the frontal and transverse planes applied through the muscles forming the pes anserine. The clinician should engage in a thorough assessment of the knee, test the stability and function of the entire kinetic chain, and make comparisons to the contralateral limb in order to elucidate the causative biomechanical deficits. To identify biomechanical deficits that need to be addressed, functional movements (e.g., gait, running, and ascending/descending a step) should be analyzed. Appropriate stretching and strengthening exercises may be found in the prior chapters regarding hamstring strains, knee osteoarthritis, patellar/quadriceps tendinopathy, and patellofemoral syndrome. These may be used in combination with knee bracing, taping, and shoe orthotics as appropriate to the deficit at hand. Therapy should advance to include exercises relevant to work-related activities and or sport-specific tasks.

SUMMARY OF BURSITIS

Knee bursitis is associated with acute or chronic external repetitive trauma and friction in occupational and sports settings, as well as with altered biomechanics. Vigilance for a septic etiology should be maintained in high-risk patients and those with suspected suprapatellar bursitis due to its communication with the knee joint. Initial conservative treatment is usually with PRICE therapy and NSAIDs, often with joint aspiration. External joint protection and activity modification are key treatments in cases with a traumatic etiology, whereas physical therapy is necessary in cases associated with biomechanical alterations. Corticosteroid injections and surgical referral may be necessary if the condition is disabling and/or refractory to conservative management.

PATELLAR INSTABILITY

INTRODUCTION

Patellar instability is a term ascribed to a clinical entity of poor patellar tracking and stability, often manifesting as the result of lateral patellar dislocation. An estimated 6 people in 100,000 in the general population suffer primary patellar dislocation, with incidence rates being disproportionately high during the second decade of life (18). Instability may result from a variety of causes that effect the conformation between the patella and the femur and the static and dynamic restraints that help maintain that conformation. Recurrent dislocations and subluxations are not uncommon, particularly in those possessing constellations of these risk factors; such patients face significant long-term sequelae including reduced functionality, low rates of return to participation in sporting activities, and increased risk of patellofemoral osteoarthritis (19,20). Given such outcomes, it is important for the clinician to be able to reliably diagnose the condition, identify the underlying etiologies, and provide appropriately directed treatment.

An understanding of the underlying pathology associated with the condition is a critical first step to this process. The stability of the relationship between the patella and the femur is governed by the complex interplay of anatomic form, soft tissue integrity, and neuromuscular function (21,22). Anatomic risk factors include those that impact lower extremity alignment and the shape of the femoral trochlea, such as patella alta, trochlear dysplasia, femoral anteversion, external tibial torsion, and genu valgum and recurvatum. These factors impact the degree to which the patella is able to engage the trochlea, particularly in extension where stability is most reliant on osseous interaction. Soft tissue abnormalities may also result in instability, and include a weakened or torn medial patellofemoral ligament, an excessively tight lateral retinaculum, and generalized connective tissue laxity. Finally, poor neuromuscular function both locally at the knee and throughout the lower quarter may also contribute. Muscular imbalance between the vastus lateralis and medialis may affect the positioning and relative distribution of force of the patella within the trochlea, and overall weakness of the quadriceps may increase instability via a reduction of the posteriorly directed force it provides to help keep the patella within the trochlea. Disruption of the normal patellofemoral dynamics may also be due to abnormalities at adjacent joints. Proximally, weakness in external femoral rotators such as the gluteus maximus may affect the orientation of the femoral trochlea relative to the patella, whereas distally tibialis posterior dysfunction may affect knee alignment via excessive levels of foot pronation.

Patients will present in various ways depending on the presence or absence of a history of traumatic events such as dislocations, and on the timeline since such events or the onset of symptoms. Those with a recent history of patellar dislocation will often describe a mechanism of injury involving direct contact or upon a sudden change of direction (such as during a cutting maneuver during sports activities). Patients will complain of significant retropatellar, medial, and lateral knee pain: retropatellar and lateral knee pain is commonly due to bone bruising from the patella contacting the more lateral aspects of the lateral condyle during the instance of dislocation, whereas medial knee pain is secondary to tearing of the medial connective tissue restraints. Other symptoms include knee swelling, weakness possibly accompanied by give-way events, and a sensation of instability during activities and toward knee extension and with often-minimal demands outside the sagittal plane. Symptoms may also present as atraumatic cases that feature slowly progressive anterior knee pain with a sensation of instability, with or without recurrent subluxations.

The physical examinationination will be notable for tenderness to palpation, effusion, reduced ROM, and pain and apprehension with strength testing. Pain may be more present in higher degrees of flexion where the extensor mechanism produces a posteriorly directed force thus compressing the contused posterior patellar surface against the femur, whereas apprehension is often prominent in positions of extension where connective tissue and osseous restraints are more important for stability. Other findings include increased patellar glide (of more than half the patellar width), increased tilt (greater than 20 degrees of elevation), a positive J-sign during patellar tracking, loss of quadriceps muscle bulk (particularly at the vastus medialis), and altered lower extremity biomechanics with malalignment and increased motion in the frontal and transverse planes (23). Crepitus during knee flexion and extension may signal the presence of an articular injury and degeneration, and is generally more commonly present in atraumatic cases.

Plain radiographs may be used in the assessment of patellar instability, and should include standard weight-bearing anterior-posterior and lateral views in extension and 45 degrees of flexion, as well as Merchant views (22). This latter view is with the knee flexed at 45 degrees over the end of the table and the beam oriented with an inclination of 30 degrees, and is used to assess for the degree of patellar tilt and subluxation, as well as trochlear dysplasia. In this view measurement can be taken of the tibial tuberosity to trochlear groove distance, where a distance greater than 20 mm is highly suggestive of the presence of instability. MRI can be useful to assess the degree of soft tissue injury and bone bruising, the presence of any cartilage damage, and the presence of osseous fragments associated with a torn medial patellofemoral ligament.

PATELLAR INSTABILITY

▪ Often the result of a primary patellar dislocation from direct contact or during cutting/twisting tasks, but may present without a history of trauma

▪ Risk factors for instability include anatomic alterations affecting patellofemoral congruity, poor integrity of the static soft tissue restraints, and disordered neuromuscular function of dynamic patellar restraints

▪ Presentation includes retropatellar, medial, and lateral knee pain, swelling, weakness, and instability, with the physical examinationination demonstrating signs of abnormal patellar tracking and altered lower extremity biomechanics

TREATMENT AND REHABILITATION

The treatment of patellar instability, particularly in the subacute phases of care after a primary patellar dislocation, has undergone significant evolution over the past several years. In light of the relatively high rates of recurrent dislocations and instability following injury, surgical stabilization of the injured medial patellofemoral ligament and/or release of the lateral retinaculum have commonly been employed. However, this has demonstrated inconsistent results in terms of stability, long-term functional improvements, or reduced risk of patellofemoral osteoarthritis (24–27). These and other procedures that seek to reestablish the integrity of static restraints and to improve patellofemoral joint anatomy still play a significant role in management of this condition, particularly in cases with osteochondral fragments accompanying medial patellofemoral ligament injury and those with significant levels of anatomic malalignment and/or dysplasia; however, in the absence of these exceptions the primary means of treatment is via conservative measures.

Initial management of patellar instability in the subacute phase after a traumatic event typically begins with PRICE treatment with particular emphasis on protection and compression. Often a short course (1–2 weeks) of immobilization in a long-legged splint is beneficial in conjunction with a compressive wrap (28); however, progression to mobilization and onward to rehabilitation is encouraged as soon as feasible to prevent weakness and atrophy of the musculature. Those cases which present with a history of chronic instability and subluxation usually do not require immobilization, but may benefit from rest and activity modification, icing, compression, and elevation along with regular oral analgesics in order to improve pain control and discomfort prior to the initiation of a rehabilitation program.

Therapeutic Modalities

Although there is some sporadic and limited evidence for the use of ultrasound therapy and iontophoresis in other causes of anterior knee pain, these modalities have limited value and little support for use in patellar instability. Electrical stimulation techniques are often used for patellar instability, particularly in the subacute phase in an attempt to overcome arthrogenic inhibition of the surrounding musculature. Although little evidence-based support for this exists specific to patellar instability, some support does exist for its use as well as that of cryotherapy in overcoming arthrogenic inhibition in related clinical entities such as after anterior cruciate ligament (ACL) reconstruction (29–31).

Manual Therapy

Joint mobilization may be useful for edema control and maintenance/restoration of ROM in the subacute phase, with some weak evidence supporting the use of soft tissue mobilization such as medial patellar gliding to stretch the lateral retinaculum and massage to stimulate the vastus medialis of the quadriceps during more intense therapy as a means of improving patellar stability and tracking (32).

Therapeutic Exercises

Physical therapy often centers on strengthening of the quadriceps musculature, with preferential targeting of the vastus medialis over the vastus lateralis to improve medial tracking and stability in the absence of competent medial static restraints. Stability of the adjacent segments and joints should also be evaluated and targeted for strengthening and neuromuscular education as necessary. This is particularly true of the hip and core to minimize excess transverse and frontal plane motion in order to provide appropriate stability and positioning of the femoral trochlea throughout engagement with the patella. Stretching exercises may also be of

use depending on the presence of any muscular imbalance, and may be particularly useful with the tensor fascia lata and iliotibial band complex, which possess connective tissue that incorporates into the lateral retinaculum. These may be used in combination with manual therapy, modalities, and orthotics as appropriate to the deficit at hand. Exercises in the initial phases after a primary dislocation should be limited with regards to knee flexion, as higher degrees of flexion increases the posteriorly directed compressive forces and thus may exacerbate pain. After initiation of therapy with open-chain and isometric exercises, therapy may advance to include higher degrees of knee flexion, closed kinetic chain exercises, and then finally exercises relevant to activities of daily living, the patient's occupation, and/or sport.

Orthotics

The efficacy of knee braces with patellar stabilization features remains somewhat controversial and lacks a robust

SUMMARY OF PATELLAR INSTABILITY

Patellar instability may present as the outcome of a traumatic lateral patellar dislocation or in patients with chronic symptoms without traumatic cause. Patellar stability is affected by biomechanical deficits that alter the relationship between the patella and femoral trochlea as a result of anatomic, soft tissue, and/or neuromuscular abnormalities. Initial conservative treatment is usually with PRICE therapy, with immobilization generally being reserved for the subacute period following traumatic dislocations. Therapy is centered on improving the dynamic restraints acting through the patella as well as the entire lower quarter dynamic stability. Rehabilitation may also include electrical stimulation and cryotherapy to improve joint activation, soft tissue mobilization to release oppositional structures and stimulate the surrounding musculature, and bracing and orthotics to improve mechanical stability and alignment. Consideration for surgical procedures should be reserved for cases with osteochondral fragments accompanying medial patellofemoral ligament injury and those with significant levels of anatomic malalignment and/or dysplasia, or cases refractory to nonoperative management.

evidence-based support (33,34). However, these are commonly employed in practice, with various levels of anecdotal success in improving stability, joint proprioception, and patient confidence. Taping may be of similar use, although this may be limited by the availability of skilled practitioners to provide repeated applications. Orthotics at adjacent joints may be considered based on the findings of a thorough lower quarter examination (e.g., use of arch supports in patients with excessive pes planus to improve frontal plane alignment).

REFERENCES

1. Jensen LK, Eenberg W. Occupation as a risk factor for knee disorders. *Scand J Work Environ Health*. 1996;22(3):165–1 75.
2. Aaron DL, Patel A, Kayiaros S, Calfee R. Four common types of bursitis: diagnosis and management. *J Am Acad Orthop Surg*. 2011;19(6):359–367.
3. Myllymaki T, Tikkakoski T, Typpö T, Kivimäki J, Suramo I. Carpet-layer's knee. An ultrasonographic study. *Acta Radiol*. 1993;34(5):496–499.
4. van Gennip S, van Bokhoven SC, van den Eede E. Pain at the knee: the Morel-Lavallee lesion, a case series. *Clin J Sport Med*. 2012;22(2):163–166.
5. Cea-Pereiro JC, Garcia-Meijide J, Mera-Varela A, Gomez-Reino JJ. A comparison between septic bursitis caused by *Staphylococcus aureus* and those caused by other organisms. *Clin Rheumatol*. 2001;20(1):10–14.
6. Mysnyk MC, Wroble RR, Foster DT, Albright JP. Prepatellar bursitis in wrestlers. *Am J Sports Med*. 1986;14(1):46–54.
7. McCarthy EM, Murphy CL, Doran MF, Cunnane G. Infrapatellar bursitis: an occupational legacy. *J Clin Rheumatol*. 2011;17(1):49–50.
8. Kamper L, Haage P. Images in clinical medicine. Infrapatellar (corrected) bursitis. *N Engl J Med*. 2008;359(22):2366.
9. Kolman BH, Daffner RH, Sciulli RL, Soehnlen MW. Correlation of joint fluid and internal derangement on knee MRI. *Skeletal Radiol*. 2004;33(2):91–95.
10. Schapira D, Nahir M. Suprapatellar pouch rupture or extension into the thigh tissue in rheumatoid disease. *Ann Rheum Dis*. 1986;45(9):791.
11. Dragoo JL, Abnousi F. Disorders of the suprapatellar pouch of the knee. *Knee*. 2008;15(5):348–354.
12. Helfenstein M, Jr. Kuromoto J. Anserine syndrome. *Rev Bras Reumatol*. 2010;50(3):313–327.
13. Handy JR. Anserine bursitis: a brief review. *South Med J*. 1997;90(4):376–377.
14. Rennie WJ, Saifuddin A. Pes anserine bursitis: incidence in symptomatic knees and clinical presentation. *Skeletal Radiol*. 2005;34(7):395–398.
15. Hemler DE, Ward WK, Karstetter KW, Bryant PM. Saphenous nerve entrapment caused by pes anserine bursitis stress fracture of the tibia. *Arch Phys Med Rehabil*. 1991;72(5):336–337.
16. Larsson LG, Baum J. The syndrome of anserina bursitis: an overlooked diagnosis. *Arthritis Rheum*. 1985;28(9):1062–1065.
17. Brookler MI, Mongan ES. Anserina bursitis. A treatable cause of knee pain in patients with degenerative arthritis. *Calif Med*. 1973;119(1):8–10.
18. Fithian DC, Paxton EW, Stone ML, et al. Epidemiology and natural history of acute patellar dislocation. *Am J Sports Med*. 2004;32(5):1114–1121.
19. Atkin DM, Fithian DC, Marangi KS, et al. Characteristics of patients with primary acute lateral patellar dislocation and their recovery within the first 6 months of injury. *Am J Sports Med*. 2000;28(4):472–479.
20. Smith TO, Song F, Donell ST, Hing CB. Operative versus non-operative management of patellar dislocation. A meta-analysis. *Knee Surg Sports Traumatol Arthrosc*. 2011;19(6):988–998.
21. Andrish J. The biomechanics of patellofemoral stability. *J Knee Surg*. 2004;17(1):35–39.
22. Colvin AC, West RV. Patellar instability. *J Bone Joint Surg Am*. 2008;90(12):2751–2762.
23. Smith TO, Davies L, O'Driscoll ML, Donell ST. An evaluation of the clinical tests and outcome measures used to assess patellar instability. *Knee*. 2008;15(4):255–262.
24. Sillanpaa PJ, attila VM, Mäenpää H, et al. Treatment with and without initial stabilizing surgery for primary traumatic patellar dislocation. A prospective randomized study. *J Bone Joint Surg Am*. 2009;91(2):263–273.
25. Palmu S, Kallio PE, Donell ST, Helenius I, Nietosvaara Y. Acute patellar dislocation in children and adolescents: a randomized clinical trial. *J Bone Joint Surg Am*. 2008;90(3):463–470.
26. Christiansen SE, Jakobsen BW, Lund B, Lind M. Isolated repair of the medial patellofemoral ligament in primary dislocation of the patella: a prospective randomized study. *Arthroscopy*. 2008;24(8):881–887.
27. Nakagawa K, Wada Y, Minamide M, Tsuchiya A, Moriya H. Deterioration of long-term clinical results after the Elmslie-Trillat procedure for dislocation of the patella. *J Bone Joint Surg Br*. 2002;84(6):861–864.
28. Maenpaa H, Lehto MU. Patellar dislocation. The long-term results of nonoperative management in 100 patients. *Am J Sports Med*. 1997;25(2):213–217.
29. Currier DP, Ray JM, Nyland J, et al. Effects of electrical and electromagnetic stimulation after anterior cruciate ligament reconstruction. *J Orthop Sports Phys Ther*. 1993;17(4):177–184.
30. Snyder-Mackler L, Delitto A, Stralka SW, Bailey SL. Use of electrical stimulation to enhance recovery of quadriceps femoris muscle force production in patients following anterior cruciate ligament reconstruction. *Phys Ther*. 1994;74(10):901–907.
31. van Grinsven S, van Cingel RE, Holla CJ, van Loon CJ. Evidence-based rehabilitation following anterior cruciate ligament reconstruction. *Knee Surg Sports Traumatol Arthrosc*. 2010;18(8):1128–1144.
32. Wu LS. Evaluation and manipulative therapy of patellar malalignment: a clinical review and preliminary report. *J Manipulative Physiol Ther*. 1991;14(7):428–435.
33. Shellock FG, Mink JH, Deutsch AL, et al. Effect of a patellar realignment brace on patellofemoral relationships: evaluation with kinematic MR imaging. *J Magn Reson Imaging*. 1994;4(4):590–594.
34. Muhle C, Brinkmann G, Skaf A, Heller M, Resnick D. Effect of a patellar realignment brace on patients with patellar subluxation and dislocation. Evaluation with kinematic magnetic resonance imaging. *Am J Sports Med*. 1999;27(3):350–353.

Lateral Ankle Sprains

James F. Wyss, Amrish D. Patel, Peter P. Yonclas, and Elizabeth Kennedy

INTRODUCTION

Lateral ankle sprains are one of the most commonly encountered musculoskeletal injuries and possibly the most common injury in sports. They can be traumatic or nontraumatic in nature. Nearly 50% of all ankle sprains in the United States occur during athletic activities, especially during basketball activities (1). The classic mechanism of injury involves excessive inversion on an already plantar flexed ankle. The anatomical structures most commonly involved include the anterior talofibular (ATFL), followed by calcaneofibular (CFL), and then posterior talofibular ligaments (PTFL) Figure 31.1. Grade I (mild) sprains typically involve overstretch or minor ATFL tears, grade II (moderate) sprains involve partial or complete ATFL tear with overstretch or minor CFL tears, and grade III (severe) sprains involve complete rupture of the ATFL and CFL with possible partial PTFL tears (2). After an ankle sprain, the individual will report the sudden onset of lateral ankle pain, swelling, and difficulty bearing weight on the involved lower limb after "rolling" their ankle while playing sports or walking on uneven terrain (e.g., sloped surface, curb, step, etc.). Initial management will always include a detailed history and physical examination.

Key elements of the physical examination include inspection, palpation, neurovascular examination, and a detailed ankle exam with ligamentous testing (e.g., talar tilt and anterior drawer test). Joints both proximal (e.g., knee) and distal (e.g., subtalar joint, midfoot) to the ankle require a quick screen to avoid missing concomitant pathology. The anterior drawer test primarily checks the ATFL (anterior displacement ≥ 5mm is considered positive). The talar tilt test primarily checks the CFL by applying an inversion stress to the ankle (a positive test is a >10° side to side difference).

Ankle and/or foot radiographs are commonly utilized to rule out fracture and the Ottawa ankle rules are commonly used to determine if an ankle and/or foot radiograph is warranted. In adults, ankle radiographs are indicated to rule out fracture if pain is present in the malleolar zones and tenderness is present at the distal malleoli or if there is an inability to bear weight. Foot radiographs are indicated if midfoot pain is present and if tenderness is present at the navicular bone or tuberosity of the fifth metatarsal or if there is an inability to bear weight (3). Once the diagnosis is confirmed and concomitant injuries (e.g., fracture, dislocation, high ankle sprain, or neurovascular injury) are ruled out, the grade of the injury must be determined (grade I–III) and then a comprehensive rehabilitation program is planned based on the severity of the injury.

THE REHABILITATION PROGRAM

A structured and supervised rehabilitation program is important for faster recovery and return to sports (4). Initial management follows the PRICE protocol with ankle

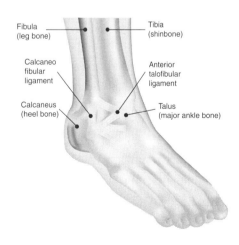

FIGURE 31.1: Ankle anatomy.

LATERAL ANKLE SPRAINS

▦ This injury has a very high prevalence and commonly occurs during athletic participation

▦ Mechanism of injury usually involves excessive inversion on an already plantar-flexed ankle

▦ Key elements of the physical examination: inspection, palpation, neurovascular, detailed foot & ankle exam with ligamentous testing

▦ The injury must be graded (I–III, mild–severe) to plan the rehabilitation program

▦ Ottawa ankle rules should be implemented when deciding if ankle and/or foot radiographs are necessary

TABLE 31.1: Phases of Rehabilitation

Phase I: Decrease pain and swelling (PRICE protocol)

Phase II: Restore ROM and normal arthrokinematics

Phase III: Strength training

Phase IV: Neuromuscular control and proprioceptive training

Phase V: Functional or sport-specific training

braces (e.g., aircast, lace up ankle braces) and/or assistive devices (e.g., cane or crutches) to protect the joint. Walking boots have also been utilized because they allow early but controlled mobilization to prevent some adverse effects of disuse. Ice applications, compressive garments, and elevation of the limb help reduce swelling. Although the PRICE protocol is important, progression through the remaining phases of rehabilitation (Table 31.1) shouldn't be excessively delayed since recent literature suggests that an early and accelerated rehabilitation program results in better short term outcomes for grades I–II lateral ankles sprains (5). The institution of an ankle injury prevention program before rehabilitation is complete is especially important with lateral ankle sprains since the rate of recurrence may be higher than 70% (6).

Therapeutic Modalities

The early application of ice, ice, and more ice is the best way to explain this section (7). Even grade I lateral ankle sprains tend to produce a great deal of swelling, therefore, immediate and continued applications of ice are very important. Ice can be applied for 20 minutes and repeated nearly hourly for the first 24 hours. Athletic trainers commonly utilize equipment that can provide compression and ice applications together, and this equipment is now available for home use (e.g., Game Ready®). The routine use of ice applications is considered standard of care;

however, the routine use of NSAIDs has been debated since animal studies have identified potential negative effects on ligament healing (8). Studies have assessed the application of electrical stimulation with ice versus ice applications alone, and there was no added benefit (9). Applications of hot packs or ultrasound are rarely necessary, unless swelling has resolved and range of motion (ROM) is still restricted. In these cases heat modalities can be applied and then active and passive stretching of a structure such as the Achilles tendon can be performed immediately after the application of heat.

Manual Therapy

The role of manual therapy for lateral ankle sprains is controversial. Some argue that transverse or deep friction massage facilitates healing and desired collagen fiber alignment but early and controlled P/AROM probably accomplishes the same goal (10). Joint mobilizations of the tibio-fibular joints, talocrural, or subtalar joint are occasionally performed. These techniques are helpful if ROM is restricted during rehabilitation phase II. Talocrural joint mobilizations have been shown to improve active ankle dorsiflexion and short term ankle function (11,12). Greene et al showed that the addition of a talocrural (anterior to posterior) mobilization, in addition to the PRICE protocol, after ankle inversion injuries lead to pain-free ankle dorsiflexion and improved stride speed in fewer treatments (11).

Therapeutic Exercise

Most patients experience a resolution of pain and swelling just by following the PRICE protocol. The following phases of rehabilitation are especially important for preventing chronic pain, disability, and recurrent injuries. Restoring ROM, strength, proprioception, and eventually progressing to functional, even sport-specific activities can be challenging. The patient needs an excellent physical therapist or athletic trainer to safely return them to their prior functional level and to prevent recurrent lateral ankle sprains.

Restoring ROM requires passive range of motion (PROM), active assistive range of motion (AAROM) and active range of motion (AROM) exercises. Valuable home exercises include ankle alphabets (Figure 31.2) and ankle circles. Flexibility exercises should include self and assisted stretching for the gastrocnemius and soleus. Isometric exercises should begin early in the rehabilitation program to prevent disuse atrophy. Resistive ROM exercises should begin once ROM and flexibility has been restored. These include the use of ankle weights or resistance bands to gradually increase strength (Figure 31.2). Strengthening begins in single planes and progresses to multiplanar exercises for functional strengthening. Ankle evertors and dorsiflexors are probably the most important muscle groups to strengthen. These are the muscle groups that can control or restrict inversion and plantarflexion moments that can cause recurrent lateral ankle sprains. Once full weight bearing is tolerated, exercises can progress from open chain to closed kinetic chain exercises and eventually progress to functional and/or sport-specific activities.

Exercises to improve neuromuscular control and proprioception should begin once ROM has been restored and strength has improved. They can begin in a seated position, with partial weight-bearing and progress to upright activities with full weight-bearing. Options include single leg stance exercises on variable surfaces with the eyes open or closed, and progressive wobble board training from seated AROM to single leg balance activities while performing functional activities (Figure 31.3). These exercises appear to be the key to restoring a preinjury level of function and for preventing recurrent ankle sprains (13–15).

In addition, gait and possibly running analysis should be completed and any identified biomechanical abnormalities should be addressed. Abnormalities in gait can lead to muscle imbalances and eventually to overuse injuries if ignored. Kinetic chain analysis should also occur with special attention being paid to the hips and trunk. Prior research has suggested altered proximal muscle function following severe unilateral ankle sprains (16). Therefore, key core muscles such as the gluteus maximus, gluteus medius, transverse abdominis, and quadratus lumborum should be analyzed and treated if dysfunction is present.

Aerobic exercises also need to be incorporated into the program. These exercises are necessary to prevent cardiopulmonary deconditioning and maintain muscular endurance; early on the use of a stationary bike can provide AROM for the ankle, knees, and hips. As tolerance to weight bearing improves, various cross trainers, ellipticals, treadmills, and steppers can be utilized to restore prior functional level.

Specialized Techniques

Hydrotherapy tubs can provide hydrostatic pressure in addition to cryotherapy to enhance the PRICE protocol, although its potential benefits have not been properly studied for lateral ankle sprains. Aquatic therapy, including aquatic treadmill use or performing sport specific activities in the pool have been utilized by professional basketball players to prevent the secondary effects of

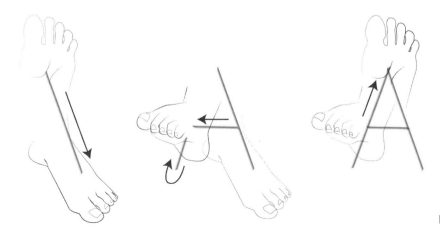

FIGURE 31.2: Ankle alphabets.

disuse. Kinesiology taping has become very popular and probably has indications for use in the recovery from lateral ankle sprains, but this technique remains unproven.

Supportive Devices

The use of tape or lace up ankle braces for athletic participation after initial ankle sprain is supported by the literature (15). A recent systematic review concluded that both tape and braces reduced the number of ankle sprains but neither type of ankle support was found to be superior to the other (17). Therefore, either option

is appropriate and can be based on patient preference and access to resources, such as a skilled athletic trainer who can properly tape the ankle before athletic participation.

Home Exercise Program

Home exercise programs (HEPs) begin on day one of rehabilitation and continue after the program is completed to prevent recurrent injuries. There is no substitute for good patient education and when done properly it promotes patient compliance with the program and positively influences outcomes.

The early HEP consists of following the PRICE protocol, PROM, and AROM exercises such as ankle alphabets (Figure 31.4). Eventually resistive exercises are incorporated to help restore strength. Once the patient is tolerating full weight bearing and has restored their ROM and strength, their balance should be challenged with single leg stance activities. These activities can be done when doing simple household chores such as washing dishes or brushing teeth. They begin in single leg stance with an extended knee and neutral ankle positioning and eventually progress to uneven surfaces (e.g., foam), performing them with eyes closed and incorporating knee flexion and ankle plantarflexion movements to further challenge balance and neuromuscular control.

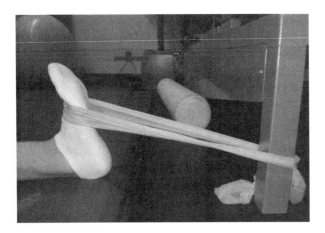

FIGURE 31.3: Ankle dorsiflexor strengthening with resistance band.

FIGURE 31.4: Proprioceptive exercises: single leg stance activities on progressively unstable surfaces from a to c.

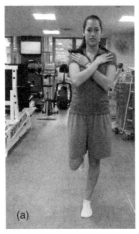 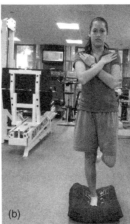 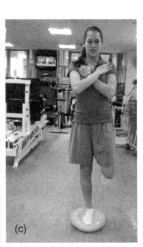

(a) (b) (c)

SUMMARY

Lateral ankle sprains are one of the most commonly encountered musculoskeletal injuries, and are especially common in the active, athletic population. Rehabilitation of these injuries should follow a logical progression through the phases of rehabilitation, but recent literature does support an early and accelerated rehabilitation program for grade I–II lateral ankle sprains. The literature supports the use of tape or lace up ankle braces after initial ankle sprain to prevent recurrent ankle sprains with return to athletic participation (15). Neuromuscular retraining and proprioceptive exercises appear to be the key to successful rehabilitation and the prevention of recurrent ankle sprains; therefore, they should be included in the HEP.

SAMPLE CASE

A 17-year-old male suffered his first left lateral ankle sprain 3 days ago. He has no significant past medical or surgical history and he denies any significant prior musculoskeletal or sports injuries. He is the starting center on his high school varsity basketball team and has plans to play in college. Ankle radiographs from the emergency department were negative for fracture. His physical examination is significant for antalgic gait, mild left lateral ankle swelling, no ecchymosis, tenderness to palpation at the distal lateral malleoli, positive anterior drawer test suggesting mild laxity. The remainder of his ankle examination revealed decreased ankle DF (- 5°) and his neurovascular exam was intact.

 SAMPLE THERAPY PRESCRIPTION

Discipline: Physical therapy.

Diagnosis: Left lateral ankle sprain (grade I).

Problem list: abnormality of gait with reduced ankle dorsiflexion (DF).

Precautions: Weight bearing as tolerated (WBAT).

Frequency of visits: 2 to 3x/week.

Duration of treatment: 3 to 4 weeks; or 8 to 12 total visits used at the therapist's discretion.

Treatment:

1. *Modalities:* cryotherapy (ice pack, ice bath, ice massage)

2. *Manual therapy:* talocrural (anterior to posterior) joint mobilization to restore ankle DF, and please assess subtalar joint and distal tibio-fibular joint motion

3. *Therapeutic exercise:* A/AA/PROM to restore DF, stretching (self-stretching, therapist assisted stretching) including gastroc/soleus stretching, strengthening/progressive resistive exercise (PRE) including dorsiflexor and evertor strengthening, balance/proprioceptive training, neuromuscular reeducation, aerobic and conditioning exercises

4. *Specialized treatments:* gait and kinetic chain analysis, correct trunk or lower limb biomechanical dysfunction, such as gluteus maximus or medius weakness, if present. Aquatic therapy if available

5. *Patient education:* HEP, include ankle injury prevention program

Goals: Decrease pain and swelling; restore ankle ROM/flexibility then restore strength, improve balance/proprioception, safely return to functional activities (e.g., sport, hobbies, work), and prevent recurrent ankle injuries.

Reevaluation: In 2 to 4 weeks by referring physician, unless return to play is being considered prior to scheduled follow-up, then earlier physician reevaluation should be arranged.

REFERENCES

1. Waterman BR, Owens BD, Davey S, Zacchilli MA, Belmont PJ. The epidemiology of ankle sprains in the United States. *JBJS*. 2010;92:2279–2284.
2. Wolfe MW, Uhl TL, McCluskey LC. Management of ankle sprains. *Am Fam Physician*. 2001;63:93–104.
3. Stiel I. Ottawa ankle rules. *Can Fam Physician*. 1996;42:478–480.
4. van Rijn RM, van Ochten J, Luijsterburg PA, van Middelkoop M, Koes BW, Bierma-Zeinstra SM. Effectiveness of additional supervised exercises compared with conventional treatment alone in patients with acute lateral ankle sprains: systematic review. *BMJ*. 2010;341:c5688.
5. Bleakley CM, O'Connor SR, Tully MA, et al. Effect of accelerated rehabilitation on function after ankle sprain: randomised controlled trial. *BMJ*. 2010;340:c1964.
6. Yeung MS, Chan KM, So CH, Yuan WY. An epidemiological survey on ankle sprain. *Br J Sports Med*. 1994;28(2):112–116.
7. Coté DJ, Prentice Jr WE, Hooker DN. Comparison of three treatment procedures for minimizing ankle sprain swelling. *Phy Ther*. 1988;68(7):1072–1076.
8. Warden SJ, Avin KG, Beck EM, DeWolf ME, Hagemeier MA, Martin KM. Low-intensity pulsed ultrasound accelerates and a nonsteroidal anti-inflammatory drug delays knee ligament healing. *Am J Sports Med*. 2006;34(7):1094–1102.
9. Michlovitz SL, Smith W, Watkins M. Ice and high voltage pulsed stimulation in treatment of acute lateral ankle sprains. *Orthop Sports Phys Ther*. 1988;9(9):301–304.
10. Safran MR, Benedtti RS, Bartolzzi AR, et al. Lateral ankle sprains: a comprehensive review part 1: etiology, pathoanatomy, histopathogenesis and diagnosis. *Med Sci Sports Exerc*. 1999;31(7):S429-S437.
11. Green T, Refshauge K, Crosbie J, Adams R. A randomized controlled trial of a passive accessory joint mobilization on acute ankle inversion sprains. *Phys Ther*. 2001;81(4):984–994.
12. Bleakley CM, McDonough SM, MacAuley DC. Some conservative strategies are effective when added to controlled mobilisation with external support after acute ankle sprain: a systematic review. *Aust J Physiother*. 2008;54(1):7–20.
13. Mohammadi F. Comparison of 3 preventive methods to reduce the recurrence of ankle inversion sprains in male soccer players. *Am J Sports Med*. 2007;35(6):922–926.
14. Zech A, Hübscher M, Vogt L, Banzer W, Hänsel F, Pfeifer K. Neuromuscular training for rehabilitation of sports injuries: a systematic review. *Med Sci Sports Exerc*. 2009;49:1831–1841.
15. Verhagen EA, Bay K. Optimising ankle sprain prevention: a critical review and practical appraisal of the literature. *Br J Sports Med*. 2010;44(15):1082–1088.
16. Bullock-Saxton JE. Local sensation changes and altered hip muscle function following severe ankle sprain. *Phys Ther*. 1994;74(1):17–28; discussion 28–31.
17. Dizon JM, Reyes JJ. A systematic review on the effectiveness of external ankle supports in the prevention of inversion ankle sprains among elite and recreational players. *J Sci Med Sport*. 2010;13(3):309–317.

Chronic Ankle Instability

Daniel Herman, Eric Magrum, and Jay Hertel

INTRODUCTION

Lateral ankle sprains are one of the most common musculoskeletal injuries that occur during adolescence and adulthood. These injuries typically occur as a result of a plantar-flexion, inversion mechanism and involve injury to the anterior talofibular ligament (ATFL) and, in more severe injuries, the calcaneofibular ligament (CFL). While lateral ankle sprains are often thought to be minor injuries without long term consequences, there is considerable evidence to the contrary. It is widely recognized that the most common predisposition to an ankle sprain is a history of previous ankle sprain (1). Nearly three-quarters of patients recovering from an ankle sprain still suffer from at least one symptom two years post-injury, and almost half of these patients report perceived instability in addition to at least one additional persistent symptom (2). It has been estimated that between 15 and 45 percent of ankle sprain patients report a lack of full recovery three years after ankle sprain (3). Persistent symptoms after ankle sprain have been associated with diminished health-related quality of life (2) as well as diminished levels of physical activity over their lifespan (4). Additionally, there is mounting evidence linking the history of single severe ankle sprains and repetitive ankle sprains with an increased risk of ankle osteoarthritis (5).

Chronic ankle instability (CAI) is a term that has been used to describe the collection of symptoms that affects individuals who do not fully recover from lateral ankle sprain. Pathological laxity due to ligamentous injury will result in mechanical instability of the ankle, while altered proprioception due to mechanoreceptor changes will trigger sensorimotor deficits. These deficits manifest clinically as repetitive bouts of ankle instability and lingering symptoms that exist for more than 1 year after initial ankle sprain. Symptoms may include pain,

swelling, weakness, and the perception of the ankle giving way during functional activities. Patients with CAI also self-report diminished functional abilities (6,7).

Key elements of the physical examination include an objective examination including manual assessment of foot and ankle arthrokinematics and biomechanical assessment that progressively loads the kinetic chain. Ankle specific self-assessment outcome tools such as the Foot and Ankle Disability Index (FADI) or the Foot and Ankle Ability Measure (FAAM) are important tools to consider using. The clinician should also remain alert to symptoms and physical exam findings consistent with commonly associated conditions, such as osteochondral defects, impingement syndrome, and peroneal tendon dysfunction.

The specific deficits associated with CAI can be categorized into functional instability and/or mechanical instability with deficits of both present in most patients. Mechanical instability is most commonly exhibited as pathological laxity (8). Insufficiency of the ATFL will result in increased laxity with the anterior drawer maneuver (anterior displacement ≥5 mm), while insufficiency of the CFL will be associated with increased inversion talar tilt ($>10°$ difference with the contralateral ankle). An important aspect of mechanical instability that is often overlooked by clinicians is that of arthrokinematic restrictions. While the ankle may be lax with anterior drawer translation and inversion talar tilt, there may be restriction in arthrokinematic and osteokinematic motion in other directions. Specifically, restricted dorsiflexion range of motion ($<20°$ while standing with the knee extended) is often seen in patients with CAI. This restriction is frequently associated with diminished posterior glide of the talus on the tibia. Likewise, restricted glide of the proximal and distal tibiofibular joints is also commonly seen. Clinicians must also be cognizant of potential restriction of arthrokinematic motion at the subtalar and midtarsal joints as well in patients with CAI.

Individuals with CAI have been shown to have a variety of functional deficits including impaired proprioception, diminished motor neuron pool excitability, slowed stretch reflex reactions, diminished strength, poorer balance, and altered mechanics during walking, running, cutting, and jumping activities (7). The cause of this array of deficits is thought to be due to the same sensorimotor etiology as opposed to individual causes. Alterations in the central nervous system are thought to alter neuromuscular control of the chronically unstable ankle.

CHRONIC ANKLE INSTABILITY

- This condition is a common sequela of lateral ankle sprains

- CAI consists of both mechanical instability and restriction of the ankle and altered sensorimotor function

- Symptoms may include pain, swelling, weakness, and ankle "giving way" during functional activities for more than one year after the initial lateral ankle sprain

- Determination of the mechanical and functional limitations is the key to planning the rehabilitation program

- Commonly associated conditions with CAI that must be considered: osteochondral defects, impingement syndrome, and peroneal tendon dysfunction

REHABILITATION

The major focus of rehabilitation for CAI is to address the key components of the mechanical deficits and functional instability that present following a comprehensive evaluation of the athlete as previously detailed. Accurate identification of altered arthrokinematics and sensorimotor deficits is the central driving force behind the rehabilitation plan. This evaluation framework allows the clinician to formulate a specific and individualized treatment program.

Therapeutic Modalities

There are no substantive evidence-based recommendations available regarding the use of modalities such as ultrasound with CAI; rather, the mainstays of treatment include manual therapy, therapeutic exercise, and external supports as detailed below.

Manual Therapy

Mechanical instability deficits that are addressed through a rehabilitation program are arthrokinematic restrictions including limited talocrural joint dorsiflexion and altered joint position of the distal tibia-fibula joint and/or tibiotalar joint (9,10). Manual therapy to address the positional faults at the distal tibia-fibula and tibiotalar joints have been demonstrated in the literature through various techniques to improve the arthrokinematics and joint position with resultant range of motion and sensorimotor improvements (11). Improving dorsiflexion range of motion through articular, myofascial, or soft tissue mobilization techniques as well as passive and dynamic stretching (Figure 32.1) should be part of a comprehensive treatment program.

Therapeutic Exercise

Functional instability has been defined as a patient presenting with one or more of the following: neuromuscular deficits, proprioceptive deficits, strength deficits, and/or impaired postural control. A recent review by Holmes described the evidence for evaluating and addressing these deficits (12).

Strengthening of the ankle musculature is commonly prescribed as a part of a comprehensive rehabilitation program. Controversy exists throughout the literature regarding the most effective strengthening program for the patient with CAI. Strength deficits have been described for ankle invertors and evertors, both concentrically and eccentrically, at a variety of speeds. Deficits have also been proposed regarding activation, timing, endurance, and co-contraction of antagonistic muscle groups throughout the literature. This results in some difficulty making specific evidence-based recommendations. The benefits discussed in the literature include improved joint position sense and improved activation and timing of peroneal muscles to decrease the risk of recurrent ankle sprain. The best available evidence suggests that closed kinetic chain eccentric

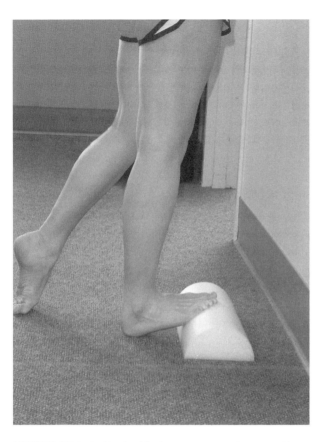

FIGURE 32.1: Ankle dorsiflexion (gastrocnemius) stretching.

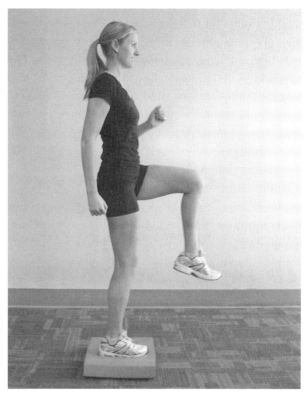

FIGURE 32.2: Balance training: single leg balance task on foam surface.

strengthening of the invertors should be part of the rehabilitation program. Secondary to the lack of evidence, it is recommended that functional and dynamic strengthening of the invertors, evertors, intrinsic foot musculature, and proximal hip musculature be part of a comprehensive program (12).

Proprioceptive deficits include frontal, greater than sagittal plane joint position sense limitations. Multistation proprioceptive exercise training has been shown to improve joint position sense, muscle reaction times, postural sway, and self-reported ankle stability (13). A multistation approach utilizes a variety of balance equipment and tasks to improve the ability of the ankle to accept and accommodate to progressive loads. The equipment and tasks include single and multiplanar equipment; different surfaces; modification of visual input; static activities progressing to dynamic activities; and sport-specific tasks (Figures 32.2–32.4). Strengthening of the ankle, primarily invertors and evertors, has been shown to improve joint position sense, although the link between proprioceptive and strength gains needs to be further studied.

Neuromuscular deficits are defined as the unconscious activation of dynamic restraints to maintain stability. Inconsistencies in the literature exist with regards to the adequacy of peroneal muscle response latency to protect the joint from excessive loading; as a result, current theory emphasizes preprogrammed feed forward synergistic mechanisms of stabilization. Rehabilitation exercises should emphasize the subconscious ability to stabilize the ankle while landing on various surfaces with the ankle in a variety of positions, especially facilitating a more dorsiflexed and everted position at initial contact.

Postural control deficits may be a combination of impaired proprioception and neuromuscular control. Deficits can be clinically assessed with functional tests such as the Star Excursion Balance Test (SEBT) (14). The evidence supports improving postural control deficits through a comprehensive balance training program that emphasizes the dynamic stabilization after perturbations such as predictable and unpredictable changes in direction, landing from a hop, and dynamic reaching tasks and

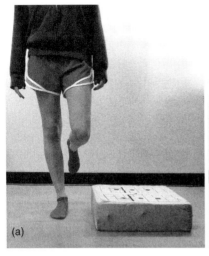
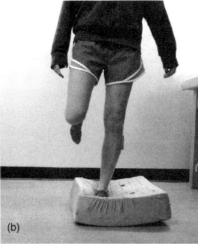

FIGURE 32.3: Dynamic hopping → Balancing activities from stable to unstable surface. Part a represents starting position, part b finishing position.

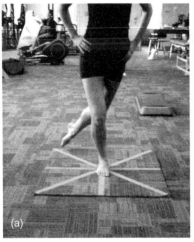
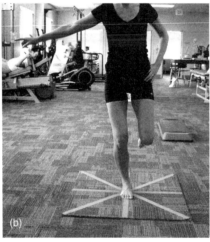

FIGURE 32.4: Strengthening and balance training. (a) Controlled reaching around "star" with foot. (b) Controlled reaching around "star" with hand.

may prove more beneficial than more traditional balance training programs (15).

Supportive Devices

Orthotics

In an extensive review of the literature regarding foot orthotic intervention in the CAI population, the authors concluded that the use of foot orthotics has been shown to improve functional impairments such as neuromuscular control, somatosensory feedback, and reduced muscle load as the mechanism for successful use of orthotic management (16). Another group demonstrated improvements in dynamic postural control with the use of custom biomechanical orthotics and concluded that the evidence suggests that orthotics may be used in conjunction with a rehabilitation program (17).

Taping

A recent systematic review concluded that taping is effective at reducing the incidence of recurrent injury in the CAI population (18). The mechanism by which taping reduces incidence is still unknown. Mechanical ankle instability appears to improve with taping (19). CAI subjects report improved perception of stability, confidence, and reassurance with dynamic postural stability measures without demonstrating improved performance with various taping techniques (20).

Bracing

Ankle bracing in the CAI literature is inconclusive. Inconsistencies and conflicting evidence exist secondary to discrepancies in methods, definitions, measurement, and assessment techniques. Authors have looked at the ability of ankle braces to improve the dynamic postural index, and directional stability and concluded that there was no difference between braced and unbraced conditions during a jump landing task (21). A numbers needed to treat analysis of the existing evidence concluded that ankle bracing may be more effective at reducing the recurrence of injury in an already injured population (22). However, most clinical guidelines recommend prophylactic ankle braces, secondary to increased proprioception, mechanical stability, decreased injury risk, and cost effectiveness (23).

Home Exercise Program

Home exercise programs (HEPs) should start at the beginning of the rehabilitation process and continue in a progressive fashion throughout the period of patient care with an appropriate transition to a maintenance program upon discharge. Early HEP should include range of motion exercises designed to reinforce the gains secondary to manual therapy in reestablishing appropriate arthrokinematics. Evaluation for and instruction in the use of appropriate foot orthotics and ankle braces will help with patient functionality early in the rehabilitation course and will facilitate patient participation with later progression to therapeutic home exercises. Resistance exercises should be incorporated to restore normal strength in a progressive fashion, beginning with single joint open-chain exercises and progressing to closed-chain and multijoint exercises. With restoration of normal ankle joint arthrokinematics and improved strength throughout the kinetic chain, increasing challenges should be incorporated to address proprioceptive, postural, and neuromuscular deficits. As detailed in prior chapters, many home exercises can be integrated into activities of daily living or leisure activities to improve patient compliance and to decrease the burden of the program.

SUMMARY

CAI is a common sequela of lateral ankle sprains, resulting in mechanical and sensorimotor deficits that may cause pain, swelling, weakness, and diminished functionality. A comprehensive rehabilitation prescription for the patient presenting with CAI would include manual therapy to address the arthrokinematic limitations, including restoration of ankle dorsiflexion range of motion; and a comprehensive exercise program incorporating strengthening, proprioceptive, neuromuscular, and dynamic stabilization techniques. Mechanical stability may be enhanced with ankle bracing or taping during functional activities in an effort to prevent recurrent ankle sprains.

SAMPLE CASE

A 20-year-old male presents with a chief complaint of left ankle joint instability. He reports suffering a significant ankle injury 2 years prior while participating in high school soccer during which he "rolled" his ankle. X-rays at that time were negative. Since the time of injury, he states that he has been "frustrated" with his inability to attain acceptable athletic performance even with lower levels of play such as college intramurals, and describes subjective weakness and sensations of "giving way," even with normal activities of daily living. His examination is notable for a lack of significant tenderness to palpation, restricted ankle dorsiflexion range of motion, mild multiplanar strength asymmetries at the ankle with manual muscle testing, poor proximal and distal dynamic control in single-leg stance and squat, and a positive anterior drawer sign. No significant evidence of an osteochondral lesion or peroneal tendon dysfunction is present.

 SAMPLE THERAPY PRESCRIPTION

Discipline: Physical therapy.

Diagnosis: Left CAI, with both mechanical and functional instability.

Problem list: Decreased ankle DF, ankle strength, and proprioception.

Precautions: WBAT.

Frequency of visits: 2 to 3x/week.

Duration of treatment: 4 to 6 weeks.

Treatment:

1. *Manual therapy:* talocrural, tibiotalar, and distal tibia-fibula joint mobilization, with particular attention to improving ankle dorsiflexion range of motion

2. *Therapeutic exercise:* passive and active range of motion exercises; multiplanar strengthening exercises at the ankle joint; proximal muscle strengthening and dynamic control; progressive

postural, proprioceptive, and neuromuscular training; advancement to sport-specific activities

3. *Orthotics/bracing:* external ankle support for therapeutic sessions and home use, evaluation for orthotics

4. *Patient education:* HEP, including injury prevention program

Goals: (a) restore normal ankle arthrokinematics; (b) restore lower extremity strength and address imbalances; (c) address proprioceptive, postural, and neuromuscular deficits; (d) incorporate sports and occupational-specific tasks with safe return to activities.

Reevaluation: In 4 to 6 weeks by referring physician.

REFERENCES

1. Beynnon BD, Murphy DF, Alosa DM. Predictive factors for lateral ankle sprains: A literature review. *J Athl Train.* 2002;37(4):376–380.
2. Anandacoomarasamy A, Barnsley L. Long term outcomes of inversion ankle injuries. *Br J Sports Med.* 2005;39(3):e14.
3. van Rijn RM, van Os AG, Bernsen RM, Luijsterburg PA, Koes BW, Bierma-Zeinstra SM. What is the clinical course of acute ankle sprains? A systematic literature review. *Am J Med.* 2008;121(4):324–331.
4. Verhagen RA, de Keizer G, van Dijk CN. Long-term follow-up of inversion trauma of the ankle. *Arch Orthop Trauma Surg.* 1995;114(2):92–96.
5. Valderrabano V, Hintermann B, Horisberger M, Fung TS. Ligamentous posttraumatic ankle osteoarthritis. *Am J Sports Med.* 2006;34(4):612–620.
6. Hertel J. Functional anatomy, pathomechanics, and pathophysiology of lateral ankle instability. *J Athl Train.* 2002;37(4):364–375.
7. Hertel J. Sensorimotor deficits with ankle sprains and chronic ankle instability. *Clin Sports Med.* 2008;27(3):353–370.
8. Hubbard TJ, Hertel J. Mechanical contributions to chronic lateral ankle instability. *Sports Med.* 2006;36(3):263–277.
9. Wikstrom EA, Hubbard TJ. Talar positional fault in persons with chronic ankle instability. *Arch Phys Med Rehabil.* 2010;91(8):1267–1271.
10. Hubbard TJ, Hertel J. Anterior positional fault of the fibula after sub-acute lateral ankle sprains. *Man Ther.* 2008;13(1):63–67.
11. Hoch MC, McKeon PO. Joint mobilization improves spatiotemporal postural control and range of motion in those with chronic ankle instability. *J Orthop Res.* 2011;29(3):326–332.
12. Holmes A, Delahunt E. Treatment of common deficits associated with chronic ankle instability. *Sports Med.* 2009;39(3):207–224.
13. Eils E, Rosenbaum D.A multi-station proprioceptive exercise program in patients with ankle instability. *Med Sci Sports Exerc.* 2001;33(12):1991–1998.
14. Hertel J, Braham RA, Hale SA, Olmsted-Kramer LC. Simplifying the star excursion balance test: analyses of subjects with and without chronic ankle instability. *J Orthop Sports Phys Ther.* 2006;36(3):131–137.
15. McKeon PO, Ingersoll CD, Kerrigan DC, Saliba E, Bennett BC, Hertel J. Balance training improves function and postural control in those with chronic ankle instability. *Med Sci Sports Exerc.* 2008;40(10):1810–1819.
16. Richie DH Jr. Effects of foot orthoses on patients with chronic ankle instability. *J Am Podiatr Med Assoc.* 2007;97(1):19–30.
17. Sesma AR, Mattacola CG, Uhl TL, Nitz AJ, McKeon PO. Effect of foot orthotics on single- and double-limb dynamic balance tasks in patients with chronic ankle instability. *Foot Ankle Spec.* 2008;1(6):330–337.
18. Dizon JM, Reyes JJ.A systematic review on the effectiveness of external ankle supports in the prevention of inversion ankle sprains among elite and recreational players. *J Sci Med Sport.* 2010;13(3):309–317.
19. Hubbard TJ, Cordova M. Effect of ankle taping on mechanical laxity in chronic ankle instability. *Foot Ankle Int.* 2010;31(6):499–504.
20. Delahunt E, McGrath A, Doran N, Coughlan GF. Effect of taping on actual and perceived dynamic postural stability in persons with chronic ankle instability. *Arch Phys Med Rehabil.* 2010;91(9):1383–1389.
21. Gribble PA, Taylor BL, Shinohara J. Bracing does not improve dynamic stability in chronic ankle instability subjects. *Phys Ther Sport.* 2010;11(1):3–7.
22. Olmsted LC, Vela LI, Denegar CR, Hertel J. Prophylactic ankle taping and bracing: A numbers-needed-to-treat and cost-benefit analysis. *J Athl Train.* 2004;39(1):95–100.
23. Wikstrom EA, Arrigenna MA, Tillman MD, Borsa PA. Dynamic postural stability in subjects with braced, functionally unstable ankles. *J Athl Train.* 2006;41(3):245–250.

Achilles Tendinopathy

Gerard A. Malanga, Alon Terry, and Heather Sleece

INTRODUCTION

Achilles tendinopathy is a common clinical condition that is characterized by pain and swelling in the posterior ankle. It is most often encountered in recreational and competitive athletes, although it does occur in the nonathletic population as well. The gastrocnemius and soleus muscles merge to form the Achilles tendon, which inserts on the posterior surface of the calcaneus. The Achilles tendon, the strongest tendon in the body, is subject to loads of up to 10 times body weight during activities such as running and jumping (1,2,3) and the development of tendinopathy is felt to be secondary to overuse and repetitive loading (4,5). Top-level runners are most at risk with an annual incidence of 7% to 9% (6). Pain in the area of the Achilles tendon can occasionally be secondary to an acute inflammatory process involving the tendon sheath or bursa, which is known as paratenonitis or retrocalcaneal bursitis. Much more commonly, however, chronically painful Achilles tendons demonstrate tendinosis rather than inflammation on histological review. It is thought that excessive loading over time leads to collagen degeneration and fiber disorientation within the tendon (7).

Intrinsic risk factors for Achilles tendinopathy include decreased ankle dorsiflexion (DF) range of motion (ROM), abnormal subtalar ROM, decreased plantarflexion (PF) strength, excessive foot pronation, and poor tendon vascularity (8,9). Extrinsic factors that may predispose individuals to develop Achilles tendinopathy include changes in training intensity, training on irregular or slanted surfaces, poor footwear, and prior injury (10). Noninsertional and insertional tendinopathy appear to be distinct clinical entities and have differing success rates with conservative treatment protocols. (Figure 33.1) Noninsertional tendinopathy accounts for 66% of all patients with Achilles tendinopathy (11) and generally occurs 2 to 6 cm proximal

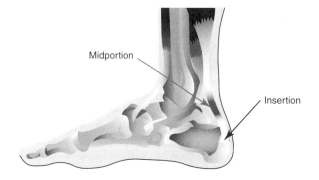

FIGURE 33.1: Achilles tendinopathy/tendinitis.

to the calcaneal insertion, which correlates with a zone of hypovascularity of the tendon (4). The classic presentation of this condition includes morning stiffness and a gradual onset of pain during activity.

Key elements of the physical examination include inspection, palpation, ROM, strength, and gait analysis looking for the above-mentioned intrinsic risk factors. Pain with palpation 2 to 6 cm proximal to the Achilles tendon insertion that moves with ankle DF and PF is indicative of noninsertional tendinopathy, while pain over the midline posterior calcaneus indicates insertional tendinopathy. If the site of maximal tenderness is adjacent to the tendon attachment, retrocalcaneal bursitis must be considered (12). In the case of paratenonitis, the site of pain will stay fixed with ankle DF and PF.

Achilles tendinopathy is typically a clinical diagnosis, but imaging can be helpful in clarifying the nature of the injury, including the location and severity of the tendinopathy. Plain radiographs are not routinely recommended in all cases but can reveal an abnormal intratendinous calcification or ossification around the Achilles insertion on the calcaneus. Ultrasound evaluation can reveal increased anterior-posterior (AP) thickness of > 6mm that is usually asymmetric, as well as focal hypoechoic areas that correspond to areas of degeneration (4). Ultrasound also allows for visualization of calcification, cortical irregularity, and neovascularization, as well as assessment of the retrocalcaneal bursa. Magnetic resonance imaging (MRI) is able to distinguish intra-tendinous from para-tendinous pathology, clarify the location and severity of the pathology, and rule out Achilles tendon tear or concomitant pathology (e.g., posterior tibial tendinopathy). Those patients with chronic noninsertional Achilles tendinopathy will show thickening and intratendinous signal changes without evidence of edema of the tendon (13).

ACHILLES TENDINOPATHY

- Common condition among athletes involved in running and jumping sports that is associated with overuse and repetitive loading of the Achilles tendon

- Chronic Achilles tendinopathy is associated with noninflammatory collagen degeneration and fiber disorientation

- Noninsertional Achilles tendinopathy is the most common form and usually affects the tendon 2 to 6 cm proximal to the Achilles insertion

- Achilles tendinopathy is largely a clinical diagnosis, but imaging such as ultrasound and MRI can be helpful in demonstrating the extent and nature of the pathology

THE REHABILITATION PROGRAM

It is essential that an individual who presents with Achilles tendinopathy be treated with a comprehensive rehabilitation program as early as possible to avoid further pain and disability. A patient who presents with an acute exacerbation of tendinosis or with a physical examination consistent with paratenonitis should initially be treated according to the PRICE principles with protection, relative rest, ice, compression, elevation, and historically nonsteroidal anti-inflammatory therapy. Recent research has questioned the role of nonsteroidal anti-inflammatory medications and

has even suggested potential negative effects on tendon healing (14). Evaluation and correction of biomechanical problems or training errors that may be contributing to increased stress on the tendon should be identified and addressed. An example includes the use of foot orthotics to control excessive foot pronation. Therapeutic exercises should initially include stretching of the lower limb, especially the gastrocnemius-soleus complex as well as other muscle length deficits identified on analysis of the kinetic chain. Progressive eccentric strengthening of the gastrocnemius-soleus complex is the cornerstone of the rehabilitation program and is supported by recent scientific evidence that has suggested both short and long term effectiveness for treating chronic Achilles tendinosis pain (25–28). This should be the primary form of strengthening until the pain level has decreased significantly, at which point the individual can advance to concentric strengthening. Once an individual is pain free, with restored ROM, strength, and proprioception, then the final phase of rehabilitation may commence; and this includes agility exercises, plyometrics, and return to previous activity level.

Therapeutic Modalities

The most commonly used modality for the treatment of Achilles tendinopathy is ice, particularly in the acute phase. Ice, in the form of a cold pack or ice massage, provides both an analgesic and anti-inflammatory effect (15). Ice can be used in the clinic and should be used after any recreational activities or a full day of prolonged weight-bearing.

Many other modalities have been used to treat Achilles tendinopathy but there is a lack of quality scientific evidence to support their use. While in vitro studies have demonstrated a theoretical benefit of therapeutic ultrasound in tendon healing by inducing tenocyte migration, two meta-analyses did not reveal any clinical improvement compared to placebo (16–17).

Low-level laser therapy (LLLT) has also been utilized in the treatment of tendinopathy. At the cellular level this treatment is thought to increase collagen production and decrease both matrix metalloproteinases as well as neovascularization. One recent randomized controlled trial (RCT) found that patients who received LLLT in combination with an eccentric strengthening program did better than those who performed exercises only (18), but this study had a small sample size, making it difficult to draw firm conclusions. Another study with a small sample size, seven patients, revealed improved pain threshold immediately after treatment with no long-term follow-up (19). This treatment remains poorly validated and at this time is not routinely recommended.

Multiple RCTs have looked at the efficacy of low energy extracorporeal shockwave therapy (ESWT) for Achilles tendinopathy. While not fully understood, it is believed that this treatment inhibits pain receptors and stimulates soft tissue healing. Two of these studies found no improvement compared to placebo and one found that ESWT plus eccentric strengthening was better than eccentric strengthening alone (20–22). One retrospective study did show positive results utilizing a single high-energy dose of ESWT compared to other conservative treatments (23).

Given the lack of consistent evidence, these additional therapeutic modalities such as ultrasound, LLLT, and ESWT are not currently recommended, particularly if their use takes time away from other components of the therapeutic program.

Manual Therapy

Many therapists perform transverse friction massage across the site of pathology at the Achilles tendon despite there being insufficient evidence to supports its routine use. The purpose of this treatment is to cause mild inflammation that will promote a normal healing response. It can also serve a mechanical role to release adhesions between newly formed collagen and adjacent structures, thereby improving soft tissue mobility (24). Transverse friction massage is typically an uncomfortable manual technique for the patient. The patient lies prone and the therapist uses their hands to apply a moderate amount of pressure perpendicularly to the Achilles tendon. Usually it is coupled with passive range of motion exercises for the ankle. Duration of treatment is about 5 to 10 minutes, with the duration and intensity of treatment based on the patient's tolerance. This treatment may be performed in conjunction with eccentric strengthening and should theoretically lead to more organized and elastic tendon structure during the remodeling phase of tendon healing, but this theory hasn't been proven or supported by the literature. Therefore, the scientific validation of transverse friction massage requires further basic science and clinical research.

As mentioned in prior chapters of this section, talocrural joint mobilizations may be utilized to help restore ankle ROM, especially ankle DF. Subtalar or tibio-fibular joints may also be assessed and if restricted, joint mobilizations may be utilized to address this problem, and in theory restore normal arthrokinematics.

Therapeutic Exercise

During the early phases of rehabilitation relative rest is important and the patient must avoid any exacerbating activities. Weight-bearing activities, such as walking or standing may require limitations through the use of an assistive device (e.g., cane or crutches) and may require some form of immobilization, such as a walking boot. However, prolonged immobilization is discouraged as it is associated with many adverse effects including muscle atrophy and soft tissue contracture. Low impact activities such as cycling, swimming, or aquatic exercises may be utilized to maintain cardiopulmonary fitness while limiting the amount of stress on the Achilles tendon.

Optimization of lower extremity ROM is an important part of the initial therapeutic program (phase II). Particular attention, should be paid to the gastrocnemius-soleus complex and deficits in length need to be corrected or at least improved. Stretching of the hip and thigh musculature, such as the hip flexors, quadriceps, rectus femoris, and hamstrings, should also be performed, since decreased length of these muscles could be contributing to impaired lower limb biomechanics. Calf stretching should be done with the knee straight to target the gastrocnemius (Figure 33.2) and with the knee bent to target the soleus (Figure 33.3), as this muscle does not cross the knee joint. Prolonged Achilles tendon stretching can also be accomplished by using an incline and the position can be held for 30 to 40 seconds. A subtalar neutral position should be maintained during the stretch to avoid excessive

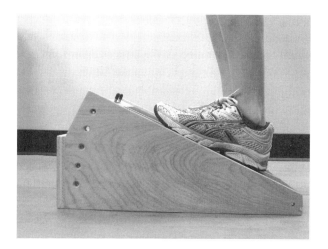

FIGURE 33.2: Gastrocnemius stretch.

Note: Knee should be maintained in extension during the stretch.

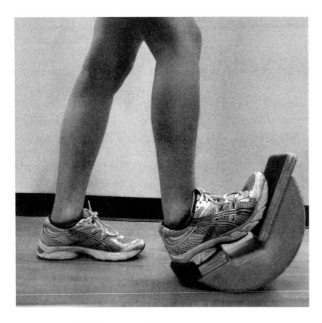

FIGURE 33.3: Soleus stretch.

pronation, which occurs as a compensatory movement pattern when the Achilles tendon is shortened.

Eccentric exercise, described as a technique of elongating a tendon during a simultaneous voluntary muscle contracture, has become the cornerstone of treatment for not only Achilles tendinopathy, but for chronic tendinopathy in general. Multiple studies have demonstrated both structural changes within the tendon as well as decreased pain and improved function with eccentric strengthening (22, 25–28). Athletic individuals with noninsertional tendinopathy have been shown to respond better to eccentric strengthening protocols than sedentary individuals or those with insertional tendinopathy. Many different eccentric strengthening protocols have been described in the literature. Alfredson et al

developed an eccentric training program that consists of 3 sets of 15 heel drops that are performed twice daily for 12 weeks and has been proven effective at short and longer term follow up (27,28). These exercises should be initiated once the patient is able to tolerate them; prior to that time, the acute phase may be treated by the PRICE principles, ROM, exercises, and gentle isometric exercises to maintain ROM and strength until eccentric strengthening can be tolerated.

The progression of eccentric exercises will be patient specific and will depend largely on the severity of pain and pain tolerance. They may begin with heel drops on the floor and progress to utilization of an incline or a step (Figure 33.4). When treating insertional Achilles tendinopathy, eccentric exercises may produce better results if they are performed in a more restricted ROM with DF to neutral position only, as seen in Figure 33.4a (29). The speed of eccentric lengthening should also be transitioned from slow to medium to fast as the individual progresses with the program. Weight can be added to increase difficulty once the individual is able to tolerate a fast eccentric load (28). Throughout the program, the individual should be performing three sets of 15 repetitions, preferably twice a day. The exercises should at least elicit strain across the tendon, while some experts have recommended that these exercises should elicit pain or discomfort, and when the exercises are no longer painful the eccentric training program should be advanced.

Once the individual is able to tolerate eccentric strengthening, strengthen other lower limb muscle groups, such as the hip extensors, hip abductors, and quadriceps. Once pain free, the athlete can progress to proprioceptive, balance training (Figure 33.5), and plyometric exercises. Exercises such as double limb jumping on a firm surface or trampoline, single limb jumping, jumping rope, jogging,

FIGURE 33.4a: Eccentric heel drops to the floor.

FIGURE 33.4b: Eccentric heel drops on a step.

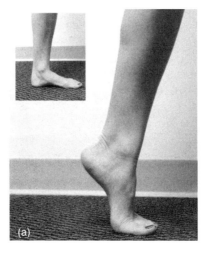
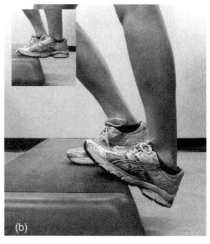

(a) (b)

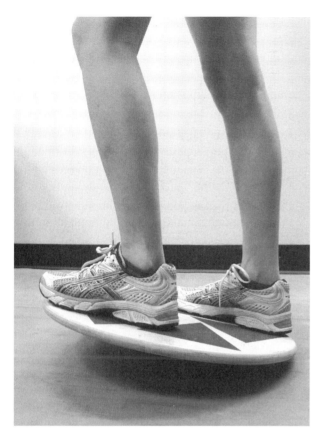

FIGURE 33.5: Balance/proprioception exercise with wobble board.

and ultimately running should be trialed. This progression will typically range from 4 to 6 weeks depending on how long the patient has been symptomatic, how compliant the patient is with the home exercise program, and whether the patient presented with insertional or noninsertional Achilles tendinopathy.

Supportive Devices

While there is no scientific evidence supporting their use, orthotics are widely utilized in the conservative treatment of Achilles tendinopathy. Heel lifts, typically 12 to 15 mm in height are often trialed to decrease the rate and range of eccentric loading on the tendon. It is important to use this only as a temporizing treatment as prolonged use of a heel lift will only perpetuate tightness of the gastroc-soleus complex. Individuals with excessive foot pronation are subject to high levels of torque across the Achilles tendon, at a site proximal to its insertion. Correction of

pronation is accomplished with either a medial wedge or a rigid arch support. It may be advisable to first trial taping techniques to stabilize the calcaneus, and the subtalar joint and to decrease foot pronation. If this intervention results in decreased pain with ambulation, then the patient is likely to benefit from a trial of foot orthotics (25).

Home Exercise Program

The home exercise program should begin immediately. With an acute exacerbation or with paratenonitis, the PRICE protocol should be followed daily. A stretching program should be taught on day one and should be performed daily, as tolerated by the patient, with prolonged stretches of 30 to 40 seconds per repetition. Once eccentric exercises are added to the rehabilitation program, the patient should be educated on how to perform them safely and independently, and they should be encouraged to perform them on a daily basis. Increasing the intensity of the exercise should be done first in therapy and then at home once the patient has demonstrated proper technique. It is important that the patient knows to pull back from any exercises that are causing significant pain. Eccentric strengthening and stretching should be continued indefinitely to help prevent recurrence. The patient should also be educated about appropriate footwear and told to progress future training programs gradually (e.g., avoid increasing mileage, modify running surfaces, and avoid hills if symptomatic).

SUMMARY

Achilles tendinopathy is a common injury in runners and other weekend warriors. Typically patients will seek treatment once the injury becomes chronic and begins to impact their daily or recreational activities. Achilles tendinopathy can be classified as insertional or noninsertional. Those with noninsertional tendinopathy have a greater likelihood of responding well to conservative treatment. Treatment for Achilles tendinopathy will include, but is not limited to, initial modification of recreational activities, and assessment of gait and footwear. A lower limb stretching program will be implemented to reduce excessive loading of the tendon. Eccentric exercises will be initiated to facilitate remodeling of damaged tissue and progressed according to patient tolerance. Transverse friction massage can be utilized to magnify the effects of the eccentric strengthening, although the literature does not definitively support its use as an adjunctive treatment. A modified, low impact aerobic activity program should be implemented to maintain cardiopulmonary endurance and to prevent weight gain during a period of relative inactivity. Plyometric activities will be introduced when the patient can tolerate eccentric exercises with resistance. Once sport- specific activities are reintroduced, it is important to analyze the athlete's technique to address any movement impairments that could predispose them to reinjury.

SAMPLE CASE

A 45-year-old executive and mother of three recently decided to get back in shape. In college she was on the cross country team but since graduation she has not had much time to run. Over the past 3 months she has been running 5 days a week. She initially started by running a mile per day and has worked her way up to five miles a day and a weekly 10 mile run on the weekend. She runs primarily on asphalt and has been using the same running shoes for 3 years. She developed pain over the right posterior ankle that has progressed from morning stiffness, to pain with running, and now pain with walking, which has worsened over the last 6 weeks. Physical examination reveals a tender nodule proximal to the right Achilles insertion that moves with ankle DF and PF. Ankle DF is limited to neutral with pain on the right and + 10 degrees of ankle DF on the left. She is unable to perform a full heel raise on the right secondary to pain.

 SAMPLE THERAPY PRESCRIPTION

Discipline: Physical therapy.

Diagnosis: Right Achilles Tendinopathy, noninsertional.

Problem list: reduced ankle DF.

Precautions: WBAT.

Frequency of visits: 2 to 3x/week.

Duration of treatment: Acute cases may respond to fewer visits (4–6) and chronic cases may need 10 to 12 visits spread out over longer duration (6–12+ weeks).

Treatment:

1. *Therapeutic Modalities:* cryotherapy PRN (ice pack, ice bath, ice massage)

2. *Manual therapy:* transverse friction massage to right Achilles tendon and talocrural joint mobilizations to help restore ankle DF. Assess subtalar joint and distal tibio-fibular joint motion, address if restricted

3. *Therapeutic exercise:* A/AA/PROM to restore DF, stretching (self stretching, therapist assisted stretching) including gastroc/soleus stretching, eccentric strengthening of gastrocnemius-soleus muscles, balance/proprioceptive training, neuromuscular reeducation, plyometrics, aerobic and conditioning exercises

4. *Specialized treatments:* biomechanical analysis of gait and the kinetic chain. Orthotics/heel lift. Taping or strapping to correct excessive pronation

5. *Patient education:* home exercise program. Modify training program, discuss appropriate intensity, progression of distance, running surface, footwear

Goals: Decrease pain and swelling; restore ankle ROM/flexibility then restore strength, improve balance/proprioception, safely return to functional activities (e.g., sport, hobbies, work) and prevent recurrent injuries.

Reevaluation: In 4 weeks by referring physician.

REFERENCES

1. Williams SK, Brage M. Heel pain-plantar fasciitis and Achilles enthesopathy. *Clin Sports Med.* 2004;23:123–144.
2. Soma CA, Mandelbaum BR. Achilles tendon disorders. *Clin Sports Med.* 1994;13:811–823.
3. Clement DB, Taunton J, Smart GW. A survey of overuse running injuries. *Physician Sports Med.* 1981;9:47–58.
4. Hennessy MS, Molloy AP, Sturdee SW. Noninsertional Achilles Tendinopathy. *Foot Ankle Clinic.* 2007;12(4):617–641.
5. Leadbetter WB. Cell-matrix response in tendon injury. *Clin Sports Med.* 1992;11:533–578.
6. Lysholm J, Wiklander J. Injuries in runners. *Am J Sports Med.* 1987;15,168–171.
7. Movin T, Gad A, Reinholt FP, Rolf C. Tendon pathology in long-standing achillodynia. Biopsy findings in 40 patients. *Acta Orthop Scand.* 1997;68(2):170–175.
8. Garcia C, Martin RL, Houck J, et al. Achilles pain, stiffness, and muscle power deficits: achilles tendinitis. Clinical practice guidelines linked to the international classification of functioning, disability, and health from the orthopaedic section of the American Physical Therapy Association. *J Orthop Sports Phys Ther.* 2010;40(9):A1–A26.
9. McCrory JL, Martin DF, Lowery RB, et al. Etiologic factors associated with Achilles tendinitis in runners. *Med Sci Sports Exerc.* 1999;31:1374–1381.
10. Longo UG, Ronga M, Maffulli N. Achilles tendinopathy. *Sports Med Arthrosc.* 2009;17(2):112–126. Review.
11. Kvist M. Achilles tendon injuries in athletes. *Sports Med.* 1994;18:173–201.
12. Solan M, Davies M. Management of insertional tendinopathy of the Achilles tendon. *Foot Ankle Clinic.* 2007;12(4):597–615.
13. Khan, KM, Forester, BB, Robinson, J. Are ultrasound and magnetic resonance imaging of value in assessment of Achilles tendon disorders? A two year prospective study. *Br J Sports Med.* 2003;37(2):149–153.
14. Dimmen S, Engebretsen L, Nordsletten L, et al. Negative effects of parecoxib and indomethacin on tendon healing: an experimental study in rats. *Knee Surg Sports Traumatol Arthrosc.* 2009;17(7):835–839.
15. Sharma P, Maffulli N. Understanding and managing Achilles tendinopathy. *Br J Hosp Med.* 2006;67:64–67.
16. Beckerman H, Bouter LM, van der Heijdan, et al. Efficacy of physiotherapy for musculoskeletal disorders: What can we learn from research? *Br J Gen Pract.* 1993;43:73–77.
17. Gam AN, Johannsen F. Ultrasound therapy in musculoskeletal disorders: a meta-analysis. *Pain.* 1995;63:85–91.
18. Stergioulas A, Stergioula M, Aarskog, R, et al. Effects of low-level laser therapy and eccentric exercises in the treatment of recreational athletes with chronic Achilles tendinopathy. *Am J Sports Med.* 2008;36(5):881–887.
19. Bjordal J, Lopes-Martins R, Iversen W. A randomized, placebo controlled trial of low level laser therapy for activated Achilles tendinitis with microdialysis measurement of peritendinous prostaglandin E2 concentrations. *Br J Sports Med.* 2006;40(1):76–80.
20. Costa M, Shepstone L, Donel, et al. Shock wave therapy for chronic Achilles tendon pain: a randomized placebo-controlled trial. *Clin Orthop Relat Res.* 2005;440:199–204.
21. Rasmussen S, Christensen M, Mathiesen I, et al. Shockwave therapy for chronic Achilles tendinopathy: a double-blind, randomized clinical trial of efficacy. *Acta Orthop.* 2008;79(2):249–256.
22. Rompe JD, Furia J, Maffulli N. Eccentric loading versus eccentric loading plus shock-wave treatment for midportion achilles tendinopathy: a randomized controlled trial. *Am J Sports Med.* 2009;37(3):463–470.
23. Furia J. High-energy extracorporeal shock wave therapy as a treatment for chronic noninsertional Achilles tendinopathy. *Am J Sports Med.* 2008;36(3):502–508.
24. Davidson CJ, Ganion LR, Gehlsen GM, et al. Rat tendon morphologic and functional changes resulting from soft tissue mobilization. *Med Sci Sports Exerc.* 1997;29:313–319.
25. Ohberg L, Lorentzon R, Alfredson H. Eccentric training in patients with chronic Achilles tendinosis: normalized tendon structure and decreased thickness at follow up. *Br J Sports Med.* 2004;38:8–11.
26. Mafi, N, Lorentzon R, Alfredson, H. Superior short-term results with eccentric calf muscle training compared to concentric training in a randomized prospective multicenter study on patients with chronic Achilles tendinosis. *Knee Surg Sports Traumatol Arthrosc.* 2001;9(1):42–47.
27. Alfredson H, Pietila T, Johnsson P, et al. Heavy-load eccentric calf muscle training for the treatment of chronic Achilles tendinosis. *Am J Sports Med.* 1998;26(3):360–366.
28. van der Plas A, de Jonge S, de Vos RJ, et al. A 5-year follow-up study of Alfredson's heel-drop exercise programme in chronic midportion Achilles tendinopathy. *Br J Sports Med.* 2012;46(3):214–218.
29. Jonsson P, Alfredson H, Sunding K, Fahlström M, Cook J. New regimen for eccentric calf-muscle training in patients with chronic insertional Achilles tendinopathy: results of a pilot study. *Br J Sports Med.* 2008;42(9):746–749.
30. Houglum PA. *Therapeutic Exercise For Musculoskeletal Injuries.* 3rd ed. Champaign, IL: Human Kinetics; 2010.

Posterior Tibial Tendinopathy

Deena Casiero, Tracey A. Viola, and Giselle Aerni

INTRODUCTION

The tibialis posterior muscle is found in the deep posterior compartment of the calf (1,2). The tendinous portion of this muscle travels behind the medial malleolus, and quickly changes direction which leads to a watershed area (1–5). It then inserts on the navicular tuberosity, cuneiforms, and second through fourth metatarsals (1). The primary functions of the musculotendinous unit are dynamic stabilization of the medial arch, inversion, and plantar flexion of the foot (1–5). With dysfunction of tibialis posterior, other tendons and ligaments of the ankle complex become weak (3). Tibialis posterior tendon dysfunction can be acute and/or inflammatory (tendonitis) or chronic and degenerative (tendinosis) (1,6,7). While believed to be common, the exact incidence is unknown (2). While the focus of this chapter is on inflammatory tendonitis, most of the techniques discussed can also be applied to the chronic form of this condition, posterior tibial tendinosis.

Inflammatory tendonitis typically presents as pain upon starting an activity, which improves while warming up, but worsens again with sustained activity (8). Pain also worsens when the tendon is stretched, or the muscle contracts against resistance (8). Patients presenting with an acute injury may have pain and/or swelling around the tendon, weakness or loss of function, including inability to walk the usual distances.

Key elements of the physical examination include tenderness to palpation of the tendon usually behind the medial malleolus, weakness and pain with resisted foot adduction or ankle inversion, reduced stride length and speed, or loss of the medial longitudinal arch (1–4,5,7,9), inability to perform a single leg heel raise and the "too many toes" sign. This sign is considered to be present when the examiner observes the patient from behind and more than the two lateral toes are seen. This occurs because of the valgus position of heel, flattening of the

medial longitudinal arch, and forefoot abduction (1–4,9). These biomechanical problems help explain why posterior tibial tendon dysfunction is associated with adult acquired flatfoot deformity (AAFD), although there is no consensus on whether it is the cause or consequence of AAFD.

The diagnosis is typically based on the clinical examination, although MRI studies are indicated if there is clinical suspicion for tendon rupture or additional pathology, such as osteochondral lesions. Ultrasound examination is another valuable imaging tool and can further characterize the extent of the tendon pathology and allows assessment of concomitant tendinopathy or bursopathy.

POSTERIOR TIBIAL TENDINOPATHY

- Common condition but exact incidence is unknown

- Tibialis posterior tendon dysfunction can be acute and/or inflammatory (tendonitis) or chronic and degenerative (tendinosis)

- Mechanism of injury can be acute or chronic, and due to overuse

- Key elements of the physical exam include: inspection, palpation for pain along the posterior tibialis tendon, pain during resisted inversion and plantar flexion and neurovascular testing, inability to perform single leg heel raise and "too many toes" sign

- Imaging is usually not indicated, unless tendon rupture or additional pathology is suspected

REHABILITATION PROGRAM

Conservative treatment goals in rehabilitation include symptom control and elimination, reduction of pain and inflammation, improvement of foot kinematics, and prevention of progression (6). Specific techniques will be discussed below, however it is common to use the PRICE protocol in acute inflammatory processes (3,8,10) to limit swelling, inflammation, hemorrhage, and pain (10). PRICE is an acronym for protection, rest, ice, compression, and elevation. Also, oral nonsteroidal anti-inflammatory drugs (NSAIDs) are commonly recommended in the acute setting (2,3,8). However, steroid injections are controversial due to the theoretical risk of tendon rupture (1,3,6).

After an acute injury the healing process occurs in multiple stages (Table 34.1). One to 3 weeks after injury is considered the proliferation phase. During this phase, the focus of a rehabilitation program should be on ankle support and stabilization while fibroblast invasion occurs along with collagen deposition (10). During weeks 3 to 4 maturation of collagen and the formation of scar tissue occurs. This phase is called the maturation phase (10). The rehabilitation goals during this phase should be gentle stretching and mobilization of the ankle joint in all directions. Four to eight weeks post injury the newly laid collagen should be strong enough to endure everyday stresses and the rehab program should begin to load the tendon progressively (10). During this recovery phase the patient may begin a return to play protocol. The practitioner should remember that the final maturation and remodeling of the ankle soft tissue structures might take up to 6 to 12 months (10). Unfortunately, many of the above mentioned treatment recommendations do not come from high quality randomized, controlled trials, but rather a matter of consensus opinion and observation.

Supportive Devices

As mentioned above, the initial components of PRICE include protection and rest. In the case of posterior tibialis tendonitis, this topic warrants early consideration, and will be discussed prior to other components of the rehabilitation program. Protection and rest can be achieved via orthotics and/or immobilization (6). Immobilization of the ankle can be achieved with a walking boot or below the knee walking cast (1,6). However, different authors have various recommendations on the duration of immobilization ranging from 2 to 6 weeks, 4 to 8 weeks, 6 to 8 weeks, or up to 2 to 3 months (1–6). After initial immobilization, if there is improvement in symptoms, you can progress to custom orthotics or arch support (1,2,4).

Braces and orthoses are used in an attempt to limit the progression of hindfoot valgus and AAFD (1–4,6,11). They act to hold the calcaneus in a neutral position, support the medial arch, prevent further deformity, and reduce symptoms (1–4,7). The purpose is to "alleviate stress on the tibialis posterior; to make gait more efficient by holding the hindfoot fixed; and thirdly to prevent progression of deformity" (3). The importance of the orthoses is further explained by the following: In patients with a normal arch, the tibialis posterior is selectively activated with barefoot resisted foot adduction. However, in patients with an arch deformity, arch supporting orthoses and shoes are required to selectively target the tibialis posterior during exercises (7). Ankle-foot orthoses have also been demonstrated to reduce pain and improve function in patients with this condition (6).

There does not appear to be consensus on when to choose a foot versus an ankle-foot orthotic, or when to choose a custom rather than a prefabricated orthotic. In one study, ankle-foot orthoses were used if pain had persisted for more than 3 months, and a foot orthotic was used for pain lasting less than 3 months (9). Proper supportive footwear, either in the form of lace up shoes, boots, or running

TABLE 34.1: Stages of Healing

Acute	Proliferation	Maturation	Recovery	Remodeling
Immediately after injury Acute inflammatory response	1 to 3 weeks Fibroblast invasion Collagen deposition	3 to 4 weeks Collagen maturation Final scar tissue formation	4 to 8 weeks Exposure of new collagen to normal stresses	6 to 12 months Final maturation and remodeling
Rest Ice Compression Elevation	Ankle support Immobilization	Gentle stretching Mobilization	Begin return to play protocol	Continue activities

shoes with motion control, are also recommended for isolation of posterior tibial tendon, as noted above (1,3,6,11). Therefore, a reasonable approach is if simple orthotics and shoes can not control mechanics or pain progresses despite their use, ankle-foot orthoses can then be used (6). Use of orthotics can then be combined with exercises to "unload" the tendon and strengthen the ankle (11).

Therapeutic Modalities

As described above, ice is commonly used in the acute setting, however little research exists to support its use (1). Ice is believed to reduce inflammation, possibly by reducing blood flow and the metabolic rate, which in turn may reduce swelling and inflammation (5,6). NSAIDs are also commonly used to control symptoms; specifically pain, swelling, and inflammation (4,6). However, there is concern both in acute and chronic settings about blocking the inflammatory process with NSAIDs. Acutely it may be detrimental to healing, and chronically there is not an active inflammatory process (6).

Ultrasound use varies practitioner to practitioner. Its use is not supported by the literature for this condition, but it has been used in other tendon disorders (5,6). Additional studies are needed to investigate potential benefits, but it is theorized to have a "thermal and mechanical effect on the target tissues resulting in an increased local metabolism, circulation, extensibility of connective tissue and tissue regeneration" (6). Conversely, Rees et al states there is little evidence supporting its efficacy (5). No additional studies were discovered to give recommendations on the use of other thermal modalities or electrical stimulation in the setting of posterior tibial tendinopathy.

Manual Therapy

Various soft tissue and massage techniques have been suggested as therapy in tendon and muscle disorders, however evidence is lacking in support of their use (1). Recommendations for deep tissue massage, friction massage, and soft tissue mobilization have been found in the literature. However, there is no evidence for improvements in outcomes such as pain or function (6). Friction massage was explored in a Cochrane review, where two randomized, controlled trials showed no efficacy (5). Recommendations for joint mobilization of the ankle (talo-crural) and subtalar joint also exist in textbooks and in theory may be beneficial for restoration of normal joint range of motion (ROM) and arthrokinematics, especially ankle dorsiflexion, but definitive evidence to support their use is lacking.

Therapeutic Exercise

As acute symptoms are resolving and the tendon begins to heal, passive stretching of the calf musculature (Figure 34.1), especially the gastrocnemius/soleus, is recommended (4,6,11). In posterior tibialis dysfunction, the calcaneus is held in a valgus position, leading to shortening of calf musculature, which is why these stretches are an important part of the rehabilitation program (7).

Once a ROM and flexibility program has been implemented and improvement has been demonstrated, it is important to progress to strengthening exercises for the tibialis posterior (6,8). Many patients can have diffuse ankle weakness after an injury, leading to recommendations for a complete ankle strengthening program while maintaining flexibility (2,6,9). Home exercise programs or formal physical therapy can achieve this goal, but it is most important that patients be educated in regards to their condition, the length of treatment, and use of orthotics and exercise programs (6,7). A model has been proposed for this called the EdUReP model. The acronym stands for patient Education, Unloading of the tendon (orthoses), followed by Reloading of the tendon (exercises), and Prevention of future injury (7,12). Written protocols highlighting the above components for patients will likely be helpful (11).

There are many types of exercises which can be employed to strengthen the entire ankle complex. Strengthening of the posterior tibialis, peroneals, anterior tibialis, and gastroc-soleus complex can be achieved by using resistance bands (Figure 34.2), along with

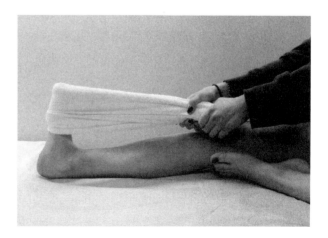

FIGURE 34.1: Calf stretches.

functional activities such as heel raises (Figure 34.3) and toe walking (9).

Concentric and eccentric exercises have been studied, and when combined with orthoses, have been shown to reduce pain and improve function (6). Eccentric exercises provide a larger load to the tendon with less muscle activation, and are performed by active lengthening of tendon (5,7). Kulig et al. found that activation of the posterior tibialis muscle was best accomplished by

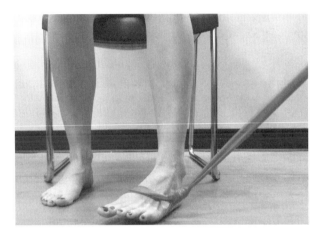

FIGURE 34.2: Resisted foot adduction for selective posterior tibialis strengthening.

resisted foot adduction exercises (Figure 34.2), although heel raises and foot supination exercises also showed good muscle activation when measured by MRI (13). For this reason, an eccentric exercise for the posterior tibialis would be active resistance of foot abduction (7) and concentric exercises would include active foot adduction against resistance (5). Resistance bands are commonly used for these progressive resistive exercises (PREs) (11).

Three different studies have compared strengthening programs. In a study by Alvarez et al, there was a three-treatment phase protocol consisting of orthoses and progressive strengthening. Patients were educated and given a home exercise program including resistance band exercises (dorsiflexion, inversion and eversion performed eccentrically), which progressed to heel raises, toe walking, and heel cord stretching. This treatment program resulted in statistically significant improvements in pain scores, ability to painlessly perform single leg heel raise, increase in distance ambulated, and concentric and eccentric strength in inversion, eversion, plantar, and dorsiflexion (9). In a study by Kulig et al, a 10 week program of orthotics, progressive eccentric tendon exercises and calf stretching, both performed twice daily, showed significant improvements in function both initially and at

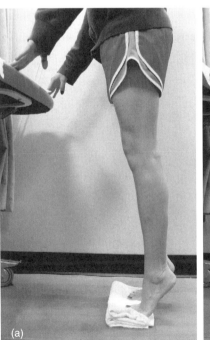
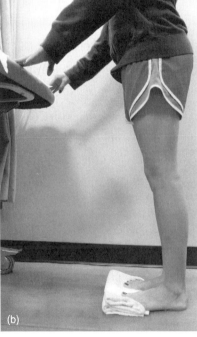

FIGURE 34.3: Stand facing a wall with only your toes on a rolled or folded towel (a). Use the wall for balance, perform a heel raise (b), then slowly lower yourself down to the starting position.

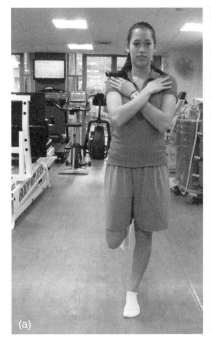 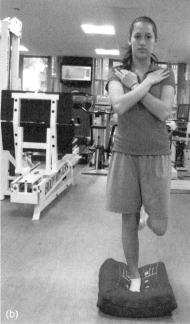 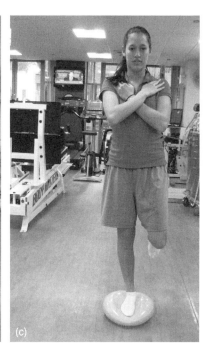

FIGURE 34.4: Proprioceptive exercises: single leg stance activities on progressively unstable surfaces from a to c.

6 months post treatment (11). Another study by the same lead author compared a 12 week program of orthoses and stretching (O+S), O+S plus eccentric exercises, and O+S plus concentric exercises. They found that foot functional index scores decreased and pain after 5 minute walk test significantly decreased in all groups, while the eccentric exercise group showed the greatest improvements (7). Therefore, there is good, quality research that supports the use of orthotics combined with an exercise program, and eccentric exercises targeted at the posterior tibialis may be most effective. Once strength is restored, proprioceptive (Figure 34.4) and eventually functional training exercises can be utilized to complete the rehabilitation program.

Specialized Techniques

There have been suggestions in the literature for the use of tape to support the medial-longitudinal arch maintenance, which would simulate the use of foot orthoses, but no formal study has investigated this treatment. Therefore, we are unable to make any firm conclusions regarding the use of kinesiology taping for posterior tibial tendinopathy.

SUMMARY

Posterior tibialis tendonitis or tendinopathy is thought to be a common condition, however the exact incidence is unknown. While the PRICE protocol and NSAIDs are commonly used, there is little evidence to support their use. Therapeutic modalities, such as ultrasound or even cryotherapy, and manual therapy techniques require further investigation to determine their roles. The best available evidence supports the use of orthotics, stretching of the calf musculature, and progressive ankle strengthening exercises, especially eccentric exercises, for the treatment of posterior tibial tendinopathy.

SAMPLE CASE

A 36-year-old female presents with medial ankle pain over the past 3 weeks. She has no significant past medical history or past surgical history, and her only medication is a levonorgestrel intrauterine device. She is an ICU nurse who has been training for her second marathon. She does not recall any specific traumatic or inciting event, but notes that the pain is aggravated with prolonged walking and standing. She is frustrated because the pain has significantly affected her training regimen, since she is unable to run properly and has worsening pain the longer she runs. Physical examination is notable for medial ankle swelling and tenderness to palpation along posterior tibial tendon, most severe behind the medial malleolus. She has pain with active or resisted inversion and passive eversion of her foot. She is able to perform a single-leg heel rise only twice on the affected side (pain-limited) versus 20 times on the unaffected side. Neurovascular exam is unremarkable.

SAMPLE THERAPY PRESCRIPTION

Discipline: Physical therapy.

Diagnosis: Posterior tibialis tendonitis.

Problem list: Pain limited strength and ROM.

Precautions: Weight-bearing as tolerated (WBAT).

Frequency of visits: 2 to 3x/week.

Duration of treatment: 1 month, but may require up to 2 to 3 months of treatment.

Treatment:

1. *Modalities:* Cryotherapy PRN

2. *Manual therapy:* none

3. *Therapeutic exercise:* Passive stretching of gastrocnemius/soleus complex and gentle posterior tibialis tendon stretch to tolerance. PREs for the ankle and foot (abductors/adductors, dorsiflexors/plantarflexors, invertors/evertors). Eccentric exercises for the posterior tibialis. Progress to proprioceptive exercises (e.g., single leg stance activities) and other functional activities, even sport-specific activities as condition improves

4. *Specialized treatments:* consider trial of taping for medial arch support, if beneficial consider pre-fabricated orthotic for arch support.

5. *Patient education:* Home exercise program.

Goals: Decrease pain and swelling. Improve strength for inversion, eversion, plantar and dorsiflexion. Improve ability to perform single leg heel rise without pain.

Reevaluation: In 4 to 6 weeks by the referring physician.

REFERENCES

1. Edwards MR, Jack C, Singh SK. Tibialis posterior dysfunction. *Curr Orthop.* 2008;22:185–192.
2. Gluck GS, Heckman DS, Parekh SG. Tendon disorders of the foot and ankle, Part 3. *Am J Sports Med.* 2010;38(10):2133–2144.
3. Kohls-Gatzoulis J, Angel JC, Singh D, Haddad F, Livingstone J, Berry G. Tibialis posterior dysfunction: A common and treatable cause of adult acquired flatfoot. *BMJ.* 2004;329:1328–1333.
4. Geideman WM, Johnson JE. Posterior tibial tendon dysfunction. *J Orthop Sports Phys Ther.* 2000;30(2):68–77.
5. Rees JD, Wilson AM, Wolman RL. Current concepts in the management of tendon disorders. *Rheumatology.* 2206;45:508–521.
6. Bowring B, Chockalingam N. Conservative treatment of tibialis posterior tendon dysfunction—a review. *The Foot.* 2010; 20:18–26.
7. Kulig K, Reischl SF, Pomrantz AB, et al. Nonsurgical management of posterior tibial tendon dysfunction with orthoses and resistive exercise: A randomized controlled trial. *Phys Ther.* 2009;89(1):26–37.
8. Sherman KP. The foot in sport. *Br J Sports Med.* 1999;33:6-13.
9. Alvarez RG, Marini A, Schmitt C, Saltzman CL. Stage I and II posterior tibial tendon dysfunction treated by a structured nonoperative management protocol: an orthoses and exercise program. *Foot Ankle Int.* 2006;27(1):2–8.
10. Renstrom PAFH, Konradsen L. Ankle ligament injuries. *Br J Sports Med.* 1997;31:11–20.
11. Kulig K, Lederhaus ES, Reischl S, Arya S, Bashford G. Effect of eccentric exercise program for early tibialis posterior tendinopathy. *Foot Ankle Int.* 2009;30(9):877–885.
12. Davenport TE, Kulig K, Matharu Y, Blanco CE. The EdUReP model for nonsurgical management of tendinopathy. *Phys Ther.* 2005;85:1093–1103.
13. Kulig K, Burnfield JM, Requejo SM, Sperry M, Terk M. Selective activation of tibialis posterior: evaluation by magnetic resonance imaging. *Med Sci Sports Exerc.* 2004;36(5):862–867.

Plantar Fasciitis

Carly Day, Stuart Willick, and Kim Cohee

INTRODUCTION

Plantar fasciitis is a common cause of foot pain in both active and sedentary individuals. It is estimated that one million patient visits per year are due to plantar fasciitis. Of these, 62 percent presented to primary care providers and 31 percent to orthopedic surgeons. The peak age of incidence is between 40 and 60 years old (1). Risk factors for plantar fasciitis include obesity, work-related weight bearing, reduced ankle dorsiflexion, and pes planus (2,3). The condition can also be seen frequently in runners and jumping athletes. The plantar fascia is composed of the central plantar aponeurosis surrounded by weaker medial and lateral components. It serves to protect the plantar aspect of the foot, support the longitudinal arches of the foot, and assist in dynamic shock absorption. The plantar aponeurosis originates posteriorly on the medial tubercle of the calcaneus and divides distally to enclose the digital flexor tendons (4). Histologically, plantar fasciitis demonstrates myxoid degeneration and collagen necrosis similar to tendinopathy (5). For this reason, some practitioners now prefer to use the term plantar fasciopathy.

Patients with plantar fasciitis often report the gradual onset of medial, plantar heel pain that is worse first thing in the morning. Early in the disease process they will note a decrease in pain with activity and as the condition progresses the pain may increase with continued weight-bearing activity.

Key elements of the physical examination include inspection of foot type (e.g., pes planus), palpation, range of motion (ROM), and a thorough neurovascular examination. Patients usually demonstrate tenderness to palpation at the medial tubercle of the calcaneus and possibly along the proximal, medial region of the plantar fascia. Pain typically increases with passive dorsiflexion of the toes or when the patient actively plantarflexes the ankle while standing (6).

Evaluation with radiographs rarely affects the decision making but should be considered in patients who fail initial conservative management. Heel spurs occur in 15% of asymptomatic subjects and 65% of symptomatic subjects (3), and their clinical relevance continues to be debated. Ultrasound of the plantar fascia shows a thickened, hypoechoic region. Magnetic resonance imaging is not necessary, but it can be used to rule out other causes of heel pain if the history or examination is atypical, as well as ruling out plantar fascia rupture.

PLANTAR FASCIITIS

- Common musculoskeletal problem with peak incidence between 40 and 60 years old

- Usually presents as plantar heel pain that is worse with the first few steps in the morning

- Physical examination should include inspection of the medial longitudinal arch while standing, palpation of the medial tubercle of the calcaneus, ankle ROM to assess for reduced dorsiflexion, and a neurovascular examination to rule out other causes

- Advanced imaging studies such as MRI or ultrasound may not be necessary, but can be used to rule out other sources of heel pain

THE REHABILITATION PROGRAM

The natural history of plantar fasciitis is very favorable, with prior research suggesting that 80 percent of patients will have resolution of symptoms in 12 months (7). Initial treatment involves ice, nonsteroidal anti-inflammatories (NSAIDs), and activity modification, although there are no randomized controlled trials evaluating these common treatments in isolation. The patient can also be referred to a physical therapist to be treated with the strategies described in the remainder of this chapter.

Therapeutic Modalities

Traditional modalities such as ultrasound, laser, and electrical stimulation have been studied. Small studies suggest laser irradiation and ultrasound were no better than placebo in patients with plantar fasciitis (8). Iontophoresis with 4% dexamethasone was shown to provide greater improvement of symptoms at 2 weeks, but no difference versus placebo at 4 weeks (9). Therefore, this may be of some benefit to athletes who need a quicker return to activity. Cryotherapy, such as use of an ice pack, ice bath, or ice massage, remains an option for symptomatic management of the condition, although research has not specifically investigated its effectiveness for treating plantar fasciitis. Some physical therapists (PTs) also recommend freezing a golf ball, placing it on the floor, and rolling the plantar aspect of the foot over it with self-applied pressure to their tolerance. Therefore, it serves as a home modality and a form of self-massage. Overall, the evidence is very limited for or against the use of therapeutic modalities to treat plantar fasciitis.

A less traditional modality, extracorporeal shock wave (ECSW) therapy has been proposed to inhibit pain receptors and stimulate healing of soft tissues (10). Many studies suggest there is no significant difference in pain relief from ECSW therapy compared to placebo (10–13). However, there is one randomized controlled trial that shows improvement of pain, but not in activity level, in patients undergoing ECSW therapy versus placebo at 8 weeks (14).

Manual Therapy

Manual therapy is not a routine treatment for plantar fasciitis and lacks good quality evidence to support its use. Massage and soft tissue mobilization may provide the patient with symptomatic relief. Counter-strain (positional release) techniques have been shown to improve pain for 48 hours but the effect did not persist at 6 days (15). In a randomized controlled trial, chiropractic adjustments of the foot and ankle combined with stretching demonstrated similar improvement in plantar fasciitis symptoms compared to orthotics in the majority of outcome measures (8). There

is anecdotal evidence that suggests improved subtalar and mid-foot mobility may help relieve symptoms associated with plantar fasciitis. In addition, a stretching program, discussed in detail in the next section, may be complemented by joint mobilizations to improve ankle dorsiflexion ROM.

Therapeutic Exercise

Stretching is a very important aspect of plantar fasciitis rehabilitation. When compared to controls, patients with plantar fasciitis have significantly restricted ankle/foot ROM (16). Working with a physical therapist assures that stretches are being performed correctly and that improvement in muscle length and joint mobility is occurring at an appropriate rate.

Cadaver studies demonstrate that maximal stretch is obtained with combined ankle and metatarsophalangeal (MTP) dorsiflexion. Stretching in mid-tarsal abduction or forefoot varus did not improve the stretch (17). Randomized controlled trials have confirmed the effectiveness of plantar specific stretching compared to various other treatments (18–20). This stretch should be performed in a seated position with the affected leg crossed over the contralateral leg. One hand should be placed distal to the MTP joints and pull the toes into dorsiflexion with the other hand palpating the plantar fascia to confirm appropriate stretch. Additional stretch may be accomplished by applying counter-traction on the heel (Figure 35.1). Patients should hold this stretch for 10 seconds, repeat it 10 times, and perform this routine three times daily. Other common exercises include

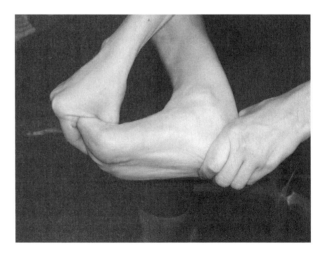

FIGURE 35.1: Optimal plantar fasciitis stretching technique.

self-massage with a golf ball or tennis ball (Figure 35.2) and Achilles tendon stretching using a wall or stairs (21,22).

Therapeutic exercises should also include strengthening exercises, especially of the intrinsic foot muscles. These muscles are optimally exerted using short foot exercises. These are accomplished by standing on a towel and using the muscles on the plantar aspect of the foot to bring the towel closer without significantly curling the toes (Figure 35.3). Electromyography (EMG) data demonstrates that short foot exercises lead to greater activation of the abductor hallucis when compared to toes curls. Also, the standing position is better than sitting (23). In addition to ankle and foot strengthening, kinetic chain analysis may reveal other biomechanical problems such as proximal muscle weakness or poor neuromuscular control of core muscles (e.g., weakness of the hip abductors, extensors, or external rotators). Addressing lower limb biomechanical dysfunction through the use of therapeutic exercises appears logical, but the body of literature doesn't definitely support this approach.

Specialized Techniques

Foot orthoses are commonly used to treat plantar fasciitis. They can provide arch support and/or elevate and cushion the heel. Most evidence suggests that prefabricated orthoses are just as effective as custom molded inserts for symptomatic treatment of plantar fasciitis (24,25). Magnetic coils in the insoles have also been utilized, but have not been proven to provide any additional benefit (26,27).

Night splinting of the affected foot is commonly performed in patients with plantar fasciitis. The goal is to decrease passive plantar flexion during sleep and to prevent the plantar fascia and Achilles tendon from shortening. The maintained length should decrease pain with the first step in the morning. Some splints provide additional MTP dorsiflexion with a toe wedge. Studies show mixed results with two crossover studies demonstrating benefit (28,29) but a larger trial showing no benefit when adding night splints to standard conservative therapy (30). A recent randomized, controlled study showed that dynamic night splints provide significant improvement in pain and function at 12 weeks (31). Patients often complain of discomfort and difficulty sleeping with night splints which negatively affects patient compliance. This may explain the mixed results seen in prior research studies.

Low-Dye taping is a option for the treatment of plantar fasciitis and appears to provide early pain reduction. The taping is thought to provide a supinating force to decrease subtalar pronation during gait (32). There does appear to be a positive effect of low-Dye taping in reducing pain during the first week of treatment (33,34). Calcaneal taping also provides a decrease in pain when compared to sham taping or stretching at one week (35).

Acupuncture is a another complementary treatment occasionally used for plantar fasciitis. In one study, patients noticed improvement in morning pain and overall pain at 1 month when receiving treatment at acupoint PC7 compared to placebo acupoint Hegu (LI4) (36).

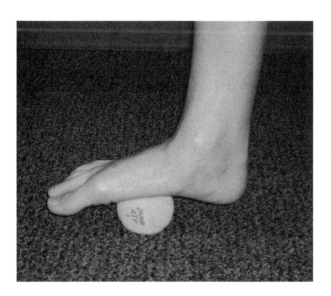

FIGURE 35.2: Self-massage with tennis ball.

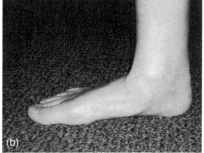

FIGURE 35.3a: Normal foot.

FIGURE 35.3b: Short foot exercise for intrinsic foot muscle strengthening.

SUMMARY

Plantar fasciitis is a very common cause of plantar heel pain. Typical presentation includes plantar heel pain that is worse with the first few steps in the morning. Initial treatment should include ice, NSAIDs, and activity modification. The patient may then work on plantar fascia and Achilles stretching as well as self-massage and strengthening exercises. Other treatment options to consider are foot orthoses, night splints, and ECSW therapy. The natural history of plantar fasciitis is very favorable and the majority have clinical improvement within 12 months. Patients rarely require surgical management (37).

SAMPLE CASE

A 42-year-old female nurse presents to clinic complaining of 1 month of right heel pain. She states that the pain is worse in the morning and then usually improves over the course of the day. Recently, it has started to bother her at work. She denies any trauma to her feet and does not have any contralateral symptoms. A review of systems is otherwise negative and she has no medical problems. The patient is taking occasional anti-inflammatory medications for pain. Physical examination demonstrates a moderately overweight female. The right foot has no swelling and there is tenderness to palpation at the medial tubercle of the calcaneus. Strength and sensation are intact but the patient has decreased passive ankle dorsiflexion bilaterally.

 SAMPLE THERAPY PRESCRIPTION

Discipline: Physical therapy.

Diagnosis: Right plantar fasciitis.

Problem list: Decreased ankle dorsiflexion.

Precautions: None.

Frequency of visits: 1x/week.

Duration of treatment: 4 to 6 weeks.

Treatment:

1. *Modalities:* cryotherapy and possibly iontophoresis

2. *Manual therapy:* Massage or soft tissue mobilization (STM), myofascial release (MFR), positional release to plantar fascia if needed for additional symptomatic management; joint mobilization if needed to complement ROM exercises

3. *Therapeutic exercise:* Active/active-assisted and passive range of motion (A/AA/PROM) exercises, stretching of plantar fascia and Achilles tendon, strengthening of the lower limb and intrinsic foot musculature. Kinetic chain evaluation

4. *Specialized treatments:* trial low-Dye taping, if beneficial consider prefabricated foot orthoses

5. *Patient education:* home exercise program

Goals: Decrease pain and increase ROM. Increase tolerance of work activities. Progressive return to exercise.

Reevaluation: In 4 to 6 weeks by referring physician if not improved.

REFERENCES

1. Riddle DL, Schappert SM. Volume of ambulatory care visits and patterns of care for patients diagnosed with plantar fasciitis: A national study of medical doctors. *Foot Ankle Int.* 2004;25(5):303–310.
2. Riddle DL, Pulisic M, Pidcoe P, Johnson RE. Risk factors for plantar fasciitis: A matched case-control study. *JBJS.* 2003;85:872–877.
3. Prichasuk S, Subhadrabandhu T. The relationship of pes planus and calcaneal spur to plantar heel pain. *Clin Orthop Relat Res.* 1994;306:192–196.
4. Moore KL, Agur AMR, Dalley AF. *Essential Clinical Anatomy,* 3rd ed. Philadelphia, PA: Lippincott Williams & Wilkins; 2006.
5. Lemont H, Ammirati KM, Usen N. Plantar fasciitis: A degenerative process (fasciosis) without inflammation. *J Am Podiatr Med Assoc.* 2003;93(3):234–237.
6. Cole C, Seto C, Gazewood J. Plantar Fasciitis: evidence-based review of diagnosis and therapy. *Am Fam Physician.* 2005;72(11):2237–2242.
7. Buchbinder R. Plantar fasciitis. *NEJM* 2004;350(21):2159–2166.
8. Stuber K, Kristmanson K. Conservative therapy for plantar fasciitis: A narrative review of randomized controlled trials. *J Can Chiropr Assoc.* 2006;50(2):118–133.

9. Gudeman SD, Eisele SA, Heidt RS, Colosimo AJ, Stroupe AL. Treatment of plantar fasciitis by iontophoresis of 0.4% dexamethasone: A randomized, double-blind, placebo-controlled study. *AJSM*. 1997;25(3):312–316.

10. Speed CA, Nichols D, Wies J, Humphreys H, Richards C, Burnet S, Hazleman BL. Extracorporeal shock wave therapy for plantar fasciitis: A double blind randomised controlled trial. *J Ortho Research*. 2003;21(5):937–940.

11. Buchbinder R, Ptasznik R, Gordon J, Buchanan J, Prabaharan V, Forbes A. Ultrasound-guided extracorporeal shock wave therapy for plantar fasciitis: A randomized controlled trial. *JAMA* 2002;288(11):1364–1372.

12. Chuckpai B, Berkson EM, Theodore GH. Extracorporeal shock wave for chronic proximal plantar fasciitis: 225 patients with results and outcome predictors. *J Foot Ankle Surg*. 2009;48(2):148–155.

13. Haake M, Buch M, Schoellner C, et al. Extracorporeal shock wave therapy for plantar fasciitis: randomized controlled multicentre trial. *BMJ*. 2003;327:75.

14. Ogden JA, Alvarez R, Levitt R, Cross GL, Marlow M. Shock wave therapy for chronic proximal plantar fasciitis. *Clin Orthop Relat Res*. 2001;387:47–59.

15. Wynne MM, Burns JM, Eland DC, Conatser RR, Howell JN. Effect of counterstrain on stretch reflexes, Hoffman reflexes, and clinical outcomes in subjects with plantar fasciitis. *JAOA*. 2006;106(9):547–556.

16. Kibbler WB, Goldberg C, Chandler TJ. Functional biomechanical deficits in running athletes with plantar fasciitis. *AJSM*. 1991;19(1):66–71.

17. Flannigan RM, Nawoczenski DA, Chen L, Wu H, DiGiovanni BF. The influence of foot position on stretching of the plantar fascia. *Foot Ankle Int*. 2007;28(7):815–822.

18. Digiovanni BF, Nawoczenski DA, Lintal ME, et al. Tissue-specific plantar fascia-stretching exercise enhances outcomes in patients with chronic heel pain: A prospective, randomized study. *JBJS*. 2003;85:1270–1277.

19. Digiovanni BF, Nawoczenski DA, Malay DP, et al. Plantar fascia-specific stretching exercise improves outcomes in patients with chronic plantar fasciitis: A prospective clinical trial with two-year follow-up. *JBJS*. 2006;88:1775–1781.

20. Rompe JD, Cacchio A, Weil L, et al. Plantar fascia-specific stretching versus radial shock-wave therapy as initial treatment of plantar fasciopathy. *JBJS*. 2010;92:2514–2522.

21. Brukner P, Khan K. *Clinical Sports Medicine*, 3rd ed. Australia: McGraw-Hill; 2006.

22. Young CC, Rutherford DS, Niedfeldt MW. Treatment of plantar fasciitis. *Am Fam Physician*. 2001;63(3):467–474.

23. Jung Dy, Ki, MH, Koh EK, Kwon OY, Cynn HS, Lee WH. A comparison in the muscle activity of the abductor hallucis and the medial longitudinal arch angle during toe curl and short foot exercises. *Phys Ther Sport*. 2011;12(1):30–35.

24. Baldassin V, Gomes CR, Beraldo PS. Effectiveness of prefabricated and customized foot orthoses made from low-cost foam for noncomplicated plantar fasciitis: A randomized controlled trial. *Arch Phys Med Rehabil*. 2009;90:701–706.

25. Landorf KB, Keenan A-M, Herbert RD. Effectiveness of foot orthoses to treat plantar fasciitis: A randomized trial. *Arch Intern Med*. 2006;166:1305–1310.

26. Caselli MA, Clark N, Lazarus S, Velez Z, Venegas L. Evaluation of magnetic foil and PPT Insoles in the treatment of heel pain. *J Am Podiatr Med Assoc*. 1997;87(1):11–16.

27. Winemiller MH, Billow RG, Laskowski ER, Harmsen WS. Effect of magnetic versus sham-magnetic insoles on plantar heel pain: long-term follow-up. *Foot Ankle Int*. 1994;15:97–102.

28. Powell M, Post WR, Keener J, Wearden S. Effective treatment of chronic plantar fasciitis with dorsiflexion night splints: a crossover prospective randomized outcome study. *Foot Ankle Int*. 1998;19:10–18.

29. Batt ME, Tanji JL, Skattum N. Plantar fasciitis: a prospective randomized clinical trial of the tension night splint. *Clin J Sport Med*. 1996;6(3):158–162.

30. Probe RA, Baca M, Adams R, Preece C. Night splint treatment for plantar fasciitis: A prospective randomised study. *Clin Orthop*. 1999;368:190–195.

31. Sheridan L, Lopez A, Perez A, John MM, Willis FB, Shanmugam R. Plantar fasciopathy treated with dynamic splinting: A randomized controlled trial. *J Am Podiatr Med Assoc*. 2010;100(3):161–165.

32. Russo SJ, Chipchase LS. The effect of low-Dye taping on peak plantar pressures of normal feet during gait. Australian Journal of Physiotherapy 2001; 47: 239–244.

33. Landorf KB, Radford JA, Keenan A-M, Redmond AC. Effectiveness of low-Dye taping for the short-term management of plantar fasciitis. Journal of the American Podiatric Medical Association 2005; 95(6): 525–530.

34. Radford JA, Landorf KB, Buchbinder R, Cook C. Effectiveness of low-Dye taping for the short-term treatment of plantar heel pain: A randomised trial. BMC Musculoskeletal Disorders 2006; **7:**64 doi:10.1186/1471-2474-7-64.

35. Hyland MR, Webber-Gaffney A, Cohen L, Lichtman PT. Randomized controlled trial of calcaneal taping, sham taping, and plantar fascia stretching for the short-term management of plantar heel pain. *J Orthop Sports Phys Ther*. 2006;36(6):364–371.

36. Zheng SP, Yip T-P, Li Q-S. Acupuncture treatment for plantar fasciitis: A randomized controlled trial with six months follow-up. *Evid Based Complement Alternat Med*. 2011;2011:154108.

37. Davis PF, Severud E, Baxter DE. Painful heel syndrome: Results of nonoperative treatment. *Foot Ankle Int*. 1994;15(10):531–535.

Other Ankle Disorders

Rosalyn T. Nguyen, Elizabeth T. Nguyen, and Smita Rao

INTRODUCTION

Other important ankle conditions that commonly affect athletes and active individuals include high ankle sprains, medial gastrocnemius muscle injuries as well as peroneal tendon disorders.

HIGH ANKLE SPRAINS

High ankle sprains, which represent approximately 10% of all ankle sprains, refer to injuries to the tibiofibular syndesmosis ligaments (1). Syndesmosis sprains are seen in various sports, including skiing, football, soccer, and hockey (2). A historically underdiagnosed condition, high ankle injuries present more indolently than other common ankle sprains, but tend to be more disabling due to the limited blood supply and difficulty maintaining the ankle immobilized to facilitate healing (3,4). As a result, rehabilitation and recovery often occur over a more protracted period of time. The classic mechanism of injury, as highlighted in Table 36.1, is forced external rotation of the tibia with excessive dorsiflexion and eversion of the ankle. Patients typically

TABLE 36.1: Summary of the Key Clinical Features and Diagnostic Approach for High-Ankle Sprains, Medial Gastrocnemius Strains, and Peroneal Tendinopathies

	High ankle sprains	Medial gastrocnemius strains (tennis leg)	Peroneal tendinopathy
Key points	• Represents 10% of all ankle sprains • Develops indolently • Recovery takes place over a more prolonged period of time	• Common in middle aged, weekend warriors • Most frequent site of injury is the musculotendinous junction	• Can be associated with chronic lateral ankle pain and instability • Most common site of pain is posterior to the lateral malleolus
Mechanism of injury	• Forced external rotation of the tibia with excessive ankle dorsiflexion and eversion	• Eccentric contraction with knee in extension and ankle in dorsiflexion	• Repetitive or forced ankle inversion injuries, supinated foot biomechanics, sudden dorsiflexion of a plantarflexed-inverted foot
Key elements of the physical exam	• Tenderness along the distal tibiofibular joint and anterior tibiofibular ligament • Swelling may not be present • Squeeze test positive • External rotation stress test positive	• Swelling and tenderness to palpation at the site of injury • Intact Achilles tendon • Painful passive dorsiflexion and active plantarflexion • Difficulty performing single-leg toe raises on the affected side	• Swelling and tenderness along the tendon • Pain with active eversion and dorsiflexion against resistance
Imaging	• X-ray if high suspicion of associated fractures	• Ultrasound or MRI to assess extent of tear, associated fluid collection and/or hematoma	• Ultrasound or MRI to assess for fluid, tendon thickening, and/or tears

report pain with ambulation, particularly during the push-off phase of gait (4).

Key elements of the physical exam for syndesmosis injuries, as well as for gastrocnemius strains and peroneal tendon disorders, include inspection, palpation, range of motion (ROM), strength, neurovascular testing, and gait analysis. Palpation of the distal tibiofibular joint, including the anterior tibiofibular ligament, may reveal tenderness. Swelling may not be present. The entire length of the tibia and fibula should be palpated to evaluate for a proximal fibula fracture, or Maisonneuve fracture, which is associated with syndesmosis injuries (1). ROM may be globally decreased. The squeeze test is positive when pain is elicited distally at the syndesmosis upon compression of the tibia and fibula at the mid-calf. The external rotation stress test is positive when dorsiflexion and external rotation of the foot triggers pain. Radiographs may be useful in evaluating the extent of injury, as high ankle sprains may be associated with medial malleolar fractures. Imaging may reveal widening of the tibiofibular clear space, which may necessitate surgery (5). Conservative management and rehabilitation is appropriate for grade I–II injuries. Grade III–IV injuries and associated injuries (e.g., dislocation, fracture, ligament rupture, and/or neurovascular compromise) require surgical intervention. Inaccurate diagnosis may delay recovery and contribute to chronic ankle pain and instability (6). Several studies have demonstrated a large variation in time required for return to play. One study of hockey players found that return to full activity ranged from 0 to 137 days, with a mean of 45 days (7).

MEDIAL GASTROCNEMIUS INJURIES

Injury to the medial head of the gastrocnemius muscle is commonly termed "tennis leg" for its prevalence in this sport. Calf muscle injuries most often affect the medial gastrocnemius muscle, as this particular area is subject to the greatest amount of tension. Tennis leg is frequently seen in the middle aged and periodically active patient, or "weekend warrior" (8,9). This injury occurs in activities that involve a sudden shift in direction, such as tennis, hill running, sprinting, jumping. Tennis leg has also been reported to occur in namaz praying (10). The most common site of injury is the musculotendinous junction, although strains or tears may occur at any point along the gastrocnemius muscle or tendon (11). Concurrent injury of the soleus muscle or lateral head of the gastrocnemius is less common. Isolated injury of the plantaris

or soleus tendon is rare and may be clinically indistinguishable from tennis leg (12,13). Furthermore, tennis leg may resemble a proximal Achilles tendinopathy (12). The mechanism of injury is eccentric contraction of the gastrocnemius muscle with the knee in full extension and ankle in dorsiflexion (8,9). Patients usually complain of sudden proximal calf pain associated with a snapping sensation, along with swelling within the initial 24 to 48 hours (11,12). Physical exam reveals significant swelling and tenderness to palpation at the site of injury, as well as a potential palpable defect in the medial muscle belly proximal to the musculotendinous junction. The Achilles tendon, on the other hand, should be intact on palpation (9). Patients may also exhibit pain on passive dorsiflexion and active plantarflexion, along with weak plantarflexion and difficulty performing single-leg toe raises on the affected side (8,11). Imaging with ultrasound or MRI is useful in assessing the severity of the tear and excluding other diagnoses (such as deep venous thrombosis). Imaging is also helpful in evaluating the presence of a fluid collection and/or an adjacent hematoma, a poor prognostic factor (11,12). Delayed complications of tears include contractures, scarring, muscle herniation, and eventual functional impairment (11). In one study, mean time for return to baseline activity level was found to be 6 to 7 weeks (12,14).

PERONEAL TENDON DISORDERS

Peroneal tendon disorders include peroneal tendonitis and tenosynovitis, tendon subluxation or dislocation, and tendon tears. They are frequently underdiagnosed etiologies of chronic lateral ankle pain and instability. The peroneal tendons have multiple avascular zones associated with corresponding areas of tendinopathy. The peroneus brevis has an avascular zone at the fibular groove and the peroneus longus at the curve around the lateral malleolus and around the cuboid (15). Repetitive overuse or prolonged activities, especially after a period of relative inactivity, can result in tendon disorders. These disorders include inflammation of the tendon or tendon sheath, interstitial injury, calcification, or thickening of the sheath (16,17). Chronic ankle instability and trauma, including ankle inversion sprains, pressure or tensile forces, and ankle fractures, can also predispose patients to peroneal tendon dysfunction (16,17). Partial or longitudinal split tears occur in the peroneus brevis more commonly than in the peroneus longus (18). Associated risk factors for tears include tendon subluxation, ankle inversion injuries with lateral ankle instability, injury at the fibular groove with superior peroneal retinacular laxity, tendon hypovascularity, and a shallow peroneal groove (16,19–21). The sports associated with tendon subluxation and ruptures include skiing, gymnastics, football, ice-skating, and soccer (17).

Symptoms of peroneal tendon injuries include pain and swelling posterior to the lateral malleolus and lateral ankle or hindfoot. Some may experience a sensation of lateral ankle instability. Decrease in subtalar motion and difficulty walking on uneven ground is possible (17). Snapping or popping may occur with evidence of tendon subluxation during active eversion or ambulation (16). Physical exam findings include tenderness along the peroneal tendons, posterior to the fibula and lateral malleolus and distally along the lateral aspect of the calcaneus (16,22). Foot alignment should be evaluated for the presence of hindfoot varus. Active eversion and passive inversion may elicit pain (17,22). Peroneus longus tendinopathy can result in pain with resisted plantarflexion or passive dorsiflexion of the first ray. Diminished first ray plantar flexion may be seen in peroneus longus tears (16,23,24). The peroneal tunnel compression test assesses for peroneus brevis tears. With the patient seated and knee flexed, the examiner applies pressure over the superior peroneal retinaculum at the retro-malleolar groove. A positive test elicits pain upon resisted dorsiflexion and eversion of a plantar flexed and inverted foot. Assessing the integrity of the lateral ligamentous complex (e.g., anterior drawer and talar tilt tests) is also important, as lateral ankle instability may contribute to peroneal dysfunction. Ultrasound, MRI, or a local anesthetic injection can help confirm the diagnosis (17). MRI remains the standard imaging study to visualize peroneal tendon disorders, evaluate for injuries to the superior peroneal retinaculum, and assess the structural anatomy of the retro-malleolar groove. Ultrasound can detect fluid in the tendon sheath, tendon thickening, tendon tears, and dynamic subluxation (16,25).

THE REHABILITATION PROGRAM

The rehabilitation program should be well structured, tailored to accommodate each patient's needs, and closely supervised by trained health care professionals. While some rehabilitation programs utilize temporal milestones to determine the patient's readiness for progression, other programs use functional criteria (26–28). Both temporal and criterion-based programs include phases similar to the five phases outlined in this book: an acute, post injury phase, followed by a sub-acute phase seeking to restore strength and weight-bearing function, and a final return-to-sports phase (29). Of note, the rehabilitation program discussed in this chapter applies to all three ankle conditions unless otherwise stated.

A key factor for optimal recovery is maintaining interval assessments of the patient to ensure he or she is progressing well. The primary objectives of rehabilitation in the acute, post-injury phase are to afford pain relief, control swelling, facilitate healing, and address co-existing impairments (2). Consequently, the PRICE protocol (protection, relative rest, ice, compression, elevation), along with adequate analgesia, remains an important early intervention. Another important part of treatment is identifying and addressing the underlying etiology. Extrinsic risk factors include repetitive overuse, training errors, tobacco use, poorly fitting footwear, or medication associations. Intrinsic factors include foot alignment and myotendinous imbalances (22).

Anti-inflammatory medications may be helpful, although their use in tendon disorders is currently under study, as animal studies have suggested that these medications may affect tendon healing (30). Judicious use of corticosteroid injections to the tendon sheath may be an option, but the risk of potential tendon rupture is a concern (16). New and innovative treatments are currently undergoing research. Studies are underway to assess the efficacy of platelet-rich plasma and topical nitrates, which are gaining more attention and are currently being used in sports medicine clinics (22).

Joint protection in the form of crutches for immediate nonweight bearing and/or a walking boot may be useful. Duration of immobilization should be limited but will largely depend on the severity of the ankle injury, while keeping in mind the potential complications of prolonged disuse (3). Ice, compression wraps, and elevation are effective in reducing edema. Once pain and edema control are optimized, patients undergo the second phase of passive and active stretching and ROM exercises. Early weight bearing should be initiated safely and as tolerated (29). Graduated weight-bearing and progression of therapeutic exercise is predicated on the absence of pain during these activities. This is followed by progressive strength training in the third phase. Individuals begin with isometric training, followed by concentric and finally eccentric exercises. Patients subsequently transition to balance and gait training to prevent development of compensatory mechanisms, which may promote secondary injuries (3). Once individuals achieve pain-free ambulation, they are gradually reintroduced into functional, sport-specific exercises. Maintenance of cardiovascular fitness is imperative throughout the rehabilitation course (4) and can be accomplished with the use of aquatic therapy and low impact aerobic activities. Patients are cleared for return to full sport-specific activity once they achieve full and symmetric ROM and strength, and are able to undergo a full practice session without swelling or pain (3). If the patient fails conservative management or has chronic, recurrent instability or tendon rupture, surgery may be indicated (17,22,31). In syndesmosis sprains, continued surveillance for limited talo-crural dorsiflexion, anterior impingement, and/or heterotopic ossification within the interosseous membrane is recommended.

CAVEATS AND CONSIDERATIONS

While syndesmotic sprains are common in the athletic population, objective evidence to guide decision making in the form of high quality clinical trials investigating specific rehabilitation strategies in this population are lacking. Consequently, general guidelines from other ligament injuries guide the overall structure of the rehabilitation program and return to sport criteria. It is crucial to note that syndesmotic sprains typically require a longer recovery period compared to classic lateral ankle sprains, and rehabilitation should be based on the severity of injury and the demands of the athlete (32).

Therapeutic Modalities

As with most other ankle sprains, cryotherapy is paramount during the early treatment phase in reducing edema. This may be in the form of ice packs, ice massage, and/or cold whirlpool therapy. Combination ice and compression pumps are also useful in minimizing edema (29). Additional modalities utilized to manage pain include transcutaneous electrical nerve stimulation (TENS), ultrasound, iontophoresis, and phonophoresis (4,22), but often cryotherapy is the only modality required to control pain and swelling. Medical acupuncture may also be considered as an adjunct therapy for improved pain management (4).

Manual Therapy

Massage techniques can help with the mobilization of interstitial fluid (9). Manual therapy in the form of joint mobilization may be useful to address pain and/or limited ankle dorsiflexion (33). Posterior talo-crural glides, as well as distal and proximal tibio-fibular joint glides may be indicated in restoring ankle ROM. A recent case report on peroneal injuries indicated that manual therapy in the form of a Maitland grade III lateral calcaneal glide may offer pain relief (34). Additionally, deep transverse friction massage can be administered by the physical therapist to help break up scar tissue (35), but evidence is lacking to support the benefits of this manual therapy technique.

Therapeutic Exercise (With Discussion of Supportive Devices)

In the first few days, the PRICE protocol should be instituted. Joint protection with a splint, cast, or boot immobilizer is appropriate for severe injuries. Less rigid immobilization using a semi-rigid brace (e.g., Aircast, Summit, NJ), stirrup, or ankle taping may be applied for minor injuries (29). Crutches maintain the patient's non-weight bearing status during this period. A walking boot is often prescribed to facilitate a short period of ankle immobilization and assist with progressive weight bearing as tolerated (4).

For syndesmotic sprains, braces with rotational control may be particularly useful (e.g., Malleoloc Brace, Bauerfield Inc., Kennesaw, GA) (32). Similarly, taping may be used for less severe injuries to reduce external rotation. Care should be taken when using orthotic devices to ensure that proximal straps do not squeeze the upper leg and cause distal tibiofibular joint separation (29).

In medial gastrocnemius injuries, bracing the ankle in a position of maximal dorsiflexion for 7 to 10 days may increase the rate of healing, decrease scarring, and maintain normal muscle tension (9,36). For partial or complete ruptures, one article demonstrated that early compression with neoprene cast sleeves (compared to elastic bands) for the first 2 to 4 weeks may promote rapid healing, decrease the extent of hemorrhage, and facilitate early ambulation (8).

For hindfoot varus alignment in peroneal tendon injuries, a lateral heel wedge may be recommended to help realign and off-load the painful peroneal tendons. For forefoot valgus alignment, a lateral forefoot post may be helpful (16).

In phase II, patients engage in ankle ROM exercises, initially within pain-free arcs. Initiating passive and active stretching during this period improves and maintains flexibility. Stretching addresses restrictions in ankle dorsiflexion, which are often noted in individuals

2

with a history of ankle instability. Pedaling on a stationary bicycle or bicycle ergometer may be used to maintain ankle ROM, as well as improve endurance and strength (29). Exercises that can easily be performed in the home setting include towel stretches and drawing the alphabet in the air several times per day (4).

When pain and swelling subside and full ROM is achieved, the patient is ready to progress to the third phase. This phase includes partial weight bearing and strength training. For syndesmosis injuries and tennis leg, a heel lift (1–2 cm) or posterior splint may be used to reduce pain, improve ambulation, and prevent excessive dorsiflexion during the mid-stance phase of walking (12). This is especially important in syndesmosis sprains, as talo-crural joint dorsiflexion results in separation of the distal tibiofibular joint as the wider part of the talus glides posteriorly into the ankle mortise. Heel lift height may be reduced as ambulation progresses.

Patients begin with open chain exercises (e.g., eversion resistance exercises for peroneal injuries) using low resistance bands, cords, or ankle weights performed in all ranges of motion. Concomitantly, bilateral weight bearing activities may be instituted (such as standing on foam or layers of toweling), with progression to unilateral activities. These tasks are followed by closed chain exercises that may include calf raises, calf presses, dumbbell squats, lunges, and step-ups (Figure 36.1) (4,29,37). Progression involves increasing the number of repetitions, increasing resistance and weights, adding step-up height, and incorporating eccentric exercises. Eccentric exercise is the modality of choice particularly in individuals with tendinopathy; however, in peroneal tendinopathy, objective evidence specifically examining the efficacy of eccentric exercise is not available (38).

Individuals advance to the fourth phase of proprioceptive and balance training once they are able to ambulate pain-free and without an antalgic gait pattern. Unilateral stance exercises focus on proprioception, with the free leg moving between flexion, extension, abduction, and adduction (4). The basic strengthening exercises mentioned above (dumbbell squats, lunges, and step-ups) incorporate more challenging proprioceptive exercises, using stability disks, domes (e.g. BOSU fitness ball, Canton, OH), wobble boards, or trampolines (Figure 36.1). A device that may be utilized during this phase is the biomechanical ankle platform system (BAPS) board, which focuses on ROM and strengthening, as well as proprioceptive training (4). Seated BAPS board exercises are performed initially, followed by standing exercises (Figure 36.2). As pain improves,

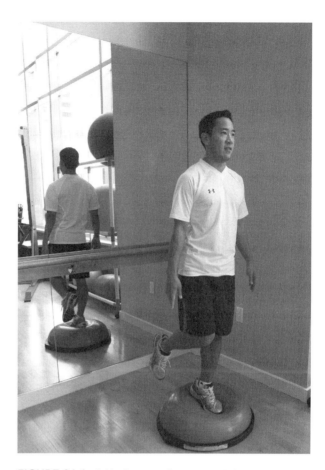

FIGURE 36.1: Calf raises may incorporate balance and proprioceptive training with the use of a Bosu ball. Position the Bosu ball with the dome up. Stand with both feet in the center of the dome. Slowly rise up on your toes as high as you can, contracting your calf muscles. Hold this position for 1 to 2 seconds before slowly lowering the heels. Perform these exercises first with both legs together, then with one leg raised off the dome. As you advance, you can also use dumbbells in each hand for extra weight.

additional weights are added to the BAPS board as tolerated. The Star Excursion Balance Test (SEBT) can be used as an assessment tool, injury predictor, or therapeutic exercise (Figure 36.3). The patient is asked to reach along a premarked "STAR" and the distance covered by the injured and noninjured lower extremity is measured. As therapeutic exercise, the SEBT can be combined with a resistance band and/or performed in front of a mirror for visual feedback.

The final phase involves further gait training and functional sport-specific drills with the goal of returning to full preinjury activity. In addition to continuing the above exercises at a more intense pace, patients begin functional

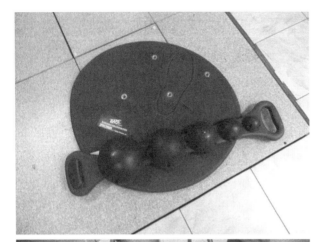

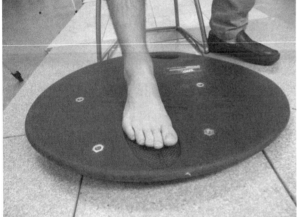

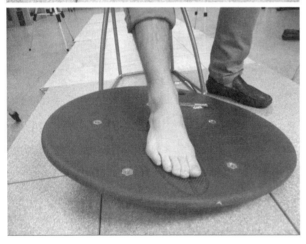

FIGURE 36.2: The biomechanical ankle platform system (BAPS) board with hemispherical attachments (top). In the early stages of rehab, the board should be used with a small hemispherical attachment and the patient nonweight bearing and seated (middle). The use of a larger hemispherical attachment allows the patient to progress through more ROM (bottom). As the patient progresses, the BAPS board can be used for weight bearing and single leg stance exercises. Weights can also be added to increase difficulty.

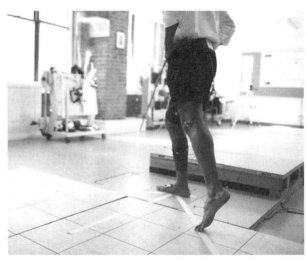

FIGURE 36.3: The Star Excursion Balance Test (SEBT) can be used as an assessment tool, injury predictor, or therapeutic exercise. The patient is asked to reach along a premarked "STAR" and the distance covered by the injured and noninjured lower extremity is measured. As a therapeutic exercise, the SEBT can be combined with a resistance band to make it more challenging and/or performed in front of a mirror for visual feedback.

training (e.g., jumping rope and shuffling) and advance to sport-specific agility drills (29). Therapeutic exercises progress from unilateral low impact activities toward high impact activities such as running, cutting, jumping, and hopping. For football players, this phase would involve high intensity interval training and agility drills that include figure-8s and lateral slides. Plyometrics (e.g., single leg and lateral hops) are incorporated toward the final weeks of rehabilitation with the goal of improving power (29).

Several studies discussed implementing functional criteria for return to sports, comprised of pain free completion of agility drills. These drills may include lateral hopping, sprinting, cutting, or figure-8s (29). Following full integration into all drills without functional limitation, athletes are deemed able to fully participate. In order to prevent ankle ligament injuries, semi-rigid braces have been recommended in high-risk sporting activities, however the efficacy of these devices specific to the prevention of syndesmotic sprains has not been evaluated (39).

Specialized Techniques

Ankle taping may be helpful, although there is no clear evidence supporting its efficacy in regards to the acceleration of healing. Shoes should be assessed and modifications made as necessary (e.g., to decrease calcaneal fibular impingement in peroneal tendon injuries) (17,22). Soft tissue techniques such as trigger point release and/or functional mobilization may be indicated to improve muscle and fascia extensibility. For injuries necessitating surgical intervention, post-operative scar mobility can be improved using scar mobilization techniques.

Home Exercise Program

A home exercise program (HEP) during and beyond completion of the formal rehabilitation program helps prevent exacerbation and recurrence of the condition. The PRICE protocol should be instituted with acute exacerbations. Proper exercise form and biomechanics should be reviewed during physical therapy. Exercises that provoke significant pain should be modified and avoided. Ankle pumps and ankle circles are initially prescribed. Calf stretches, with the knee flexed and extended, are strongly recommended. As patients recover ROM, they may progress to resisted plantarflexion and weight bearing activities. Bilateral and then unilateral heel raises with resistance should be added in the later stages, followed by balance exercises (e.g., using the wobble board if accessible, or other uneven surfaces such as foam or folded towels). Advancement of the program should be supervised by the physical therapist during formal sessions and tolerated well before continuing with these at home. The HEP during the return to sports phase (phase V) should include plyometric exercises (e.g., hopping and jumping).

SUMMARY

Syndesmosis, medial gastrocnemius, and peroneal tendon injuries are fairly common conditions in athletes. Syndesmosis injuries present more indolently and may result in significant debility and prolonged time lost from sports. Medial gastrocnemius injuries, or tennis leg, tend to occur in the middle aged, periodically active individual, and may resemble proximal Achilles tendon strains. Peroneal tendon disorders are often underdiagnosed, can be associated with chronic ankle instability, and should be on the differential diagnoses of lateral ankle pain.

A comprehensive rehabilitation program is imperative for all three conditions in order to achieve full functional recovery. In the acute phase, patients should focus on rest, ice, compression, and elevation 2 to 3 times daily. Activity modification will also be necessary while symptomatic. For syndesmosis sprains, bracing with rotational control and heel lifts may help prevent excessive rotation and dorsiflexion. In tennis leg, early ankle bracing in a position of maximal dorsiflexion with early compression may improve healing and decrease scarring. For peroneal tendon injuries, lateral ankle instability should be corrected to avoid overworking the peroneals. A lateral heel wedge may be helpful in some cases to protect and unload the tendon.

Therapeutic exercise initially includes ankle circles and ankle pumps as tolerated, along with bicycle ergometry for ROM and conditioning. Joint mobilization may help improve ankle ROM. Deep transverse friction massage and soft tissue techniques may be implemented but remain unproven treatments. As patients regain full ROM and weight-bearing ability, emphasis is placed on achieving normal gait patterns. Open chain resistive exercises using resistance bands, with progression to bilateral followed by unilateral heel raises is recommended. The return to sports phase should include multidirectional hopping, jumping, and landing on stable and unstable surfaces. Ensuring that patients achieve adequate rehabilitation is critical in order to avoid reinjury and development of chronic strains and sprains (36).

SAMPLE CASE

A 27-year-old male hockey player presented with a chief complaint of acute onset left ankle pain after falling on the ice that same day during practice. He landed on his left side, twisting his left ankle. The patient experienced immediate sharp ankle pain, rated an intensity of 8/10, which significantly limited his ability to ambulate. He localized his symptoms to the dorsum of his foot, approximately at the level of the talar dome. He denied hearing a snap or pop. Pain occurred with weight bearing and with push-off. Physical exam revealed no significant ankle swelling. Tenderness was present along the anterior ankle. Active and passive ranges of motion were pain free with the exception of dorsiflexion and external rotation, which was painful in the region of the anterior tibiofibular ligament. The squeeze and external rotation stress tests reproduced the patient's ankle pain. Left ankle x-rays were unremarkable for fractures or abnormal widening of the tibiofibular clear space. The patient was diagnosed with a grade I sprain of the distal tibiofibular syndesmosis.

 SAMPLE THERAPY PRESCRIPTION

Discipline: Physical therapy.

Diagnosis: Syndesmosis sprain (aka high ankle sprain).

Problem list: Pain limited ankle dorsiflexion and reduced ankle strength.

Precautions: Weight bearing as tolerated (WBAT).

Frequency of visits: 2 to 3x/week.

Duration of treatment: 4 to 8 weeks.

Treatment:

1. *Modalities*: Cryotherapy with leg elevation (ice pack, ice bath, ice massage), compression (ace bandage wraps)

2. *Manual therapy*: Grade I talo-crural distraction for pain relief in the sub-acute stage and grade II talo-crural mobilization to maintain joint play. With continued improvement in pain-free ROM and ability to bear weight, apply grade III talo-crural posterior glides and tibio-fibular glides to restore arthrokinematics at the ankle complex

3. *Therapeutic exercise*: Active/active assisted/ passive range of motion to restore dorsiflexion, stretching, progressive resistance exercises, strengthening, proprioceptive training, neuromuscular reeducation, aerobic and conditioning exercises

4. *Specialized treatments*: Brace or walking boot, avoid straps that may cause widening of the syndesmosis. Heel lift once able to weight bear to limit dorsiflexion. May add medial longitudinal arch support to limit excessive internal rotation during stance phase

5. *Patient education*: HEP, strict adherence to PRICE protocol in acute phase, advise on proper orthotics and footwear, discuss activity modification, and appropriate intensity and duration of training program

Goals: Decrease pain and swelling, restore ankle ROM and flexibility, progressive restoration of strength, improve balance and proprioception, return to functional activities safely, prevention of recurrent injuries.

Reevaluation: In 4 weeks by referring physician or sooner if complications arise.

REFERENCES

1. Wolfe MW, Uhl TL, McCluskey LC. Management of ankle sprains. *Am Fam Physician*. 2001;63(1):93–105.
2. Lin CF, Gross ML, Weinhold P. Ankle syndesmosis injuries: anatomy, biomechanics, mechanism of injury, and clinical guidelines for diagnosis and intervention. *J Orthop Sports Phys Ther*. 2006;36(6):372–384.
3. Chinn L, Hertel J. Rehabilitation of ankle and foot injuries in athletes. *Clin J Sport Med*. 2010;29(1):157–167.
4. Pajaczkowski JA. Rehabilitation of distal tibiofibular syndesmosis sprains: a case report. *Journal of the Canadian Chiropractic Association*. 2007;51(1):42–49.
5. Nielson JH, Gardner MJ, Peterson MG, et al. Radiographic measurements do not predict syndesmotic injury in ankle fractures: an MRI study. *Clin Orthop Relat Res*. 2005;436:216–221.
6. Brosky T, Nyland J, Nitz A, et al. The ankle ligaments: consideration of syndesmotic injury and implications for rehabilitation. *J Orthop Sports Phys Ther*. 1995;21(4):197–205.
7. Wright RW, Barile RJ, Surprenant DA, et al. Ankle syndesmosis sprains in national hockey league players. *Am J Sports Med*. 2004;32(8):1941–1945.
8. Kwak HS, Lee KB, Han YM. Ruptures of the medial head of the gastrocnemius ("tennis leg"): clinical outcome and compression effect. *Clin Imaging*. 2006;30(1):48–53.
9. Saglimbeni AJ, Ertl JP, Francisco T. Medial gastrocnemius strains. *Medscape Reference*. 2009 Aug. Retrieved August 30, 2011 from http://emedicine.medscape.com.
10. Yilmaz C. Rupture of the medial gastrocnemius muscle during namaz praying. *Comput Med Imaging Graph*. 2008;32(8):728–731.

11. Shah JR, Shah BR, Shah AB. Pictorial essay: Ultrasonography in "tennis leg." *Indian Journal of Radiology and Imaging.* 2010;20(4):269–273.

12. Russel AS, Crowther S. Tennis leg—a new variant of an old syndrome. *Clin Rheumatology*, 2011;30(6):855-857.

13. Campbell, JT. Posterior calf injury. *Foot Ankle Clin.* 2009;14(4):761–771.

14. Shields CL Jr, Redix L, Brewster CE. Acute tears of the medial head of the gastrocnemius. *Foot Ankle.* 1985;5(4):186–190.

15. Petersen W, Bobka T, Stein V, et al. Blood supply of the peroneal tendons: injection and immunohistochemical studies of cadaver tendons. *Acta Orthop Scand.* 2000;71(2):168–174.

16. Heckman D, Reddy S, Pedowitz D, et al. Operative treatment for peroneal tendon disorders. *J Bone Joint Surg.* 2008;90:404–418.

17. Glazerbrook MA. Tendon disorders in the lower extremity. In: Johnson DH, Pedowitz RA, eds. *Practical Orthopaedic Sports Medicine and Arthroscopy.* Philadelphia, PA: Lippincott Williams & Wilkins; 2007:894–896.

18. Dombek MF, Lamm BM, Saltrick K, et al. Peroneal tendon tears: a retrospective review. *The J Foot Ankle Surg.* 2003;42(5):250–258.

19. Sobel M, Geppert MJ, Olson EJ, et al. The dynamics of peroneus brevis tendon splits: a proposed mechanism, technique of diagnosis, and classification of injury. *Foot Ankle.* 1992;13(7):413–422.

20. Dombek MF, Orsini R, Mendicino RW, et al. Peroneus brevis tendon tears. *Clin Podiatr Med Surg.* 2001;18(3):409–427.

21. Squires N, Myerson MS, Gamba C. Surgical treatment of peroneal tendon tears. *Foot Ankle Clin.* 2007;12(4):675–695, vii.

22. Simpson M, Howard T. Tendinopathies of the foot and ankle. *Am Fam Physician.* 2009;80(10):1107–1114.

23. Schnirring-Judge M, Perlman MD. Chronic ankle conditions. In: Banks AS, Downey MS, Martin DE, et al. eds. *Mcglamry's Comprehensive Textbook of Foot and Ankle Surgery*, Volume 1, 3rd Ed. Philadelphia, PA: Lippincott Williams & Wilkins; 2001:1110.

24. McCormick J. Athlete with overuse foot and ankle injuries. In: Busconi J, Stevenson JH, eds. *Sports Medicine Consult: A Problem-Based Approach to Sports Medicine for the Primary Care Physician.* Philadelphia, PA: Lippincott Williams & Wilkins; 2009:215.

25. Bianchi S, Delmi M, Molini L. Ultrasound of peroneal tendons. *Semin Musculoskelet Radiol.* 2010;14(3):292–306.

26. Brosky JA, Nyland JA, Nitz AJ, et al. The ankle ligaments: consideration of syndesmotic injury and implications for rehabilitation. *J Orthop Sports Phys Ther.* 1995;21(4):197–205.

27. Nussbaum ED, Hosea TM, Sieler SD, et al. Prospective evaluation of syndesmotic ankle sprains without diastasis. *Am J Sports Med.* 2001;29(1):31–35.

28. Gerber JP, Williams GN, Scoville CR, et al. Persistent disability associated with ankle sprains: a prospective examination of an athletic population. *Foot Ankle Int.* 1998;19(10):653–660.

29. Williams GN, Jones MH, Amendola A. Syndesmotic ankle sprains in athletes. *Am J Sports Med.* 2007;35(7):1197–1207.

30. Dimmen S, Engebretsen L, Nordsletten L, et al. Negative effects of parecoxib and indomethacin on tendon healing: an experimental study in rats. *Knee Surg Sports Traumatol Arthrosc.* 2009;17(7):835–839.

31. Frey C, Donatelli R. Chronic lateral ankle pain. In: Griffin LY, eds. *Essentials of Musculoskeletal Care*, 3rd Ed. Rosemont, IL: American Academy of Orthopaedic Surgeons; 2005:608.

32. Press CM, Gupta A, Hutchinson MR. Management of ankle syndesmosis injuries in the athlete. *Curr Sports Med Rep.* 2009;8(5):228–233.

33. Hoch MC, McKeon PO. The effectiveness of mobilization with movement at improving dorsiflexion after ankle sprain. *Sports Rehab J.* 2010;19(2):226–232.

34. Hensley CP, Emerson Kavchak AJ. Novel use of a manual therapy technique and management of a patient with peroneal tendinopathy: A case report. *Man Ther.* 2012;17:84–88.

35. Kolodin EL, Vitale T. Foot disorders. In: DeLisa JA, Gans BM, Walsh NE, eds. *Physical Medicine and Rehabilitation: Principles and Practice*, Volume 1. Philadelphia, PA: Lippincott Williams & Wilkins; 2005:877–878.

36. Bylak J, Hutchinson MR. Common sports injuries in young tennis players. *Sports Med.* 1998; 26(2):120–132.

37. Silvestri PG, Uhl TL, Madaleno JA, et al. Management of syndesmotic ankle sprains. *Athletic Therapy Today.* 2002;7(5):2–3.

38. Rompe JD, Nafe B, Furia JP, et al. Eccentric loading, shock-wave treatment, or a wait-and-see policy for tendinopathy of the main body of tendo Achillis: a randomized controlled trial. *Am J Sports Med.* 2007;35(3):374–383.

39. Handoll HH, Rowe BH, Quinn KM, et al. Interventions for preventing ankle ligament injuries. *Cochrane Database Syst Rev.* 2001;(3):CD000018.

Cervical Facet Arthropathy

Brett A. Gerstman, Sean Hampton, and David E. Fish

INTRODUCTION

Neck pain is the second most common musculoskeletal complaint among the general population (1). The prevalence of zygapophyseal (facet) mediated pain in patients with chronic neck pain has been estimated to be between 25% to 65% (2–4). The cervical facet joints are diarthrodial joints formed by the articulation of the superior articular process (SAP) of the caudal vertebrae with the corresponding inferior articular process (IAP) of the cephalad vertebrae. Each facet joint is surrounded by a fibrous capsule and richly innervated by the medial branches of the cervical dorsal rami above and below.

Many diagnostic terms have been used to describe painful and pathological conditions of the cervical facets and these include cervical facet arthropathy, cervical facet syndrome, cervical facet dysfunction, and facet mediated pain. Cervical facet arthropathy results from either traumatic or, more commonly, degenerative processes. Traumatic causes include fracture and/or dislocation injuries and whiplash disorders. Degenerative facet arthropathy may be caused by an age-related primary degenerative processes such as osteoarthritis (5) or secondarily from cervical disc disease (6,7).

Patients with facet arthropathy will primarily complain of axial neck pain exacerbated with extension and/or rotation, and possible radiation of pain into the occiput, shoulder, scapula, and proximal upper arm (Figure 37.1) (8). Neurological symptoms, such as numbness, tingling, or weakness in the upper limbs should be absent (9).

Key elements of the physical examination include inspection, palpation, range of motion (ROM), and neurologic testing. Patients with cervical facet mediated pain often develop a forward-head posture to offload the posterior elements. This forward head posture is commonly accompanied by rounded shoulders (humeral internal rotation and scapular protraction) (10). Point tenderness may be noted throughout the axial cervical spine, occiput and

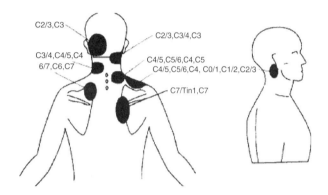

FIGURE 37.1: Referred pain distributions for the zygapophyseal joints from C0-1 to C7-T1 and the dorsal rami from C3 to C7.

Source: Reproduced with permission of the International Association for the Study of Pain® (IASP®). The figure may not be reproduced for any other purpose without permission.

cervical paraspinal musculature, and the osseous structures may be examined best in the supine position with the paraspinal muscles more relaxed. Cervical ROM may be preferentially limited in extension due to pain and neurologic testing should be normal. There are no validated physical examination maneuvers to evaluate for cervical facet dysfunction; however, special tests should be performed to rule out other pathologic processes such as cervical radiculopathy. Cervical quadrant testing can reveal facet arthropathy or dysfunction if all other cervical spine ROM testing is negative for eliciting the patient's complaints. This is a maneuver that involves maximal extension, lateral flexion and then ipsilateral rotation, thereby maximally narrowing the facet joint on the convex side of the cervical spine being tested.

Diagnostic testing may include plain radiographs with flexion and extension views to look for instability or fractures. Advanced imaging (CT or MRI) is not necessary, unless you are attempting to rule out neurologic involvement. When considering the diagnosis of facet mediated pain, relief of pain after injections of local anesthetic into the facet joint or blocking its corresponding medial branch with patient blinding is thought by some to be diagnostic (11–13).

CERVICAL FACET ARTHROPATHY

▦ Cervical facet mediated pain has a high prevalence in individuals with chronic axial neck pain

▦ It may result from either degenerative processes or trauma such as whiplash

▦ Patients complain of axial neck pain exacerbated with extension and/or rotation and possible radiation of pain into the occiput, shoulder, scapula, and upper arm

▦ Key findings on physical examination include forward-head posture, abnormal scapular alignment, point tenderness along cervical spinal musculature and normal neurologic examination

▦ Radiographs with flexion-extension views may confirm the presence of facet arthrosis and local anesthetic blocks may help support the diagnosis of cervical facet mediated pain

THE REHABILITATION PROGRAM

Therapeutic exercise is widely utilized as part of comprehensive conservative management of neck pain. There are no studies examining the benefit of physical therapy specifically on cervical facet arthropathy, facet mediated pain, or facet dysfunction, but there is a growing body of literature demonstrating the benefits of comprehensive therapy in the treatment of chronic mechanical neck pain (14,15). The goals of therapy should include decreasing local inflammation, pain, muscle tension, and ROM of affected facet levels while increasing, ROM of hypomobile cervical and thoracic spine segments and normalizing strength of cervical, thoracic, scapular, and core stabilizing musculature. Special attention should be given to optimizing the patient's spinal posture and ergonomics to limit the strain across the facet joints and pain recurrence in the future.

Therapeutic Modalities

Despite mixed support of its use in the literature (16–18), modalities are widely used in conjunction with other therapeutic techniques during the acute phase of rehabilitation. *They are primarily used to treat the overlying myofascial component of the patient's pain rather than the primary underlying facet dysfunction.* Cryotherapy is thought to be beneficial by decreasing local inflammation, inhibiting local muscle spasm overlying the facets, and also having direct anti-nociceptive effects (19,20). Deep heat in the form of ultrasound has a growing amount of literature supporting its use in treating myofascial pain (21). Despite common use of electrical stimulation (both interferential and TENS), there are no strong studies supporting its use (22,23). No studies have been used specifically for facet syndrome with sympathetic therapeutic stimulation (STS), but this mode of electrical stimulation has been found to be effective in the management of chronic cervical pain syndromes. The treatment consists of bilateral application of interferential stimulation through the upper extremities intersecting and crossing four separate currents at the level of the cervical and upper thoracic sympathetic chain ganglia.

Manual Therapy

In the acute phase of rehabilitation, manual therapy is commonly employed to decrease myofascial tension, increase muscle length, and decrease pain. Manual techniques include joint soft tissue mobilization, neural tissue mobilization, mobilization with movement, myofascial release, muscle energy and strain/counter strain techniques. Hypertonic and shortened muscles that are targeted include the sub-occipital muscles, cervical paraspinals, sternocleidomastoids, scalenes, upper trapezius, levator scapula, and pectoralis major and minor muscles. Attention should also be devoted to normalizing accessory and physiological movements at nonaffected hypomobile segments. In the early phase of treatment, mobilization to the unaffected cervical and thoracic hypomobile segments may be effective at relieving tension and pain in the affected levels of arthropathy. As the patient progresses to the subacute and chronic stage, a more direct approach to treatment of the affected levels can commence. Joint and soft tissue mobilization techniques can be performed with more vigor to accelerate the recovery in the subacute and chronic phases. The literature is mixed regarding the benefit of manual therapy. Multiple studies have confirmed the benefit of manual therapy in the acute phase of rehabilitation (24,25), but long term benefits have only been found when manual therapy was used in a multimodal approach that included exercise and mobilization (26,27). Specific manual therapy techniques with or without therapeutic exercise have not been studied in a subset of patients experiencing neck pain due to facet arthropathy.

Therapeutic Exercise

The evidence of associating mechanical neck pain and cervical muscular dysfunction has been widely accepted. Combining exercise and manual therapy has been shown to be the most effective treatment for mechanical neck pain (28). Therapeutic exercises for cervical facet arthropathy as well as most all problems arising from the cervical spine involve a combination of stretching (Figures 37.2-37.4) and strengthening of the cervical spine, upper thoracic, shoulder, and scapular muscles as well as core strengthening exercises. These exercises should continue to follow the phases of rehabilitation. Pain reduction, and restoration of ROM and flexibility with stretching

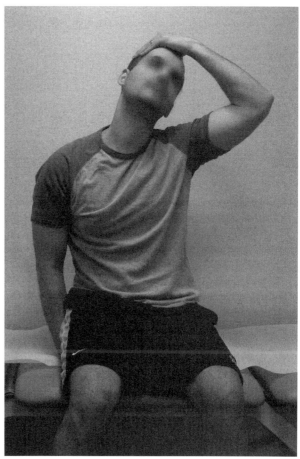

FIGURE 37.3: Scalene muscle self-stretch.

and mobility exercises should always precede aggressive strength training.

Therapeutic exercises to address muscular impairments need to be commenced early and should be pain free (29). Exercises at low loads (20%) have been shown to be more effective than moderate to maximal loads (50%–100%) at selective activation of the deep cervical muscles (30). The common muscles that need to be strengthened include the deep craniocervical flexor muscles, deep lower cervical extensors, cervical rotators, middle and lower trapezii, latissimus dorsi, and core stabilizers. In a study of patients with unilateral neck pain it was found that patients had significantly decreased trapezius strength on the affected side (31).

Strength training may begin with isometric strengthening in positions that do not overload the weak muscle groups. These are then followed by active and resistive strengthening of the affected weak muscles. As the patient's individual weaknesses resolve, the exercise program should begin to involve the other non-affected cervical paraspinal,

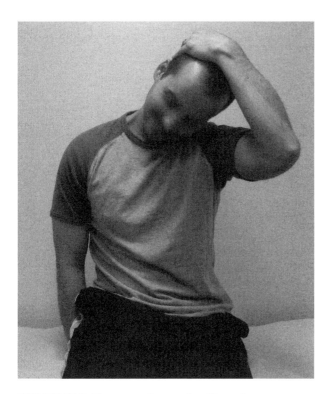

FIGURE 37.2: Upper trapezius muscle self-stretch.

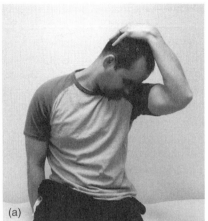
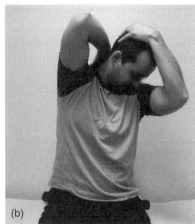

FIGURE 37.4: Levator scapulae muscle self-stretch.

core, and upper quadrant muscles. Strengthening in functional or sport-specific positions are essential for returning patients to a normal level of function in life, work, and sport activities.

Specialized Techniques

Postural Training
Anterior and posterior load distributions on the cervical spine are impacted by the posture and alignment of the cervicothoracic spine (32). Studies have shown that the angle of cervical lordosis will increase in response to increased thoracic kyphosis over time. Those with increased thoracic kyphosis had an increased incidence of neck pain compared to those with decreased kyphosis (33,34). Postural changes are commonly due to a change in muscular activation of the upper trapezii, levator scapulae, lower trapezii, latissimus dorsi, and cervical extensors, therefore, a rehabilitation program must address appropriate facilitation and inhibition of these muscle groups (35). Often patients with facet pain exhibit poor scapular awareness and control of scapular orientation during open and closed upper limb activities. Simple correction of this positional fault by scapular repositioning, and muscle reeducation as well as corrective taping can help reduce pressure and ultimately pain from the involved facets and surrounding soft tissues. Patients who report specific repetitive upper limb activities or poor postures or positions as an exacerbating factor should engage in a treatment program focused on postural correction. The

clinician should focus on confirming the painful posture, position, or upper limb activity and then correct it in an attempt to alleviate their symptoms. This gives the treating clinician further evidence that the facet pain is in part related to posture, position, or activity and confirms to the patient that postural awareness is critical to resolving their neck pain (36).

Taping
Numerous taping techniques have been found beneficial for reduction in muscle tension and pain and postural reeducation. The focus of taping is to unload tension on the cervical paraspinals as well as the upper trapezii and levator scapulae muscles. Kinesiology taping can be used to facilitate or inhibit muscles that are found to be essential in decreasing stress on the involved facet joints. Taping the scapulae into proper position can reduce tension on the upper trapezius and levator scapulae and thus across the cervical spine. Further studies need to be performed to prove the efficacy of taping for cervical facet arthropathy as well as other conditions of the cervical spine. However, taping remains an option and may be a useful adjunctive treatment during the patient's rehabilitation program.

Breathing Education
Often patients with cervical facet arthropathy will exhibit poor breathing mechanics, especially if the patient also has pulmonary disease. Patient education to avoid overuse

of accessory breathing muscles can help to decrease repetitive compressive forces applied to the cervical spine during inspiration. Simple diaphragmatic breathing techniques can be taught and incorporated into the patient's daily life.

Home Exercise Program

No therapy program will be effective without the patient performing many of these exercises on their own outside of the clinic. Patients are given combinations of stretching, strengthening, and mobilization exercises that have been proven to be effective at relieving pain and increasing ROM during the treatment sessions in the office. Clear and detailed instructions must be given to the patient regarding these exercises and postural and ergonomic adjustments that should be made to their workplace, car, and home. Instructions should also be provided in proper ergonomic setup for participation in hobby or sports activities. This will limit their pain and decrease muscle and joint strain as well as prevent pain recurrence.

SUMMARY

Cervical facet joint mediated pain and arthropathy is a common cause of mechanical, axial neck pain. The initial phase of rehabilitation should be focused on decreasing local inflammation, pain, and muscle tension. As the patient's symptoms improve during therapy, muscular imbalances and deficits in ROM should be addressed with appropriate ROM, flexibility, and strengthening exercises that consist of isometrics, progressive resistive exercises, as well as dynamic stabilization of the spine and scapulothoracic region. The use of modalities, manual therapy, and taping can play an important role in maximizing the benefits of therapy. Special attention should be given to optimizing the patient's spinal and scapulothoracic posture as well as ergonomics to limit the strain across the facet joints and pain recurrence in the future.

SAMPLE CASE

A 67-year-old male presents with complaint of aching axial neck pain for 6 months with associated decrease in ROM and periscapular pain. He denies upper limb numbness, paresthesias, or weakness. He denies bowel or bladder dysfunction and gait ataxia. He has no significant past medical history (PMH)/past surgical history (PSH)/medications (Meds)/Allergies. ROS is unremarkable and he denies prior history of neck pain. X-rays were negative for fracture but found evidence of multilevel degenerative disc disease and facet arthropathy. Physical examination findings are significant for forward head posture, mild point tenderness along cervical paraspinal and upper trapezius muscles, and cervical ROM preferentially decreased in extension. Strength testing revealed weakness and poor recruitment of the bilateral lower trapezii, lower cervical extensors, deep neck flexors, and lower abdominals. Neurologic examination was normal and Spurling's test was negative.

 SAMPLE THERAPY PRESCRIPTION

Discipline: Physical therapy.

Diagnosis: Cervical facet arthropathy with pain and decreased ROM.

Problem list: Forward head and shoulder posture.

Precautions: Avoid cervical hyperextension.

Frequency of visits: 2 to 3x/week.

Duration of treatment: 4 to 6 weeks for a total of 10 to 12 visits

Treatment:

1. *Modalities:* cryotherapy, ultrasound, STS may be utilized for symptom management

2. *Manual therapy:* joint and neural tissue mobilization, soft tissue mobilization, myofascial release, mobilization with

movement, muscle energy and strain/counter strain techniques

3. *Therapeutic exercise:* A/AA/PROM and flexibility exercises for the cervical spine to restore pain-free ROM, pain free isometric strengthening of weakened muscles progressing to resistive and functional strengthening programs. Strengthening of deep neck flexors, lower trapezius, rhomboids and postural correction exercises, such as chin tucks and scapular retractions

4. *Specialized treatments:* taping, breathing education, static and dynamic postural correction, movement reeducation

5. *Patient education:* HEP, breathing, ergonomics, sleep hygiene, self-taping may be considered if effective

Goals: Decrease local inflammation, pain, muscle tension and improve ROM of affected facet levels. Increase ROM of shortened muscles, hypomobile cervical and thoracic segments and improve strength of cervical, thoracic, and scapular stabilizing muscles. Improve static and dynamic posture.

Reevaluation: In 4 to 6 weeks by referring physician.

REFERENCES

1. Ferrari R, Russell AS. Regional musculoskeletal conditions: neck pain. *Best Pract Res Clin Rheumatol.* Feb;17(1):57–70
2. Aprill C, Bogduk N. The prevalence of cervical zygapophyseal joint pain. A first approximation. *Spine.* 1992;17:744–747.
3. Manchikanti L, Boswell MV, Singh V, Pampati V, Damron KS, Beyer CD. Prevalence of facet joint pain in chronic spinal pain of cervical, thoracic, and lumbar regions. *BMC Musculoskelet Disord.* 2004;5:15.
4. Barnsley L, Lord SM, Wallis BJ, Bogduk N. The prevalence of chronic cervical zygapophysial joint pain after whiplash. *Spine.* 1995;20(1):20-25; discussion 26.
5. Fletcher G, Haughton VM, Ho K, Yu S. Age-related changes in the cervical facet joints: studies with cryomicrometry, MR, and CT. *AJR Am J Roentgenol.* 1990;154:817–820.
6. Butler D, Trafimow JH, Andersson GB, McNeill TW, Huckman MS. Discs degenerate before facets. *Spine.* 1990;15:111–113.
7. Fujiwara A, Tamai K, Yamato M, et al. The relationship between facet joint osteoarthritis and disc degeneration of the lumbar spine: an MRI study. *Eur Spine J.* 1999;8:396–401.
8. Dwyer A, Aprill C, Bogduk N. Cervical zygapophyseal joint pain patterns. I: A study in normal volunteers. *Spine (Phila Pa 1976).* 1990;15(6):453–457.
9. Fukui S, Ohseto K, Shiotani M, et al. Referred pain distribution of the cervical zygapophyseal joints and cervical dorsal rami. *Pain.* 1996;68:79–83.
10. Malanga G, Nadler S, eds. *Musculoskeletal Physical Examination: An Evidence Based Approach.* Philadelphia, PA: Elsevier Mosby; 2006.
11. Sehgal N, Dunbar EE, Shah RV, Colson J. Systematic review of diagnostic utility of facet (zygapophysial) joint injections in chronic spinal pain: an update. *Pain Physician.* 2007; 10(1):213–228.
12. Lord SM, Barnsley L, Bogduk N. The utility of comparative local anesthetic blocks versus placebo-controlled blocks for the diagnosis of cervical zygapophysial joint pain. *Clin J Pain.* 1995;11(3):208–213.
13. Bogduk N, ed. Cervical medial branch blocks. In: Bogduk N, ed. *Practice Guidelines for Spinal Diagnostic And Treatment Procedures*, 1st ed. San Fransisco, CA: International Spine Intervention Society; 2004:112–137.
14. Kay TM, Gross A, Goldsmith C, Santaguida PL, Hoving J, Bronfort G; Cervical Overview Group. Exercises for mechanical neck disorders. *Cochrane Database Syst Rev.* 2005; (3):CD004250.
15. Gross AR, Goldsmith C, Hoving JL, et al. Conservative management of mechanical neck disorders: a systematic review. *J Rheumatol.* 2007;34(5):1083–1102.
16. (16) Chiu TT, Hui-Chan CW, Chein G. A randomized clinical trial of TENS and exercise for patients with chronic neck pain. *Clin Rehabil.* 2005;19(8):850–860.
17. Hubbard TJ, Denegar CR. Does cryotherapy improve outcomes with soft tissue injury? *J Athl Train.* 2004;39(3):278–279.
18. French SD, Cameron M, Walker BF, Reggars JW, Esterman AJ. A Cochrane review of superficial heat or cold for low back pain. *Spine (Phila Pa 1976).* 2006;31(9):998–1006.
19. Mac Auley DC. Ice therapy: how good is the evidence? *Int J Sports Med.* 2001;22(5):379–384.
20. Swenson C, Swärd L, Karlsson J. Cryotherapy in sports medicine. *Scand J Med Sci Sports.* 1996;6(4):193–200.
21. Srbely JZ, Dickey JP. Randomized controlled study of the antinociceptive effect of ultrasound on trigger point sensitivity: novel applications in myofascial therapy? *Clin Rehabil.* 2007;21(5):411–417.
22. Chiu TT, Hui-Chan CW, Chein G. A randomized clinical trial of TENS and exercise for patients with chronic neck pain. *Clin Rehabil.* 2005;19(8):850–860.
23. Kroeling P, Gross A, Goldsmith CH, et al. Electrotherapy for neck pain. *Cochrane Database Syst Rev.* 2009;(4):CD004251.
24. Hoving JL, de Vet HC, Koes BW, et al. Manual therapy, physical therapy, or continued care by the general practitioner for patients with neck pain: long-term results from a pragmatic randomized clinical trial. *Clin J Pain.* 2006;22(4):370–377.
25. Miller J, Gross A, D'Sylva J, et al. Manual therapy and exercise for neck pain: A systematic review. *Man Ther.* 2010;(22):334–354.
26. Griffiths C, Dziedzic K, Waterfield J, Sim J. Effectiveness of specific neck stabilization exercises or a general neck exercise program for chronic neck disorders: a randomized controlled trial. *J Rheumatol.* 2009;36(2):390–397.
27. Kay TM, Gross A, Goldsmith C, et al. Exercises for mechanical neck disorders. *Cochrane Database Syst Rev.* 2005; (3):CD004250.

28. Gross AR, Goldsmith C, Hoving JL, et al. Conservative management of mechanical neck disorders: a systematic review. *J Rheumatol.* 2007;34:1083–1102.

29. Falla D, Farina D, Dahl MK, Graven-Nielsen T. Muscle pain induces task-dependent changes in cervical agonist/antagonist activity. *J Appl Physiol.* 2007;102:601–609.

30. O'Leary S, Falla D, Jull G, Vicenzino B. Muscle specificity in tests of cervical flexor muscle performance. *J Electromyogr Kinesiol.* 2007;17:35–40.

31. Petersen, SM, Wyatt, SN; Lower trapezius muscle strength in individuals with unilateral neck pain. *J Orthop Sports Phys Ther.* 2011;41:260–265.

32. Kumaresan S, Yoganandan N, Pintar FA. Posterior complex contribution to the axial compressive and distractive behavior of the cervical spine. *J Musculoskeletal Res.* 1998;2:257–265.

33. Falla D, Jull G, Russell T, Vicenzino B, Hodges P. Effect of neck exercise on sitting posture in patients with chronic neck pain. *Phys Ther.* 2007;87:408-417.

34. Szeto GP, Straker L, Raine S. A field comparison of neck and shoulder postures in symptomatic and asymptomatic office workers. *Appl Ergon.* 2002;33:75–84.

35. Szeto GP, Straker LM, O'Sullivan PB. EMG median frequency changes in the neck-shoulder stabilizers of symptomatic office workers when challenged by different physical stressors. *J Electromyogr Kinesiol.* 2005;15:544–555.

36. Jull G, Sterling M, Falla D, Treleaven J, O'Leary S. *Whiplash, Headache, and Neck Pain: Research- Based Directions for Physical Therapies.* Edinburgh, UK: Elsevier; 2008.

Cervical Disc Pathology

Benjamin D. Levy

INTRODUCTION

The cervical intervertebral discs have a structure that allows them to support axial loads while providing adequate range of motion (ROM) in multiple planes. However, the versatility of these structures also predisposes them to injury. It is estimated that 20% of chronic neck pain may be due to cervical intervertebral disc disruption (1). As in lumbar intervertebral discs, cervical discs are comprised of an outer annulus fibrosus and an inner nucleus pulposus. They differ in the additional lateral structural support received by the uncinate processes found in the cervical spine from C3-7. The cervical discs are innervated from a branch of the ventral primary ramus, the sinuvertebral nerve, and the gray ramus (1). Histologic examination reveals the greatest densities of pain fibers and mechanoreceptors in the posterolateral aspect of the annulus fibrosus; no pain fibers enter the nucleus pulposus (1,2). Disruption of the annulus fibrosus can be a significant pain generator that can radiate to the occiput, neck, shoulder, or arms, though the exact mechanism of this radiation is still unclear (3,4). Furthermore, bilateral radiation of pain has been noted when performing provocative discography (5). Following disruption of the annulus, the disc may be deformed or herniated.

The pertinent history of cervical discogenic pain may vary widely. Pain onset may be insidious due to degenerative disc disease, or may be abrupt in traumatic disc disruption such as that which occurs in whiplash injuries. Acute cervical disc disruption has also been described in weight lifters who forcefully forward flex their neck during heavy lifts (6). Patients may complain of primarily axial neck pain with referral patterns as described above (5). Further complicating the picture is that cervical zygapophyseal-mediated pain may refer with very similar patterns (7).

Key elements of the physical examination include inspection, palpation, range of motion (ROM), a complete cervical spine examination with neurological evaluation, shoulder examination to rule out alternative or concomitant pathology, and provocative maneuvers (e.g., Spurling's maneuver, dural tension testing). Cervical ROM may be restricted due to pain. If upper limb pain, numbness, or weakness predominates, than cervical radiculopathy should be considered. Pain relief with an abducted arm (Bakody's sign) may also suggest radiculopathy (8). Hyperreflexia and/or weakness in the upper or lower limbs or upper motor neuron signs such as a Hoffman's sign, ankle clonus, or spasticity should prompt an evaluation for cervical myelopathy. While not sensitive, the Spurling maneuver is specific for cervical radiculopathy (4).

It may be difficult to distinguish cervical discogenic pain from cervical myofascial pain on physical examination. Both entities can show paramidline tenderness with a normal neurological examination (1). Theoretically, pain with palpation over a spinous process connotes discogenic pain rather than myofascial, though there may be overlap between the two conditions and this finding. Diagnostic imaging can also be difficult to interpret, as one study found that 36% of asymptomatic volunteers had focal annular tears and disc protrusions on magnetic resonance imaging (9). Furthermore, cervical degeneration on plain radiographs has been shown not to correlate well with patients' symptoms (10).

Given the limitations of history, physical examination, and imaging modalities, provocative discography can help establish the diagnosis of discogenic pain, and can correlate well with symptoms in 50% to 78% of patients (7). Importantly, if a control disc is not injected, the procedure can have up to a 50% false positive rate (7). Ultimately, the diagnosis of cervical discogenic pain hinges upon the clinician's skillful history taking, physical

CERVICAL DISC PATHOLOGY

■ Discogenic pain may account for 20% of all chronic neck pain

■ Pathogenesis may be traumatic or degenerative and can range from annular tears to disc extrusion with sequestration

■ Physical examination may show midline and paramidline posterior spinal tenderness and reduced cervical ROM with normal neurological examination

■ Plain radiography and MRI may be helpful, but may not correlate well with the clinical symptoms

■ Diagnostic provocative discography can assist the clinician in making the proper diagnosis, but it is only considered after an extensive course of conservative care has failed to provide a reduction in pain and disability

examination, prudent use of imaging, and judicious application of interventional diagnostic procedures.

THE REHABILITATION PROGRAM

As the diagnosis of cervical discogenic pain is often difficult to prove, its treatment must address the specific symptoms and functional deficits of each patient. Because of the wide variation of nonoperative treatment protocols for cervical discogenic pain, there is little consensus in the literature regarding the optimal approach. The rehabilitation program or phases of rehabilitation should follow similar tenets of other chapters in this text. The first phase of rehabilitation should include adequate pain control and relative rest. This can be achieved with nonsteroidal anti-inflammatories (NSAIDs) if not contraindicated. If there is concomitant cervical myofascial pain, centrally acting muscle relaxants such as cyclobenzaprine, metaxalone, or methocarbamol may be helpful. As the nucleus pulposus is an immune privileged site, more significant disc herniation can trigger local inflammation (11). When cervical radiculopathy is also present, a rapid taper of oral steroids or fluoroscopically guided cervical epidural steroid injection may be beneficial.

Restriction in cervical ROM and relative rest should also be instituted in the acute phase of rehabilitation (4). While not a true immobilizing orthosis, a soft cervical collar can provide some relative restriction in cervical ROM, valuable proprioceptive feedback, and localized warmth that may improve acute pain. Wearing a soft cervical collar for sleeping can improve comfort and allow for a better night's rest during a period of acute neck pain. Once pain has decreased, the cervical collar should be discontinued promptly to avoid physical or psychological dependence.

Once pain has improved to a more tolerable level, ROM can progressively be restored. Following restoration of ROM, resistance exercises can be used to restore neck musculature strength. Finally, activity and sport-specific training can return the patient to their prior level of functioning.

Therapeutic Modalities

As previously noted, cervical discogenic pathology often has secondary myofascial pain. If this is identified in the history and physical examination, the myofascial component may respond well to moist heat. Therapeutic ultrasound has been used as a deep heating modality for neck pain in some studies, though usually in conjunction with therapeutic exercise (12). Effectiveness of these modalities for long-term benefit is lacking in the literature. Heat can act as an analgesic and facilitate stretching exercises (1). Transcutaneous electrical nerve stimulation (TENS) may be helpful to some patients to facilitate the therapeutic exercise program, though a standard protocol defining pulse width, frequency, and amplitude has not been established. In one randomized multicenter prospective single-blinded trial, TENS was compared to manual therapy for nonspecific mechanical neck pain. The authors found the two interventions to be equally effective in relieving neck pain 1 month after treatment initiation, though efficacy waned after treatment was stopped for 6 months (13). However, no adverse events were reported.

A recent meta-analysis showed low level laser therapy (LLLT) to be an effective and safe treatment for nonspecific mechanical neck pain (14). However, the effect was found to be dose-dependent. Two protocols that were found to be effective employed a wavelength of 830 nm continuous wave mode with average output of 300 mW. Joules per point treated was 9 and time per point treated was 30 seconds. An average of 11 points were treated twice per week for 7 weeks. Further research is required before LLLT is routinely recommended for the treatment of neck pain and more specifically for discogenic neck pain.

Manual Therapy

Soft tissue mobilization and manual or mechanical traction have been two important adjuvant therapies that should be trialed for benefit in the conservative treatment of cervical discogenic pain. The methods of soft tissue mobilization have included myofascial release, muscle energy, trigger point techniques, and Swedish massage (15,16). No one method has been shown to be superior to another, though patients have reported greater benefit in acute and chronic neck pain when manual therapies are combined with therapeutic exercise (12).

Manual traction may provide relief to patients with cervical discogenic pain. It is usually done by the physical therapist with the patient lying supine. The cervical spine is placed in flexion, and then an axial distraction is applied. The exact degree of cervical flexion and distraction force applied vary widely (17–19). Some suggest that flexion between 20 to 30 degrees may obtain better outcome by stretching posterior cervical musculature and by increasing spacing between the posterior aspects of the vertebral bodies (19). Forces applied during manual traction are inexact and difficult to measure. However, radiographically detectable change in intervertebral spaces was identified between 11 and 21 kilograms of force (20). Others have suggested that force be applied that is approximately 10% to 20% of the patient's body weight (17). While there is no absolute maximum force, 55kg has been shown to cause C5-6 disc rupture (20). A mere 4.5 kg has been shown to cause separation of the atlanto-occipital and atlantoaxial joints (20). A trial of manual cervical traction is recommended to assess for the patient's response before starting a program of mechanical traction. Mechanical traction requires frequent patient monitoring to ensure the treatment is reducing neck pain and/or radicular symptoms and is discussed in further detail in the specialized treatment section of this chapter. Some patients who respond very well to manual and/or mechanical traction can subsequently be prescribed home cervical traction units. As such, extreme care must be taken to evaluate patients for instability at these levels if underlying rheumatologic or connective tissue diseases are suspected prior to the prescription of any traction.

Spinal manipulation and mobilization are commonly utilized by physical therapists and chiropractors for the treatment of neck pain. A great deal of controversy surrounds cervical spine manipulation due to potentially serious complications, including injury to the vertebrobasilar system and subsequent stroke. Review of the literature has associated rotatory cervical spine manipulation (high velocity, low amplitude) with the more serious complications and has lead the authors of this review to advise against this type of spinal manipulation (21). Lower grade mobilizations of the cervical spine offer potential benefits with a lower risk of complications. Prior reviews have found the efficacy of manipulation/mobilization to be inconclusive for acute neck pain and moderate evidence to support short term pain reduction for chronic neck pain. The authors acknowledge that future trials need to examine these treatments for well defined subsets of patients (22).

Therapeutic Exercise

Manual therapy and modalities used in isolation have been shown to be less effective than when combined with a proper exercise regimen (12). There is no specific protocol for discogenic pain, but a therapeutic algorithm addressing nonradicular neck pain has been described (16). The cervical paraspinals, scalenes, levator scapulae, and upper trapezii should be stretched. This can be facilitated with moist heat or manual traction (4). Following stretching, active ROM of the cervical spine and isometric strengthening exercises can be performed in flexion (Figure 38.1), extension, lateral rotation (Figure 38.2), and lateral side-bending (Figure 38.3). As mentioned in the chapter on Cervical Facet Arthropathy, neuromuscular reeducation and then strengthening of the deep neck flexors is as important to consider since many patients present with a muscular imbalance of tight suboccipital and upper cervical spine extensors (e.g., paraspinals) and weakened deep neck flexors. Postural exercises including chin tucks (Figure 38.4) and scapular retraction (Figure 38.5) can help restore proper cervical positioning. If the patient has referral of neck pain to the occiput, shoulders, or arms, a trial of McKenzie centralizing techniques may be helpful (23).

Following restoration of cervical ROM and strength, activity-specific rehabilitation can proceed. Review of work-related biomechanics and ergonomics may help prevent reinjury. Sports-related trauma, such as falls with hyperflexion of the neck, and weight-lifting with the neck flexed can also injure the cervical discs (6,24). In addition to reviewing sports-specific safe practices and proper use of safety equipment, proper timing of return-to-play must be considered. While there are no evidence-based guidelines

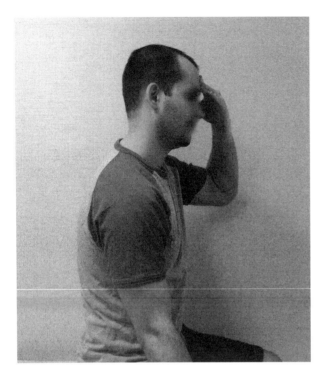

FIGURE 38.1: Isometric cervical flexion exercise.

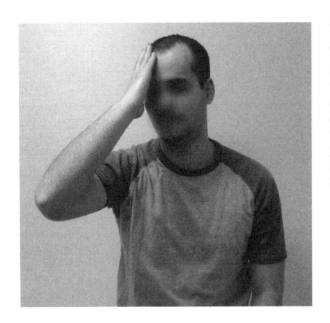

FIGURE 38.2: Isometric cervical lateral rotation.

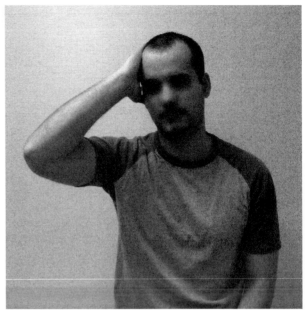

FIGURE 38.3: Isometric cervical lateral side bending.

for return-to-play after cervical discogenic pathology, an athlete can be considered for return to play when he or she has completed rehabilitation with pain-free cervical spine ROM and full strength in sports-specific activities (4).

Specialized Techniques

While manual traction may be helpful, a physical therapist may not be able to generate the consistent force necessary to achieve pain relief. Under the direction of a physician and physical therapist, mechanical traction may be of additional benefit. While Cochrane Review of mechanical traction for neck pain did not find definitive evidence to support or refute this technique, Zylbergold et al found some improvement in cervical pain and ROM specifically with intermittent cervical traction (18,19). However, there was a 33% rate of participant drop-out (19). Her protocol utilized neck care education, moist heat for 15 minutes, neck ROM exercises, isometric neck strengthening, and intermittent mechanical traction for 15 minutes. The traction was performed with 25 degrees of cervical flexion. The distraction force used was 11 kg and was applied for 10 second intervals with 10 seconds of rest in between. Care must be taken to ensure that the traction device is properly fitted to the patient as improper strap may cause ipsilateral facial palsy (25). While computerized traction units are available, there

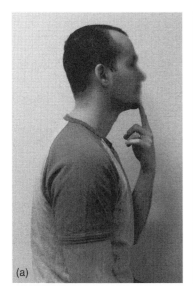
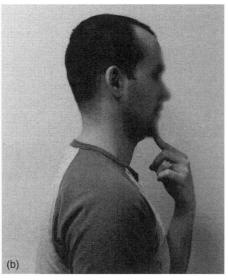

FIGURE 38.4: (a) Starting position for chin tuck. (b) Final position of chin tuck.

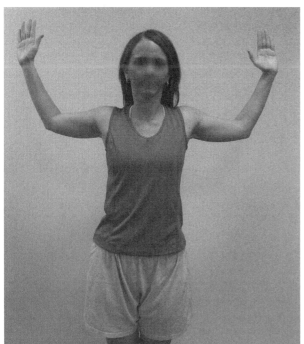

FIGURE 38.5: Scapular retraction exercise.

are no studies available to comment on their efficacy at the time of this chapter's publication.

Home Exercise Program

The home exercise program (HEP) should be instituted at the onset of rehabilitation, and should reflect each phase of rehabilitation as the patient progresses. The patient should be educated on proper performance of cervical active ROM, isometric strengthening and postural exercises. The stretching and strengthening programs are vital parts of the HEP. An emphasis should be made on injury prevention. As mentioned in the manual therapy section, a home cervical traction unit may be beneficial if the patient is found to be traction responsive in therapy or during initial evaluation by the physician (26). The use of home cervical traction should be trialed by the therapist in clinic and the patient should be educated thoroughly on use of the device.

SUMMARY

Cervical disc pathology can be a nebulous and elusive clinical entity, which makes its accurate diagnosis and subsequent treatment difficult. While evidenced-based rehabilitation of this disorder is not well-defined, the basic tenets of rehabilitation that apply to other musculoskeletal injuries are pertinent and can guide the clinician toward a successful outcome. In addition, prudent use of modalities that have some evidence of efficacy, such as LLLT and cervical traction, may accelerate recovery. Emphasis on stepwise progression through relative rest, ROM restoration, isometric strengthening, postural training, activity-specific training, and institution of a practical HEP can guide the patient to successful improvement in function.

SAMPLE CASE

A 60-year-old male was shoveling snow last week and felt progressive onset of midline lower neck pain without radiation. He denied any upper or lower limb numbness, tingling, or weakness. He had no bowel or bladder incontinence. He has no other pertinent past medical, surgical, or social history. He had been examined by his primary care physician, who found the patient to have localized pain with Spurling maneuver and tenderness over the lower cervical paraspinals. His neurological examination was normal. An MRI was ordered, which showed mild disc bulging at C4-5 and C5-6 and a small central protrusion with annual tear at C6-7 without any significant facet arthropathy or central or neural foraminal stenosis.

SAMPLE THERAPY PRESCRIPTION

Discipline: Physical therapy.

Diagnosis: C6-7 discogenic pain with overlying cervical myofascial pain.

Precautions: Avoid extreme cervical flexion, avoid overhead lifting with flexed neck, avoid Valsalva.

Frequency of visits: 2 to 3x/week.

Duration of treatment: 3 to 4 weeks; for a total of 8 to 12 visits used at the therapist's discretion.

Treatment:

1. *Modalities:* Moist heat for up to 15 minutes as needed before stretching or manual therapy. Trial of TENS if patient's pain is poorly controlled or trial of LLLT may be considered with the following settings:

- Wavelength 830 nm
- Continuous wave mode with average output of 300 mW
- ~9 Joules per point treated; ~30 seconds per point treated

- May treat 10 to 20 points per treatment for up to 12 treatments if beneficial

2. *Manual therapy:* Soft tissue mobilization with myofascial release to cervical paraspinals, levator scapulae, scalenes, and upper trapezii. Trial of supine manual cervical traction with 20 to 30 degrees of cervical flexion and low grade spinal mobilization

3. *Therapeutic exercise:* Cervical A/AAROM and isometric strengthening exercises in flexion, extension, lateral rotation, and lateral sidebending. Strengthening and if needed neuromuscular reeducation of the deep cervical flexors. Postural correction exercises, scapular retractions, chin tucks

4. *Specialized treatments:* Consider trial of mechanical traction if limited or no response to manual traction. Consider short term use of home unit if it provides relief. Ergonomic evaluation and education on protection of cervical spine with activities

5. *Patient education:* HEP

Goals: Decrease pain; restore cervical ROM, flexibility and strength. Safely return to functional activities (e.g., sport, hobbies, work) and prevent recurrent injuries.

Reevaluation: In 4 weeks by referring physician.

REFERENCES

1. Braddom RL, Chan L, Harrast MA. *Physical Medicine & Rehabilitation*, 4th ed. Philadelphia, PA: Saunders/Elsevier; 2011.
2. Mendel T, Wink CS, Zimny ML. Neural elements in human cervical intervertebral discs. *Spine (Phila Pa 1976)*. 1992;17(2):132–135.
3. Garvey TA, Transfeldt EE, Malcolm JR, Kos P. Outcome of anterior cervical discectomy and fusion as perceived by patients treated for dominant axial-mechanical cervical spine pain. *Spine (Phila Pa 1976)*. 2002;27(17):1887–1895; discussion 1895.
4. Scherping SC, Jr. Cervical disc disease in the athlete. *Clin Sports Med.* 2002;21(1):37–47, vi.
5. Slipman CW, Plastaras C, Patel R, et al. Provocative cervical discography symptom mapping. *Spine J.* 2005;5(4):381–388.

6. Lefavi R, Smith D, Deters T, Lander J, Serrato J, McMillan JL. Lower cervical disc trauma in weight training: Possible causes and preventive techniques. *National Strength and Conditioning Association Journal.* 1993;15(2):34–36

7. Manchikanti L, Dunbar EE, Wargo BW, Shah RV, Derby R, Cohen SP. Systematic review of cervical discography as a diagnostic test for chronic spinal pain. *Pain Physician.* 2009;12(2):305–321.

8. Beatty RM, Fowler FD, Hanson EJ, Jr. The abducted arm as a sign of ruptured cervical disc. *Neurosurgery.* 1987;21(5):731–732.

9. Ernst CW, Stadnik TW, Peeters E, Breucq C, Osteaux MJ. Prevalence of annular tears and disc herniations on MR images of the cervical spine in symptom free volunteers. *Eur J Radiol.* 2005;55(3):409–414.

10. Marchiori DM, Henderson CN. A cross-sectional study correlating cervical radiographic degenerative findings to pain and disability. *Spine (Phila Pa 1976).* 1996;21(23):2747–2751.

11. Wang J, Tang T, Yang H, et al. The expression of Fas ligand on normal and stabbed-disc cells in a rabbit model of intervertebral disc degeneration: a possible pathogenesis. *J Neurosurg Spine.* 2007;6(5):425–430.

12. Miller J, Gross A, D'Sylva J, et al. Manual therapy and exercise for neck pain: A systematic review. *Man Ther.* 2010;15:334–354.

13. Escortell-Mayor E, Riesgo-Fuertes R, Garrido-Elustondo S, et al. Primary care randomized clinical trial: manual therapy effectiveness in comparison with TENS in patients with neck pain. *Man Ther.* 2011;16(1):66–73.

14. Chow RT, Johnson MI, Lopes-Martins RA, Bjordal JM. Efficacy of low-level laser therapy in the management of neck pain: a systematic review and meta-analysis of randomised placebo or active-treatment controlled trials. *Lancet.* 2009;374(9705):1897–1908.

15. Haraldsson BG, Gross AR, Myers CD, et al. Massage for mechanical neck disorders. *Cochrane Database Syst Rev.* 2006;3:CD004871.

16. Wang WT, Olson SL, Campbell AH, Hanten WP, Gleeson PB. Effectiveness of physical therapy for patients with neck pain: an individualized approach using a clinical decision-making algorithm. *Am J Phys Med Rehabil.* 2003;82(3):203–218; quiz 219–221.

17. Chiu TT, Ng JK, Walther-Zhang B, Lin RJ, Ortelli L, Chua SK. A randomized controlled trial on the efficacy of intermittent cervical traction for patients with chronic neck pain. *Clin Rehabil.* 2011;25:814–822.

18. Graham N, Gross A, Goldsmith CH, et al. Mechanical traction for neck pain with or without radiculopathy. *Cochrane Database Syst Rev.* 2008(3):CD006408.

19. Zylbergold RS, Piper MC. Cervical spine disorders. A comparison of three types of traction. *Spine (Phila Pa 1976).* 1985;10(10):867–871.

20. Saunders HD. Use of spinal traction in the treatment of neck and back conditions. *Clin Orthop Relat Res.* 1983(179):31–38.

21. Assendelft WJ, Bouter LM, Knipschild PG. Complications of spinal manipulation: a comprehensive review of the literature. *J Fam Pract.* 1996;42(5):475–480.

22. Bronfort G, Haas M, Evans RL, Bouter LM. Efficacy of spinal manipulation and mobilization for low back pain and neck pain: a systematic review and best evidence synthesis. *Spine J.* 2004;4(3):335–356

23. Schenk R, Bhaidani T, Melissa B, Kelley J, Kruchowsky T. Inclusion of mechanical diagnosis and therapy (MDT) in the management of cervical radiculopathy: A case report. *J Man Manip Ther.* 2008;16(1):e1–8.

24. Ecker TM, Kleinschmidt M, Martinolli L, Zimmermann H, Exadaktylos AK. Clinical presentation of a traumatic cervical spine disc rupture in alpine sports: a case report. *Scand J Trauma Resusc Emerg Med.* 2008;16:14.

25. So EC. Facial nerve paralysis after cervical traction. *Am J Phys Med Rehabil.* 2010;89(10):849–853.

26. Swezey RL, Swezey AM, Warner K. Efficacy of home cervical traction therapy. *Am J Phys Med Rehabil.* 1999;78(1):30–32.

Cervical Radiculopathy

John M. Vasudevan, Christopher Plastaras, and Scott Becker

INTRODUCTION

Cervical radiculopathy refers to dysfunction of one or more nerve roots in the cervical spine. The term *radiculopathy* refers to any pathology at the root level, and usually involves a deficit in strength, sensation, and/or reflexes in the distribution of the nerve root. The term *radiculitis* or *radicular pain* is often used to describe nerve root irritation by an active inflammatory process or structural compression that causes pain in the dermatomal distribution of the nerve root. The frequency of cervical radiculopathy is approximately 85 per 100,000, which is less than lumbosacral radiculopathy (1). The most commonly affected roots are the seventh (60%) and sixth (25%) cervical roots (2). The causes of a radiculopathy may be mechanical (e.g., compression by a herniated intervertebral disc, stenosis of the neural foramen, an osteophyte as the root exits the neural foramen) or chemical (inflammatory mediators such as prostaglandin E2, IL-6, nitric oxide, etc.) (3,4). Fortunately, a majority of patients with neck pain—whether from muscular strain, facet joint injury, or radiculopathy—will experience improvement of symptoms with conservative treatment. The challenge to practitioners of musculoskeletal medicine is to effectively reduce pain, restore function, and prevent further or recurrent injury with conservative care.

The cervical spine consists of seven vertebra and eight nerve roots. Unlike the thoracic or lumbosacral spine, the cervical nerve roots exit *above* their respective vertebra, with the eighth nerve exiting between the C7 and T1 vertebra. The cervical roots arise from dorsal and ventral rootlets within the spinal canal, and the root then exits via lateral neural foramen, which are bordered by the uncovertebral joint anteromedially and zygapophysial (or facet) joint posterolaterally. Intervertebral discs begin at the C2-C3 level and all levels caudal, and consist of a tough outer annulus fibrosis and gelatinous inner nucleus pulposus.

There are many potential etiologies of cervical radiculopathy, but the two most common are disc herniations and degenerative conditions of the spine. Disc herniations are more common in younger patients, and patients over 50 are more likely to have osteophyte formation (5). Disc herniations may cause mechanical compression or chemical irritation. Research has demonstrated that the release of chemicals from the nucleus pulposus through the annular tear can cause an inflammatory reaction (3,4). Osteophytes from degenerative disorders of the spine may cause compression of the nerve within or just beyond the foramen.

A thorough history is essential to both identify radiculopathy and exclude differential diagnoses. In the event of a traumatic onset of symptoms, it is important to ask about the mechanism of injury. Trauma involving extension, lateral bending, and rotation toward the affected side all reduce space in the neural foramen. Sustained end-range positioning of the cervical spine (e.g., while sleeping) is also a potential mechanism of injury. A compressive force in flexion or extension may cause a disc herniation. A traction injury may occur if the head is suddenly flexed and bent away from the affected side (6). In patients without trauma or insidious onset, it is important to rule out malignancy or vasculopathy.

Regardless of cause, patients should be asked to describe the presence, location, quality, and progression of pain, and whether there is tingling, numbness, or weakness in the neck, arm, or both. Pain may be described either as neuropathic (i.e., severe burning, electrical, stinging pain) or a dull ache, thought to be related to whether the dorsal (sensory) or ventral (motor) rootlets are more primarily involved, respectively (7). Symptoms often follow the dermatome (innervated skin), myotome (innervated muscle), or sclerotome (tissues developing from the embryologic mesodermal layer) distribution. Clinical presentation of symptoms may include overlap of pain referral patterns. When determining a rehabilitation strategy, it may be helpful to distinguish whether the symptoms are intermittent or constant in nature. As a general rule, but with some exceptions, mechanical issues tend to be more intermittent in nature, while chemical issues tend to be more constant. Cervical myelopathy must not be missed and usually presents with complaints of bilateral upper limb or lower limb weakness, gait instability, incoordination, or bowel/bladder incontinence.

The differential diagnosis of neck pain is extensive. Additional disorders related to the spine include cervical zygapophysial (facet) arthropathy, discogenic pain, and cervical myelopathy. Other tissues to consider are the muscles and ligaments of the neck, which may include active trigger points as a primary or secondary cause of pain. Just as pathology in the neck may refer to the shoulder, it is also possible for shoulder pathology, including rotator cuff and biceps tendinopathies, labral tears, or glenohumeral osteoarthrosis to refer to the neck. Visceral pain originating from the heart (left arm), gallbladder (right shoulder), spleen (left shoulder), diaphragm (either shoulder), or thoracic aorta (upper thoracic back) must also be considered (8).

Key elements of the physical examination include inspection, palpation, postural evaluation, active range of motion (AROM), strength, reflex, sensation examination, and special test. Inspect for atrophy of neck, periscapular, and upper limb muscles and for postural deficits including forward head posture. AROM of the cervical spine in all planes should be observed for asymmetries and reproduction of pain. Palpate for muscle spasm or trigger points to evaluate for muscular imbalances. Sensory examination should include dermatomes C5-T1, and a peripheral nerve examination (e.g., median vs. radial vs. ulnar) can help distinguish radiculopathy from brachial plexopathy or peripheral neuropathy. Reflexes may be diminished in radiculopathy and can be tested at the biceps (C5), brachioradialis (C6), triceps (C7), pronator teres (C6-7), and deep finger flexors (C8). Common muscles and sensory testing points evaluated in an upper limb screen are as summarized in Figure 39.1 and Figure 39.2. Brisk reflexes or a positive Hoffman or Babinski sign may indicate upper motor neuron pathology.

Special tests can also be performed to attempt to confirm cervical radiculopathy. Neural compression is suggested by a positive Bakody sign, which patients may demonstrate

Middle Deltoid	C5, C6
Biceps	C5, C6
Extensor Carpi Radialis Longus	C6, C7
Triceps	C6, C7, C8
Flexor Digitorum Profundus	C8, T1 (Digits 2/3=Median, Digits 4/5=Ulnar)
Abductor Digiti Minimi/1ˢᵗ Dorsal Interosseous	C8, T1 (Ulnar)
Abductor Pollicis Brevis	C8, T1 (Median)
Note: Dominant root underlined.	

FIGURE 39.1: Key muscles and roots involved in cervical radiculopathy.

C4	Over the acromioclavicular joint
C5	Halfway between biceps tendon and lateral epicondyle
C6	Dorsal proximal phalanx of thumb (radial); Palmar thumb (median)
C7	Dorsal proximal phalanx of long finger (radial); Palmar long finger (median)
C8	Dorsal proximal phalanx of little finger (ulnar)
T1	Halfway between biceps tendon and medial epicondyle

FIGURE 39.2: Key dermatomal sensory testing points in cervical radiculopathy.

spontaneously and is defined by relief of pain when the arm is passively abducted and the patient's hand is resting on the back of the head. Spurling's test reproduces pain with the neck extended and then rotated toward the affected side with axial compression. In the author's experience, even gentle positioning at end range of motion during Spurling's test can reproduce radicular symptoms. A positive axial traction test, which produces relief of symptoms with 10 to 15 kg traction, suggests foraminal root compression. These three tests have poor sensitivity (26%–64%) but good specificity (80%–100%) (9,10). A positive L'Hermitte's sign, in which an electric-like sensation is produced with neck flexion, is suggestive but not specific since it may also be seen in malignancy and multiple sclerosis.

When cervical radiculopathy is suspected, plain radiographs are not needed but if trauma is suspected then x-rays with anteroposterior, lateral, oblique, flexion/extension, and open-mouth views may help rule out fractures and gross instability. Decreased intervertebral disc space height is consistent with degenerative disc disease. Magnetic resonance imaging (MRI) has been the preferred advanced imaging modality for several years, since it offers a much finer resolution of soft tissue in the neck and spine without the ionizing radiation and associated health risk associated with computerized tomography (CT). However, CT may be preferred for assessing bony pathology or if MRI is contraindicated (e.g., pacemaker, foreign metal bodies). It should be noted, however, that anatomic abnormalities can be found by MRI in up to 20% of asymptomatic patients (11). Cervical radiculopathy may be suspected and diagnosed clinically and does not initially mandate imaging studies, but should be considered if the condition is refractory to conservative treatment, when looking for structural changes or the etiology of the radiculopathy, to rule out alternative or concomitant pathology, or for planning interventional or surgical procedures.

Electrodiagnostic studies, which include nerve conduction studies (NCS) and electromyography (EMG), offer assessment of nerve and muscle physiology where other modalities focus on anatomical abnormalities. This procedure is most sensitive and specific when ordered at least 21 to 28 days after onset of symptoms in order to capture most abnormalities. EMG/NCS is also a useful tool for distinguishing among several suspected pathologies (e.g., radiculopathy vs. plexopathy, concurrent peripheral nerve injury) (12).

CERVICAL RADICULOPATHY

- ▪ Cervical radiculopathy is a common condition, although less common than lumbosacral radiculopathy

- ▪ The most commonly affected roots are the seventh (60%) and sixth (25%) cervical roots

- ▪ The cause can be mechanical or chemical radiculopathy, and common etiologies include cervical disc herniation and degenerative conditions of the spine

- ▪ Patients complain of neck pain that radiates in a dermatomal pattern

- ▪ Key findings on physical examination include any or all of the following: decreased sensation in dermatomal pattern, weakness in a myotome, diminished reflexes, and a positive Spurling's maneuver

- ▪ MRI is the imaging modality of choice for radiculopathy of nontraumatic onset; in the case of trauma, x-rays or CT scan may be warranted to quickly assess for bony pathology

THE REHABILITATION PROGRAM

The first step in managing cervical radiculopathy is pain control. Relative, but not complete, rest can help reduce motions and positions that provoke pain. Although there are no studies that have directly evaluated the effect of rest on neck pain, it is known that strength is lost at a rate of 1% to 4% per day with complete bed rest (13). Medications such as NSAIDs or steroids may reduce pain related to inflammation, and tramadol has been shown to be as effective as low-dose opioids for analgesia (14). Chronic opioid use is not supported by evidence-based practice guidelines and is independently associated with worse clinical outcomes after surgery (15).

Cervical orthoses, such as a soft cervical collar, have been shown to decrease neck pain by increasing proprioception and limiting movement. However, evidence suggests that early mobilization, whether performed with a physical therapist or at home, results in a greater degree of pain reduction than a brace and rest by 8 weeks (16,17).

Therapeutic Modalities

Modalities such as ice or heat can be prescribed for use in therapy or at home to assist with pain control. It is important to limit application of heat or ice to 20 minutes at a time, with at least 20 minutes between applications, to prevent damage to the skin. Heat sources should not be placed between the patient and a surface (e.g., bed, chair) since the heat does not dissipate as effectively and can damage skin more rapidly. These modalities have limited evidence in the literature regarding long term benefits but can be used for symptom control.

Transcutaneous electrical nerve stimulation (TENS) applies electrical current (currents usually less than 100 mA with pulse rates ranging 2–200 Hz) to peripheral nerves through electrodes on the skin to reduce pain. The proposed mechanism of action of high-dose TENS is the gate-control theory of pain, in which depolarization of larger sensory nerves overrides the input of smaller nociceptive nerve fibers (18). Low-dose TENS, also known as acupuncture like TENS, is believed to release endogenous opioids. TENS may be used in therapy and if found to be beneficial, a home TENS unit may be prescribed. A meta-analysis found weak evidence to suggest that TENS is superior to placebo, but not to other interventions used for neck pain (19).

Ultrasound is a deep heating modality that can only be administered in therapy sessions. Ultrasound is contraindicated in patients experiencing acute symptoms (may exacerbate inflammatory response) or with a history of laminectomy (potential to damage the spinal cord) (6). Evidence is limited to support its use for short or long term beneficial effects.

Although cervical traction has been used for decades to relieve neural tension, there is no consensus or sufficient evidence to recommend a particular weight, angle of neck flexion, and mode (continuous vs. intermittent). However, a common arrangement cited in the literature places the patient supine, with the neck flexed to 24° and intermittent traction with 30 lbs of force over 20 minutes; this has been shown to maximize radiologic separation at the C5-C6 and C6-C7 levels (Figure 39.3a) (20).

Manual Therapy

After pain has been adequately controlled to allow some passive and active movement, the next step is to mobilize the patient using one or more exercise paradigms. The approach favored by the authors, with a high degree of reproducible systemized assessment and exercise prescription, is the McKenzie Mechanical Diagnosis and Treatment (MDT), first developed by Robin McKenzie (21). The MDT approach has become one of the most widely used therapies for the treatment of low back pain (22,23). Manual therapy, when based upon the principles of MDT, is believed to be a more effective means of achieving symptomatic relief than other therapeutic approaches because it is thought to actually produce a mechanical change in the spine which then leads to a reduction in symptoms. Other therapeutic interventions,

such as opioid therapy, may only mask the symptoms while not addressing their underlying cause. As such, those other treatments can lead to a higher rate of symptom recurrence, greater dependence on medical care, and higher expenditures.

Other manual therapies which can be used to reduce pain and mobilize the patient include techniques of strain/counterstrain and soft tissue/nerve mobilization. Strain/counterstrain (SCS) is a technique developed by Dr. Lawrence Jones in 1955 and further elaborated upon in his book *Strain and Counterstrain* (24). It involves identifying the muscle which is in spasm (thus being the pain generator) and positioning it in a shortened length in an effort to enable it to relax aberrant reflexes which produce the muscle spasm. Holding this position from between 90 seconds to 5 minutes can allow the muscle to change from spasm to normal resting tone. The therapist then slowly brings the patient out of this position which then allows the body to reset the muscle to a normal level of tension and function more optimally, thus enabling an increase in range of motion and function. An example of SCS technique is shown in (Figure 39.3b). Support for SCS was recently shown in a study done in 2006, which showed that SCS was effective in reducing pain in the upper trapezius of symptomatic subjects (25). Soft tissue mobilization (STM), myofascial release (MFR), and nerve mobilization are other "manual therapies" where the therapist attempts to reduce pain and restore normal function by mobilizing muscle, fascia, and/or the nervous system. By implementing STM and MFR techniques one can reduce any restrictions in the muscle or fascia which can be causing abnormal responses from the nervous system. Neural mobilization, a concept developed by David Butler and described in his book *Mobilization of the Nervous*

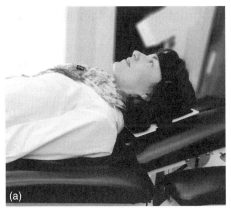
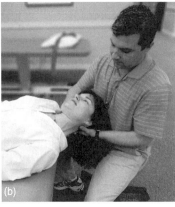

FIGURE 39.3: Physical Therapy Techniques. These pictures illustrate the equipment and appropriate set up for cervical traction (a) and an example of Strain and Counterstrain technique (b).

System, employs techniques to mobilize the peripheral nerves focusing on identifying and freeing up any areas where the nerves may become compressed and irritated within various parts of the body (26).

Patients may also seek massage therapies. Several techniques exist, and they all involve compression, stimulation, and mobilization of soft tissue. There is weak evidence to suggest that massage may improve circulation and release of serotonin and oxytocin while decreasing feelings of pain, anxiety, and depression, but a significant effect has not been demonstrated (27). Contraindications to massage include unstable fractures, severe hypertension, fever, contagious skin condition, and malignant tumors. These soft tissue techniques are beneficial to treat muscle spasm and tension related to guarding and protecting the underlying injury. However, the focus of treatment still remains on reducing nerve root irritation through activity modification and restoring function through therapeutic exercises.

Therapeutic Exercise

We consider the hallmark of therapy for cervical radiculopathy to be the MDT method, which is based upon the concept of *centralization* (28). Centralization is the phenomenon whereby radiating symptoms originating from the spine and referring distally are caused to move proximally toward the midline of the spine as a result of the performance of certain repeated movements or the adoption of certain positions (28). Once identified, these positions and movements can be used to abolish the radicular symptoms. Avoidance of positions and movements that cause peripheralization throughout the day is also very important.

The most accepted explanation for the centralization phenomenon suggests that displaced nuclear material from the disc migrates intradiscally and thus reduces pressure on the nerve root exiting from a particular level in the spine (21). Through repeated movements or positions, one could "mechanically" cause the disc material to migrate in the opposite direction and, in turn, reduce the mechanical and chemical irritation on the nerve root and abolish the radicular symptoms. While research investigating this "disc model" is limited and has mostly focused on the lumbar spine, there are several investigations which support the theory (29,30,31). In the lumbar spine, it has been reported that centralization by the McKenzie Method correlated to lumbar disc mediated pain as defined by positive discography (32). Studies

involving the mechanics of the cervical spine are even more scarce, but more recent work supports the "disc model" of pain in the neck as well (33,34). In particular, it was found in a porcine model that repeated cervical flexion induces disc prolapse and that the displaced nucleus can be directed back toward the center of the disc with other active and passive movements and positions (34). An additional study examined a group of patients with neck and radicular pain and found that a posture of sustained flexion significantly increased peripheral pain and root compression (as measured by H-reflex amplitude). Yet, repeated retractions significantly decreased both the pain and nerve root compression (35). These clinical findings suggest that there might be an anatomic change occurring in humans, as reported in the porcine model (34).

Clinical studies suggest that MDT can be helpful in treating cervical pain (36,37). One study investigated 77 patients with neck pain in a prospective, randomized clinical trial randomizing to treatments administered by five McKenzie Method trained physical therapists (36). Treatment groups included general exercise (neck ROM, patient specific, 2x/week for 8 weeks), MDT (McKenzie protocol, 8 weeks), and a control group (lowest level of ultrasound to turn indicator lights on); 70 patients (93%) were available for 12-month follow-up. All three groups showed significant improvement in pain intensity and Neck Disability Index. In all, 79% reported that they were better or completely restored after treatment although 51% reported constant and daily pain. When compared with the control group, the MDT group had a tendency toward greater improvement for pain intensity at 3 weeks and for Neck Disability Index at 6-month follow-up. Significant improvement in Distress and Risk Assessment Method scores were shown only in the MDT group. Although all three groups had similar recurrence rates, at 12 months, the MDT group showed a tendency toward *fewer visits for additional health care*. This finding is consistent with a study that found that the centralization phenomenon in lumbar spine patients with sciatica portended a more favorable outcome at 1, 2, 3, and 12 months, and that centralization was a very good predictor of not requiring surgery (38).

After adequate pain control and restoration of ROM has occurred, the final step is a functional rehabilitation program tailored to the patient to restore proper spinal mechanics and prevent recurrence of symptoms. The program begins by maximizing range of motion and proper posture. Cervicothoracic stabilization helps to correct cervical lordosis, normalize segmental loading, open the neural foramen and the thoracic outlet, and restore muscle balance. The goal of these exercises is to decrease pain and dependence on other medications, modalities, and therapies. Exercises progress from supine to seated to standing, isometric to concentric, and static to dynamic/functional. Isometric exercises of neck flexion, extension, lateral bending, and rotation are performed first. Program exercises include supine isometric head lift, prone head lift, prone "butterflies," seated/standing rowing, and posture and positioning. Overactive muscles are stretched and underactive muscles are strengthened to achieve muscular balance. Scapulothoracic muscles should be addressed concurrently, including the trapezius, serratus anterior, rhomboid, and rotator cuff muscles (6). Popular treatment approaches for restoring cervical and scapulothoracic function are described elsewhere (39,40). Examples of key exercises are illustrated in (Figure 39.4 a-e). Applying strengthening programs to overall postural correction and translation to functional activities is a key education point. Allowing ergonomic corrections to the workplace, evaluation of daily activities, and training in correct postures is vital to treatment and prevention of future exacerbations.

Specialized Techniques

Nearly 42% of patients have used CAM therapies within the past year (41), making CAM less "alternative" than the name suggests. Practitioners of musculoskeletal medicine must not only ask their patients which CAM therapies they may have already pursued, but also understand the evidence base for these therapies.

Nearly 11% of adults who use CAM have tried chiropractic care, in which spinal manipulative therapy (SMT) is a major component in an overall functional reactivation program. The goals of SMT are to reduce pain by restoring dysfunctional joint mechanics and reducing mechanical stress on the adjacent tissues (42). Contraindications to SMT include spinal instability, infection, myelopathy, or vertebral artery stenosis. A 2004 Cochrane Review found that SMT and exercise were superior to no treatment (43). Some literature suggests that SMT alone (without exercise) may be superior, but the evidence is weak (44). Care must be taken and proper patient selection considered when recommending cervical spine manipulation as high velocity low amplitude manipulations have been

shown to be associated with craniocervical arterial dissections (45).

Yoga, Tai Chi Chuan (Tai Chi), and Acupuncture are derivatives of Eastern Medicine that have seen increasing popularity in the United States in recent decades. Yoga has several methods that all emphasize postural restoration, flexibility and strengthening, and mental emphasis on relaxation and meditation. There is no direct study of the effect of Yoga on neck pain, but there is evidence that Yoga may reduce pain and disability in chronic low back pain, as well as improve mood (46,47). Tai Chi is an ancient Chinese martial art consisting of five separate schools that focuses on slow, controlled, continuous movements coordinated with breathing, resulting in motion meditation. Tai Chi is generally safe, and while it is unlikely to worsen musculoskeletal conditions, there is little evidence that it improves the pathologic progression of these conditions (48). However, while there is no direct study on the effect on neck pain, Tai Chi can reduce fear of falling and improve body stability (49). Acupuncture consists of several heterogeneous methods of using fine needles along defined points and meridians to restore balance of chi (or qi) energy in the body. Acupuncture is regarded as a safe treatment modality with very few serious complications reported in the literature; fatigue and soreness or bleeding at insertion sites are the most common adverse effects (50). A full discussion of acupuncture is beyond the scope of this chapter, but there is evidence—often with poor methodology, however—to suggest short-term improvement of pain compared to sham or no treatment (51,52,53,54,55,56).

Home Exercise Program

The home exercise program (HEP) should be instituted at the onset of rehabilitation, and should reflect each phase of rehabilitation as the patient progresses. The patient should be educated on the principle of "centralization" and the repeated movements that centralize symptoms. After learning to centralize symptoms, education on proper performance of cervical active ROM, isometric and postural correction exercises without peripheralizing symptoms should be emphasized. Centralization, stretching, and strengthening exercises are vital parts of the HEP. An emphasis should be made on injury prevention. Finally, a home cervical traction unit may be beneficial if the patient is found to be traction responsive in therapy or during initial evaluation by the physician (57).

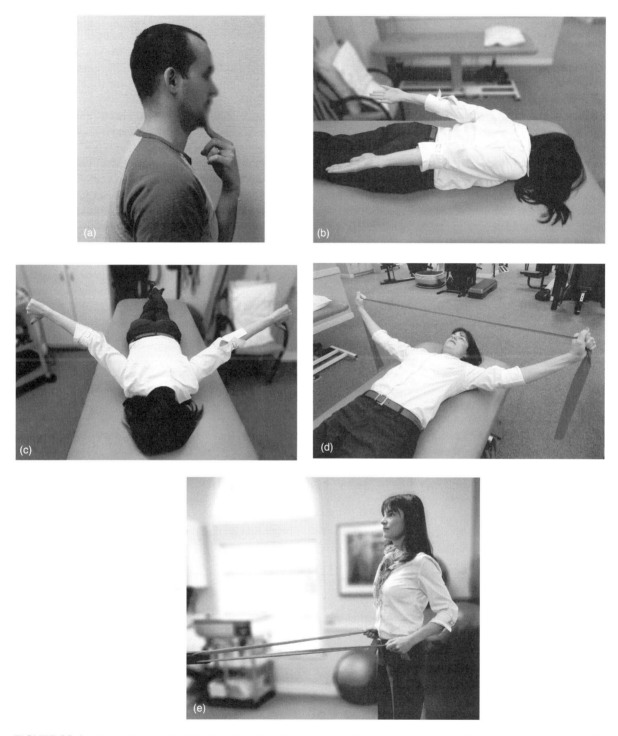

FIGURE 39.4: Cervicothoracic Stabilization Exercises. These pictures illustrate common exercises that may be incorporated in a home exercise program designed to improve cervical and scapulothoracic posture and muscle balance: sitting cervical retraction (a), prone scapular retraction (b), prone butterflies (c), supine abduction pullout (d), and standing row with resistance band (e).

SUMMARY

Cervical radiculopathy has several possible presentations based on mechanism of onset, radiation of symptoms, and clinical presentation. A thorough examination of sensation, reflexes, strength, and special tests can help confirm suspected pathology. Imaging, such as plain radiographs, may be necessary to rule out acute bony pathology, but MRI is the imaging modality of choice to assess for the etiology of cervical radiculopathy. Electrodiagnostic studies can help localize the level and severity of the injury. Evidence-based treatments are not well defined, however; the principles of rehabilitation, such as the phases of rehabilitation, can be followed for safe and effective treatment. Once pain is addressed, allowing the patient to participate in therapy, the concept of centralization is a key element to recovery. McKenzie MDT is a method of evaluation to determine directional preference to help guide treatment. Modalities, though evidence is limited, may help patients tolerate the therapy program. Mechanical traction for home use may also help enhance recovery. A strengthening program and postural correction exercises with emphasis on return to functional activities should be the key focus of the HEP.

SAMPLE CASE

R.S. is a 37-year-old construction worker who experienced a sudden onset of lancinating neck pain radiating into his left arm after throwing a bag of concrete over his left shoulder 4 weeks ago. The neck pain radiates down the lateral aspect of his left arm and forearm, into the thumb. He also has weakness when trying to reach to his left side or bring objects toward him. He denies any associated weight loss, angina, lower limb weakness, balance problems, or bowel/bladder incontinence.

R.S. has a medical history of hypertension, and no past surgical history. His family history is significant for diabetes, coronary artery disease, and osteoarthritis. He is a 1-pack-per-day smoker and drinks 2 to 3 beers on weekends. There is no personal or family history of cancer. On physical examination, he has decreased ROM with neck flexion, extension, and lateral bending and rotation to the left side. Strength examination of the upper and lower limbs is normal with the exception of 4/5 strength of the left elbow flexors and wrist extensors. Sensation is normal with the exception of decreased light touch and pinprick along the palmar and dorsal aspects of the left thumb and second digit. Reflexes are normal except 1+ at the left brachioradialis. Hoffman and Babinski signs are negative.

Spurling's test is positive with the head turned to the left side, and pain is relieved using Bakody's sign. MRI of the cervical spine demonstrates left para-central C5-6 disc protrusion and left C5-6 foraminal stenosis, without evidence of spinal cord edema.

 SAMPLE THERAPY PRESCRIPTION

Discipline: Physical therapy—evaluate and treat.

Diagnosis: Left C6 radiculopathy with strength deficit due to left para-central C5-6 disc protrusion and left C5-6 foraminal stenosis.

Precautions: Avoid ultrasound during period of acute inflammation; initially avoid manual mobilization at pathologic segment; monitor for progression of weakness.

Frequency of visits: 1 to 2x/week.

Duration of treatment: 3 to 4 weeks.

Treatment:

1. *Modalities:* cryotherapy or superficial heat

2. *Manual therapy:* Mechanical Diagnosis & Treatment (McKenzie Method), MFR, cervical traction (see specialized treatment section)

3. *Therapeutic exercise:* MDT method to be applied to early ROM exercises and positioning

to facilitate centralization of symptoms; A/AA/PROM to pain tolerance to restore flexion, extension, rotation, lateral bending, and cervical retractions; gentle stretching; functional cervicothoracic postural training; ergonomic assessment; strengthening exercises for neck and left upper limb; scapulothoracic stabilization; progressing from isometric to concentric, static to dynamic

4. *Specialized treatments:* trial of manual traction first, if beneficial consider intermittent cervical traction at 30 lbs force and 24° flexion for 20 minutes; may issue home unit for purchase if helpful

5. *Patient education:* HEP with progression to gym program; discuss exercise progression with personal trainer if appropriate

Goals: Decrease pain; restore cervical ROM/ flexibility; restore strength; safely return to functional activities (e.g., sport, hobbies, work) and prevent recurrent injury.

Reevaluation: In 4 weeks by referring physician.

REFERENCES

1. Malanga GA. Cervical radiulopathy: evaluation and management. *Medicine & Science in Sports & Exercise.* 1997;29(7):236–245.
2. Radhakrishnan K, Litchy WJ, O'Fallon WM, et al. Epidemiology of cervical radiculopathy: a population-based study from Rochester, Minnesota, 1976–1990. *Brain.* 1994;117:325–335.
3. Furusawa N, Baba H, Miyoshi N, et al. Herniation of cervical intervertebral disc: immunohistochemical examination and measurement of nitric oxide production. *Spine.* 2001;26(10):1110–1116.
4. Kang JD, Stefanovic-Racic M, McIntyre LA, et al. Toward a biochemical understanding of human intervertebral disc degeneration and herniation. Contributions of nitric oxide, interleukins, prostaglandin E2, and matrix metalloproteinases. *Spine.* 1997;22(10):1065–1073.
5. Gore DR, Sepic SB, Gardner GM. Roentgenographic findings of the cervical spine in asymptomatic people. *Spine.* 1986;11(6):521–524.
6. De Palma MJ, Slipman CW. Common neck problems. In: Braddom RL, Chan L, Harrast MA et al, eds. *Physical Medicine & Rehabilitation*, 4th ed. Philadelphia, PA: Saunders; 2011:787–815.
7. Bogduk N. *Medical Management of Acute Cervical Radicular Pain: An Evidence Based Approach.* Newcastle, UK: International Spine Intervention Society; 1999.
8. Ness TJ. Visceral pain: a review of experimental studies. *Pain.* 1990;41:167–234.
9. Ellenberg MR, Honet JC, Treanor WJ. Cervical radiculopathy. *Arch Phys Med Rehabil.* 1994;75:342–352.
10. Viikari-Juntura E, Porras M, Laasonen EM. Validity of clinical tests in the diagnosis of root compression in cervical disk disease. *Spine.* 1989;14:253–257.
11. Boden SD, McCowin PR, Davis DO, et al. Abnormal magnetic resonance scans of the cervical spine in asymptomatic subjects. *J Bone Joint Surg Am.* 1990;72:1178–1184.
12. Wilbourn AJ, Aminoff MJ. The electrodiagnostic examination in patients with radiculopathies. *Muscle Nerve.* 1998;21:1612–1631.
13. Spitzer WO. Scientific monograph of the Quebec Task Force on Whiplash-Associated Disorders: redefining 'whiplash' and its management. *Spine.* 1995;20(suppl):1–73.
14. Nemat A, Richeimer SM. Pharmacologic therapies for neck pain. *Phys Med Rehabil Clin N Am.* 2003;14:629–641.
15. Lawrence JTR, London N, Bohlman NH, et al. Preoperative narcotic use as a predictor of clinical outcome. *Spine.* 2008;33(19):2074–2078.
16. Mealy K, Brennan H, Fenelon GC. Early mobilization of acute whiplash injuries. *BMJ.* 1986;292:656.
17. McKinney LA. Early mobilisation and outcome in acute sprains of the neck. *BMJ.* 1989;299:1006.
18. Melzack R, Wall PD. Pain mechanisms: a new theory. *Science.* 1965;150:971–979.
19. Kroeling P, Gross AR, Goldsmith CH. A Cochrane review of electrotherapy for mechanical neck disorders. *Spine.* 2005;30(21):E641-E648.
20. Colachis SC. A study of tractive forces and angle of pull on vertebral interspaces in the cervical spine. *Arch Phys Med Rehabil.* 1965;46(12):820.
21. McKenzie R. *The Lumbar Spine: Mechanical Diagnosis and Therapy.* Waikanae, New Zealand: Spine Publications; 1981.
22. Battie M, Cherkin DC, Dunn R, Ciol MA, Wheeler KJ. Managing low back pain: attitudes and treatment preferences of physical therapists. *Phys Ther.* 1994;74(3):219–226.
23. Foster N, Thompson KA, Baxter GD, Allen JM. Management of nonspecific low back pain by physiotherapists in Britain and Ireland. *Spine.* 1999;24(13):1332–1342.
24. Jones LH. *Strain and Counterstrain.* Newark, OH: American Academy of Osteopathy; 1981.
25. Meseguer A, et al. Immediate effects of the Strain/Counterstrain Technique in local pain evoked by tender points in the upper trapezius muscle. *Journal of Bodywork and Movement Therapies.* 2006;9(3),112–118.
26. Butler D. *Mobilization of the Nervous System.* London, UK: Churchill Livingston; 1991.
27. Binesh N, Cohen RM, Moser FG, et al. Does massage therapy affect brain metabolites? *The Internet Journal of Alternative Medicine.* 2008;5(2).
28. McKenzie R. *The Cervical and Thoraric Spine: Mechanical Diagnosis and Therapy.* Waikanae, New Zealand: Spinal Publications; 1990.
29. Adams MA, Hutton WC. Prolapsed intervertebral disc: a hyperflexion injury. *Spine.* 1982;7(3):184.
30. Schnebel B, Simmons W. A digitizing technique for the study of movement of intradiscal dye in response to flexion and extension of the lumbar spine. *Spine.* 1998;13:3.

31. Alexander LA, Hancock E, Agouris I, Smith FW, MacSween A. The response of the nucleus pulposus of the lumbar intervertebral discs to functionally loaded positions. *Spine*. 2007;32:1508–1512.

32. Young S, Aprill C, Laslett M. Correlation of clinical examination characteristics with three sources of chronic low back pain. *Spine J*. 2003;3:460–465.

33. Skrzpiec D, Hancock E, Agouris I, Smith FW, MacSween A. The internal mechanical properties of cervical intervertebral discs as revealed by stress profilometry. *Eur Spine J*. 2007;16(10):1701–1709.

34. Scannell JP, McGill SM. Disc prolapse: evidence of reversal with repeated extension. *Spine*. 2009;34(4):344–350.

35. Adbulwahab SS, Sabbahi M. Neck retractions, cervical root decompression, and radicular pain. *JOSPT*. 2000;30(1):4–12.

36. Kjellman K, Oberg B. A randomized clinical trial comparing general exercise, McKenzie Treatment and a control group in patients with neck pain. *J Rehabi Med*. 2002;34(4):183.

37. Rathore S. Use of McKenzie Cervical Protocol in the treatment of radicular neck pain in a machine operator. *J Can Chiropr Assoc*. 2003;47(4):291–297.

38. Skytte L, May S, Petersen P. Centralization: its prognostic value in patients with referred symptoms and sciatica. *Spine (Phila Pa 1976)*. 2005;30(11):E293-E299.

39. Gary Gray Institute (website). http://www.grayinstitute.com/articles.aspx?Article=14. Last accessed 1 May 2011.

40. Burkhard SS, Morgan CD, Kibler WB. The disabled throwing shoulder: spectrum of pathology Part III: the SICK scapula, scapular dyskinesis, the kinetic chain, and rehabilitation. *J Arthrosc Rel Surg*. 2003;19(6):641–661.

41. Miller J, Gross A, D'Sylva J, et al. Manual therapy and exercise for neck pain: a systematic review. *Man Ther*, 2010;15:334–354.

42. Plasteras C, Schran S, Kim N. Complementary and Alternative Treatment for Neck Pain: Chiropractic, Acupuncture, TENS, Massage, Yoga, Tai Chi, and Feldenkrais. *Phys Med Rehabil Clin N Am*. 2011;22(3):521–537, ix.

43. Gross AR, Hoving JL, Haines TA, et al. Cervical Overview Group. A Cochrane review of manipulation and mobilization for mechanical neck disorders. *Spine*. 2004;29:1541–1548.

44. Gross A, Miller J, D'Sylva J, et al. Manipulation or mobilization for neck pain: a Cochrane review. *Man Ther*. 2010;15:315–333.

45. Albuquerque F, Hu YC, Dashti SR, et al. Craniocervical arterial dissections as sequelae of chiropractic manipulation: patterns of injury and management. *Neurosurgery J*. 2011;115(6):1197–1205.

46. Williams K, Steinberg L, Petronis J. Therapeutic application of iyengar yoga for healing chronic low back pain. *Int J Yoga Ther*. 2003;13:55–67.

47. Woolery A, Myers H, Sternlieb B, Zeltzer L. A yoga intervention for young adults with elevated symptoms of depression. *Altern Ther Health Med*. 2004;10:60–63.

48. Yeh G. Commentary on the Cochrane review of Tai Chi for rheumatoid arthritis. Explore, 2008;4(4):275–277.

49. Chen KM, Snyder M. Research-based use of Tai Chi/Movement Therapy as a nursing intervention. *J Holist Nurs*. 1999;17:267.

50. Ernst E, White AR. Prospective studies of the safety of acupuncture: a systematic review. *Am J Med*. 2001;110:481–485.

51. Birch S, Jamison R. Controlled trial of Japanese acupuncture for chronic myofascial neck pain: assessment of specific and nonspecific effects of treatment. *Clin J Pain*. 1998;14:248–255.

52. White PF, Craig WF, Vakharia AS, et al. Percutaneous neuromodulation therapy: does the location of electrical stimulation effect the acute analgesic response? *Anesthesia Analgesic*. 2000;91:949–954.

53. Irnich D, Behrens N, Molzen H, et al. Randomized trial of acupuncture compared with conventional massage and "sham" laser acupuncture for treatment of chronic neck pain. *BMJ*. 2001;322:1574–1578.

54. Vickers AJ. Statistical re-analysis of four recent randomized trials of acupuncture for pain using analysis of covariance. *Clin J Pain*. 2004;20(5):319–323.

55. White P, Lewith G, Prescott P, et al. Acupuncture versus placebo for the treatment of chronic mechanical neck pain. *Ann Int Med*. 2004;141:920–928.

56. He D, Veiersted KB, Hostmark AT, et al. Effect of acupuncture treatment on chronic neck and shoulder pain in sedentary female workers: a 6-month and 3-year follow-up study. *Pain*. 2004;109(3):299–307.

57. Swezey RL, Swezey AM, Warner K. Efficacy of home cervical traction therapy. *Am J Phys Med Rehabil*. 1999;78(1):30–32.

Other Cervical Spine Disorders

Brian Domenic Wishart, Heather Roehrs Galgon, and Gina M. Benaquista DeSipio

INTRODUCTION

Neck pain is a common problem with 30% to 50% of the population experiencing some form of it every year. The cervical spine, like the shoulder, was designed for mobility, which in turn leaves it susceptible to injury. The chapters in this section reviewed common injuries to the cervical spine, including cervical radiculopathy, cervical facet syndrome, and discogenic pain. The focus of this chapter is to address sprains and strains, involving noncontractile and contractile elements respectively, which can result in a diverse set of symptoms, including but not limited to, neck pain, facial pain and cervicogenic headaches, and whiplash related injuries. These injuries often co-exist in the aforementioned cervical spine injuries. Not all injuries will require healthcare professionals and only 2% to 11% of people will experience pain that limits activity (1). Cervical sprains/strains are seen in all ages with a peak incidence between ages 35 and 55. Often these injuries can linger for a period of time if not addressed.

Several risk factors have been identified for persistent cervical pain and include previous neck pain, low back pain, or headaches; poor self-rated health; and psychological health disorders. Smoking and second hand smoke exposure have been shown to be associated with neck pain while exercise has been associated with a better prognosis and thought to be protective. Interestingly, several studies have been unable to demonstrate or associate common disc and vertebral degeneration as a risk factor or the cause of neck pain symptoms (2,3).

Cervical sprain/strain is defined as injury to the soft tissues of the neck including the muscles, tendons, fascia, and ligaments (4) and can occur from trauma, overuse, or neuromuscular imbalances. Specific focal pathology is not always identified in patients with complaints of sprain/ strains of the neck, even after a thorough clinical and radiographic examination (see Table 40.1). Cervical soft tissue injury can occur from any acceleration/deceleration of the unrestrained head resulting in excessive flexion and extension or rotation of the cervical spine. This is classically seen in "whiplash," but can occur during contact sports or any type of trauma. A complete understanding of the cervical spine anatomy is important to the diagnosis and treatment of cervical pathology. Damage to any or all of the superficial muscles, anterior or posterior deep muscles, the suboccipital triangle, the levator scapulae, intervertebral discs, the zygapophysial joints, the brachial plexus, or any of the ligaments can be potential causes of pain in these types of injuries and all should be addressed (5).

As with other injuries, cervical sprains/strains follow a natural course during the healing process. Most of the signs and symptoms (see Table 40.2) of the injury will manifest over a few hours to days. During the acute stage, inflammation is the predominate reaction which results in swelling, erythema, heat, pain, and decreased range of motion (ROM). Typically these symptoms last from four to six days. From 14 to 21 days after the injury, the tissues enter the restorative stage during which the cervical spine tissues undergo repair and healing while the inflammatory mediators are slowly removed. Finally, after about 3 weeks, during the maintenance/return to function stage, most injured muscle fibers should be healed and the pain should be resolved, except when the tissues are being constantly stressed (see Table 40.3) (5).

Cervical sprain/strain is associated with several other disorders. Scott et al found that following whiplash injury patients showed widespread sensitivity "consistent with central nervous system hypersensitivity and ongoing tissue injury" (6). This hyperalgesia was independent of anxiety states and was likely due to alterations in pain processing mechanisms of the central nervous system. Many patients also displayed cold hyperalgesia which is a nonspecific indication

TABLE 40.1: Diagnostic Considerations in Neck Pain (7)

Imaging and Other Tests	Indication	Differential Diagnosis
X-Ray	• Suspected subluxation or fracture • Painful distracting type of injury • Loss of consciousness • Midline tenderness on spinous process • Focal neurological deficit • Injured while intoxicated by alcohol or other substance	Traumatic fracture, dislocation, subluxation, ligamentous instability
MRI	• If soft tissue or CNS pathology suspected *Caution due to high probability of unrelated findings	Myelopathy, radiculopathy
Blood Work	• Systemic symptoms (fever, chills, multiple joint involvement)	Rheumatic disease, infection, abscess, malignancy
EMG	• Correlating symptoms and anatomic pathology in difficult cases	

TABLE 40.2: Signs and Symptoms of Cervical Sprain/Strain (4,6,7)

Signs and Symptoms			
Neck pain (88–100%)	Tightness	Swelling	Tenderness
Headaches (54–66%)	Visual changes	Muscles spasm	Paraesthesia
Thoracic pain	Weakness	Dizziness	Dysphagia
Jaw pain	Lumbar pain	Fatigue	Nausea
Memory/Concentration difficulties	Positive Spurlings' Maneuver	Positive Lhermitte Sign	Anxiety and depression

TABLE 40.3: Classification Systems for Cervical Sprain/Strain (6)

Grade	Quebec Task Force	Temporal Classification
0	No complaints	
1	Neck pain, stiffness, tenderness No physical signs	< 4 days after injury
2	Neck complaints Signs limited to MSK structures	4–21 days after injury
3	Neck complaints Neurologic signs	22–45 days after injury
4	Neck complaints Fracture or dislocation	46–180 days after injury *risk for chronic symptoms
5		> 6 months after injury *considered chronic

of sympathetically maintained pain, of which, the pathophysiology is unclear. It is thought to be due to peripheral nerve injury which leads to sprouting of sympathetic fibers into nerves of the dorsal root ganglion. This cold hyperalgesia has been shown to be a feature of neuropathic pain and can lead to pain upon sympathetic nervous system activity (6).

Cervicogenic headache is a well-documented syndrome that is very common after whiplash-type injuries. One study found that 15.2% of patients experienced headaches lasting longer than 42 days after injury and 4.6% of patients went on to develop chronic daily headaches (7). Cervicogenic headache is defined by pain being perceived in the head but whose source is in the cervical region. Though the criteria for diagnosis of cervicogenic headaches are quite strict, chronic headaches attributed to whiplash injury is defined entirely by the temporal relationship between injury and the onset of headaches. As these headaches are secondary to a cervical spine injury they should be considered a subtype of cervicogenic headaches (8).

The neck has rich nociceptive innervations within many aspects including the zygapophysial joints, the intervertebral discs, the ligaments, the muscles, and the skin. These nerves refer pain to the head and face because the nociceptive afferents within the trigeminal nerve, including those from the supratentorial dura, synapse with the same second order sensory neurons in the trigeminal nucleus caudalis. This convergence of pain fibers from the trigeminal nerve, particularly the ophthalmic branch, and the upper cervical nerves results in pain from the cervical spine being perceived in the head. The zygapophysial joints, or facet joints, are thought to be the main pain generators of the neck. This is consistent with joints being a common cause of pain elsewhere in the body and the neck is no different. A second source of cervical generated pain in the head is from myofascial trigger points. There are many muscles within the neck, such as the splenius capitis, the suboccipital triangle muscles, and the trapezius, that refer pain to the head. Though these are classically considered tension-type headaches, it is reasonable to include them in the cervicogenic headache category (8).

It is important to note that cervical sprain/strain, and whiplash in particular, is a total body injury. It is the result of a traumatic incident that affects the entire neuromusculoskeletal system. It is important to obtain a complete history including a specific description of the mechanism of injury, any loss of consciousness, initial symptoms at the time of injury, and the emergency room evaluation and work up. Recognizing the interrelated connections of the body will make it clear that treating neck pain as a lone entity will not be as efficacious as treating the entire body (9).

THE REHABILITAION PROGRAM

It is important to address acute neck pain with a comprehensive and supervised rehabilitation program to avoid the development of a more chronic condition. Application of the phases of rehabilitation followed throughout this book can help guide the rehabilitation program.

This can begin with protection of the soft tissue injuries of the neck, and some patients find a soft cervical collar to be beneficial during the acute phase; however, it is not recommended for long term use. It does not provide motion control, but can provide comfort by retaining heat and serving as a reminder to restrict motion via sensory feedback which may help reduce muscle spasm (10). The optimal approach to neck injury includes an aggressive approach to controlling inflammation and thereby pain (controversial), early mobilization, and specific strength and postural training (refer to Table 40.4). Mobilization, if performed within 96 hours after an acute injury, will have more significant effect on pain reduction than immobilization or rest (11). An integral component of a rehabilitation program is functional training and postural reeducation in order to prevent future episodes or exacerbations of cervical spine pain and dysfunction. Studies have shown up to 40% of patients who sustained a whiplash injury from a motor vehicle incident or a sports injury will continue to experience pain 15 years after the injury (11).

Therapeutic Modalities

Cryotherapy should be used during the acute phase of injury to decrease pain fiber conduction, blood flow, and metabolism to the tissues thereby inhibiting the propagation of acute inflammatory cytokines. Ice should be used for no longer than 20 minutes or the "therapeutic vasoconstriction" will turn into "detrimental vasodilation" when the tissues reach $-10°$ (12). During the subacute and chronic phases, superficial heating modalities (e.g., moist heat, heat wrap therapy) can be introduced as an effective modality to raise the pain threshold and

TABLE 40.4: Phases of Rehabilitation

Phases of Rehabilitation
Phase I: Decrease pain and inflammation using ice
Phase II: Restore ROM
Phase III: Address underlying pathology (Manual techniques by a trained provider)
Phase IV: Postural and strength training
Phase V: Functional/ergonomic assessment and modification

stimulate a relaxation reflex in deeper muscles allowing for a greater stretch (12). Forms of deep heating can include ultrasound therapy but have limited literature on their benefit of recovery. Electrotherapy with transcutaneous electrical nerve stimulator (TENS) and interferential stimulation also have limited literature to support their use in soft tissue injuries.

Manual Therapy

A recent Cochrane Review indicates that manipulation and mobilization are key components of an effective multimodal approach that benefits patients with persistent neck pain and dysfunction. Patients also report greater satisfaction when manual therapies are used in conjunction with exercises (13). Techniques found to be successful in addressing nonradicular cervical spine pain include myofascial release (MFR) of the anterior, pectoralis-clavicular, and posterior cervical fascia, soft tissue "massage" to the posterior cervical muscles, and release of the occipital-atlantal (OA) joint (13). Facilitated positional release (FPR) as well as counterstrain points, especially those in the anterior cervical region, can also be effective in reducing subacute neck pain. Manual cervical traction might be beneficial in chronic neck pain where significant degenerative disease of the cervical spine is present (13).

Therapeutic Exercise

Many patients experience a significant reduction in neck pain once the acute phase of injury is over. The goal of the next phase of rehabilitation is to restore motion, increase strength, and prevent fear avoidance behaviors, which is critical to preventing chronic neck pain, or disability. Ideally the patient will have a physician, physical or occupational therapist, and/or a manual medicine

practitioner to aid in their return to pain free functioning and prevent future occurrences.

Several studies have concluded that early mobilization, including exercises, within the first 96 hours is more effective at providing pain relief at 1, 2, and 6 months after an acute whiplash injury than immobilization with a soft collar and analgesics (13). Early mobilization is also more effective at reducing pain and sick leave at 3 years after an acute whiplash injury (13). Restoring ROM should comprise gentle "pain free" active range of motion (AROM) and passive range of motion (PROM). This should include flexion, extension rotation, and side bending (SB). Once the acute pain has subsided it is safe to start gentle stretching and then advance to isometric strengthening of the cervical muscles including levator scapulae, scalenes, posterior paraspinals, deep neck flexors (anterior paraspinals), trapezius and (Figures 40.1 and 40.2).

Successful rehabilitation of neck pain must consider the structurally and anatomically connected area adjacent to the affected region. In order to maintain proper cervical mechanics it is important to have strong thoracic and scapular-thoracic muscles to ensure the region operates in a functionally sound manner. A dyskinetic scapula due to weak scapular stabilizers can create or perpetuate pain in the upper thoracic and cervical musculature. This is due to the cervical region compensating for poor scapulothoracic mechanics. As a result, in an effective rehabilitation program one should address the "phasic" muscles which are activated less frequently and tend to fatigue sooner such as the rhomboids, lower trapezius, and the mid thoracic erector spinae (Figures 40.3–40.5) (12).

Strength training should focus on muscles in the neck, shoulders, and upper back. To create an effective strengthening program, the muscles that serve as postural stabilizers, that are continuously activated at a low level (e.g., scalenes, upper trapezius, erector spinae), should be adequately relaxed before the "phasic" muscles, those that function in quick short bursts and fatigue easily, are strengthened. Strengthening of "phasic" muscles

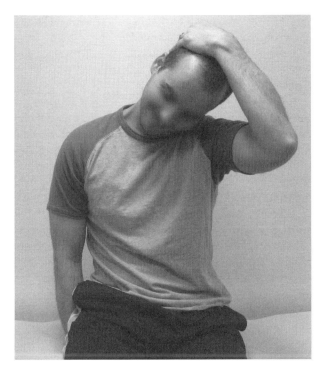

FIGURE 40.1: Trapezius stretch.

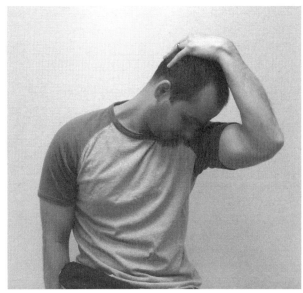

FIGURE 40.2: Levator scapulae stretch.

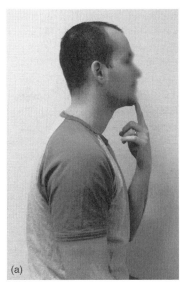
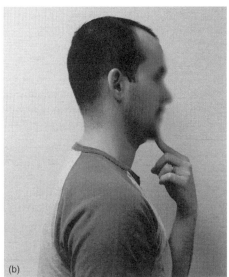

(a) (b)

FIGURE 40.3: Cervical retractions.

should occur with correct underlying posture (upon a solid foundation). Strength training should also include core stabilization in order to maintain proper posture, ensure balanced kinetic chain mechanics, and minimize dysfunction in the upper thoracic, scapular stabilizers, and cervical region.

In addition, functional and ergonomic training should be addressed. Neuromuscular training is a valuable tool

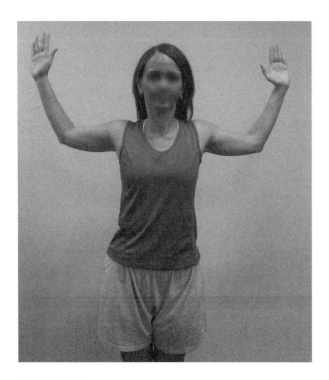

FIGURE 40.4: Scapular retraction exercise.

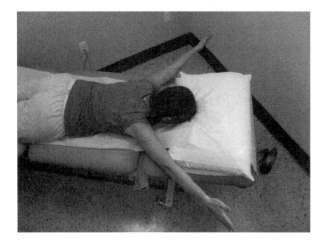

FIGURE 40.5: Lower trapezius strengthening.

used to correct poor postural mechanics. The patient should be taught to attain correct cervical-thoracic positioning and then perform ROM exercises for the neck and upper limbs. Also if there are specific concerns with the patient's work

or home environment, individualized recommendations should be made to prevent poor mechanics.

Specialized Techniques

Several alternative and complementary medicine therapeutic methods may also be considered in the treatment of neck pain. A recent study found that a series of five dry cupping treatments was both safe and effective in the treatment of chronic nonspecific neck pain (14). Acupuncture is well studied and has been shown to decrease pain intensity and improve quality of life with long term efficacy in chronic neck pain patients (15). There are several types of medical acupuncture ranging from a neuroanatomical model to traditional Chinese medicine to microacupuncture where needles are inserted into the ear, scalp, hand, or feet. A pain protocol, using auricular acupuncture, also known as battlefield acupuncture because of its use in the military, has been described with some success to produce a pain free period without use of narcotics (16).

Other techniques that can be implemented involve the use of trigger point management. Trigger points are seen as focal spots in a taut band of skeletal muscle tissue that can produce local and referred pain. They can result from acute trauma or repetitive microtrauma and can manifest as tension headache, tinnitus, or temporomandibular joint (TMJ) pain. Trigger-point injections have been shown to be an effective and almost immediate treatment modality (17). Evidence supporting the use of acupuncture and dry needling techniques are limited at best (18). The use of Botox for trigger point mediated pain in myofascial syndrome has not been proven to be an effective method of treatment (19).

Home Exercise Program

Immediately following an acute cervical sprain/strain injury, it is important to reduce inflammation with the use of ice, minimize pain (e.g., with analgesics), and continue gentle AROM exercises. Once the patient's pain is adequately controlled and the full AROM is mostly restored, a home exercise program (HEP) can be safely initiated. This includes AROM, neck stretches, and isometric strengthening in all planes of motion, while cautioning against "neck circles" or "rolling the neck" especially into extension. Specific muscles that should be addressed include deep cervical flexors, scalenes, levator scapulae, trapezius, and the pectoralis muscles. The patient should perform routine postural self-analysis to improve their own postural awareness, especially while sitting at a desk, computer or driving. Cueing oneself, for example, asking questions such as: "Am I sitting up straight?" "Are my shoulders rounded and 'hunched' toward my ears, or should I pull them back so my shoulder blades are together and down?" "Is my chin protruding forward, or do I need to bring it back into the 'tucked' position?" To prevent future neck pain and injury, a daily routine should be established that includes stretching, frequent postural corrections, and strengthening of the scapular stabilizers, deep neck flexors, and core musculature. Sometimes using a timer while at work to help remind you when it rings to correct your overall posture may be useful as well.

SUMMARY

Successful rehabilitation for cervical strain/sprain starts by decreasing pain in the acute stage using ice, analgesics, and occasionally a soft cervical collar for comfort. During the acute phase it is also important to encourage early mobilization through gentle ROM exercises as opposed to immobilization with a soft cervical collar (20). Once the pain begins to dissipate and the subacute or restorative phase begins, the patient can safely start isolated stretching and strengthening while under the supervision of a therapist or physician. To effectively prevent chronic neck pain or future aggravation, a therapeutic exercise program should be created. This individualized program should include postural and ergonomic evaluation, as well as patient education.

SAMPLE CASE

A 45-year-old male presents with increasing neck pain and decreased cervical ROM in all directions. Two days prior, he was rear ended while driving in his car; he was wearing a seatbelt. Pain began one day prior and is aching in nature, nonradiating, and not associated with new weakness or numbness. He denies loss of consciousness and reports driving himself to the emergency department evaluation, at which time x-rays and MRI was performed. He also admits to new onset headaches in the right greater than left temporal region not associated with light

hypersensitivity, nausea, or vision changes. He denies prior significant musculoskeletal or sports injuries. He has no significant past medical or surgical history or medications. He works as a software engineer for which he sits in front of a computer most of the day. He reports a sedentary life style. The x-rays from the emergency department were negative for spinal fracture or subluxation. MRI revealed (some) degenerative changes at C5-6 but were thought to be chronic. His examination is significant for decreased ROM in the cervical spine, and minimal erythema and swelling in the posterior cervical musculature. There was no tenderness to palpation along the spinous processes of the cervical spine; decreased ROM noted in bilateral rotation, sidebending and flexion. Strength and sensation intact in the upper and lower limbs bilaterally. Spurling's maneuver was negative bilaterally.

 SAMPLE THERAPY PRESCRIPTION

Discipline: Physical therapy.

Diagnosis: Cervical strain and cervicogenic headache following whiplash injury.

Precautions: safety, weight bearing as tolerated (WBAT).

Frequency of visits: 2 to 3x/week.

Duration of treatment: 4 to 6 weeks for a total of 10 to 12 visits.

Treatment:

1. *Modalities:* cryotherapy (ice pack, ice massage) acutely, then thermotherapy (hot packs or ultrasound)

2. *Manual therapy:*

   a. Acute: indirect MFR superficial cervical muscles (anterior and posterior), counterstrain

   b. Subacute or chronic: direct MFR, soft tissue massage, assess motion at OA, atlanto-axial joint (AA), C2-C7

   c. Gentle manual traction

3. *Therapeutic exercise:*

    a. AROM with passive and isometric stretching of the pectoralis muscles, upper trapezius scalenes, levator scapula, anterior and posterior cervical muscles

    b. Deep neck flexor strengthening

    c. Scapular stabilization

    d. Postural correction exercises

    e. Neuromuscular reeducation

4. *Specialized treatments:* assessment and recommendations for ergonomic positioning

5. *Patient education:* HEP, postural training

REFERENCES

1. Fejer R, Kyvik KO, Hartvigsen J. The prevalence of neck pain in the world population: a systematic critical review of the literature. *Eur Spine J.* 2006;15:834–848.
2. Hogg-Johnson S, van der Velde G, Carroll L, et al. The burden and determinants of neck pain in the general population: results of the bone and joint decade 2000-2010 task force on neck pain and its associated disorders. *Journal of Manipulative and Physiological Therapeutics.* 2008;32:S46–60.
3. Nordin M, Carragee EJ, Hogg-Johnson S, et al. Assessment of neck pain and its associated disorders: results of the bone and joint decade 2000-2010 task force and its associated disorders. *Spine.* 2008;33:S101–122.
4. Rouzier P. *The Sports Medicine Patient Advisor,* 3rd ed. Amherst, MA: SportsMed Press; 2010:6–10.
5. Malanga G, Peter J. Whiplash injuries. *Current Pain and Headache Reports.* 2005;9:322–325.
6. Scott D, Jull G, Sterling M. Widespread sensory hypersensitivity is a feature of chronic whiplash-associated disorder but no chronic idiopathic neck pain. *Clin J Pain.* 2005;21:175–181.
7. Obermann M, Nebel K, Riegel A, et al. Incidence and predictors of chronic headache attributed to whiplash. *Cephalalgia.* 2010;30(5):528–534.
8. Becker W. Cervicogenic headache: Evidence that the neck is a pain generator. *Headache Currents.* 2010;50:699–705.
9. Cisler TA. Whiplash as a total-body injury. *JAOA.* 1994;94:2.
10. Cuccurullo S. *Physical Medicine and Rehabilitation Board Review,* 2nd ed. New York, NY: Demos Medical; 2010:527.
11. Binder A. Neck pain. *Clinical Evidence.* 2008;8:1103, 1–34.
12. Steven J. *Karageanes. Principles of Manual Sports Medicine.* Philadelphia, PA: Lippincott Williams & Wilkins; 2005:49-55, 143–158.
13. Gross A, Hoving J, Haines T, et al. A Cochrane review of manipulation and mobilization for mechanical neck disorders. *Spine.* 2004;29(14):1541–1548.
14. Lauche R, Cramer H, Choi K, et al. The influence of a series of five dry cupping treatments on pain and mechanical thresholds in patients with chronic non-specific neck pain - a randomised controlled pilot study. *BMC Complementary and Alternative Medicine.* 2011;11:63, 2–30.
15. Liang Z, Zhu X, Yang X, et al. Assessment of a traditional acupuncture therapy for chronic neck pain: a pilot randomized controlled study. *Complementary Therapies in Medicine.* 2011;19(suppl 1):S26–S32.
16. Niemtzow R. Battlefield acupuncture. *Medical Acupuncture.* 2007;19(4):225–228.
17. Alvarez DJ, Rockwell PG. Trigger points: diagnosis and management. *Am Fam Physician.* 2002;65(4):653–660.
18. Toug EA, White AR, Cummings TM, Richards SH, Campbell JL. Acupuncture and dry needling in the management of myofascial trigger point pain: a systematic review and meta-analysis of randomised controlled trials. *Eur J Pain.* 2009;13(1):3–10.
19. Ho KY, Tan KH. Botulinum toxin A for myofascial trigger point injection: a qualitative systematic review. *Eur J Pain.* 2007;11(5):519–527.
20. Schnabel M, Ferrari R, Vassiliou T, Kaluza G. Randomised, controlled outcome study of active mobilisation compared with collar therapy for whiplash injury. *Emerg Med J.* 2004;21(3):306–310.

Thoracic Spine Dysfunction

Oluseun A. Olufade, Paul H. Lento, and John Walker

INTRODUCTION

Thoracic pain can either emanate from spinal structures or be referred from nearby viscera. This chapter will focus on the manual assessment and categorization of thoracic spine disorders. In order to understand this concept, the anatomy and kinesiology of the thoracic spine needs to be reviewed.

The thoracic spine is made up of 12 heart-shaped vertebrae which increase in height and width proceeding cranially to caudally. Additionally, the dorsal side of the vertebra is about 2 mm greater than the ventral side which creates the normal kyphosis associated with the thoracic spine. Motion of the thoracic spine occurs between the three-joint complex (two facet or zygapophysial joints and the corresponding intervertebral disc). The orientation of the thoracic facet joints changes cranially to caudally, with the more cranial joints oriented like the cervical facets in a coronal plane, and the more caudal joints similar to the lumbar vertebrae, oriented toward the sagittal plane. The thoracic spine is unique in that it has articulating ribs which provide protection to the underlying viscera. The first 10 ribs articulate with the thoracic vertebra at the costovertebral joint but also anteriorly through a cartilaginous junction at the costo-sternal joints. The 11th and 12th ribs are "floating" and do not have an anterior articulation. During inhalation, the thoracic spine extends while flexing during exhalation. The ribcage swings outwards during inhalation while closing in and down during exhalation.

The presence of the ribs and the orientation of the facet joints dictate motion of the thoracic spine. Greater thoracic axial rotation occurs cranially rather than caudally with even distribution during lateral bending (1). The thoracic spine is also unique in that it exhibits coupled movements. Coupled motion is seen when a vertebral segment rotation in one axis is accompanied with translation or rotation in another axis. This can be ipsilateral, contralateral, or in a mixed fashion.

The relative decreased thoracic spine mobility together with a relatively larger spinal canal diameter compared to the lumbar and cervical segments results in an overall lower incidence of symptomatic thoracic radiculopathy. With increasing age, however, physiological changes are noted in the thoracic spine which may contribute to various clinical causes of pain as well as decreased mobility. For example, the normal aging process is associated with disc degeneration which may cause symptomatic disease. Concomitant with disc degeneration, there are also bony and cartilaginous changes such as osteophytes and Schmorl's nodules. Bony compression injury in the thoracic spine may occur due to hormonal changes associated with aging as well as other metabolic and endocrinological processes.

Various structures within the thoracic spine may be the source of spinal pain. These include, but are not limited to, the costovertebral articulations, facet joints, and intervertebral disc pathology. The diagnosis of costovertebral pain is difficult to obtain as there is no specific examination for it. With that said, it can manifest as atypical chest pain. Thoracic facet mediated pain can be suspected in patients with paravertebral pain worsened by prolonged standing, hyperextension, or rotation. This is most common in the lower thoracic spine especially T11-12 (2). Although 73% of asymptomatic individuals have thoracic MRI abnormalities, symptomatic thoracic disc herniations are responsible for only 0.15% to 4% of symptomatic disc diseases within the thoracic spine (2,3,4). Distinguishing thoracic radicular pain from symptomatic rib dysfunction, or costotransverse joint-mediated pain, can create a clinical conundrum. Disc herniations, compression fractures, and a degenerative spinal cascade may also lead to symptomatic spinal stenosis; however, there is an overall lower incidence of this disorder compared to the cervical and lumbar spine. Thoracic periscapular pain, while it may be due to an underlying thoracic disorder, more commonly is referred from the cervical spine.

CLASSIFICATION TECHNIQUES

Thoracic pain can be assessed using somatic dysfunction or mechanical assessment. Somatic dysfunction evaluation is usually performed by an osteopathic physician with the aim of restoring function. The treatment principle originates from the concept of the body as a single unit with interrelating structures and function with the ability to heal itself. The diagnosis is based on palpation within the musculoskeletal system. Mechanical assessment is another way of diagnosing thoracic region pain. It is usually performed by physical therapist. Physical therapy treatments are attained to relieve impairments through improvement in mobility, functional ability, and quality of life. The intention of mechanical treatment is to identify soft tissues and joints involved and determine the extent of the damage and the ability to correct it.

McKenzie Classification

The McKenzie Classification method of categorizing thoracic spine pain utilizes mechanical assessment, often performed by a therapist with training in mechanical diagnosis and therapy (MDT). In the mechanical assessment process, patients can be categorized as having a derangement, dysfunction, or postural syndrome. A derangement is considered an anatomical displacement or disruption within a moveable joint that is best visualized during the event of a herniated intervertebral disc. A dysfunction is defined as limitation in movement due to end-range stress of shortened structures (scarring, fibrosis, nerve root adherence). Finally, a postural classification is used when normal anatomical structures have symptomatic response due to end-range stress. The assessment occurs in the sagittal, frontal, and transverse plane to determine provocative and symptom reducing movements. After completion of the assessment, an individualized treatment program is assigned to emphasize movements and positions that centralize and abolish symptoms.

Somatic Dysfunction

A somatic dysfunction is an impairment of musculoskeletal organs through the assessment of tissue texture, symmetry, restriction, and tenderness. Dysfunctions are based upon directions in which a patient has difficulty moving into and the position their spine assumes as a result of this deficiency. Somatic dysfunction is an impairment in the function of the skeletal gliding joint and myofascial structures. Dysfunction can also be associated with myofascial changes. These changes have been described as restrictive barriers that can be diagnosed by observing for tissue texture changes, asymmetry, restriction, and tenderness. Myofascial changes have been described as muscle hypertonicity, increased local tissue temperature, and hyperesthesia (5). Immobilization of soft tissue results in reduction in water, diminished fiber glide, reduction of glycosaminoglycan, and production of cross-link formation.

The goal of manual medicine in the treatment of somatic dysfunction is to restore normal range of motion (ROM) and improve the function and movement of the joints and soft tissues in the body. Muscles such as the quadratus lumborum and erector spinae can result in thoracolumbar pain. Up to 40% of patients with low back pain have been mistakenly diagnosed with thoracolumbar joint dysfunction (6).

Clinicians often refer to a manual evaluation to detect a clinical thoracic dysfunction. For example, a patient that has difficulty flexing, side bending, and rotating to the left at the T4 level will be in a right extended, side bent, rotated position. This is described as a left flexion restricted or right extended, rotated, side-bent (ERS) dysfunction (7).

Key points in the history that should be evaluated throughout the assessment process should include history of trauma, osteoporosis, malignancy, and prolonged static postures (e.g., desk job). As with any pain, a thorough evaluation of location, quality, intensity, and duration along with alleviating and exacerbating factors is required. Further inquiry to evaluate for radiculopathy should include any radiation of symptoms, areas of weakness, and sensory disturbances. Furthermore one must ask about the classic "red flags" including but not limited to changes in bowel and bladder function, balance, and gait. Finding out about unexplained weight loss, fevers, chills, or severe nocturnal symptoms can be keys to determining more severe pathology. Given the vast medical problems that can occur in any patient presenting with pain, asking about possible organ dysfunction must be included.

The *key elements of the physical examination* include inspection, palpation, ROM, sensorimotor testing, reflexes, and special tests. Inspection should start with an overall postural evaluation and extend to specifically address cervical, thoracic, lumbar spines, and the abdominal and hip musculature. Identifying any dermatomal pattern of sensory loss and also checking reflexes helps differentiate upper motor neuron from lower motor neuron pathology.

Special Tests

▨ Spurling's maneuver

▨ Seated slump test

▨ Straight leg raise

▨ "Sciatic list gait"

- Patient will lean away from herniated side to relieve pressure on disc

▨ Beevor's sign

- Indicates paralysis of the lower abdominal

Thoracic Mobility

Testing of T1-6 region dysfunction is performed by inspecting and palpating ribs I–IV with the patient in a supine position. The T3-T12 region is tested during inhalation and exhalation, while the patient is in a seated position. Decreased excursion can be caused by pulmonary disease, ankylosing spondylitis, spinal scoliosis, or muscular imbalance of the shoulder and neck. Furthermore, mobility of the thorax is examined when the examiner places one hand on the sternum and the other over the mid thoracic area. The patient is then asked to place both hands behind their neck while the examiner palpates the associated spinous process. As the patient flexes and extends the thoracic spine, the examiner evaluates the mobility between the spinous processes. Lack of spinous process separation during flexion or inability to approximate during extension is suggestive of pathologies including degenerative diseases or Scheuerman's disease in the younger population. This testing requires advanced knowledge and training in manual techniques to be performed effectively and efficiently.

Segmental Dysfunction

To evaluate thoracic segmental dysfunction, the patient places their hand posteriorly on their neck. The examiner's hand reaches across the chest to stabilize the shoulder and

tests for coupling patterns. Side bending to the right can result in the spinous process rotating to the right also. Lack of this pattern is indicative of a segmental dysfunction. Rotation of the thorax is tested in a similar position while the examiner palpates rotation of the spinous process (7).

Spring Test

The spring test can be performed to detect inter-vertebral or costo-vertebral instability. It is performed by first having the patient lie in a prone position. The examiner then places their index and middle finger on the symptomatic costo-transverse joint. A posterior to anterior force is applied to assess for difference in mobility compared to other asymptomatic joints.

Imaging for thoracic back pain can provide some insight into the underlying conditions that may be contributing to pain. X-rays can demonstrate kyphoscoliosis, and spondylosis and suggest degenerative disc disease of the thoracic spine. Imaging should be ordered if there is concern for vertebral compression fractures or rib fractures. Concern for any metastatic disease or metabolic bone disease also warrants diagnostic bone scan testing. CT scan of the thoracic spine can give further information about the bony architecture if there is concern for fracture that is not seen on x-ray. CT myelogram can be used to also assess for any vascular defects in the thoracic spine and to evaluate for central canal stenosis. MRI can also be used to assess for any soft tissue abnormalities or disc herniations that may cause nerve root compression or central canal stenosis. In the case of potential referred pain from the cervical spine such as cervical radiculopathy,

---

THORACIC SPINE DYSFUNCTION

▨ Less common than cervical and lumbar spine pathology, but still considered a common cause of back pain

▨ Key elements of the physical examination: inspection, palpation, neurovascular, detailed spine exam with dural tension testing

▨ Imaging studies may be required to rule out thoracic spine pathology such as kyphoscoliosis and vertebral compression fractures that would require a different management approach

electrodiagnostic testing can help determine if periscapular or thoracic region pain is generated from a compressed nerve root in the cervical spine.

THE REHABILITATION PROGRAM

The thoracic spine is often seen as a difficult area to treat given the rigid construct of the thoracic cage that limits motion at the vertebral segments. This leads to a diverse treatment program, which again follows the five phases of rehabilitation that is used throughout this book. If a vertebral fracture is suspected and found then bracing may be warranted until bone healing occurs and until a strengthening and mobility program can safely be started. The ultimate goal is to improve overall mobility and return to function.

Often pain can be improved or abated with the use of topical analgesics or nonsteroidal anti-inflammatory drugs (NSAIDs), oral NSAIDs, ice, or heat as warranted. Once pain is controlled, and if fracture is not present, restoration of ROM in the thoracic spine is the next step. Stretching tight muscles and strengthening postural muscles is the focus once mobility is regained. Manual therapy applied to the thoracic spine can be a very important treatment modality for restoring pain-free ROM. Incorporating functional based activities and assessing posture and scapular mobility are all crucial to a complete rehabilitation program.

Therapeutic Modalities

There is limited evidence to support the use of modalities in the treatment of thoracic back pain. However, heat can be used to help relax soft tissues before any soft tissue or joint mobilization. Cryotherapy can be used after treatments if any inflammation was elicited from treatment or exercise. Transcutaneous electrical nerve stimulator (TENS) can be used to help alleviate pain and encourage participation in exercise and possibly to decrease the use of oral analgesics. Russian stimulation may be used to help elicit muscle contraction to promote strengthening of periscapular muscles and thoracic extensors, even though evidence for its use is limited (8).

Manual Therapy

The goal of manual medicine in the treatment of somatic dysfunction is to restore normal ROM and improve function and movement of the joints as well as soft tissues in the body. Clinicians often refer to a manual evaluation to detect a clinical thoracic dysfunction. For example, a patient who has difficulty flexing, side bending, and rotating to the left at the T4 level will be in a right extended, side bent, rotated position. This is described as a left flexion restricted or right ERS dysfunction (7).

Movement Loss and Manual Treatment

A Flexion Restricted/ERS Dysfunction

Muscle energy technique (MET) can be used in ERS somatic dysfunction commonly seen at the T3-5 region and lower thoracic areas (6). There are limitations in flexion of this area because of the extension bias of these segments. It is treated by placing one hand of the examiner on the head of the patient and the other at the interspinous process and intervertebral space of the T3-4. Left side bending is then elicited by moving the patient to the right to engage the barrier. Treatment occurs with asking the patient to look backward to the right shoulder. The patient is then told to relax after 3 to 5 seconds and a translational motion to increase left flexion, side bending, and rotation is achieved.

High velocity technique (HVT) can be done to open the left facet joints with flexion-restricted patients. In a seated position, the examiner supports the head in one hand and places the other hand at the T2 spinous process. The patient is asked to slump to the left with right rotating and side bending translational movement. Then the patient is instructed to tilt left ear toward left shoulder, relax, and a graded HVT is performed with right thumb in a right to left translation direction (7).

For the lower thoracic spine (T4-12), flexion restriction treatment by MET is performed while the patient is seated with the examiner's right hand over the patient's shoulder and the left hand at the T10-11 inter-transverse space. The barrier is engaged when the examiner drops his right shoulder to introduce side bending followed by slight rotation. Then the patient is told to lift right shoulder and drop left shoulder contracting left side benders isometrically.

The HVT technique for lower thoracic spine is done in a supine position while the patient is cross-armed. The examiner's hand should stabilize the inferior transverse process of the level being treated. In order to open, for example, the left T4 facet, the patient rolls toward the examiner in contact with the T5 transverse process. Then, the examiner cradles the patient's head and upper back with slight right rotation and side bending.

Extension Restrictions (Flexed, Rotated, and Side Bent Dysfunctions)

Extension restrictions are usually seen at levels T1-2 and T11-12 while evaluating for spinous processes down the thoracic spine. For example, in T1-3 flexed, rotated, and side bent dysfunctions (FRS), MET treatment of the patient can be done in a seated or standing position in order to perform MET. The left hand of the examiner supports the head while the right hand monitors for motion and contraction at the T3-4 inter-transverse space. The examiner then rotates patient's head to the right and translates the trunk forward while asking the patient to stand erect. Translating the patient to the right barrier corrects side bending. The patient is told to look toward the left ear or the floor and relax after 3 to 5 seconds. Then, a translational motion to increase extension, right rotation, and side bending is introduced at T3 segment.

HVT treatment of T3 FRS is aimed at closing the right facet. Rotating the patient's head to the right and translating the trunk forward to introduce extension locate the restriction barrier. The rotation deficit is engaged by translating patient's head to the right with slight head rotation. The patient is asked to look to the left. At the end of an exhalation, the examiner's thumb from a right to left and slight ventral position introduces a HVT.

The extension restriction of the lower thoracic spine (e.g., T10 FRS right) can be treated in a MET fashion in a seated position by asking the patient to stick their stomach out introducing extension. Lowering the patient's left shoulder toward left buttocks with slight left rotation corrects for side bending. The patient is then told to drop the right shoulder to the left against resistance. After 3 to 5 seconds, the patient is told to relax and a translatory motion to increase extension left rotation, and side bending is introduced.

The HVT treatment for lower thoracic spine extension restriction (e.g., FRS right) is done with the patient in a prone position with the head toward the left, facing the examiner. The examiner's right hypothenar eminence presses on right T6 transverse process loading ventrally introducing left rotation. After a deep breath in and out, a HVT is applied toward the table.

Rotation/Side Bending Restrictions

There is presence of asymmetry of the thoracic spine when three or more segments are involved in motion restriction. This is because rotation and side bending of a particular thoracic level occurs in opposite direction of the vertebrae. For example, a patient can have rotation and side bending restriction of T1-4 and this can be treated by MET by introducing right side bending followed by left rotation of the patient's head to T3-4 segments while keeping the spine neutral. The patient is then told to tilt left ear toward their left shoulder, relax after 3 to 5 seconds, and translationary motion to increase right side bending followed by left rotation to new T3 barrier is introduced. HVT treatment of the rotation and side bending restriction is another option of treatment.

MDT for the thoracic spine is based on the theory that repeated movements and prolonged positions result in the altering and often damaging of ligaments, soft tissues, and intervertebral discs that is often the basis of the MDT, also known as a McKenzie approach. Under this treatment concept, patients undergo a detailed assessment of how movements and positions affect symptoms. For example, a patient who presents with increased or radicular symptoms with thoracic flexion and reduction or centralization of symptoms with thoracic extension will be placed on a repeated extension program until symptoms are resolved. After symptoms are considered stable, reintroduction of formerly provocative movements will be restored (9).

Therapeutic Exercises (Figures 41.1-41.6)

Although mechanical or manual treatment is beneficial in correcting many underlying thoracic spinal conditions, it is prudent that a therapeutic exercise program that includes flexibility and strength training is done. An important goal of therapeutic exercise for the thoracic spine is to improve mobility and dynamic stability through the use of strengthening exercises and abdominal breathing (10).

Dr. Vladimir Janda developed the principle of crossed syndrome, the imbalance of tight and weak muscles resulting in forward pelvic tilt, increased lumbar lordosis, and hip flexion. A similar phenomenon, proximal crossed syndrome, is when tightness of neck and scapula muscles causes protraction and elevation of the shoulder. It is important to have flexibility of the thoracic spine to allow for proper balancing of force from the upper and lower limbs and head and neck and to allow for efficient use of energy. Special attention should be paid to muscles such as the hip flexors and latissimus dorsi, which are often shortened.

Thoracic spine posture needs to be stressed with all therapeutic exercise. The effect of poor posture in symptomatic patients is often overlooked during the assessment and treatment of the thoracic spine. Prolonged positions such as forward head and rounded shoulders may result in progressive overstretching of ligaments, muscles, and other soft tissues. Also affected by slouched and kyphotic postures are the intervertebral discs that are more susceptible to posterior herniations in these positions. Whether as the source or contributing factor to thoracic pain, postural assessment is imperative to recovery in the thoracic spine. Good positioning and mobility of the pelvis is important in the posture of the thoracic spine. Correction of forward head posture and forward rounded shoulders can also decrease compressive forces across the thoracic spine (Figure 41.2). Strengthening of the posterior chain to promote thoracic spine extension will also improve posture. Paying specific attention to these common postural deficits is another key component of the therapeutic exercise program.

An example of therapeutic exercises for the treatment of thoracic region pain is the sphinx exercise. It is the repetition of full extension to full flexion of the thoracolumbar spine. Extension of the thoracic spine can be improved by having a patient assuming a cat-camel position with their hand or forearms on the floor (Figure 41.1). Head nodding in this position increases the efficacy of this treatment (6).

In addition to the sphinx exercises, Swiss ball exercises are another example of therapeutic exercise used for thoracic pain. This requires continuous adjustment of

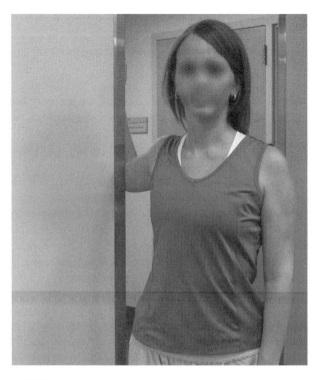

FIGURE 41.2: Unilateral pectoralis muscle stretch.

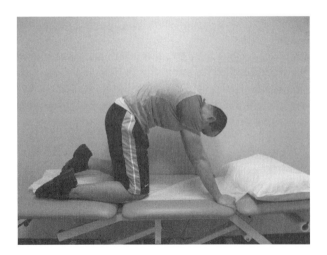

FIGURE 41.1: Cat–camel exercise, angry cat position for increasing thoracic spine flexion is demonstrated.

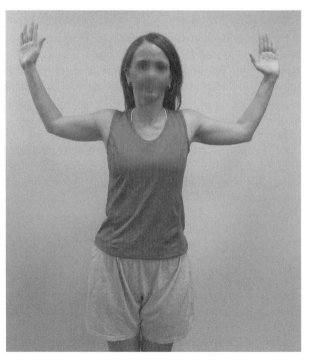

FIGURE 41.3: Scapular retraction exercise.

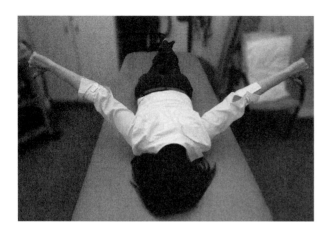

FIGURE 41.4: Prone flys or "T" for scapular strengthening of the rhomboids, middle trapezius, cervical, and thoracic extensors.

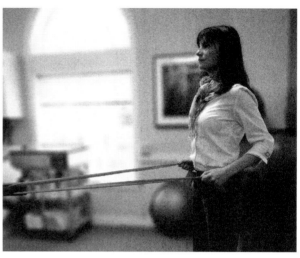

FIGURE 41.5: Standing scapular retractions or rows with resistance bands.

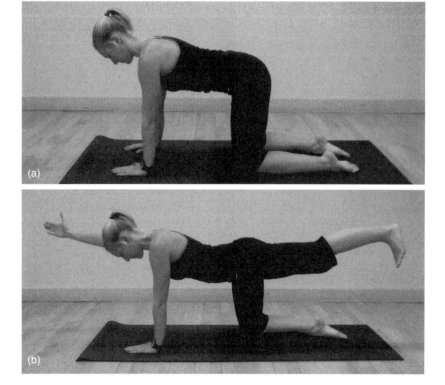

FIGURE 41.6: (a) Quadruped position. (b) Quadruped stabilization exercise with alternate upper and lower extremity lifts, also known as Bird dogs.

the body to maintain equilibrium while lying supine on the ball. This is achieved by increasing muscular demand required to maintain postural stability. It can be employed for patients with kyphoscoliosis by instructing activation of mid thoracic spinal muscles while supporting the abdomen on a Swiss ball (6). Foam roll exercises can be used to improve stabilization of base support in increased muscle firing. Resistance bands can also be used for scapular and thoracic spine strengthening and may help to correct postural alignment.

Respiration mechanics are also important in maintaining good posture and spinal stabilization. Breathing exercises can influence the thoracic spine by acting on muscle imbalances, body pH imbalances, and psychological factors (11). Functional breathing involves instructing the patient to feel the abdomen lift with inspiration and lower with expiration. It is started in a supine position with one hand on the upper abdomen, then progress to sitting and standing (10). It will allow for breathing without the use of accessory breathing muscles such as scalene. This exercise can eventually progress to manual resistance to the abdomen or ribcage.

Specialized Approaches

Spinal orthoses are usually used in the treatment of vertebral compression fractures and post-surgical patients but can be used in the conservative treatment of thoracic spine pain (12). Short-term bed rest, ice, heat, ultrasound, and electrical stimulation may give short term relief to thoracic pain. Brown et al showed that 77% of patients treated conservatively were able to return to their previous functional level (4).

Thoracic orthoses decrease load on the spine and intervertebral discs by increasing intra-abdominal pressure (13). Various types of thoracic orthoses such as the Knight-Taylor and Milwaukee brace can be used in the treatment of thoracic pain. Postural training supports with light weight braces that are well tolerated can be used to help promote an upright posture and improved kinesthetic awareness.

Home Exercise Program

Much of the manual therapy that may be performed in the clinic should have the effects continued by a well balanced home exercise program (HEP). The HEP should emphasize stretching of anterior chain muscle groups (e.g., pectoralis major) and strengthening of the posterior chain muscle groups (e.g., erector spinae, scapular retractors). Postural correction

exercises are part of the HEP and can be reinforced throughout the day by encouraging improved postural awareness. The progression to functional activities will be guided by the therapist in the clinic and translated to the HEP.

SUMMARY

This chapter provides you with basic anatomy of the thoracic spine and the differential diagnoses of patients that practitioners see with thoracic related pain. After ruling in/out other pathologies, manual and mechanical therapies are options in restoring the health of a restricted or painful thoracic spine. After carefully matching a patient and treatment, appropriate intervention based on the thoracic level can be introduced, if there are no contraindications. Stretching of muscles such as the hip flexors and pectoralis muscles and strengthening of the posterior chain muscles should be a focus of the HEP. Continuous exercising after therapy enables the longevity of the treatment.

SAMPLE CASE

A 64-year-old male presents with pain between his shoulder blades. He reports the pain started insidiously over the last 6 months and has been progressively worsening. He has noticed occasional pain when taking deep breaths. Also he experiences pain with upper limb activities. He denies any history of trauma, associated weakness, numbness, or tingling. He is also concerned that he has been getting shorter. Review of systems and remainder of the history were noncontributory. On physical examination he is noted to have forward rounded shoulders, forward head, and mildly increased thoracic kyphosis. There is tenderness around the thoracic paraspinals in the periscapular region. With shoulder flexion and abduction there is altered movement of the right scapula. Motor, sensory, and reflex examinations are normal. Thoracic spine X-rays reveal mild increase in thoracic kyphosis, without any significant bony or degenerative changes.

SAMPLE THERAPY PRESCRIPTION

Discipline: Physical therapy.

Diagnosis: Thoracic myofascial pain syndrome.

Precautions: Weight bearing as tolerated (WBAT), universal, avoid repeated flexion

Frequency of visits: 2 to 3x/week.

Duration of treatment: 4 weeks.

Treatment:

1. *Modalities:* ice, heat, ultrasound

2. *Manual therapy:* direct action muscle energy type to flexion, left rotation, and left side-bending

3. *Therapeutic exercise:* Swiss ball requires continuous adjustment of the body to maintain equilibrium. Foam roll exercises are used to improve stabilization of base support in increased muscle firing. Thera-band can be used to correct postural alignment. Strengthening of posterior chain muscles and stretching of anterior chain muscles. Correction of scapular dyskinesia and forward head posture.

    a. *Mechanical therapy:* Repetitive movements that reduce and abolish symptoms of mechanical origin.

    b. *Posture:* awareness and correction of prolonged positions that produce or contribute to diagnosis.

4. *Specialized treatments:* thoracic orthotics as necessary

5. *Patient education:* HEP

Goals: Restore and increase ROM, flexibility, and strength. Ability to function in a pain free manner.

Reevaluation: In 4 weeks by referring physician.

REFERENCES

1. Dvorak J, Dvorak V. Structural examination and functional treatment of the thoracic spine and ribs. *Musculoskeletal Manual Medicine*, 2nd ed. Thieme Medical Publishers; 1990:393–424.
2. O'Connor RC, Andary MT, Russo RB, DeLano M. Thoracic radiculopathy. *Phys Med Rehabil Clin N Am.* 2002;13: 623–644.
3. Wood KB, Garvey TA, Gundry C, Heithoff KB. Magnetic resonance imaging of the thoracic spine. Evaluation of asymptomatic individuals. *J Bone Joint Surg Am.*1995;77(11):1631–1638.
4. Brown CW, Deffer PA, Akmakjian J, Donaldson DH, Brugman JL. The natural history of thoracic disc herniation. *Spine.* 1992;17(Suppl 6):S97–667102.
5. Ellis JJ, Johnson SJ. Myofascial considerations in somatic dysfunction of the thorax. In: Flynn TW. *Thoracic Spine and Rib Cage: Musculoskeletal Evaluation and Treatment.* Boston, MA: Butterworth-Heinemann; 1996:287–310.
6. De Franca. Manipulation techniques for key joints. In: Liebenson C. *Rehabilitation of the Spine*, 2nd ed. Lippincott William & Wilkins; 2007:487–510.
7. Flynn TW. Direct treatment for the thoracic spine and rib cage: muscle energy, mobilization, high-velocity thrust. In: Flynn TW. *Thoracic Spine and Rib Cage: Musculoskeletal Evaluation and Treatment.* Boston, MA: Butterworth-Heinemann; 1996:171–210.
8. Ward A, Shkuratova N. Russian electrical stimulation: the early experiments. *Phys Ther.* 2002;82(10):1019–1030.
9. Greenmann EP. The manipulative prescription. In: *Principles of Manual Medicine*, 1st ed. Baltimore, MD: Williams & Wilkins; 1984:39–48.
10. Carriere B. Therapeutic exercises and self-correction programs. In: Flynn TW. *Thoracic Spine and Rib Cage: Musculoskeletal Evaluation and Treatment*, Boston, MA: Butterworth-Heinemann; 1996:287–310.
11. Walkowski S, Baker R. Osteopathic manipulative medicine: a functional approach to pain. In: Leonard T, et al. *Pain Procedures in Clinical Practice*, Elsevier Saunders; 2011:
12. Moore DP, Tilley E, et al. Spinal orthoses in rehabilitation. In: Braddom RL, Ed. *Physical Medicine and Rehabilitation.* Philadelphia, PA: Saunders/Elsevier, 2007:369–380.
13. Uustal H, Baerga E. Prosthetics and orthotics. In: Cuccurullo SJ. *Physical Medicine and Rehabilitation Board Review.* New York, NY: Demos; 2002:409–488.

X. LUMBAR

Lumbar Facet Arthrosis/Spondylosis

Stacey Franz, Neeti Bathia, and Meredith K. Sena

INTRODUCTION

Low back pain (LBP) accounts for greater than 50% of all spinal pain (1). Furthermore, the lumbar zygapophysial joints, also known as facet or z-joints, have been identified as the pain generator in 15% to 45% of patients with chronic LBP (1–3); though causes of chronic LBP may also be multifactorial. The facet joints form the posterolateral articulations of the spinal canal, in which the inferior articulating process of the cephalad vertebrae meets with the superior articular process of the caudal vertebrae. Although they assist with axial weight bearing, their primary role is to limit motion between vertebrae. During extension, these joints may bear anywhere from 16% to 70% (in the case of spondylosis) of the compressive axial load (4–6). These joints also help limit hyperflexion and excessive torsion, thereby limiting rotational forces on the intervertebral disc (7).

While various entities may lead to facet-mediated pain (e.g., articular fractures, meniscoid entrapment), this chapter will focus solely on facet spondylosis, also known as facet degeneration or spinal arthritis. This condition is likely due to repetitive strain and/or low-grade trauma over time that results in wearing down of the articular hyaline cartilage, development of subchondral bone cysts, osteophyte formation, and/or synovial cyst formation. Nociceptive signals from the joint capsule are carried by the medial branches of the dorsal rami and autonomic nerve fibers, thus pathology involving these joints can result in pain (8–10). Furthermore, the subchondral bone of degenerative lumbar facet joints contains substance P, a neuropeptide associated with inflammation and pain (11).

The diagnosis of facet-mediated pain is one of exclusion or is confirmed with diagnostic injections; currently there is not a clearly defined pathway for defining facet-mediated pain (2,12–15). Despite this, however, the practitioner should still perform a thorough history and physical examination.

Key elements of the physical examination include but are not limited to inspection, palpation, range of motion (ROM), provocative or special tests, and a neurologic examination. It is well documented, via intra-articular provocative injections, that lumbar facet-mediated pain can cause both axial and lower limb pain (16–19). One researcher documented an association between facet-mediated pain with groin or thigh pain, paraspinal tenderness, and reproduction of pain during extension-rotation maneuvers (20), theoretically because maximal pressure on these joints occurs in extension. Complaints of symptoms common to degenerative processes in other joints, such as stiffness, increased pain and stiffness upon waking in the morning, and improved mobility with physical activity are reasonable to expect (21). However, no studies to date have successfully identified reproducible findings unique to the group of patients who respond to facet joint injections (2,12–14).

Pathognomonic findings don't exist on diagnostic imaging to denote facet pathology as the etiology of one's LBP, as the presence of an anatomic abnormality of a facet joint on imaging does not indicate that the joint is an active pain generator. Plain radiographs, including oblique films, are generally recommended as a means to rule out other possible sources of LBP. While MRI or CT scan may demonstrate facet joint arthropathy, this is nondiagnostic; lumbar facet arthropathy has been documented on CT scans in greater than half of all individuals 40 years of age or older (22). In addition, the absence of degenerative or pathologic facet joint changes on imaging does not exclude the potential for lumbar facet-mediated pain (23–25).

Given the suboptimal diagnostic value of the history, physical examination, and imaging when evaluating facet-mediated pain, diagnostic facet injections are often utilized to differentiate facet-mediated pain from other possible etiologies. Specifically, diagnostic intra-articular injections or medial branch blocks can be used in the diagnostic work-up (26–28). Due to the high rate of false positives, however, it is essential that such injections be performed in accordance with a comparative anesthetic paradigm.

To our knowledge, there are not yet any studies in the medical literature which evaluate the efficacy of non-interventional management of LBP caused specifically by z-joint dysfunction; this is likely secondary to the difficulty with stratifying patients for conservative treatments. The current consensus is that early, noninterventional management of z-joint pain conform to standards of care for the treatment of chronic LBP (29). These treatments include use of oral nonsteroidal anti-inflammatory (NSAID) and analgesic medications, exercise therapy and rehabilitation, manual medicine, activity modification, and cognitive behavioral therapy (29). Manual medicine and exercise therapy are discussed in more detail below. Evidence supporting the efficacy of long-term use of NSAID medication for the management of chronic LBP is scant, and long-term use of NSAID medication should be undertaken with great care, given the wide range of potential side effects (30).

Should these initial conservative measures fail, or should a patient's pain level be so severe as to make usage of these conservative measures difficult, interventional spine procedures may be considered. The two main procedures currently utilized are intra-articular corticosteroid injections and medial branch blocks with progression to radiofrequency denervation of the medial branches of the dorsal rami, which supply nociceptive sensory output from the z-joints. Observational and uncontrolled studies of z-joint intra-articular corticosteroid injections have shown transient beneficial effects (generally up to 3 months) (31), but more rigorous randomized controlled trials (RCTs) have not uniformly demonstrated their lasting efficacy (29,32,33). Medial branch blocks with progression to radiofrequency denervation is considered the gold standard of care, as more robust evidence in the form of randomized controlled trials support its efficacy (34–36). As compared with intra-articular injections, this procedure may afford the patient 8 to 10 months relief, with a possibility for the pain to return pending nerve regeneration. The most common complications of this treatment are transient, localized burning pain and self-limiting back pain (2.5%), although rare occurrences of local burns and motor weakness have been reported (37).

LUMBAR FACET ARTHROSIS/SPONDYLOSIS

░ The lumbar zygapophysial joints, also known as the facet or z-joints, form the posterolateral articulations of the spinal canal

░ Nociceptive signals from the joint capsule are carried by both the medial branches of the dorsal rami and autonomic nerve fibers

░ Facet spondylosis, also known as facet degeneration, is likely due to repetitive strain over time and can result in wearing of the articular cartilage, development of subchondral bone cysts, osteophyte formation, and synovial cyst formation

░ Diagnosis of facet mediated pain remains challenging, as the diagnosis is one of exclusion or confirmed with diagnostic injections (via comparative anesthetic paradigm)

░ Imaging is nondiagnostic, as facet arthropathy is often found on lumbar imaging and the absence of facet pathology does not exclude facet-mediated pain

░ Various researchers have been unable to identify findings unique to the group of patients who respond to facet injections. Yet, there is some evidence that individuals with facet-mediated pain present with axial and lower limb pain, paraspinal tenderness, and reproduction of pain during extension-rotation maneuvers

░ Treatment may include NSAIDs, analgesic medications, manual medicine, activity modification, cognitive behavioral and interventional procedures, if warranted

THE REHABILITATION PROGRAM

A comprehensive physical therapy (PT) program can be effective in managing pain and improving functional activity tolerance in people with lumbar facet arthrosis. The focus of PT for patients with this diagnosis is on decreasing pain, increasing ROM by decreasing musculoskeletal restrictions, and improving core strength. Emphasis is placed on the home exercise program (HEP), with the inclusion of postural and body mechanics education (1). The five phases of rehabilitation can also be utilized in the management of patients with facet mediated LBP.

Therapeutic Modalities

There is little evidence to support the use of therapeutic modalities for patients with lumbar facet arthrosis. Many practitioners continue to use therapeutic ultrasound, and patients often report decreased pain after such treatments (38). In addition, moist heat and/or use of a home transcutaneous electrical stimulation (TENS) unit may decrease or modulate one's pain and empower patients with the ability to manage their pain at home. The goal of any modality is to allow patients to participate in their therapeutic exercise program and improve their overall functional level.

Manual Therapy

Patients with lumbar facet spondylosis may present with restriction at the spinal level and/or the muscular level. Physical therapists may use spinal mobilization, spinal manipulation, and soft tissue mobilization techniques to reduce these restrictions and restore the patient's functional ROM while decreasing pain (39–41). The use of spinal manipulation, specifically, is controversial, as some studies have shown benefit (42,43), while one study showed no significant difference when compared with sham treatment (44).

Spinal mobilization at the restricted level can decrease inflammation and improve mobility of adjacent vertebral levels. Traditional mobilizations can be performed using a grading system of I to V, determined by the depth and amount of oscillation, with grade V equivalent to a high velocity low amplitude manipulation. Sustained natural apophyseal glides (SNAGs) are an example of dynamic mobilizations, in which vertebral mobilizations are performed while the patient is moving, as a means to restore normal spinal motion during functional activity. Patients can be educated and instructed in self SNAG techniques to be completed at home.

Soft tissue mobilization can be performed in the form of massage (40), trigger point release, strain-counterstrain, or instrument assisted techniques (i.e., Graston Technique).

Finally, for a patient who presents with radicular symptoms due to neural irritation, nerve glides may be effective in increasing neural mobility (45). The patient can be instructed in self-administration of these techniques at home. While these treatments are frequently utilized and provide needed pain relief to patients, the evidence to support their use is limited and conflicting, therefore, well-designed studies are needed to further clarify the role of manual therapy in the treatment of facet mediated LBP.

Therapeutic Exercise

Current research points to exercise as the most effective noninvasive treatment for lumbar spondylosis (38,46). Exercise should include cardiovascular activity, core muscle strengthening, extensibility training, and education in body mechanics and ergonomics. The therapist's main goal with exercise prescription is to educate the patient on proper technique, ensuring appropriate muscle facilitation and avoidance of compensatory patterns and helping the patient avoid fear of movement.

Considering the patient's weight-bearing tolerance and comorbidities, cardiovascular exercise can be performed in the weight-bearing or nonweight-bearing position and should be low impact. Depending on the patient's activity tolerance, strengthening and extensibility exercises can be performed in supine, side-lying, prone, or quadruped position, progressing to sitting, then standing on even surfaces, and finally standing on uneven surfaces. Emphasis is on controlled exercises through contraction of the core muscles, such as the transversus abdominis (Figure 42.1), obliques, multifidus (Figure 42.2), pelvic floor, and hip musculature while completing movements of the upper and/or lower limbs (Figure 42.3). The patient is educated on how to carry over the core muscle contraction while performing daily activities such as during walking, transfers, lifting, and completing household chores (1,46,47). Patient education should also include advice on maintaining a healthy lifestyle, which includes a healthy diet, good sleep hygiene, and smoking cessation if this issue needs to be addressed, since nicotine and smoking have been speculated as risk factors for degenerative disease of the spine (48).

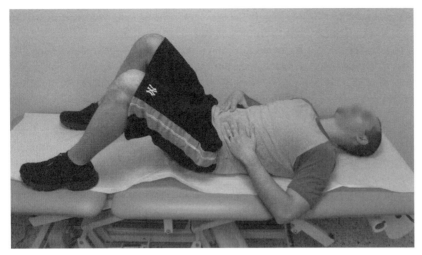

FIGURE 42.1: Abdominal draw-in maneuver.

Lay on your back, with knees bent and feet flat on floor. Place your fingers on the muscles just below your belly button then contract those muscles by pulling them down and away from your fingers. Keep your upper abdominal muscles, back muscles, and hip muscles relaxed. Hold this position for 5 seconds making sure you continue to breathe.

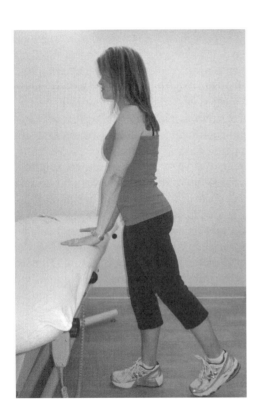

FIGURE 42.2: Multifidus strengthening.

Stand with your hands resting on a table. Perform the abdominal draw-in maneuver and kick one leg back slightly, making sure not to arch your back or twist your pelvis. Repeat on other leg, and continue alternating legs.

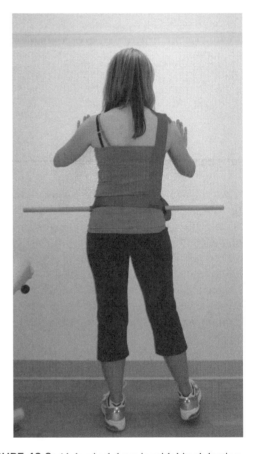

FIGURE 42.3: Abdominal draw-in with hip abduction.

Stand facing the wall with hands supported on wall. Perform abdominal draw-in maneuver and kick one leg out to the side, keeping your hips level and toes pointed straight ahead, making sure not to twist or tilt your pelvis. Repeat on the other side, and continue alternating legs. In this picture a dowel attached at the level of the pelvis is used to monitor pelvic stability. If the dowel raises or lowers on one side when you move your leg, then you are not keeping your hips level.

Specialized Techniques

Aquatic therapy can be useful for patients with poor weight-bearing tolerance or decreased land-based exercise tolerance. Patients may benefit from the buoyancy that the water provides enabling them to perform cardiovascular, strengthening, and extensibility exercises in the pool without increased pain (49,50).

Taping techniques may also be useful in decreasing LBP associated with lumbar spondylosis. The benefits of these taping techniques range from providing support, to decreasing muscle tension, to acting as a reminder for postural correction.

Qi Gong, a form of martial arts, is also an effective program in reducing pain, increasing extensibility, and increasing strength. In addition, Qi Gong promotes relaxation and improves concentration and circulation (51). Tai chi is also considered to be an effective exercise program that can improve strength and balance. Recently a RCT of tai chi exercise resulted in decreased pain and disability in patients with LBP, therefore, the authors concluded that tai chi can be considered a safe and effective intervention for chronic LBP symptoms (52). Since this is the first RCT on tai chi for LBP, further research is necessary to confirm their results.

Home Exercise Program

Patient education is critical to ensuring a positive outcome. With the encouragement of a physical therapist, patients need to take ownership of their pain and understand that their compliance with a comprehensive HEP can determine the effectiveness of their treatment. Patients should be shown that they are able to move without pain and to learn to not avoid movement because of fear of pain. Patients should be instructed to perform their HEP daily and incorporate their body mechanic and ergonomic training into their activities of daily living (1).

SUMMARY

The lumbar facet joints are a possible and common pain generator in patients with LBP. Wear and tear or stress to the joints over time can lead to lumbar spondylosis. Diagnosis is not clearly defined but rather is one of exclusion

or via confirmation with diagnostic injections. Yet, imaging is recommended to rule out other possible causes of LBP. Treatment may include NSAIDs, analgesic medications, manual medicine, activity modification, cognitive behavioral and interventional procedures, if warranted. Current research, however, points to exercise as the most effective noninvasive treatment for spondylosis. A well-balanced PT regimen may include therapeutic exercise, supplemented by therapeutic modalities, manual therapy, and a HEP. Furthermore, exercise should emphasize core strengthening, with attention to the abdominal muscles, multifidus, pelvic, and hip musculature.

SAMPLE CASE

The patient is a 45-year-old male who presents with LBP of 6 months duration without a clear inciting or traumatic event preceding the onset of pain. Pain is described as deep aching pain in the bilateral low back in a band-like distribution, located above the belt line, worse with standing or walking or when moving from sit-to-stand, and improved with sitting. Work-up and treatment to date are unremarkable. Past medical, family, and social histories are unremarkable. Review of systems (ROS) is unremarkable, including no history of gastrointestinal (GI) ulcer, gastroesophageal reflux disease (GERD), GI bleed, coronary artery disease, hypertension, or renal disease. He denies any allergies. Examination is notable for well-appearing male in no acute distress, functional active range of motion (AROM) lumbar spine with pain at end-range extension and bilateral oblique extension, some tenderness over the bilateral lower lumbar paraspinals, negative provocative testing (bilateral straight leg raise [SLR], Gaenslen's, and FABER's tests), normal neurologic exam, and unremarkable inspection of the lumbar spine. Lumbar x-rays (anteroposterior [AP], lateral, bilateral obliques) were obtained and demonstrate no fractures, listhesis, or osseous destruction. MRI lumbar spine w/o contrast reveals narrowed disc space

SAMPLE THERAPY PRESCRIPTION

Discipline: Physical therapy.

Diagnosis: LBP due to lumbar facet arthrosis, spondylosis at L5-S1.

Precautions: Avoid lumbar hyperextension and hyperextension/rotation.

Frequency of visits: 2 to 3x/week.

Duration of treatment: 12 visits.

Treatment:

1. *Modalities:* ice versus moist heat prn pain; consider TENS prn pain modulation

2. *Manual therapy:* spinal mobilization and/or manipulation, soft tissue mobilization

3. *Therapeutic exercise:* emphasis on lower limb extensibility and core strengthening (including the abdominal muscles, multifidus, and hip musculature)

4. *Specialized techniques:* consider taping techniques for postural correction

5. *Patient education:* HEP, including education in SNAGs

Goals: Decrease pain, increase ROM, increase core strength, and safely return to functional activities.

Reevaluation: In 4 weeks by referring physician.

REFERENCES

1. Manchikanti L, Boswell MV, Singh V, et al. Prevalence of facet joint pain in chronic spinal pain of cervical, thoracic, and lumbar regions. *BMC Musculoskelet Disord.* 2004;5(1):15.
2. Schwarzer AC, Aprill CN, Derby R, et al. Clinical features of patients with pain stemming from the lumbar zygapophysial joints: Is the lumbar facet syndrome a clinical entity? *Spine.* 1994;19(10):1132–1137.
3. Schwarzer AC, Wang SC, Bogduk N, et al. Prevalence and clinical features of lumbar zygapophysial joint pain: a study in an Australian population with chronic low back pain. *Ann Rheum Dis.* 1995;54:100–106.
4. Adams MA, Hutton HC. The effect of posture on the role of the apophyseal joints in resisting intervertebral compressive forces. *J Bone Joint Surg Br.* 1980;62B:358–362.
5. Dunlop RB, Adams MA, Hutton WC. Disc space narrowing and the lumbar facet joints. *J Bone Joint Surg Br.* 1984;66B:706–710.
6. Yang KH, King AI. Mechanism of facet load transmission as a hypothesis for LBP. *Spine.* 1984;9:557–565.
7. Adams MA. The mechanical function of the lumbar apophyseal joints *Spine.* 1983;8:327–330.
8. Ashton IK, Ashton BA, Gibson S J, et al. Morphological basis for low back pain: the demonstration of nerve fibers and neuropeptides in the lumbar facet joint capsule but riot in the ligamentum flavum. *J Orthop Res.* 1992;10:72–78.
9. Giles LG, Hasrvey AR. Immunohistochemical demonstration of nociceptors in the capsule and synovial folds of human zygapophysial joints. *Br J Rheumatol.* 1987;26:362–364.
10. Giles LGF, Taylor JR. Innervation of the lumbar zygapophysial joint folds. *Acta Orthop Scand.* 1987;58:43–46.
11. Beaman DN, Graziano GP, Glover RA, et al. Substance P innervation of lumbar spine facet joints. *Spine.* 1993;18:1044–1049.
12. Schwarzer A, Derby R, Aprill C, et al. Pain from the lumbar zygapophysial joints: a test of two models. *J Spinal Disord.* 1994;7:331 336.
13. Revel ME, Listrat VM, Chevalier XL, et al. Facet joint block for LBP: identifying predictors of a good response. *Arch Phys Med Rehabil.* 1992;73:824–828.
14. Jackson RP, Jacobs RR, Montesano PX. Facet injection in LBP: a prospective statistical study. *Spine.* 1988;13:966–971.
15. Jackson RP. The facet syndrome: Myth or reality? *Clin Orthop.* 1992;121:ll0–121.
16. Hirsch C, Ingelmark B, Miller M. The anatomical basis for low back pain. *Acta Orthop Scand.* 1963;33:1 17.
17. Marks R. Distribution of pain provoked from lumbar facet joints and related structures during diagnostic spinal infiltration. *Pain.* 1989;39:37–40.
18. McCall IW, Park, WM, O'Brien JP. Induced pain referral from posterior lumbar elements in normal subjects. *Spine.* 1979;3:441–446.
19. Mooney V, Robertson J. The facet syndrome. *Clin Orthop.* 1976;115:149–156.
20. Helbig T, Lee CK: The lumbar facet syndrome. *Spine.* 1988;13:61–64.
21. Eisentein SM, Parry CR. The lumbar facet arthrosis syndrome. *J Bone Joint Surg Br.* 1987;69B:3–7.
22. Wiesel SW, Tsourmas N, Feffer HL, Citrin CM, Patronas N. A study of computer assisted tomography I: The incidence of positive CAT scans in an asymptomatic group of patients. *Spine.* 1981;9:549–551.
23. Carrera GF, Williams AL. Current concepts in evaluation of the lumbar facet joints. *CRC Crit Rev Diagn Imaging.* 1984;21:85–104.
24. Lippitt AB. The facet joint and its role in spine pain: management with facet joint injections. *Spine.* 1984;9:746–750.
25. Raymond J, Dumas J, Lisbona R. Nuclear imaging as a screening test for patients referred for intra-articular facet block. *J Can Assoc Radiol.* 1984;35:291–292.
26. Marks R, Houston T. Facet joint injection and facet nerve block-a randomized comparison in 86 patients. *Pain.* 1992;49:325–328.
27. Dreyfuss P, Schwarzer A, Lau P, Bogduk P. The target specificity of lumbar medial branch and L5 dorsal ramus nerve blocks:

ACT study. *Presented at the 3rd Annual Scientific Meeting of the International Spinal Injection Society*, September 23, 1995, New Orleans, LA.

28. Bogduk N. Back pain: Zygapophysial blocks and epidural steroids. In: Cousins MJ, Bridenbaugh PO, eds. *Neural Blockade in Clinical Anaesthesia and Management of Pain*, 2nd ed. Philadelphia, PA: Lippincott; 1989:935–954.

29. van Kleef M, Vandelderen P, Cohen S, Lataster A, Van Zundert J, Mekhail N. Pain originating from the lumbar facet joints. *Pain Practice.* 2010;10(5):459–469.

30. Airaksinen O, Brox JI, Cedraschi C, et al. European guidelines for the management of chronic nonspecific low back pain. *Eur Spine J.* 2006;15(suppl. 2):S192–300.

31. Pneumaticos SG, Chatziioannou SN, Hipp JA, Moore WH, Esses SI. Low back pain: prediction of short-term outcome of facet joint injection with bone scintigraphy. *Radiology.* 2006;238:693–698.

32. Carette S, Marcoux S, Truchon R, et al. A controlled trial of corticosteroid injections into facet joints for chronic low back pain. *N Engl J Med.* 1991;325:1002–1007.

33. Varlotta GP, Lefkowitz TF, Schweitzer M, et al. The lumbar facet joint: a review of current knowledge: part II: diagnosis and management. *Skeletal Radiol.* 2011;40:149–157.

34. Gallegher J, Vadi PLP, Wesley JR. Radiofrequency facet joint denervation in the treatment of low back pain—a prospective controlled double-blind study to assess its efficacy. *Pain Clinic.* 1994;7:193–198.

35. van Kleef M, Barendse GA, Kessels F, Voets HM, Weber WE, de Lange S. Randomized trial of radiofrequency lumbar facet denervation for chronic low back pain. *Spine.* 1999;24:1937–1942.

36. Nath S, Nath CA, Pettersson K. Percutaneous lumbar zygapophysial (facet) joint neurotomy using radiofrequency current, in the management of chronic low back pain: a randomized double-blind trail. *Spine.* 2008;33:1291–1297.

37. Kornick C, Kramarich SS, Lamer TJ, Todd Sitzman B. Complications of lumbar facet radiofrequency denervation. *Spine.* 2004;29:1352–1354.

38. Goren A, Yildiz N, Topuz O, Findikoglu G, Ardic F. Efficacy of exercise and ultrasound in patients with lumbar spinal stenosis: a prospective randomized controlled trial. *Clin Rehabil.* 2010;24(7):623–631.

39. Bronfort G, Haas M, Evans R, Leeinenger B, Triano J. Effectiveness of manual therapies: the UK evidence report. *Chiropr Osteopat.* 2010;18:3.

40. Furlan AD, Brosseau L, Imamura M, Irvin E. Massage for low back pain: a systematic review within the framework of the Cochrane Collaboration Back Review Group. *Spine.* 2002;17:1896–1910.

41. Triano JJ, McGregor M, Hendros MA, Brennan PC. Manipulative therapy versus education programs in chronic low back pain. *Spine.* 1995;20(8):948–955.

42. Andersson GB, Lucente T, Davis AM, Kappler RE, Lipton JA, Leurgans S. A comparison of osteopathic spinal manipulation with standard care for patients with low back pain. *N Engl J Med.* 1999;341:1426–1431.

43. Giles LG, Muller R. chronic spinal pain: a randomized clinical trail comparing medication, acupuncture and spinal manipulation. *Spine.* 2003;28:1490–1502.

44. Licciardone JC, Stoll ST, Fulda KG, et al. Osteopathic manipulative treatment for chronic low back pain: a randomized controlled trial. *Spine.* 2003;28:1355–1362.

45. Ellis R, Hing W. Neural mobilization: a systematic review of randomized controlled trials with an analysis of therapeutic efficacy. *J Man Manip Ther.* 2008;16(1):8–22.

46. Tsauo JY, Chen WH, Liang HW, Jang Y. The effectiveness of a functional training programme for patients with chronic low back pain-a pilot study. *Disabil Rehabil.* 2009;31(13):1100–1106.

47. Press J. Core strengthening. In: O'Connor, F ed. *Sports Medicine: Just the Facts.* New York, NY: McGraw-Hill; 2005:412–414.

48. Akmal M, Kesani A, Effect of nicotine on spinal disc cells: a cellular mechanism for disc degeneration. *Spine (Phila Pa 1976).* 2004;29(5):568–575.

49. Dundar U, Solak O, Evcik D, Kavunco V. Clinical effectiveness of aquatic exercise to treat chronic low back pain: a randomized controlled trial. *Spine.* 2009;(34)14:1436–1440.

50. Mamoru A, Kyosuke S, Kensei N, et al. Efficacy of aquatic exercises for patients with low-back pain. *Kurume Medical Journal.* 1999;46:91–96.

51. Vincent A, Hill J, Kruk KM, Cha SS, Bauer BA. External qigong for chronic pain. *Am J Chin Med.* 2010;38(4):695–703.

52. Hall AM, Maher CG, Lam P, Ferreira M, Latimer J. Tai chi exercise for treatment of pain and disability in people with persistent low back pain: a randomized controlled trial. *Arthritis Care Res (Hoboken).* 2011;63(11):1576–1583.

Lumbar Disc Pathology

Paul M. Cooke, Stephen Massimi, and Lee Rosenzweig

INTRODUCTION

Low back pain (LBP) is a very common problem that affects up to 80% of adults at some time during their lives, however, in only a small fraction of patients with axial LBP is a herniated disc the actual cause (1). The prevalence of symptomatic lumbar disc herniations is about 1% to 3% in Finland and Italy, depending on age and sex (2). Discogenic LBP, presenting as axial LBP, is theorized to result from irritation to nerve receptors that innervate the outer fibers of the annulus fibrosus, in the cartilaginous endplates, as well as in the periosteum of the vertebral bodies (3). Irritation can be from degenerative disc disease, annular tears, or inflammatory processes that can affect the disc. LBP with associated leg pain results from nerve root compression or chemical irritation by an intervertebral disc which may lead to pain, weakness, reflex loss, or sensory deficits.

There are three main intervertebral lumbar disc pathologies that cause LBP: degenerative disc disease, internal disc disruption, and disc herniation (4). Internal disc disruption occurs when the internal architecture of the disc is disrupted but its external surface remains essentially normal (5). It is characterized by degradation of the nucleus pulposus and radial fissures in the annulus. Since the outer third of the annulus is innervated, tears in this region can be a source of LBP (4), and they can be seen as *high-intensity zones* on MRI (6). A disc herniation refers to disc material that extends beyond the intervertebral disc space. When disc material is displaced at more than 50% of the circumference of the intervertebral disc, it is classified as a bulge, and when it involves less than 50% of the intervertebral disc circumference it is called a herniation (7). Disc herniations can then be sub-classified into either a protrusion when the distance of the edges

of the herniated material is less than the distance of the edges at its base, or an extrusion when the distance of the edges of the herniated material is greater than the distance of the edges at its base (4).

Discogenic lumbar pain classically presents with axial LBP that is nonradiating, that is worse during spinal flexion with or without rotation, prolonged sitting, or with Valsalva maneuvers (e.g., coughing, sneezing), although in some patients discogenic pain may be worse during extension or side bending and this depends on the site of disc pathology. Although most patients with lumbar disk herniation present with LBP radiating into the legs (commonly referred to as sciatica), patients may also present with nonradiating pain in either the back or the legs, or with purely sensory and/or motor deficits (8). Symptoms that increase the specificity of radicular symptoms caused by lumbar disk herniation include pain that is worse in the leg than in the back; a typical dermatomal distribution of neurologic symptoms; and pain that is worse with the Valsalva maneuver (9).

Over 95% of lumbar disc herniations occur at the L4-5 and L5-S1 levels (10,11), and more commonly occur in people 55 years of age or older (12,13). Posterolateral, or para-central, disc herniations are the most common because the annulus fibrosus may be weaker in this location and there is poor secondary support from the posterior longitudinal ligament, which is tapered and narrower in the lower lumbar spine. Posterolateral discs can affect the nerve root as it descends in the lateral recess or just before it enters the neural foramen. Far lateral or extraforaminal herniations can affect the nerve root as it exits the neural foramen, and central disc herniations may affect any part of the cauda equina depending on the level (4). Pain may start abruptly after an activity or it may develop insidiously. Risk factors for lumbar disc herniation include flexion and twisting and other repetitive motions, sedentary occupations, prolonged driving of motor vehicles (14), obesity, and cigarette smoking (15,16).

Initial management will always include a detailed history and physical examination. *Key elements of the physical examination* include inspection, palpation, range of motion (ROM), a thorough neurologic examination including assessment of strength, sensation, and reflexes, and provocative tests such as dural tension testing (e.g., the passive straight-leg-raise (SLR) test, seated slump test). The SLR test is commonly used as an aid for the diagnosis of lumbar disc herniations. It has a relatively high sensitivity but widely varying specificity (17) and thus there is little recognition that a negative passive SLR test may be of greater diagnostic value than a positive one (18). However, a positive crossed SLR test (pain elicited with contralateral hip flexion) is more specific for lumbar disk herniation, and it complements the sensitive uncrossed SLR test (8). Combining positive test results (forward flexion, SLR test, hyper-extension test, and slump test) will increase the specificity of the physical examination (17).

Note that sciatic pain is not specific for lumbar disk herniation, and many other common conditions may cause radiating pain similar to sciatica (8). Included in the differential diagnosis of LBP are mechanical lesions (degenerative changes, herniated discs, spinal stenosis, spondylolisthesis, synovial cysts); systemic diseases such as primary neural or bone tumors, sciatic neuropathy, metastatic cancer, serious infections, and inflammatory spondyloarthropathies; and visceral diseases that may present with back pain as a chief symptom but that do not involve the spine (e.g., nephrolithiasis, endometriosis, and aortic aneurysm) (19).

The timing and modality of imaging is based on risk factors for serious spinal disease, the patient's clinical progress, and the characteristics of the imaging modality (8). Imaging tests should be reserved for patients in whom an alternative diagnosis is suspected (e.g., patients with signs of systemic disease or with a known history of cancer), or for patients who have neurologic abnormalities suggesting a herniated disc and who have not responded to 3 to 4 weeks of conservative therapy (19). Suspected discogenic LBP that is refractory to conservative care also warrants an MRI. Since 25% to 30% of asymptomatic individuals will have a lumbar intervertebral disc herniation on imaging studies (20,21), imaging findings are most useful when carefully correlated to findings on the physical examination.

Most symptomatic disc herniations result in clinical manifestations, such as pain, weakness, reflex loss, and sensory deficits that resolve with conservative management alone (22). In the absence of cauda equina syndrome or a rapidly progressive neurologic deficit, virtually all patients with a suspected disc herniation should be treated conservatively for 6 weeks (19). Several nonsurgical treatments have been proven effective in improving symptoms of lumbar disk herniation and should be considered first-line in the first 6 weeks of conservative management (8). For 90% of patients with lumbar disk herniation, acute sciatica starts to improve within 6 weeks and resolves by 12 weeks with conservative care (23). It is estimated that only 5% to 22% of patients with persistent radicular symptoms will ultimately require surgery (24,25). In a prospective study comparing surgical and conservative therapies, there was a benefit of surgery noted at one year follow-up, but not later (26). Moreover, more than 60% of the nonoperated patients had a favorable outcome (27). Interestingly, large and migrated herniations tend to spontaneously decrease to a greater extent than protrusions or small contained herniations (28), and evidence has shown that even patients with extensive herniations are good candidates for a conservative treatment approach (27). It has been demonstrated that a longer course of conservative management before surgery (i.e., averaging more than 18 weeks in one randomized controlled trial) did not alter the incidence of adverse outcomes as a result of waiting longer before surgery (29). Patients should be informed that the expected amount of pain and disability 2 years after surgery will be indistinguishable from the pain 2 years after prolonged conservative management (8).

THE REHABILITATION PROGRAM

A brief period of relative rest is acceptable in the acute phase prior to starting PT (4), however prolonged bed rest greater than three days is not indicated as it may contribute to muscle deconditioning (30) and has not been shown to reduce disability from LBP (31). Patients should be encouraged to stay active and avoid activities that exacerbate their pain (e.g., lifting, repetitive bending and twisting, and prolonged sitting). In the acute phase, analgesic medications, non-steroidal anti-inflammatories, and other therapeutic modalities may be helpful to decrease pain prior to initiating a PT program (4).

A PT program that utilizes MDT for the treatment of discogenic LBP has been shown to result in high rates of patient satisfaction, recovery from neurologic deficits, and

LUMBAR DISC PATHOLOGY

▦ Discogenic LBP results from irritation to nerve receptors that innervate the outer fibers of the annulus fibrosus, the cartilaginous endplates, and/or the periosteum of the vertebral bodies

▦ Lumbar radiculopathy results from nerve root irritation or compression by an intervertebral disc, which may lead to pain, weakness, reflex loss, or sensory deficits in the legs

▦ 95% of herniated discs occur at the L4-5 and L5-S1 levels

▦ Most patients with discogenic LBP have directional preferences that reproducibly either ameliorate or aggravate their clinical symptoms. These directional preferences are often used to guide physical therapy (PT) programs, known as mechanical diagnosis and therapy (MDT)

▦ Imaging should be reserved for patients in whom an alternate diagnosis is suspected or who have not responded to 3 to 4 weeks of conservative therapy

▦ In the absence of cauda equina syndrome or a rapidly progressive neurologic deficit, the vast majority of patients with a suspected disc herniation should be treated conservatively for several weeks

▦ Most cases of lumbar disc herniation are self-limited and resolve with conservative treatment

▦ Early mobilization is helpful, and patients should avoid prolonged bed rest and also avoid activities that exacerbate their symptoms

return to employment and a low rate of surgical intervention (27). An appropriate exercise prescription, education regarding why the exercises should help, and realistic expectations should increase compliance with this treatment (32). PT should begin with patient education on proper body biomechanics for lifting, sitting, and standing postures.

Since the location of the disc herniation typically dictates which lumbar spine movements increase or reduce pain, a single set of exercises or cookbook approach will not be effective for all patients with discogenic LBP. Thus, a patient's clinical picture should guide the design of his or her PT program (4). For most patients, including up to 50% of patients with chronic LBP (33–35), directional characteristics can be found that reproducibly either ameliorate or aggravate a patient's clinical symptoms (36). Evidence supports the notion that if a preferred direction of trunk movement that reduces LBP symptoms can be found during examination, then exercises in this preferred direction and appropriate symptom-driven postural strategies can reduce LBP and improve function (37–40). This concept is the basis for a PT program guided by directional preference, also referred to as MDT or the McKenzie method (41). The assessment of directional preference using the McKenzie method that was developed by physical therapist Robin McKenzie can help identify appropriate rehabilitation exercises, which for most patients are not flexion but extension exercises (42), which can be attributed to the central or para-central location of most disc herniations.

Therapeutic Modalities

Heat and cold are often used in the treatment of LBP. There is moderate evidence that continuous heat wrap therapy reduces pain and disability in the short term, and that the addition of exercise to heat wrap therapy further reduces pain and improves function. However there is insufficient evidence to make recommendations about the application of cold treatment to LBP (43), although this modality is safe and often aids to reduce pain and inflammation in many patients. Therapeutic ultrasound and transcutaneous electrical nerve stimulation (TENS) may provide short-term benefit (44,45) and may be used early in the treatment course, but haven't been shown to alter long term outcomes.

Research on mechanical traction is conflicting. One uncontrolled study found that traction, ultrasound, and low level laser (LLLT) therapies were all effective in the treatment of patients with acute lumbar disc herniation based on MRI and clinical parameters (46). A systematic review concluded that the addition of mechanical traction to medication and electrotherapy was effective, but that mechanical traction was occasionally associated with adverse events, such as increased pain, anxiety, lower limb weakness, and fainting which were all reported in trials using traction (47), while another systematic review concluded that traction is not effective (48).

Manual Therapy

Studies evaluating spinal manipulation for lumbar disk herniation have had conflicting results. One study comparing manipulation with sham manipulation found that manipulation significantly improved pain (49). While an exercise based approach is the conventional primary physical treatment of lumbar disc pathology, manual therapies may be useful in selected patients, but may be reserved for therapists who have received specific training in manual therapy and patients not responding to therapeutic exercise. Patients with LBP due to discogenic pathology also frequently seek out or receive manual therapy from massage therapists, chiropractors, and osteopathic physicians. Overall, the evidence tends to be lower quality and conflicting for the use of these treatments in the setting of LBP, and it is even more difficult to draw conclusions about the effectiveness of these treatments in the subset of patients with discogenic LBP.

Therapeutic Exercise

MDT is an individualized program that is based on directional preference and will begin with movements that patients can do with little pain, then progress to include additional planes of motion in order to improve function and decrease pain. In general, extension based programs may be more appropriate for central or para-central disc herniations, whereas neutral or flexion based programs may be more effective for foraminal herniations. But this is a simplistic view of MDT, or the McKenzie method, which requires advanced training to properly make a mechanical diagnosis and formulate a therapy program to centralize and reduce symptoms.

In addition to MDT, hip/trunk and lower limb mobility exercises must be included and improvements should be made before transitioning to a core strengthening program. Gentle trunk mobility exercises may be utilized, including flexion and extension cycles to reduce joint stiffness and relax elastic structure resulting in lower joint loads during subsequent movements (50).

Careful attention needs to be paid to the patient's gait and postural examination. A flat back posture (decreased lumbar lordosis) is often associated with short hamstrings, and increased lumbar lordosis is often associated with tight hip flexors (32). In these cases, exercises to correct these postural and muscular imbalances can help reduce chronic strain on the spinal structures. Postural control has repeatedly been found to be altered in patients with chronic LBP compared to healthy controls (51). Patients should be instructed to develop improved core, biomechanical, and postural awareness, and then incorporate this improved awareness into their daily activities. Flexible hips and knees are required to adopt postures that protect the low back (23), thus it is imperative that hip and knee mobility exercises (Figures 43.1 and 43.2) are included if ROM deficits are present in order to facilitate spine-conserving postures (50).

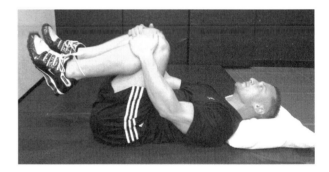

FIGURE 43.1: Double knee to chest stretch.

Lie on your back with your knees bent and your feet flat on the floor. Gently pull one knee toward your chest and hold for 20 seconds and then relax. Repeat this with the other leg. This exercise can also be performed by pulling both knees to the chest at the same time. Do not pull any of the stretches into pain. Perform 3 to 5 repetitions.

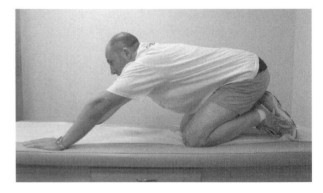

FIGURE 43.2: Quadruped rocking back to heels.

On your hands and knees, slowly rock back toward your heels, keep your back flat, not allowing it to arch. Hold for 10 seconds. Perform 10 repetitions.

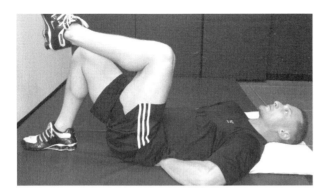

FIGURE 43.3: Abdominal stabilization exercise with single leg hip flexion in supine.

Lie on your back and contract your abdominal muscles pressing your back down against the floor or mat, lift one leg with the knee bent toward your chest. Lower the leg slowly while keeping your abdominals contracted and your back flat against the floor or mat. Alternate legs. Perform 10 repetitions.

Core strengthening, lumbo-pelvic stability programs may be initiated early in the program for the purpose of neuromuscular reeducation of the transverse abdominis and multifidus. Then patients should learn to perform gentle limb movements during core muscle contraction (32) (Figure 43.3). Exercises may be gradually advanced, with the goal of maintaining optimal spine stabilization during increasing challenges to the body. The therapeutic program should aim to improve muscle strength and endurance by incorporating exercises that limit compressive forces on the spine, which has been demonstrated as a mechanism of injury (50). The patient will focus on training specific muscles, beginning with anterior abdominal exercises while maintaining the spine in neutral posture, then lateral muscle exercises for the quadratus lumborum and lateral abdominal wall muscles, and then a trunk extensor program (50). The ultimate goal is for the patient to perform high-level activities without pain, such as work and sports, while maintaining spinal stability (52).

The strengthening and stability program should be systematic, gradual, and progressive, and should emphasize endurance training (i.e., longer duration and lower-effort) before strengthening. There is evidence indicating that endurance training has more protective value than strength training alone, especially when considering that back injuries can occur during activities with seemingly low-level demands, and that the risk of injury from motor control error may occur (53). Thus strength gains should not be over-emphasized at the expense of endurance (50).

Proprioceptive exercises that enhance neural and motor control have been recognized as an important element of therapy for discogenic LBP (54). A sensorimotor stimulation program that incorporates training on semi-unstable surfaces, such as an exercise ball, wobble, or rocking board, can specifically activate the gluteal muscles and improve pelvic control by training the body to handle unexpected perturbations. Activation of the gluteus maximus and gluteus medius helps to provide improved stabilization of the pelvic girdle and in turn will help in the protection of the low back against injury (54).

The final phase of rehabilitation attempts to incorporate the gains made in postural awareness, lower limb mobility, and spinal stability into functional exercises that may include weights, pulleys, and advanced closed chain exercises such as lunges with a diagonal punch. If the patient is an athlete, return to play criteria should be followed and sport-specific activities are added prior to return to sport (52).

Specialized Techniques

Many consider the McKenzie method or MDT that was previously discussed in this chapter to be a specialized technique. Dr. Shirley Sahrman teaches an approach that focuses on identification and correction of movement impairment syndromes (55) and Dr. Vladimir Janda has emphasized a neuromuscular reeducation approach to treating LBP (56), while both have recommended the correction of muscular imbalances. Similar exercises that incorporate these concepts have been discussed in the therapeutic exercise section of this chapter.

In addition, there is mixed evidence supporting the efficacy of aquatic exercise for the treatment of discogenic LBP. One study suggests that aquatic backward locomotion exercise is as beneficial as progressive resistance exercise for improving lumbar extension strength in patients after lumbar discectomy surgery (57). What is clear is that patients with axial load sensitivity may be good candidates for aquatic therapy, which takes advantage of water buoyancy to reduce axial load. In the acute phase, many patients are able to tolerate exercise in warm water better than on land, in part due to the buoyancy effect of water, as well as the relaxing effect from the proprioceptive input and support of the warm water. Aquatic therapy facilitates low load and low impact exercise for the spine. Freestyle swimming may exacerbate symptoms in the early stages of recovery due to the spinal extension and twisting that are involved. If this is the case, a patient may better tolerate stationary aquatic exercises, such as standing in a pool and performing abdominal sets, leg and arm movements, or treading water with a vest, all of which are effective adjuncts to land based exercises.

Supportive Devices

The routine use of lumbar corsets for LBP is not supported by the literature (58), and should not be considered as an alternative exercise-based therapies. Prolonged bracing may lead to abdominal and trunk musculature weakness due to disuse atrophy.

Home Exercise Program

Patient adherence to a well-planned home exercise program (HEP) is an important component of an effective rehabilitation program for discogenic LBP. Thorough patient education that includes an explanation of the rationale behind the exercises will improve patient compliance and help to prevent further injury.

The early HEP focuses on core and postural awareness and proper spinal biomechanics. Exercises to improve flexibility in the hips and knees are included to facilitate proper spinal biomechanics. Core strengthening exercises are then incorporated, which may include isometric flexion and extension cycles guided by directional preference, to achieve improved control throughout the newly established ROM. The core strengthening regimen will then advance to incorporate gentle limb movements while maintaining core muscle contraction with neutral spine alignment. The patient may practice proprioceptive exercises with the goal of improving pelvic control and spine stabilization during advanced activities.

Patients should be instructed on a general conditioning program that includes cardiovascular training or low impact aerobic exercise (e.g., walking), which has been shown to improve outcomes in patients with LBP, and helps to prevent future injury (59).

Although patients may see a physical therapist three times per week, there is some evidence that low back exercises are most beneficial when performed daily (60). This underscores the importance of a HEP.

SUMMARY

LBP related to intervertebral disc pathology is common. Axial LBP from discogenic sources incudes annular tears or herniations and limb pain may be from disc protrusions or extrusions causing nerve root irritation. In the absence of red flags, a six week course of conservative treatment including PT is indicated prior to ordering imaging tests or a surgical referral. A rehabilitation program must be individualized to each patient's clinical picture, and should follow a logical progression through the phases of rehabilitation. Modalities such as the application of heat, ultrasound, or TENS have been shown to be beneficial adjuncts to therapeutic exercise. MDT or the McKenzie method should guide the initial phases of therapy, along with a gentle hip mobility program and then spine stabilization program. Key elements of the PT program include core awareness, postural re-training, knee and hip mobility, as well as neuromuscular re-training and proprioceptive exercises to enhance pelvic stability. A HEP should include a general exercise program that incorporates cardiovascular training for general conditioning and improved muscular endurance in an attempt to prevent further injury.

SAMPLE CASE

A 36-year-old male without significant past medical or surgical history presents with lower lumbar pain that radiates down the lateral left leg to the ankle. He reports that his symptoms began one week prior after lifting weights at the gym. Review of systems is unremarkable. He has been taking ibuprofen intermittently for pain with little relief. His examination is significant for limited lumbar flexion that reproduces his left sided lower lumbar pain, a positive left SLR test, subtle left extensor hallucis longus weakness (5-/5), and decreased sensation at the first web space of the left foot. Deep tendon reflexes were normal.

SAMPLE THERAPY PRESCRIPTION

Discipline: Physical therapy.

Diagnosis: Discogenic LBP with left-sided L5 radiculopathy.

Precautions: Weight bearing as tolerated (WBAT).

Frequency of visits: 2 to 3x/week.

Duration of treatment: 4 to 6 weeks (or an alternative is to provide a total of 8–12 visits that may be used at the therapist's discretion).

Treatment:

1. *Modalities:* heat, cold, ultrasound, and/or TENS if not tolerating therapeutic exercise

2. *Manual therapy:* lumbar spine manipulation/mobilization (optional, if indicated and if appropriately trained physical therapist is available)

3. *Therapeutic exercise:* postural awareness and re-training, core strengthening starting with a therapeutic program of directional preference (i.e., McKenzie program) and gentle spine stabilization, with progression to restoring lumbar spine motion in all planes, hip and knee flexibility to facilitate neutral spine posture, proprioceptive and balance exercises

4. *Specialized treatments:* biomechanical analysis of gait and the kinetic chain; aquatic therapy (optional, if available may be utilized during initial phases of rehabilitation)

5. *Patient education:* proper biomechanics, HEP

Goals: Decrease pain, improve core and lower limb ROM, as well as strength and endurance, correct postural problems, improve balance/proprioception, safely return to functional activities, prevent further back injuries.

Reevaluation: In 4 to 6 weeks by referring physician.

REFERENCES

1. Waddell G. *The Back Pain Revolution*. London, UK: Churchill Livingstone Press; 1998.
2. Andersson G. Epidemiology of spinal disorders. In: Frymoyer JW, Ducker TB, Hadler NM, et al, eds. *The Adult Spine: Principles and Practice*. New York, NY: Raven Press; 1997:93–141.
3. Mayer HM. Discogenic low back pain and degenerative lumbar spinal stenosis—how appropriate is surgical treatment? *Schmerz*. 2001;15(6):484–491.
4. Barr KP, Harrast MA. Low back pain. In: Braddom RL. *Physical Medicine and Rehabilitation*, 3rd ed. Philadelphia, PA: Elsevier; 2007:911–912.
5. Bogduk N. *Clinical Anatomy of the Lumbar Spine and Sacrum*. Edinburgh, UK: Churchill Livingstone; 1997.
6. Aprill C, Bogduk N. High-intensity zone: a diagnostic sign of painful lumbar disc on magnetic resonance imaging. *Br J Radiol*. 1992;65(773):361–369.
7. Fardon DF, Milette PC. Nomenclature and classification of lumbar disc pathology. Recommendations of the Combined Task Forces of the North American Spine Society, American Society of Spine Radiology, and American Society of Neuroradiology. *Spine*. 2001;26(5):E93-E113.
8. Gregory DS, Seto CK, Wortley GC, Shugart CM. Acute lumbar disk pain: navigating evaluation and treatment choices. *Am Fam Physician*. 2008;78(7):835–842; 844.
9. Vroomen PC, de Krom MC, Wilmink JT, Kester AD, Knottnerus JA. Diagnostic value of history and physical examination in patients suspected of lumbosacral nerve root compression. *J Neurol Neurosurg Psychiatry*. 2002;72(5):630–634.
10. Deyo RA, Loeser JD, Bigos SJ. Herniated lumbar intervertebral disk. *Ann Intern Med*. 1990;112(8):598–603.
11. Spangfort EV. The lumbar disc herniation. A computer-aided analysis of 2,504 operations. *Acta Orthop Scand Suppl*. 1972;142:1–95.
12. Friberg S, Hirsch C. Anatomical and clinical studies on lumbar disc degeneration. *Acta Orthop Scand*. 1949;19:222–242.
13. Schultz A, Andersson G, Ortengren R, et al. Loads on the lumbar spine. *J Bone Joint Surg Am*. 1982;64:713–720.
14. Fraser RD. Chymopapain for the treatment of intervertebral disc herniation. A preliminary report of a double blind study. *Spine*. 1982;7:608–612.
15. Heliovaara M. Body height, obesity, and risk of herniated lumbar intervertebral disc. *Spine*. 1987;12:469–472.
16. Kelsey JL, Githens PB, O'Conner T, et al. Acute prolapsed lumbar intervertebral disc. An epidemiologic study with special reference to driving automobiles and cigarette smoking. *Spine*. 1984;9:608–613.
17. van der Windt DA, Simons E, Riphagen II, et al. Physical examination for lumbar radiculopathy due to disc herniation in patients with low-back pain. *Cochrane Database Syst Rev*. 2010;(2):CD007431.
18. Rebain R, Baxter GD, McDonough S. A systematic review of the passive straight leg raising test as a diagnostic aid for low back pain (1989 to 2000). *Spine (Phila Pa 1976)*. 2002;27(17):E388–395.
19. Deyo RA, Loeser JD, Bigos SJ. Herniated lumbar intervertebral disk. *Annals of Internal Medicine*. 1990;112:598–603.
20. Vucetic N, Svensson O. Physical signs in lumbar disc hernia. *Clin Orthop*. 1996;333:192–210.
21. Waddell G, Main CJ, Morris EW, et al. Chronic low-back pain, psychologic distress, and illness behaviour. *Spine*. 1984;9:209–213.

22. Rhee JM, Schaufele M, Abdu WA. Radiculopathy and the herniated lumbar disc. Controversies regarding pathophysiology and management. *J Bone Joint Surg Am.* 2006;88(9):2070–2080.

23. Saal JA, Saal JS. Nonoperative treatment of herniated lumbar intervertebral disc with radiculopathy. An outcome study. *Spine.* 1989;14(4):431–437.

24. Frymoyer JW. Back pain and sciatica. *N Engl J Med.* 1988;318:291–300.

25. Weinstein JN, Lurie JD, Tosteson TD, et al: Surgical vs nonoperative treatment for lumbar disk herniation: the Spine Patient Outcomes Research Trial (SPORT) observational cohort. *JAMA.* 2006;296:2451–2459.

26. Weber H. Lumbar disc herniation. A controlled, prospective study with ten years of observation. *Spine.* 1983;8:131–140.

27. Brotz D, Kuker W, Maschke E, et al. A prospective trial of mechanical physiotherapy for lumbar disk prolapse. *J Neurol.* 2003;250:746–749.

28. Benoist M. The natural history of lumbar disc herniation and radiculopathy. *Joint Bone Spine.* 2002;69:155–160.

29. Peul WC, van Houwelingen HC, van den Hout WB, et al. Surgery versus prolonged conservative treatment for sciatica. *N Engl J Med.* 2007;356(22):2245–2256.

30. Hagen KB, Hilde G, Jamtvedt G, Winnem M. Bed rest for acute low-back pain and sciatica. *Cochrane Database Syst Rev.* 2004;(4):CD001254.

31. Deyo RA, Diehl AK, Rosenthal M. How many days of bed rest for acute low back pain? A randomized clinical trial. *N Engl J Med.* 1986;315(17):1064–1070.

32. Barr KP, Griggs M, Cadby T. Lumbar stabilization: a review of core concepts and current literature, part 2. *Am J Phys Med Rehabil.* 2007;86(1):72–80.

33. Donelson R, Aprill C, Medcalf R, Grant W. A prospective study of centralization of lumbar and referred pain: a predictor of symptomatic discs and anular competence. *Spine.* 1997;22(10):1115–1122.

34. Long A. The centralization phenomenon: its usefulness as a predictor of outcome in conservative treatment of chronic low back pain. *Spine.* 1995;20(23):2513–2521.

35. Kopp JR, Alexander AH, Turocy RH, Levrini MG, Lichtman DM. The use of lumbar extension in the evaluation and treatment of patients with acute herniated nucleus pulposus, a preliminary report. *Clin Orthoped.* 1986;202:211–218.

36. Wetzel FT, Donelson R. The role of repeated end-range/pain response assessment in the management of symptomatic lumbar discs. *Spine J.* 2003;3(2):146–154.

37. Long A, Donelson R, Fung T. Does it matter which exercise? A randomized control trial of exercise for low back pain. *Spine.* 2004;29:2593–2602.

38. Snook S, Webster B, McGorry R, Fogleman M, McCann K. The reduction of chronic nonspecific low back pain through the control of early morning lumbar flexion: a randomized controlled trial. *Spine.* 1998;23:2601–2607.

39. Spratt K, Weinstein J, Lehmann T, Woody J, Syare H. Efficacy of flexion and extension treatments incorporating braces for low-back pain patients with retrodisplacement, spondylolisthesis, or normal sagittal translation. *Spine.* 1993;18(13):1839–1849.

40. Williams M, Hawley J, McKenzie R, Van Wijmen P. A comparison of the effects of two sitting postures on back and referred pain. *Spine.* 1991;16(10):1185–1191.

41. McKenzie R. *The Lumbar Spine: Mechanical Diagnosis And Therapy.* Waikanae, New Zealand: Spinal Publications; 1981.

42. Kuritzky L. Low-back pain: consider extension education. *Phys Sportsmed.* 1997;25(1):56–64.

43. French SD, Cameron M, Walker BF, Reggars JW, Esterman AJ. A Cochrane review of superficial heat or cold for low back pain. *Spine (Phila Pa 1976).* 2006;31(9):998–1006.

44. Bloodworth DM, Nguyen BN, Garver W, et al. Comparison of stochastic vs. conventional transcutaneous electrical stimulation for pain modulation in patients with electromyographically documented radiculopathy. *Am J Phys Med Rehabil.* 2004;83(8):584–591.

45. Nwuga VC. Ultrasound in treatment of back pain resulting from prolapsed intervertebral disc. *Arch Phys Med Rehabil.* 1983;64(2):88–89.

46. Unlu Z, Tasci S, Tarhan S, et al. Comparison of 3 physical therapy modalities for acute pain in lumbar disc herniation measured by clinical evaluation and magnetic resonance imaging. *J Manipulative Physiol Ther.* 2008;31(3):191–198.

47. Hahne AJ, Ford JJ, McMeeken JM. Conservative management of lumbar disc herniation with associated radiculopathy. *Spine.* 2010;35:E488-E504.

48. Clarke JA, van Tulder MW, Blomberg SE, et al. Traction for low back pain with or without sciatica. *Cochrane Database Syst Rev.* 2007;(2):CD003010.

49. Santilli V, Beghi E, Finucci S. Chiropractic manipulation in the treatment of acute back pain and sciatica with disc protrusion: a randomized double-blind clinical trial of active and simulated spinal manipulations. *Spine J.* 2006;6(2):131–137.

50. McGill SM. Low back exercises: evidence for improving exercise regimens. *Phys Ther.* 1998;78(7):754–765.

51. Barr KP, Griggs M, Cadby T. Lumbar stabilization: core concepts and current literature, Part 1. *Am J Phys Med Rehabil.* 2005;84(6):473–480.

52. McGill S, ed: Evaluating the patient. In: *Low Back Disorders: Evidence-Based Prevention and Rehabilitation.* Champaign, IL: Human Kinetics; 2002: 223–238.

53. Luoto S, ed, Heliovaara M, Hurri H, Alaranta M. Static back endurance and the risk of low back pain. *Clinical Biomechanics.* 1995;10:323–324.

54. Bullock-Saxton JE, Janda V, Bullock MI. Reflex activation of gluteal muscles in walking. An approach to restoration of muscle function for patients with low-back pain. *Spine (Phila Pa 1976).* 1993;18(6):704–708.

55. Sahrman S: *Diagnosis and Treatment of Movement Impairment Syndromes.* 1st ed. Mosby Inc; 2002.

56. Janda V: Evaluation of muscular imbalance. In: Liebenson C, ed. *Rehabilitation of the Spine: A Practitioner's Manual,* 1st ed. Baltimore, MD: Lippincott, Williams & Wilkins; 1996:97–112.

57. Kim YS, Park J, Shim JK. Effects of aquatic backward locomotion exercise and progressive resistance exercise on lumbar extension strength in patients who have undergone lumbar diskectomy. *Arch Phys Med Rehabil.* 2010;91(2):208–214.

58. van Duijvenbode IC, Jellema P, van Poppel MN, van Tulder MW. Lumbar supports for prevention and treatment of low back pain. *Cochrane Database Syst Rev.* 2008;(2):CD001823.

59. Nutter P. Aerobic exercise in the treatment and prevention of low back pain. *Occup Med.* 1988;3:137–145.

60. Mayer TG, Gatchel RJ, Kishino N, et al. Objective assessment of spine function following industrial injury: a prospective study with comparison group and one-year follow-up. *Spine.* 1985;10:482–493.

Lumbar Radiculopathy

Frederick Bagares, Joel M. Press, and Melissa Kolski

INTRODUCTION

Lumbar radiculopathy is a very common cause of back and leg pain resulting in acute and chronic disability. It is defined as a focal neurological deficit in a specific myotomal and/or dermatomal distribution due to nerve root compression or irritation. Common complaints from the patient include low back pain with radiating pain to the lower limb, lower limb weakness, and/or sensory changes such as numbness or tingling. Men are affected more frequently than women. Men are commonly affected after age 40, whereas women are commonly affected between the ages of 50 to 60 years old.

The primary role of the spinal column is to protect the spinal cord while allowing segmental motion. There are typically five lumbar vertebrae each composed of a vertebral body, transverse process, pedicle, lamina, spinous process, and superior/inferior articulating processes. On occasion anatomic variations may exist, with the fifth lumbar vertebrae not being completely divided from the sacrum (a sacralized segment) or the first sacral vertebrae not being completely fused making the appearance of a sixth lumbar vertebrae (lumbarized sacral segment). The spinal cord lies within the spinal canal and ends at about the L1/L2 intervertebral level as the conus medullaris. The nerve roots continue and descend collectively known as the cauda equina exiting through intervertebral foramen at their corresponding levels. There are a total of 11 spinal nerves that arise from the lumbosacral spinal cord (five lumbar, five sacral, and one coccygeal). The ventral roots that arise from the ventral gray matter of the spinal cord carry primarily motor fibers. The dorsal roots carry sensory information from the periphery and extend centrally from the dorsal root ganglion (DRG). The DRG is located adjacent to the spinal cord and within the intervertebral foramen. Just distal to the intervertebral foramen, the dorsal and ventral roots join and form a mixed spinal nerve. The dorsal rami of the mixed spinal nerve innervate the paravertebral skin and musculature while the ventral rami continue on and form the lumbosacral plexus and give rise to the nerves that innervate the lower limbs.

In between each vertebral segment lies an intervertebral disc (IVD) that helps absorb compression and translates forces, allows motion between vertebral bodies, and provides nourishment to the cartilaginous endplates of the vertebral body. The biconvex IVD is composed of a firm outer ring called the annulus fibrosus with a gelatinous center called the nucleus pulposus. Both structures are composed of type I and II collagen fibers but the annulus fibrosus is predominantly type I. The annulus fibrosus has concentric layers of collagen fiber that provide stability and contain the inner substance of the disc. The inner matrix of the nucleus pulposus is comprised of chondrocytes, collagen fibers, and proteoglycans. These proteoglycans are composed of mucopolysaccharides (chondroitin sulfate, keratin sulfate, hyaluronic acid) that have the ability to imbibe water molecules and become deformable.

With respect to radiculopathy, patients can experience radicular symptoms when there is nerve root impingement or irritation as it leaves the spinal canal through the intervertebral foramen. Because the intervertebral foramen is a discrete space, any structural changes or space-occupying lesions that encroach up on this space can cause neuropathic signs and symptoms. There are several causes of lumbar radiculopathy including infection (i.e., lumbar abscess), tumors (primary vs. metastatic), and inflammatory processes. This chapter will focus on the two most common causes: herniated nucleus pulposus (HNP) and spondyloarthopathy.

The most common cause of lumbar radiculopathy under the age of 50 is a HNP. As the spine ages, the ability to absorb water decreases. This alters the internal structure of the matrix and the disc's ability to absorb force. With time, the disc begins to desiccate and degenerate predisposing it to fissures and annular tears. Often precipitated by a forward bending, twisting, and lifting event, IVD pressure increases and the once contained nucleus pulposus herniates through an annular tear. Because of the broadness of the posterior longitudinal ligament, the herniated contents most often exit posterolaterally adjacent to intervertebral foramen as the ventral and dorsal roots exit (Figure 44.1).

Over the age of 50, another common cause of lumbar radiculopathy is spondyloarthopathy, which is generally a degenerative phenomenon. As a result of the IVD degeneration, the ability to absorb force diminishes requiring the bony structures around the disc to absorb more force. Osteophytes start to form as a reaction to increased force (as described by Wolff's law). They occur within the bony vertebrae and around the zygapophyseal joint and vertebral endplates. Ligaments (i.e., ligamentum flavum) supporting the vertebrae also lose their elasticity and begin thickening and buckling. IVD height decreases as the vertebral bodies begin to approximate. As the spine loses its inherent stability, bony and ligamentous structures start to encroach upon neural structures causing stenosis within the central canal, lateral recess, and neural foramen (Figures 44.2 and 44.3).

While symptoms can begin suddenly with an inciting event (i.e., lifting a box), it is not uncommon for the patient to have an underlying history of low back pain (LBP) with a gradual progression of mild symptoms. Classically, the patient will complain of LBP with radiating symptoms down the leg and into the foot in a dermatomal pattern. The pain is often described as stabbing, burning, dull, or aching. Tingling and numbness are also common complaints. Signs and symptoms, including weakness, are dependent on the nerve root levels that are involved (Table 44.1). L1 and L2 radiculopathies are not common but typically manifest with sensation deficits over the anterolateral thigh. There may be some associated hip flexion weakness with L2 radiculopathies. L3 radiculopathies can present with weakness with hip flexion and knee extension. L4 radiculopathies present with knee extension weakness and with possible ankle dorsiflexion weakness. Functionally, the patient may complain of some leg instability/buckling with ambulation and difficulty climbing stairs. L5 radiculopathies can present with hip weakness, especially hip abductor weakness, and a foot drop. Clinically, S1 radiculopathies can present with hip, knee, and ankle weakness since the sciatic nerve innervates all the muscles in the posterior thigh and leg. Functionally,

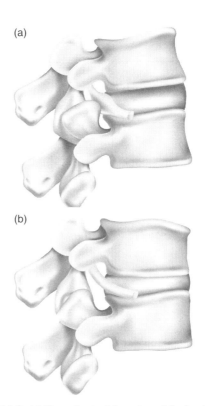

(a)

(b)

FIGURE 44.2: (a) Normal spinal foramina of the lumbar spine. (b) Degenerative spine changes causing neuroforaminal stenosis.

Source: Adapted from Ref. (31).

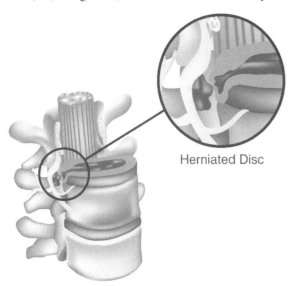

Herniated Disc

FIGURE 44.1: Example of a herniated nucleus pulposis causing nerve root impingement.

Source: Adapted from Ref. (31).

TABLE 44.1: Signs and Symptoms of Lumbar Radiculopathy by Root Level

Root Level	Distribution of Pain/Sensory Changes	Motor Weakness	Muscle Stretch Reflex Affected
L1	Inguinal region	None	None
L2	Anterolateral thigh	Hip flexion	None
L3	Anterolateral thigh	Hip flexion and adduction	Patellar
L4	Medial lower leg	Hip flexion, hip adduction, knee extension, ankle dorsiflexion	Patellar
L5	Lateral leg and dorsum of the foot	Hip abductors, ankle dorsiflexion, ankle eversion, great toe extension	Medial hamstrings
S1	Posterior thigh, leg, and plantar surface of foot	Hip extension, knee flexion, ankle plantar flexion, toe flexion	Achilles

patients may complain of difficulty with walking, stair climbing, and/or getting out of chairs.

Provocative daily symptoms with radiculopathy can be dependent on the underlying pathophysiology. With an acute herniated disc protrusion, patients often do not like forward flexion through the lumbar spine that increases posterior disc pressure causing disc contents to further irritate the nerve root. In cases of lumbar foraminal stenosis, however, patients may actually prefer a flexed position as this opens up a structurally stenotic area around the nerve root (Figure 44.3). It is thought that the increase in epidural pressures causes the pain associated with extension as opposed to direct pressure on the spinal nerves.

Key elements of the physical examination include inspection, palpation, lumbar spine examination with mechanical assessment, and neurological examination including dural tension testing. The physical examination begins as soon as the clinician meets the patient. The practitioner should pay attention to how the patient moves throughout the interview with pain behaviors and body language. The practitioner might notice an antalgic gait, hip girdle weakness, and/or difficulty with foot clearance suggesting a foot drop. On visual inspection, paravertebral musculature of the symptomatic side may appear asymmetric and there may be tenderness to palpation over the vertebral elements and the paravertebral musculature. The patient may appear to be favoring or leaning toward one side to offload the weight through the lumbar spine that may be impinging on neural structures. This compensatory maneuver to find a position of relief is called a *lateral*

shift. It is defined as a lateral displacement of the trunk in relation to the pelvis (1). It can be performed actively or involuntarily/reflexively. The reliability of detecting a lateral shift has been challenged in the literature, despite the fact that sometimes it is quite obvious to the observer (2). Static testing should include manual muscle testing,

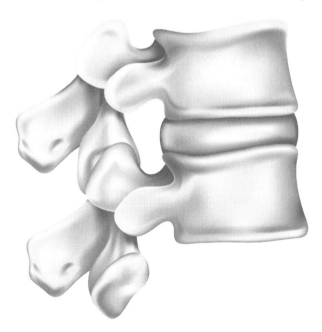

FIGURE 44.3: Flexion of the lumbar spine causing increased space within the neural foramen.

Source: Adapted from Ref. (31).

sensation testing (sampling all lumbosacral dermatomes), and muscle stretch reflexes. Dural tension signs such as seated slump and straight leg raise should reproduce familiar radiating symptoms into the leg in order to be positive.

Dynamic testing can begin while the patient is standing. To gain a general sense of lumbar motion, flexion, extension, and lumbar side glide should be assessed. To observe lumbar flexion, instruct the patient to slide their hands down their thighs and to touch their toes (Figure 44.4). This may provoke symptoms so tell the patient to use pain as their guide. The practitioner should be assessing the quality of their movement through the lumbar spine with each baseline motion. For lumbar extension have the patient place their hands in the small of their back and bend back as far as they can tolerate (Figure 44.5) Side glide may be observed to both sides with the patient keeping their shoulders parallel to their hips

and translating the pelvis to the right or left. This can give the clinician an estimation of side-bending and rotation in the lumbar spine. An unloaded assessment of lumbar extension may be performed in prone by performing a press-up and can provide some basic information about tolerance to this movement (Figure 44.6). If the clinician observes symptom alleviation, this may suggest a HNP whereas exacerbation may suggest lumbar stenosis or a foraminal HNP. The assessment described above is not a specific repeated movement examination, but it can give the physician an idea of directional preference that may help guide a therapy prescription.

Besides a complete history and physical examination, the diagnostic work-up may include plain films and/or MRI may be necessary to ensure that the patient is safe to participate in therapy if there is a clinical suspicion of an acute fracture, focal weakness, or cord compression.

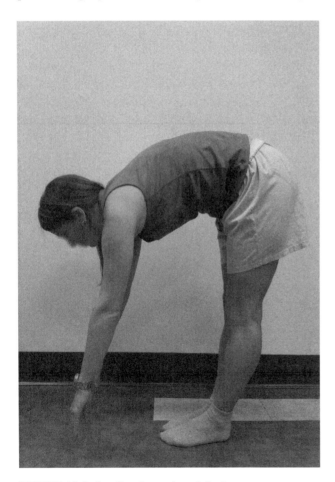

FIGURE 44.4: Standing forward trunk flexion.

Source: Adapted from www.spineuniverse.com/conditions/herniated-disc/lumbar-herniated-disc

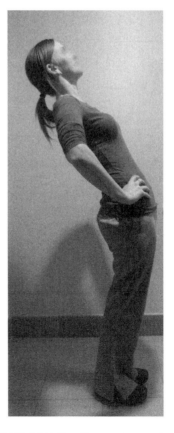

FIGURE 44.5: Standing trunk extension.

LUMBAR RADICULOPATHY

- It is estimated that between 70 and 80 percent of all Americans will have an episode of LBP in their lifetime (3).

- In 1998, total health care expenditures for LBP care were >90 billion dollars, and those suffering from LBP acquired 60% higher costs than others without LBP (4).

- Lumbar radiculopathy is a very common cause of back and leg pain.

- The most common cause of lumbar radiculopathy under the age of 50 is a HNP, and over the age of 50, is usually spondyloarthopathy, a degenerative phenomenon.

- The mechanism of injury usually involves flexion and rotation from a standing or seated position.

- Key elements of the physical examination include mechanical assessment of flexion, extension and side glide motions, and neurologic assessment including dural tension testing, motor, reflex, and sensory assessment.

- Diagnostic work up may include lumbar spine radiographs and/or MRI to ensure that the patient is safe to participate in a rehabilitation program.

- The Quebec task force concluded that the "effectiveness of LBP therapies is unproven," and it is very difficult to identify the pain generator. They recommended a classification system based on symptom location rather than tissue type (5).

- Studies show that patients treated as part of classification system do better (6,7). Subgroups respond better to one type of intervention than another (8,9,10).

Patients with suspected malignancy, cord compression, signs of infection, or bowel/bladder incontinence require a more extensive work-up and medical management before starting a rehabilitation program.

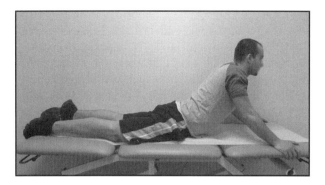

FIGURE 44.6: Prone press up or extension.

THE REHABILITATION PROGRAM

The primary and most effective treatment for lumbar radiculopathy is getting the patient involved in a physical therapy program. However, the patient may have a significant amount of pain that may need to be managed prior to participating in physical therapy. Therefore, educating the patient about their pain management options is essential. Medications such as nonsteroidal anti-inflammatory drugs (NSAIDs), oral steroids, and/or opioids may be necessary during the acute phase of a radiculopathy. If the pain is severe, transforaminal or interlaminar epidural steroid injections are also options to control pain. These medications and procedures have associated drug interactions and risks so these must be considered when making medical decisions.

A mechanical diagnosis can help to facilitate the rehabilitation process when a patient presents with a lumbar radiculopathy. Aside from looking for deficiencies in active range of motion (ROM), the therapist will begin their evaluation and determine if a directional preference exists (flexion, extension, or lateral). Matching the patient with his/her directional preference has been shown to significantly decrease pain, medication usage, and improve overall functional outcomes (6).

Therapeutic Modalities and Manual Therapy

There are several nonpharmacological therapies and modalities that are available for the treatment of LBP, including spinal manipulation, massage, exercise therapy, back schools, psychological therapies (biofeedback, progressive relaxation, cognitive behavioral therapy), interdisciplinary rehabilitation, and functional restoration (physical conditioning, work hardening, work conditioning). Complementary and alternative medicine therapies available for the treatment of LBP include acupuncture and yoga. There are relatively few trials, however, that specifically evaluate the effectiveness of these treatments and modalities in the setting of lumbar radiculopathy and conclusions from these trials are unclear due to the variation in experiment design and back pain inclusion criteria.

With regards to chronic or subacute LBP (>4 weeks), the literature supports moderate effects for psychological interventions, exercise, interdisciplinary rehabilitation, and functional restoration. The literature regarding spinal manipulation is inconclusive with respect to subacute and chronic LBP. There does not appear to be consistent and/or clinically significant differences across these therapies. For acute LBP (<4weeks), superficial heat/ice and spinal manipulation were found to have small to moderate benefit. The other noninvasive therapies (back schools, interferential therapy, low-level laser therapy, lumbar supports, transcutaneous electrical nerve stimulation (TENS), traction, and ultrasonography) have not been shown to be effective in acute, subacute, and/or chronic LBP (11).

Therapeutic Exercise

Therapeutic exercise is the key to functional recovery. While medications, manual therapy, and modalities can help to decrease pain and inflammation, progression through the remaining phases of rehabilitation is dependent on therapeutic exercise. As for ROM and lumbar radiculopathy, it has been demonstrated that patients who achieved end range lumbar extension (12) and achieved it quickly (13) had a better prognosis of avoiding surgery than patients who did not. Patients who are unable to centralize their pain were six times more likely to have surgery (14). Prognostic factors such as leg pain at onset are associated with poor outcomes and a greater likelihood of developing chronic symptoms, as well (15,16,17,18,19,20). Therefore, once patients are able to centralize symptoms and their pain is well controlled, a lower limb flexibility and spinal mobility program should be initiated to restore functional ROM. Postural training and proper spine biomechanics should also be taught and awareness gradually improved during this period of decreased pain and improved ROM.

Core strengthening and lumbar stabilization programs are another key component of the therapeutic exercise program for lumbar radiculopathy. Patients who are likely to respond to specific stabilization programs have been identified by Hicks et al (21). These patients tend to be younger (<40 years old), have an average straight leg raise greater than 91 degrees, the presence of aberrant movements such as a painful arc or catch with their movement on ascending from flexion, positive prone instability test, and the presence of a level of fear avoidance beliefs. In addition, it has been demonstrated that a "specific exercise" treatment approach directed at the lumbar multifidus and deep abdominal stabilizers may be more effective in patients with chronically symptomatic spondylolysis or spondylolisthesis, who may or may not present with lower extremity pain, when compared to general strengthening and modalities (22). Therefore, neuromuscular reeducation exercises should be included to retrain the transverse abdominis and multifidus. With improved control of these muscles the patient can gradually progress from basic to advanced core strengthening exercises in a neutral spine posture. Please refer to the chapter on Lumbar Disc Pathology for further details.

Specialized Techniques

Mechanical diagnosis and therapy (MDT) is another specialized technique that has been shown to be an effective assessment method for determining if certain patients will respond to treating themselves with directionally specific exercises. Concepts such as centralization will help the clinician and patient determine if their radiculopathy will respond to mechanical treatment.

Centralization is defined as when "pain is progressively abolished in a distal to proximal direction with each progressive abolition being retained over time until all symptoms are abolished" (23).Movements in other directions or the opposite direction can potentially cause symptoms or mechanics to worsen, as well. Centralization of leg pain has been proven to be a predictor of good outcomes (20,24,25,26,27,28). Inability to centralize symptoms is the strongest predictor of chronicity compared to a range of psychological, clinical, and demographic factors (29). Other factors such as a significantly higher percentage of leg to back pain may have a high probability of harboring an extruded disc fragment (30).

Home Exercise Program

The patient's home exercise program (HEP) begins as soon as the therapist or treating clinician assesses the impact of posture on the patient's radicular symptoms. If correction of the posture causes symptoms to centralize or move proximally into the limb, the position should be strongly encouraged and maintained throughout the day and at all times with assistance of devices such as a lumbar roll. Patient education should focus on the critical concept of centralization and the idea that the pain may increase closer to the spine or proximally in the limb as the patient improves. Education should focus on the frequency of an exercise program that moves the pain proximally. Once a day may not be frequent enough to counteract act the day-to-day postures of the patient. Repeating the HEP six to eight times a day or every couple of hours may be required to keep a patient with a radiculopathy feeling good. Then as the therapeutic exercise program progresses to lower limb flexibility exercise and core strengthening, these exercises are slowly incorporated into the HEP.

SUMMARY

Lumbar radiculopathy is a very common problem and cause of disability in the United States. The onset of symptoms can be insidious or acute in nature and extremely painful and debilitating. Acute pain management and initiation of physical therapy are the key treatments in the initial phases of the rehabilitation process. Determining a directional preference with MDT will help decrease acute pain and medication usage, set up the foundation for the patient's therapy program, and ultimately improve overall functional outcomes. After obtaining centralization of symptoms, lower limb flexibility, spinal mobility, and core strengthening exercises may be included and advanced. As we all know, LBP can be recurrent in nature, therefore, patient education, teaching of a HEP, and implementation of proper spine biomechanics and ergonomics are good preventative measures the patient can use to manage their pain and hopefully prevent recurrent LBP.

SAMPLE CASE

A 35-year-old male with a significant medical history of depression presents with a LBP. He started having back pain about 2 years ago after a lifting incident from which he "was never the same." His symptoms have been intermittent until recently. About 45 days ago he started having daily back symptoms which progressed to radiating symptoms down his right leg. The patient was seen by his primary care provider and was sent for a lumbar spine MRI and found to have an L5/S1 HNP with nerve impingement of the right L5 nerve root. He was referred for a right L5/S1 transforaminal epidural steroid injection but experienced minimal symptomatic improvement. His review of systems was positive for numbness and tingling of the right leg but otherwise unremarkable. His examination was significant for an antalgic gait with a flexed and side bent posture to the right on a flexed right knee. The patient technically did not present with a lateral shift. He has normal muscle tone and muscle strength is 5/5 bilaterally, except for weakness in right EHL plantarflexors and ankle evertors 4/5. Sensation to light touch and pin prick are decreased in the L5 distribution on the right. Seated slump and straight leg raise tests are positive on the right. Muscle stretch reflexes are decreased at the medial hamstring on the right but otherwise normal. The patient was placed in a trial of sustained prone on elbows after his symptoms peripheralized in standing. His 9/10 pain changed to 3/10. Mechanically, his limited left side glide improved significantly based on static unloaded extension on elbows followed by repeated extension in prone lying after several minutes. Left side-lying, the only posture he noted as relieving on his intake and clinical interview, had no effect. Based on the fact that intermittent distal symptoms were present down to the calf of this patient, and dynamic end ROM initially worsened his symptoms, static movements became necessary to improve the patient's lumbar mechanics, functional mobility, and pain. This ability to locate a positive movement in a specific direction can often cause symptoms to decrease, abolish, or centralize and potentially create a favorable mechanical response in other directions. The patient was initially deemed to be a "nonresponder" by his neurosurgeon.

SAMPLE THERAPY PRESCRIPTION

Evaluate and Treat: Physical therapy.

Diagnosis: Right L5-S1 HNP with R L5 radiculopathy.

Problem list: Diminished L5 reflex, lower extremity weakness, severe pain rating, and clinical history of depression.

Precautions: Universal.

Frequency of visits: Per therapist discretion, 2 to 3x/week.

Duration of treatment: 6 to 8 sessions. Please call if centralization has not occurred in this time frame.

Treatment:

1. *Modalities:* Cryotherapy (ice pack) or thermotherapy (heat pack) prn, electrical stimulation for acute lumbar pain (attempts to use positioning and movement should precede modalities)

2. *Manual therapy:* Lumbar extension posterior to anterior (PA) glide after active care has plateaued. (No manipulation on this patient example)

3. *Therapeutic exercise:* Trunk ROM (self-stretching, therapist assisted stretching) including neural mobilization within patient tolerance, core strengthening/lower extremity strengthening including plantarflexor and evertor strengthening based on current weakness, balance/proprioceptive training for new radiculopathy, pain and patient education

4. *Specialized treatments:* Mechanical Diagnosis and Therapy (MDT)

5. *Patient education:* HEP (frequency and expectations), pain mechanism, posture and positioning for pain relief at home, and avoidance of aggravating factors

Short Term Goals:

▪ In 4 to 6 visits the patient will demonstrate centralization of lower extremity radicular symptoms to allow improvements in uninterrupted sleep

▪ In 4 to 6 visits the patient will sit uninterrupted 1 hour to allow him to commute to work

▪ In 4 to 6 visits, the patient will be able to walk 6 to 8 blocks to the train station, to his daughter's school, and resume regular walking of his dog

Long Term Goals (8–12 weeks):

▪ Patient will demonstrate independence in HEP and regular performance of reductive movements

▪ Patient will return to all activities of daily living (including exercise prescription) incorporating pain management strategies as needed

Reevaluation: In 4 weeks by referring physician, please call my office before then if centralization has not occurred within 6 to 8 visits.

REFERENCES

1. McKenzie R, May S. *The Lumbar Spine Mechanical Diagnosis and Therapy,* Vol 2. Waikanae, New Zealand: Spinal Publications; 2003:24–26.
2. May S, Littlewood C, Bishop A. Reliability of procedures used in the physical examination of non-specific low back pain: a systematic review. *Aust J Physiother.* 2006;52(2):91–102.
3. Andersson G. Epidemiology of low back pain. *Acta Orthop Scand Suppl.* 1998;281:28–31.
4. Luo X, Pietrobon R, Sun SX, et al. Estimates and patterns of direct health care expenditures among individuals with back pain in the United States. *Spine.* 2004;29(1):79–86.
5. Spitzer, Le Blanc F. Scientific approach to the assessment and management of activity-related spinal disorders (The Quebec Task Force). *Spine.* 1987;12(75):P516–521.
6. Audrey L, Donelson R, Fung T. Does it matter which exercise? A randomized control trial of exercise for low back pain. *Spine.* 2004;29(23):2593–2602.
7. Fritz JM, Delitto A, Erhard RE. Comparison of classification-based physical therapy with therapy based on clinical practice guidelines for patients with acute low back pain. A RCT. *Spine.* 2003;28:1363–1372.

8. Childs JD, Fritz JM, Piva SR, et al. Clinical decision making in the identification of patients likely to benefit from spinal manipulation: a traditional versus an evidence-based approach. *J Orthop Sports Phys Ther*. 2003;33(5):259–272.

9. Childs JD, Fritz JM, Piva SR, et al. Proposal of a classification system for patients with neck pain. *J Orthop Sports Phys Ther*. 2004;34(11):686–696.

10. Haldorsen EM, Grasdal AL, Skouen JS, et al. Is there a right treatment for a particular patient group? Comparison of ordinary treatment, light multidisciplinary treatment, and extensive multidisciplinary treatment for long-term sick-listed employees with musculoskeletal pain. *Pain*. 2002;95(1–2):49–63.

11. Roger C, Huffman LH. Medications for acute and chronic low back pain: A review of the evidence for an American Pain Society/American College of Physicians Clinical Practice Guideline. *Ann Intern Med*. 2007;147:505–514.

12. Wetzel FT, Donelson R. The role of repeated end-range/pain response assessment in the management of symptomatic lumbar discs. *Spine J*. 2003;3:146–154.

13. Kopp JR, Alexander AH, Turocy RH, Levrini MG, Lichtman DM. The use of lumbar extension in the evaluation and treatment of patients with acute herniated nucleus pulposus. *Clin Orthop Relat Res*. 1986;202:211–218.

14. Skytte L, May S, Petersen P. Centralization: Its prognostic value in patients with referred symptoms and sciatica *Spine*. 2005;30:E293-E299.

15. Goertz MN. Prognostic indicators for acute low-back pain. *Spine*. 1990;15(12):1307–1310.

16. Lanier DC, Stockton P. Clinical predictors of outcome of acute episodes of low back pain. *J Fam Pract*. 1988;27(5):483–489.

17. Chavannes AW, Gubbels J, Post D, et al. Acute low back pain: patients' perceptions of pain four weeks after initial diagnosis and treatment in general practice. *J R Coll Gen Pract*. 1986;36(287):271–273.

18. Cherkin DC, Deyo RA, Street JH, Barlow W. Predicting poor outcomes for back pain seen in primary care using patients' own criteria. *Spine*. 1996;21(24):2900–2907.

19. Carey TS, Garrett JM, Jackman AM. Beyond the good prognosis. Examination of an inception cohort of patients with chronic low back pain *Spine*. 2000;25(1):115–120.

20. Werneke M, Hart DL. Centralization phenomenon as a prognostic factor for chronic low back pain and disability. *Spine*. 2001;26(7):758–765.

21. Hicks GE, Fritz JM, Delitto A, et al. Preliminary development of a clinical prediction rule for determining which patients with low back pain will respond to a stabilization exercise program. *Arch Phys Med Rehabil*. 2005;86(9):1753–1762.

22. O'Sullivan PB, Twomey LT, Allison GT. Evaluation of specific stabilizing exercise in the treatment of chronic low back pain with radiologic diagnosis of spondylolysis or spondylolisthesis. *Spine*. 1997;22(24):2959–2967.

23. McKenzie RA, May S. The intervertebral disc: the centralization phenomenon. In: McKenzie RA, ed. *The Lumbar Spine: Mechanical Diagnosis and Therapy*. Waikanae, New Zealand: Spinal Publications, 1981:22.

24. Donelson R, Silva G, Murphy K. Centralization phenomenon. Its usefulness in evaluating and treating referred pain. *Spine*. 1990;15(3):211–213.

25. Sufka A, Hauger B, Trenary M, et al. Centralization of low back pain and perceived functional outcome. *J Orthop Sports Phys Ther*. 1998;27(3):205–212.

26. Long A. The centralization phenomenon: its usefulness as a predictor of outcome in conservative treatment of chronic low back pain. *Spine*. 1995;20(23):2513–2521.

27. Werneke M, Hart DL, Cook D. A descriptive study of the centralization phenomenon, a prospective analysis. *Spine*. 1999;24(7):676–683.

28. Karas R, McIntosh G, Hall H, Wilson L, Melles T. The relationship between nonorganic signs and centralization of symptoms in the prediction of return to work for patients with low back pain *Phys Ther*. 1997;77:354–360.

29. Werneke M, Hart D. Centralization phenomenon as a prognostic factor for chronic low back pain and disability. *Spine*. 2001;26:758–765.

30. Pople IK, Griffith HB. Prediction of an extruded fragment in lumbar disc patients from clinical presentations.*Spine*. 1994;19(2):156–158.

31. Yue JJ. *The Comprehensive Treatment of the Aging Spine: Minimally Invasive and Advanced Techniques*. Philadelphia, PA: Saunders/Elsevier, 2011.

Lumbar Spondylolysis and Spondylolisthesis

Kelly Scollon-Grieve, Jill May, and Larry H. Chou

INTRODUCTION

Lumbar spondylolysis is a common cause of axial low back pain (LBP) in children and adolescents. It is defined as a defect of the pars interarticularis of the lumbar vertebrae. It occurs most frequently at the L5 level, and the etiology can be either congenital or acquired. The most commonly recognized mechanism of acquired spondylolysis is repetitive hyperextension causing axial loading of the immature spine, especially in sports such as gymnastics and football (1,2). The overall incidence has been reported to be approximately 3% to 6% of the general population (2,3). It is the most common cause of persistent LBP in young athletes (4).

Spondylolisthesis, an anterior or posterior slippage of the superior vertebrae in relationship to the inferior vertebrae, has six etiologies: *Dysplastic*, which is a congenital abnormality of the zygapophyseal joint; *Isthmic*, the most common, occurs due to a defect in the bilateral pars interarticularis either from congenital incomplete fusion or acquired stress fractures; *Degenerative* occurs in the elderly population due to facet arthrosis causing subluxation; *Traumatic* occurs after an acute fracture in a surrounding structure; *Pathological* is caused by a medical condition that can lead to local bone disease; and *Postsurgical* spondylolisthesis can occur after extensive decompression resulting in instability (1,2). This chapter will focus on acquired spondylolysis and isthmic spondylolisthesis; conditions such as degenerative spondylolisthesis require knowledge of degenerative spine conditions (such as degenerative disc disease, facet arthrosis, and even spinal stenosis).

Patients with spondylolysis or spondylolisthesis often present with unilateral or bilateral LBP that is exacerbated by extension, standing, or lying prone or supine with the lower limbs extended and relieved with flexion, sitting, and resting. The onset may be gradual or acute. A patient may also have intermittent radicular symptoms caused by nerve root irritation from the unstable segment, secondary central or foraminal stenosis, or secondary intervertebral disc pathology.

Initial management should always include a detailed history and physical examination. *Key elements of the physical examination* include inspection, palpation, lumbar spine range of motion (ROM), assessment of flexibility, a single-leg hyperextension (stork) test, and assessment of motor strength, sensation, and reflexes. The physical examination of a patient with spondylolysis or spondylolisthesis may reveal a hyperlordotic posture, localized lumbar tenderness, hamstring tightness, and/or hip flexor tightness and pain with lumbar extension and/or the single-leg hyperextension test. Patients with spondylolisthesis may also have a palpable step-off on palpation of the spinous processes.

The first step in radiologic assessment of a suspected spondylolysis or spondylolisthesis are plain radiographs with antero-posterior, lateral, and oblique views to demonstrate the typical "broken neck of the Scottie dog" appearance of a pars interarticularis defect of the lumbar vertebrae. The lateral view is used to determine the presence of a slippage of the vertebra (spondylolisthesis) and flexion/extension views are utilized to rule out instability. If the diagnosis is not clear with plain radiographs, the next step would be bone scan with or without single-photon emission computed tomography (SPECT), CT, or MRI (1–4). MRI is gaining popularity as the imaging modality of choice in adolescent athletes since diagnostic accuracy is improved with special imaging sequences, which should include fat saturation sequences to identify bone marrow edema in acute stress reactions, while avoiding radiation exposure (5,6). While most patients respond well to conservative management, the use of a bone growth stimulator in recent years has shown promise, even in refractory cases (2). However, surgery may be indicated for patients who remain symptomatic for greater than 6 months, have high-grade spondylolisthesis, or demonstrate neurological deficits (7). Management also differs for spondylolysis without a slip versus spondylolysis with a low-grade spondylolisthesis. If the latter condition exists, especially in a skeletally immature individual with bilateral pars defects, then standing lateral radiographs should be used for surveillance and repeated within 6 to 12 months to rule out progression to a high-grade spondylolisthesis (8).

THE REHABILITATION PROGRAM

The first step in developing a treatment program for spondylolysis is deciding if the fracture is acute or chronic, which most of the time can be determined by a complete history and physical examination along with imaging studies to support or rule out clinical suspicion. In an acute fracture, the goal is to promote healing and avoid nonunion. The treatment recommendation for an acute fracture in an adolescent has been

LUMBAR SPONDYLOLYSIS AND SPONDYLOLISTHESIS

▦ Lumbar spondylolysis should be suspected in adolescent athletes with persistent axial LBP

▦ Spondylolysis is more common in sports with repetitive extension motions, such as gymnastics

▦ The isthmic type of spondylolisthesis is the most common etiology and occurs due to spondylolysis

▦ *Key elements of the physical examination* include inspection, palpation, lumbar spine ROM, assessment of muscle tightness, single-leg hyperextension test, and lower limb neurovascular examination

▦ Imaging studies, such as plain x-ray, SPECT, CT, or MRI, confirm the presence of spondylolysis or spondylolisthesis and may be used to determine the acuity of the injury, which further guides management

activity restriction with or without a spinal orthosis for a minimum of 3 months, although there have been no randomized controlled trials to support or disprove the required period of activity restriction with or without bracing (7). The utility of bracing remains controversial, as does the choice regarding the best type of spinal orthosis to use if bracing is chosen. If the fracture is chronic or present in an older adult, rest and bracing can be utilized for symptomatic relief. When the patient's pain is controlled, the rehabilitation program can be initiated. The typical rehabilitation phase is 2 to 4 months with an athlete returning to sport when they are asymptomatic (8).

Therapeutic Modalities

The use of therapeutic modalities can assist in relieving the pain associated with spondylolisthesis and spondylolysis. Transcutaneous electrical nerve stimulation (TENS) has been shown to be successful in the treatment of LBP through the gate control mechanism associated with sensory level stimulation (9,10). The use of hot or cold modalities has also been shown to be effective for temporary relief of LBP.

Manual Therapy

Studies have demonstrated manual therapy techniques for patients experiencing LBP to be as effective as other treatments. Soft tissue mobilization can assist in alleviating restrictions in the soft tissues around the area of injury and attention should be paid to joints above and below the injured area, such as the thoracic spine, pelvis, and hips. Manual techniques for the correction of pelvic or lumbar spine malalignments may include muscle energy techniques, joint mobilization, or strain-counterstrain techniques to name a few (11).

Therapeutic Exercise

Therapeutic exercise should focus on improving core control through dynamic lumbar stabilization, maintaining or enhancing flexibility of the lower limbs (especially the hamstrings and hip flexor muscles), and aerobic conditioning. In cases of acute spondylolysis, therapeutic exercise should only begin after adequate rest has taken place and symptoms have resolved, although low impact aerobics (e.g., aquatic exercise, cycling) may be utilized for athletes during the period of relative rest to prevent further deconditioning. In the case of acute spondyloly-sis, a lengthy rehabilitation program is required, with 3 months of rest and then at least 2 months of physical therapy before returning to sport (8).

Lumbar spinal extension and activities that increase pain should be avoided. One of the most important tech-niques to teach the patient is abdominal bracing, or the abdominal draw-in maneuver (12). The patient should be instructed to perform this in supine, in the hook lying posi-tion, and in quadruped. The patient should be instructed to draw the umbilicus toward the spine to contract the trans-verse abdominis muscle. Alternatively, abdominal brac-ing can also be obtained with slight abdominal protrusion and activation of the transverse abdominis. This has been shown to have increased stability of the lumbar spine in static positions (13). Cues for normal breathing and relax-ing the buttocks may be necessary to avoid over-recruiting the muscles of the hips, chest, and neck. Research has also demonstrated atrophy of the lumbar multifidus in patients with both acute and chronic LBP (14). The lumbar multifi-dus can be trained either in isolation or as a co-contraction with the transverse abdominis, and should be part of the neuromuscular reeducation component of the therapeu-tic exercise program. Once control over these muscles has been mastered, the therapist can gradually introduce dynamic core strengthening, which includes movement of the limbs to further challenge the dynamic core stability with progression to more sport-specific training in athletes. As progress is made, unstable surfaces should be utilized to further challenge the core muscles and proprioception.

Specialized Techniques

A detailed postural assessment should be conducted dur-ing the initial evaluation by the physical therapist and the patient should be viewed in both the sagittal and coronal planes. A detailed critique of the entire kinetic chain is essential, but with lumbar spine conditions, it is impor-tant to focus on the resting position of the pelvis. An ante-rior pelvic tilt can reveal tight hip flexors and elongated hamstrings, while a posterior pelvic tilt with a flat back posture can expose tight hamstrings. A postural assess-ment can help to guide your interventions for therapeutic exercise and manual therapy.

Training in posture and body mechanics is essential in the management of painful lumbar spine pathology. Patients should evaluate their work station for ergonomic

risk factors as outlined by the Occupational Safety and Health Administration. Patients should be instructed in the following techniques when lifting:

- Carry the load close to your body
- Do not twist your spine when moving objects between surfaces, turn your whole body instead
- Bend at your knees, not at your back
- Use the abdominal bracing technique described above

Supportive Devices

For an acute lumbar spondylolysis or an acute stress reac-tion of the posterior elements, rest and activity restriction is very important. If LBP persists with routine activities of daily living, then supportive devices such as an anti-lordotic lumbosacral orthoses should be considered (15), although lumbosacral corsets have also been utilized with success. As previously mentioned, the type of bracing and the duration of bracing, even the period of required activity restriction, remain controversial topics.

Home Exercise Program

The home exercise program (HEP) should begin at the initiation of the rehabilitation program. It should consist of dynamic lumbar stabilization and lower limb stretch-ing. Compliance to the HEP is essential to the overall suc-cess of physical therapy treatments.

SUMMARY

Lumbar spondylolysis and spondylolisthesis are common causes of LBP and the inability to participate in sporting activities. Treatment of these conditions depends on the acuity of the condition, the severity of symptoms, and radiographic findings and may include withdrawal from sports and lumbar spinal bracing. The rehabilitation program can be initiated once the symptoms are controlled and should include a HEP, progressive core stabilization exercises, aerobic conditioning, and stretching of tight lower limb and trunk muscle groups.

SAMPLE CASE

A 14-year-old previously healthy female volleyball player has had LBP with no radicular symptoms for 1 month, since the first game of the season. She has no significant past medical, social, or medication history. Review of systems is only positive for her complaint of LBP. X-rays of her lumbar spine with anterior–posterior (AP)/lateral and oblique views were negative. MRI was obtained after her pain continued for 2 more weeks and revealed a right L5 pars interarticularis fracture. Her examination was significant for hyperlordotic posture, tight hamstrings, pain worse with lumbar spinal extension, and no palpable step-off.

 SAMPLE THERAPY PRESCRIPTION

Discipline: Physical therapy.

Diagnosis: Right L5 pars interarticularis fracture (spondylolysis), hamstring tightness.

Precautions: Weight bearing as tolerated (WBAT), avoid lumbar hyperextension.

Frequency of visits: 2 to 3x/week.

Duration of treatment: 3 to 4 weeks; or an alternative would be to provide a total of 8 to 12 visits used at the therapist's discretion.

Treatment:

1. *Modalities:* TENS and ice or heat to lumbar spine

2. *Manual therapy:* Soft tissue mobilization to address restrictions in the soft tissues of thoraco-lumbar spine and even the hips and pelvis, manual techniques for the correction of pelvic or lumbar spine mal-alignments (muscle energy techniques, joint mobilization, strain-counterstrain)

3. *Therapeutic exercise:* stretching (focus on hamstrings and hip flexors), strengthening with progressive resistive exercise (PRE), aerobic and conditioning exercises, neuromuscular reeducation of the transverse abdominis and multifidus, progressive lumbar and core stabilization exercises, balance/proprioceptive training, and sport-specific training when appropriate

4. *Specialized treatments:* biomechanical analysis of kinetic chain, postural assessment

5. *Patient education:* HEP, back school

Goals: Decrease pain, restore ROM, flexibility, strength, improve core and lumbar stabilization, safely return to functional activities (e.g., sport, hobbies, work), prevent recurrence of LBP, independence with HEP.

Reevaluation: In 4 weeks by referring physician.

REFERENCES

1. Barr KP, Harrast MA. Low back pain. In: Braddom RL, Ed. *Physical Medicine and Rehabilitation*, 3rd ed. Philadelphia, PA: Saunders Elsevier; 2007:883–972.
2. McTimoney CA, Micheli LJ. Current evaluation and management of spondylolysis and spondylolisthesis. *Curr Sports Med Rep*. 2003;2(1):41–46.
3. Standaert CJ, Herring SA. How should you treat spondylolysis in the athlete? In: MacAuley D, Best TM, Eds. *Evidenced-Based Sports Medicine*, 2nd ed. Malden, MA: Blackwell; 2007:281–300.
4. Masci L, Pike J, Malara F, et al. Use of the one-legged hyperextension test and magnetic resonance imaging in the diagnosis of active spondylolysis. *Br J Sports Med*. 2006;40(11):940.
5. Sauryo K, Katoh S, Takata Y, et al: MRI signal changes in the pedicle as an indicator for early diagnosis of spondylolysis in children and adolescents; a clinical and biomechanical study. *Spine*. 2006;31:206–211.
6. Leone A, Cianfoni A, Cerase A, Magarelli N, Bonomo L. Lumbar spondylolysis: a review. *Skeletal Radiol*. 2011;40(6):683–700.
7. Tallarico RA, Madom IA, Palumbo MA. Spondylolysis and spondylolisthesis in the athlete. *Sports Med Arthrosc*. 2008;16(1):32–38.
8. Standaert CJ, Herring SA. Expert opinion and controversies in sports and musculoskeletal medicine: the diagnosis and treatment of spondylolysis in adolescent athletes. *Arch Phys Med Rehabil*. 2007;88(4):537–540.
9. Robinson AJ. Transcutaneous electrical nerve stimulation

for the control of pain in musculoskeletal disorders. *J Orthop Sports Phys Ther.* 1996;24(4):208–226.

10. Stasinopoulos D. Treatment of spondylolysis with external electrical stimulation in young athletes: a critical literature review. *Br J Sports Med.* 2004;38:352–354.

11. Rubinstein SM, van Middelkoop M, Assendelft WJ, et al. Spinal manipulative therapy for chronic low-back pain. *Cochrane Database Syst Rev.* 2011;16(2):CD008112.

12. Richardson C, Hides J, Hodges, PW. Principles of the "segmental stabilization" exercise model. In: Richardson C, Hides J, Hodges, PW, Eds. *Therapeutic Exercise for Lumbopelvic Stabilization: A Motor Control Approach for the Treatment and Prevention of Low Back Pain,* 2nd ed. Edinburgh, UK: Churchill Livingstone; 2004:175–183.

13. Grenier SG, McGill SM. Quantification of lumbar stability by using 2 different abdominal activation strategies. *Arch Phys Med Rehabil.* 2007;88(1):54–62.

14. O'Sullivan PB, Twomey LT, Allison GT. Evaluation of specific stabilizing exercise in the treatment of chronic low back pain with radiologic diagnosis of spondylolysis or spondylolisthesis. *Spine.* 1997;22(24):2959–2967.

15. Steiner ME, Micheli LJ. Treatment of symptomatic spondylolysis and spondylolisthesis with the modified Boston brace. *Spine.* 1985;10(10):937–943.

Lumbar Spinal Stenosis

Susan Garstang

INTRODUCTION

Lumbar spinal stenosis (LSS) is a common condition, with an annual incidence of five cases per 100,000 (1) The prevalence increases with age, and is reported to be between 1.7% to 8% in the general population (2). It is the most common diagnosis leading to spinal surgery in patients over 65 years of age; approximately 1 in a 1,000 people over the age of 65 have had a laminectomy for LSS, with an estimated cost of ~$1 billion (3). The term lumbar spinal stenosis refers to narrowing of the spinal canal either centrally, laterally, or of the neural foramina. This narrowing is associated with neural compression, and clinically most often manifests with low back pain (LBP) in combination with symptoms of neurogenic claudication or radiculopathy.

LSS can affect one level or multiple levels, and can be unilateral or bilateral. In addition, spinal stenosis can be central, lateral, or foraminal. The most common level affected by LSS is L4-5, followed by L3-4, L5-S1, and L1-2 (1). Central stenosis is due to compression of the neural sac by a combination of structural changes: facet joint arthrosis and hypertrophy, bulging of the thickened ligamentum flavum, spondylolisthesis, and bulging of the intervertebral disc. Compression of the nerves in the lateral recess or foramina are often due to many of the same factors, including facet joint hypertrophy, spondylolisthesis, bulging of the intervertebral disc, as well as loss of disc height. The anterior–posterior (AP) dimension of the spinal canal can be used to subdivide LSS into relative or absolute central stenosis (1). Relative central stenosis is present if the AP diameter is between 10 to 12 mm (normal is 22–25 mm). Absolute central stenosis is present if the AP diameter is <10 mm. The lateral recess can be considered stenotic if its diameter is <2 mm (normal 3–5 mm). No definite association between the degree of narrowing and clinical symptoms has been determined (2).

LSS can be classified by etiology as either primary or secondary. Primary etiologies can be congenital or developmental. Secondary or acquired etiologies can be degenerative (e.g., spondylolisthesis or ossification of the ligamentum flavum), metabolic/endocrine (e.g., epidural lipomatosis), infectious (e.g., discitis, epidural abscess), neoplastic, rheumatologic, or posttraumatic/ postoperative (1). Occasionally the etiology is considered mixed, due to the presence of congenital stenosis that is exacerbated by secondary conditions. The differential diagnosis of LSS includes other etiologies of low back and/or legs symptoms: vascular claudication, polyneuropathy, intraspinal synovial cysts, tethered cord or spina bifida, arthrosis of the hip or sacroiliac joint, abdominal aortic aneurysm, neoplasia, or inflammatory conditions (e.g., arachnoiditis).

The clinical manifestations of LSS are often due to dynamic changes in the lumbar spine, in addition to the structural changes described above. Extension of the lumbar spine causes bulging of the ligamentum flavum and posterior protrusion of the intervertebral disc (3). In a cadaveric study, the cross-sectional area of the neural foramen decreases by 15% in extension and increases by 12% in flexion; this is associated with nerve root compression of 21% in neutral, 15.4% in flexion, and 33.3% in extension (4). These changes can be worse in patients with underlying LSS; the decrease in dural AP diameter during spinal extension goes from 9% in normals to 67% in those with LSS (5).

Classically, patients with LSS often present with LBP which can radiate into the gluteal region, groin, and legs; this is often associated with radicular pain from neural compression in the foramina and/or lateral recesses, as well as neurogenic claudication. Neurogenic claudication is a clinical syndrome characterized by pain, paresthesias, or cramping in one or both legs, brought on while walking and relieved with forward flexion or sitting. There is often little correlation between the severity of the LSS and the presenting symptoms. Approximately 90% of patients with LSS report either unilateral or bilateral leg pain. Complaints of impaired balance, weakness, or sensory loss are less common. About 65% of patients with LSS present with neurogenic claudication. Symptoms of cauda equina syndrome, while worrisome, are quite rare. Sphincter involvement in LSS is rare, as the sacral nerves are in the center of the cauda equina and thus relatively protected from compression. Thus, bowel or bladder dysfunction, especially with upper motor neuron signs, is more likely to be due to cervical or thoracic myelopathy (1). Most of the symptoms associated with LSS are position-dependent, with worsening of symptoms associated with extension or weight-bearing (axial loading) (3).

Key elements of the physical examination include determining postural and biomechanical contributions to the symptoms of LSS. Physical examination should include inspection; palpation; neurological examination with focus on abdominals, gluteal muscles, and hamstring strength; and assessment of pelvic position, along with assessment of flexibility of both one-joint and two-joint muscles (e.g., hip flexors and hamstrings). Patients often have tight hip flexors, both the iliopsoas and rectus femoris, which serve to rotate the pelvis anteriorly (3). Anterior pelvic tilt, defined as when a vertical plane through the anterosuperior iliac spines is anterior to a vertical plane through the symphysis pubis, is associated with excessive extension of lumbar spine. In addition, lengthened and weakened gluteal muscles and hamstrings lead to early recruitment of lumbar extensors, as well as increased lumbar extension. Finally, lumbar extension can be due to weakened abdominal muscles, also leading to anterior pelvic tilt. Note that in spinal stenosis the focus on hamstring assessment is more for over-lengthening and weakness than for shortening, as longer hamstrings put the pelvis in an anterior position and thus worsen lumbar lordosis. This principle must be remembered when designing a therapy program, to avoid overstretching of the hamstrings (3). The most common abnormal physical examination finding in LSS, in concert with the above findings, is decreased lumbar extension, which may be painful. Decreased or absent ankle reflexes, sensory deficits, or positive straight leg raise are found in about 50% of patients, with weakness present in 23% to 51% of patients (3).

Imaging is typically used in more symptomatic cases, when interventional procedures or surgical treatment is being considered. The purpose of imaging is to confirm the presence or absence of LSS, exclude other conditions in the differential diagnosis, and identify the most affected levels for intervention. MRI is the preferred imaging modality for LSS, as it provides improved soft-tissue contrast with no ionizing radiation. However, there is no clear evidence that the findings on MRI examination add useful information regarding prognosis or outcome of surgery, when compared to clinical findings alone. The presence and severity of stenosis on MRI also does not correlate to patients' clinical status (6), however, electrodiagnostic studies have been shown to be more predictive of symptomatic versus asymptomatic LSS than MRI (7).

Prognosis in patients with LSS is not that of continuous decline. Many patients remain functionally or symptomatically unchanged over time. In a study of conservative treatment in 32 patients over 4 years, 70% of patients were symptomatically unchanged, 15% were improved, and 15% were worse. Walking capacity improved in 37% of patients, remained unchanged in 33%, and worsened in 30% (8). Other studies have shown that 15% to 43% of patients will have improvement for 1 to 5 years when treated nonoperatively (9). Studies of surgical treatments show some benefit, but are difficult to interpret as treatment groups are often stratified based on the severity of LSS. A study of 100 patients with LSS was performed, where patients with severe symptoms were selected for surgery and those with moderate symptoms for conservative treatment (10). After 4 years, half of the conservative treatment group had excellent or fair results, as compared to 80% of the surgical treatment group. Patients who did not improve with conservative treatment were offered surgery; in this group the results of surgical treatment when delayed were no different than the initial surgical treatment group outcomes (10). Complication rates overall from surgery range from 14% to 35%, and the 10-year reoperation rate is between 10% to 23% (1). Thus, despite favorable surgical outcomes in some patients, the risks are also significant and thus a trial of conservative treatment for 3 to 6 months is warranted prior to surgical referral in most cases.

LUMBAR SPINAL STENOSIS

▪ Prevalence of up to 8% in patients over 65 years of age

▪ Classically presents with LBP and neurogenic claudication

▪ Key elements of the physical examination include inspection, palpation, neurological examination, and testing for flexibility and pelvic position

▪ Imaging should be used to confirm the diagnosis, rule out more serious conditions, and to plan further medical management (e.g., interventional spine procedures), but is not required before starting a rehabilitation program

▪ Natural history is not that of progression, but rather stabilization in many cases

▪ Despite favorable surgical outcomes in some patients, the risks are also significant and thus a trial of conservative treatment for 3 to 6 months is warranted prior to surgical referral in most cases

THE REHABILITATION PROGRAM

A variety of different treatments are commonly utilized to treat the symptoms of LSS, despite a lack of significant evidence supporting one approach over another. Treatment techniques include manual therapy, physical therapy exercises, traction, anti-lordotic spinal orthotics, behavioral therapy, and acupuncture. Pharmacologic treatments are also helpful for pain management, and may include oral medications as well as those delivered by epidural injection. Studies have shown that imaging findings correlate poorly with clinical symptoms, thus clinical presentation should be the guide to treatment planning (9).

Empirically, exercise programs favoring flexion are used, because of data showing an increase in canal size and a decrease in epidural pressure with spinal flexion. It is important to differentiate LBP from radicular leg pain and neurogenic claudication when formulating the rehabilitation program. In addition, exacerbating and alleviating factors should be elicited, to guide treatment planning.

Psychosocial factors which may affect outcomes are also important to consider, and should be assessed. General treatment should focus on muscular weakness, postural and flexibility deficits, and also address concomitant coexisting problems such as myofascial pain, as well as restrictions at joints from conditions such as hip or knee osteoarthritis.

The rehabilitation program can be divided into three phases: pain control, stabilization, and then conditioning (see Table 46.1) (9). Pain control may be achieved with oral or injectable medications such as nonsteroidal anti-inflammatory drugs (NSAIDs), oral methylprednisolone, or epidural steroids. Depending on the duration of the pain, other oral medications that modulate pain, such as tricycle antidepressants and anticonvulsants, may be useful adjuvants to treatment. Passive modalities to help with pain control and tolerance of therapy may be useful initially, including heat, ultrasound, and soft tissue mobilization. Behavior modification and education should be part of all treatments. Once pain is under control, exercise may begin with a goal of improving lumbopelvic muscular stabilization and control over proper pelvic positioning. Exercising in a neutral to flexed position, which increases the AP canal diameter (e.g., inclined treadmill or stationary bicycle) can improve cardiovascular conditioning while avoiding symptom provocation. For some patients, aquatic therapy is an excellent option and may allow for more comfortable form of cardiovascular conditioning.

Therapeutic Modalities

The use of therapeutic modalities in LSS is primarily to achieve pain relief as part of an overall management plan, and to allow patients to perform their therapeutic exercises. The literature does not contain evidence for the use of modalities in LSS, partly because studies tend to focus on LBP as

---

TABLE 46.1: Phases of Rehabilitation for Lumbar Spinal Stenosis

- Phase I: Pain control

- Phase II: Lumbopelvic stabilization and improved pelvic position

- Phase III: Conditioning

- Behavior modification and education may be included throughout the rehabilitation program.

a broad diagnostic category, and mostly look at acute or sub-acute LBP (defined as <2 months duration). There is moderate evidence in a small number of trials that heat wrap therapy provides a small, short-term reduction in pain and disability in patients with acute or sub-acute LBP. There is no convincing evidence in any studies to support the use of cryotherapy for LBP, and there is conflicting evidence to determine the differences between heat and cold for LBP (11), although many patients subjectively report that cryotherapy (e.g., gel ice pack) helps alleviate acute exacerbations of LBP. Thus, patients with LSS should be instructed to use heat if they feel that it provides symptomatic or functional benefits only.

The use of transcutaneous electrical nerve stimulation (TENS) has been studied in chronic LBP, again without specific analysis of whether patients with LSS might benefit. After 1 month of use, no significant effect of TENS was found for pain or activity level, as compared to exercises which significantly reduced both the intensity and frequency of pain, and improved activity levels (12). (Note that the beneficial effects of exercises were not sustained past 2 months, when most patients discontinued the exercises.) Thus, while TENS can be trialed in patients with LSS, and may help some individuals, the benefits should not be expected to be substantial.

The other class of therapeutic modality that has been studied in chronic LBP is spa therapy, which includes submersion in heated water without an active exercise component, unlike aquatic therapy. Note that some studies of spa therapy include balneotherapy as a type of spa therapy, which utilizes the beneficial effects of medicinal water, such as bath salts. An analysis of five randomized clinical trials of spa therapy in chronic LBP (when compared to control group with no intervention) showed significant reduction in pain scales (18–26 points on visual analogue scale) (13). Again, the generalizability of these results is difficult to judge as the cause of the LBP was not specified, and may not include significant numbers of patients with LSS. Thus, like heat modalities, this type of treatment may serve as a useful adjunct for pain control in patients who wish to participate.

Manual Therapy

Manual therapy for LBP includes spinal manipulation and spinal mobilization techniques; often these two techniques are combined both clinically and in the literature. The literature has a variety of studies of these techniques in patients with acute and chronic LBP. However, no studies specifically look at these treatments in patients with LSS. A Cochrane review of spinal manipulative therapy for LBP revealed that there was no statistically or clinically significant advantage

over general practitioner care, analgesics, physical therapy, exercises, or back school (14). Radiation of pain, study quality, profession of manipulator, and use of manipulation alone or in combination with other therapies did not affect these results. A trial of manual therapy may be still be warranted, especially in patients who have tried other therapeutic options with limited success. As mentioned in other chapters, well designed randomized controlled trials on spinal manipulation in this specific population would further clarify the proper role of spinal manipulative therapy in LSS.

Massage has also been evaluated as a monotherapy technique for subacute and chronic LBP, with inconclusive outcomes (15). Some studies show beneficial effects of massage, especially short term for pain and function (16). The type and amount of massage therapy needed, and duration of benefit is not clear; nor is the generalizability of this literature to patients with LSS. Thus, massage in combination with therapeutic exercise and patient education, as part of an overall management plan, may be beneficial.

Therapeutic Exercise

Unfortunately, the evidence basis for the treatment of LSS with therapeutic exercise is poor. The NASS guideline from 2008 states that there is insufficient evidence to support the effectiveness of physical therapy for LSS (17). However, this gap in the literature is in part due to the paucity of studies on rehabilitation for LSS, rather than a clear lack of effect of interventions. Thus, the treatment of LSS with therapeutic exercise is based on some small studies which show efficacy, and an understanding of biomechanical principles which may contribute to worsened pain with impaired function.

It is known that the diameter of the spinal canal lessens with extension and increases with flexion, thus a flexion-based program for the lumbar spine is often recommended, with avoidance of lumbar hyperextension. In a study of patients with LSS and neurogenic claudication, treating physical therapists reported in a survey that their preferred treatment plan included flexion-based exercises (82%), trunk muscle stabilizing exercises (70%), and general fitness exercises (58%) (18). Williams' flexion-biased exercises target and attempt to correct increased lumbar lordosis, paraspinal and hamstring inflexibility, and abdominal muscle weakness. These exercises incorporate single and double knee-to-chest maneuvers (Figure 46.1), hamstring and hip flexor stretches (Figures 46.2a and 46.2b), stretches for the trunk and paraspinal muscles (Figure 46.3), pelvic tilts (Figures 46.4a and 46.4b), partial sit-ups, bridges in a neutral spine posture (Figure 46.5), and squats. Lumbar stabilizing exercises are usually performed in a neutral spine position, or even with a flexion bias to control symptoms of LSS while progressing with these therapeutic exercises. Positional therapy is a technique using a wheeled walker to promote lumbar flexion with gait; this method has been shown in a case series (*n* = 52) to improve ambulation and reduce neuropathic pain (19). Anecdotally, for those patients who do not desire a wheeled walker, trialing bilateral walking sticks may also provide some benefits for functional ambulation.

Use of a treadmill for ambulation training, as part of the therapeutic program for patients with LSS, has been shown to be helpful in several studies. Traction harness-supported treadmill and aquatic ambulation to reduce compressive spine loading have been shown to improve lumbar range

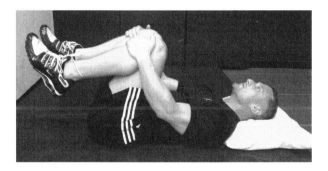

FIGURE 46.1: Double knee to chest stretch.

of motion (ROM), straight leg raising, gluteal and quadriceps femoris muscle force production, and maximal (up to 15 minutes) walking time (20). In a study comparing patients doing manual therapy, exercises, and body-weight supported treadmill walking to patients doing flexion exercises and treadmill walking, more patients in the former group recovered at 6 weeks compared with the latter group. These gains were maintained at 1 year by 62% of the manual therapy, exercise, and walking group (body weight supported) and 41% of the flexion exercise and walking group (21). Because both groups had multiple interventions, it is difficult to generalize from this study. Another study with 68 patients with LSS performed either treadmill with body weight support or cycling, twice weekly for 6 weeks. Both groups also received an exercise program consisting of heat, lumbar traction, and flexion exercises. No significant difference between the groups was found in terms of pain or disability (22).

Because of the ability to alter amount of spinal flexion with walking on a treadmill, a two-stage treadmill test can be used to assess patients with LSS. This test uses a treadmill to control walking posture, and assist in the diagnosis of LSS (23). It also has utility as an outcome measure to assess progress with therapy, specifically ambulation distance and speed. Unloading using a traction harness can also be part of the treatment of LSS; it allows for decompression of the spine, which increases spinal diameter and unloads structures such as the discs

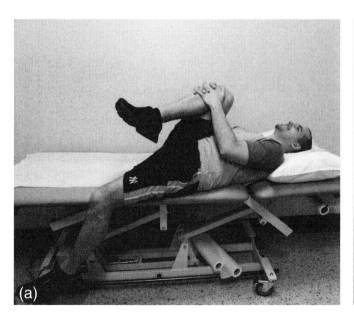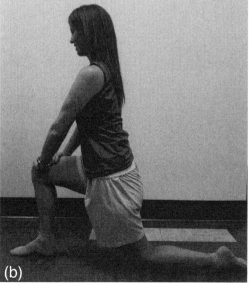

FIGURE 46.2: (a) Hip flexor stretch in supine position using gravity to assist ; (b) half-kneel position for more aggressive stretching of the hip flexors (a chair or table can be placed in front of the patient, the patient can rest their hands on this item instead of their knee and this can further assist with balance).

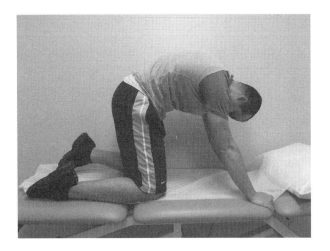

FIGURE 46.3: Angry cat stretch.

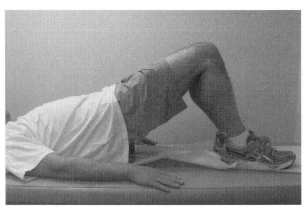

FIGURE 46.5: Bridge.

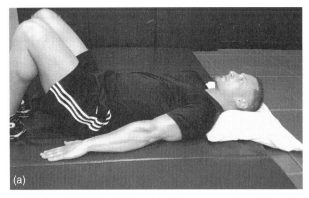

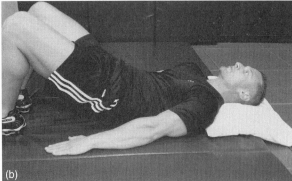

FIGURE 46.4: Pelvic tilts in the starting (a) and finishing position (b).

and facet joints. Note that pool therapy for initial ambulation may also be used for its offloading effects (23). For patients who can't tolerate treadmill walking and don't have access to a pool, cycling on a traditional stationary or recumbent bicycle may be an excellent initial alternative for cardiovascular conditioning.

Specialized Techniques

Studies have also looked to see if determining a "directional preference" in patients with LBP can be used to guide treatment (24). A directional preference is an immediate, lasting improvement in pain that results from performing repeated lumbar flexion, extension, or side-gliding/rotation tests. When directionally based treatment was used in patients with a directional preference (74% of 312 patients), this led to significant improvement in all outcomes including a rapid decrease in pain and medication use, but when the exercises given are "opposite" to directional preference (DP) or "nondirectional," then 1/3 of patients dropped out in 2 weeks (no matched subjects withdrew) (24). Note that these studies were not specific for patients with spinal stenosis, but these techniques can be used in those with LBP only and with sciatica, with exercises specifically used to decrease or eliminate lumbar midline pain, or cause referred pain to centralize (or retreat in a proximal direction).

The use of acupuncture as a therapeutic modality is gaining in popularity, yet the evidence base for its effectiveness is lagging behind. A recent review of studies on the efficacy of acupuncture in both acute and chronic LBP was performed, but the utility of acupuncture in patients with LSS was not specifically studied. The results of this analysis were that there was no evidence showing acupuncture to be more effective than no treatment. There was moderate evidence indicating that acupuncture is not more effective than trigger-point injection or TENS, and there was limited evidence that acupuncture is not more effective than placebo or sham acupuncture for the management of chronic LBP (25). Given the lack of efficacy in a chronic LBP population, and no way to know if these treatments are specifically useful for patients with LSS, recommendations for patients to pursue acupuncture should be limited.

Home Exercise Program

Patient adherence to a home exercise program (HEP) is an important way to help them get relief with the initial rehabilitation program, as well as to maintain improvements made in treatment over the long term. Patient education regarding the postural etiologies underlying symptoms in LSS should be the first element to teach. This allows the patient to immediately begin altering their gait, maybe by using a walker or walking sticks, or by stopping to rest and flexing the spine for symptomatic relief. Reinforcing the role of posture and the pelvic tilt, and giving exercises to do at home to work on lumbar stabilization and pelvic position will allow the patient to continue to improve their strength, function, and hopefully reduce pain. Finally, patients can be discharged from therapy with a set of exercises designed to stretch chronically tight muscles and strengthen weak or over-lengthened muscles, while observing improved posture and pelvic position throughout their daily tasks. The HEP can also encourage continuation of conditioning and endurance activities.

SUMMARY

LSS is a common condition, with an increasing prevalence as the population ages. Patients often present with LBP and leg pain, which may be radicular or neurogenic claudication. The symptoms of this condition are worsened with lumbar extension, thus assessment should focus on posture and pelvic position, core and lower limb strength, and flexibility. The rehabilitation program then focuses on improving mobility, and lumbopelvic stability and improving posture by correcting biomechanical factors (e.g., muscular imbalances across the pelvis) to reduce pain and improve function. Despite there being no change (or even a slow progression) with the anatomic causes underlying this condition, the course of symptoms is variable and does not correlate with imaging findings. Many patients remain stable over long periods or even improve.

SAMPLE CASE

Mrs. Jones is a 71-year-old woman with a 6 year history of progressive LBP. Her pain is located across the low back and radiates into her buttocks. She has worsening of her pain when upright, and notes that walking makes her back pain worse unless she bends forward over a shopping cart. Her legs also start to cramp and tingle, and then feel numb after she walks for a few minutes; if she leans forward or sits these sensations are relieved quickly. She denies bowel or bladder incontinence. On examination, she has an anterior pelvic tilt, limited active lumbar extension, tight hip flexors, and weak abdominals and hip extensors. Her neurological exam is normal except absent Achilles reflexes. MRI obtained at her request reveals an AP lumbar spinal canal dimension of 9 mm.

 ### SAMPLE THERAPY PRESCRIPTION

Discipline: Physical therapy.

Diagnosis: Lumbar spinal stenosis.

Problem list: Poor flexibility of the hip flexors, weak core, and poor posture (anterior pelvic tilt).

Precautions: Fall, universal. Avoid spinal extension exercises.

Frequency of visits: 2 to 3x/week.

Duration of treatment: 3 to 4 weeks.

Treatment:

1. *Modalities:* topical heat to low back and to tight muscles for 5 to 10 minutes to facilitate stretching

2. *Manual therapy:* may consider a trial of spinal mobilization/manipulation, or massage to the lumbar spine

3. *Therapeutic exercise:*

   a. *Stretching exercises:* hip flexor stretching, supine with single and double knee to chest (William's flexion exercises); hamstring stretching, supine or seated;

lumbosacral paraspinal stretching, supine and seated; and quadruped spinal flexion (angry cat stretch).

b. *Strengthening exercises:* abdominal and gluteal strengthening, recommend including pelvic tilts, bridges with neutral spine, progressive lumbopelvic stabilization exercises, mini-squats, hip abduction/extension in standing, single leg standing, lateral step-ups.

c. *Conditioning exercises:* inclined treadmill, stationary bicycle

d. *Other:* postural exercises to maintain posterior pelvic tilt in various functional positions

4. *Specialized treatments:* aquatic exercises if available and if patient is unable to tolerate land-based exercises. Trial of assistive devices (e.g., rolling walker, walking sticks) to assess for improvements in gait and walking tolerance.

5. *Patient Education:* HEP, teach proper posture and body mechanics (3).

Goals: Reduce pain, improve posture and flexibility, and improve walking distance.

Follow-up: 4 weeks with physicia n.

REFERENCES

1. Siebert E, Pruss H, Klingebiel R, Failli V, Einhaupl KM, Schwab JM. Lumbar spinal stenosis: syndrome, diagnostics and treatment. *Nat Rev Neurosci.* 2009;5(7):392–403.

2. Amundsen T, Weber H, Lilleas F, Nordal HJ, Abdelnoor M, Magnaes B. Lumbar spinal stenosis. Clinical and radiologic features. *Spine.* 1995;20(10):1178–1186.

3. Bodack MP, Monteiro M. Therapeutic exercise in the treatment of patients with lumbar spinal stenosis. *Clin Orthop Relat Res.* 2001;384:144–152.

4. Inufusa A, An HS, Lim TH, Hasegawa T, Haughton VM, Nowicki BH. Anatomic changes of the spinal canal and intervertebral foramen associated with flexion-extension movement. *Spine.* 1996;21(21):2412–2420.

5. Sortland O, Magnaes B, Hauge T. Functional myelography with metrizamide in the diagnosis of lumbar spinal stenosis. *Acta Radiol. Suppl.* 1977;355:42–54.

6. Geisser M, Haig A, Tong HC, et al. Spinal canal size and clinical symptoms among persons diagnosed with lumbar spinal stenosis. *Clin J Pain.* 2007;23(9):780–785.

7. Haig A, Geisser M, Tong HC, et al. Electromyographic and magnetic resonance imaging to predict lumbar stenosis, low-back pain, and no back symptoms. *J Bone Joint Surg Am.* 2007;89:358–366.

8. Johnsson KE, Rosen I, Uden A. The natural course of lumbar spinal stenosis. *Clin Orthop Relat Res.* 1992;279:82–86.

9. Simotas AC. Nonoperative treatment for lumbar spinal stenosis. *Clin Orthop Relat Res.* 2001;384:153–161.

10. Amundsen T, Weber H, Nordal HJ, Magnaes B, Abdelnoor M, Lilleas F. Lumbar spinal stenosis: conservative or surgical management?: A prospective 10-year study. *Spine.* 1 2000;25(11):1424–1435; discussion 1435–1426.

11. French S, Cameron M, Walker B, Reggars J, Esterman A. Superficial heat or cold for low back pain. *Cochrane Database Syst Rev.* 2006;1:CD004750.

12. Deyo RA, Walsh NE, Martin DC, Schoenfeld LS, Ramamurthy S. A controlled trial of transcutaneous electrical nerve stimulation (TENS) and exercise for chronic low back pain. *N Engl J Med.* 1990;322(23):1627–1634.

13. Pittler M, Karagülle M, Karagülle M, Ernst E. Spa therapy and balneotherapy for treating low back pain: meta-analysis of randomized trials. *Rheumatology.* 2006;45(7):880.

14. Assendelft W, Morton S, Yu E, Suttorp M, Shekelle P. Spinal manipulative therapy for low back pain. *Cochrane Database Syst Rev.* 2004;1.

15. Ernst E. Massage therapy for low back pain: a systematic review. *J Pain Symptom Manage.* 1999;17(1):65–69.

16. Furlan A, Imamura M, Dryden T, Irvin E. Massage for low-back pain. *Cochrane Database Syst Rev.* 2008;4:CD001929.

17. Watters III WC, Baisden J, Gilbert TJ, et al. Degenerative lumbar spinal stenosis: an evidence-based clinical guideline for the diagnosis and treatment of degenerative lumbar spinal stenosis. *Spine J.* 2008;8(2):305–310.

18. Comer CM, Redmond AC, Bird HA, Conaghan PG. Assessment and management of neurogenic claudication associated with lumbar spinal stenosis in a UK primary care musculoskeletal service: a survey of current practice among physiotherapists. *BMC Musculoskel Disord.* 2009;10:121.

19. Goldman SM, Barice EJ, Schneider WR, Hennekens CH. Lumbar spinal stenosis: can positional therapy alleviate pain? *J Fam Pract.* 2008;57(4):257–260.

20. Wallbom AS, Geisser ME, Haig AJ, Koch J, Guido C. Alterations of F wave parameters after exercise in symptomatic lumbar spinal stenosis. *American Journal Of Physical Medicine & Rehabilitation/Association Of Academic Physiatrists.* 2008;87(4):270–274.

21. Whitman JM, Flynn TW, Childs JD, et al. A comparison between two physical therapy treatment programs for patients with lumbar spinal stenosis: a randomized clinical trial. *Spine.* 2006;31(22):2541–2549.

22. Pua Y, Cai C, Lim K. Treadmill walking with body weight support is no more effective than cycling when added to an exercise program for lumbar spinal stenosis: a randomised controlled trial. *Aust J Physiother.* 2007;53(2):83.

23. Fritz JM, Erhard RE, Vignovic M. A nonsurgical treatment approach for patients with lumbar spinal stenosis. *Phys Ther.* 1997;77(9):962–973.

24. Long A, Donelson R, Fung T. Does it matter which exercise? A randomized control trial of exercise for low back pain. *Spine.* 2004;29(23):2593–2602.

25. van Tulder MW, Cherkin DC, Berman B, Lao L, Koes BW. The effectiveness of acupuncture in the management of acute and chronic low back pain: a systematic review within the framework of the Cochrane Collaboration Back Review Group. *Spine.* 1999;24(11):1113.

Other Lumbar Spine Disorders

Mirielle Diaz, Suzanne Gutiérrez Teissonniere, and Marcello Sarrica

INTRODUCTION

There are many other important conditions to consider when a patient complains of low back pain (LBP), including myofascial pain syndrome, nonspecific chronic low back pain (CLBP), and failed back surgery syndrome. The rehabilitation program for chronic, long-standing LBP should be focused on a multidisciplinary approach, often requiring physical, pharmacologic, and psychotherapy. The program should be individualized for each patient.

MYOFASCIAL PAIN SYNDROME

Myofascial pain syndrome has been defined by the International Association for the Study of Pain (IASP) as a regional painful condition associated with the presence of trigger points. Myofascial trigger points are loci of hyperirritability, which when subjected to mechanical pressure, give rise to characteristic patterns of referred pain (1,2). Trigger points have both a sensory and a motor component. Clinical characteristics of a trigger point includes circumscribed point tenderness of a hard nodule that is part of a palpably tense taut band of muscle fibers, patient recognition of the pain that is evoked by pressure on the tender spot as being familiar, pain referred in the pattern characteristic of the trigger points in that muscle, a local twitch response or "jump" sign, painful limitation of stretch range of motion (ROM), and weakness of that muscle (3,4). Often multiple muscles are involved. The terms trigger points and tender points are often incorrectly used interchangeably. A tender point is a widespread, nonspecific, soft tissue pain often associated with fibromyalgia, as compared to a trigger point which is a localized area within a taut band of skeletal muscle which has a characteristic nodular texture and upon palpation generates a twitch response or referral pattern as seen in myofascial pain syndrome (5). Trigger

points can be active or latent. An active trigger point is associated with spontaneous pain present without palpation, either at the site of the myofascial trigger point or remote from it. Palpation increases pain locally and usually reproduces the subject's remote pain. A latent trigger point is not associated with spontaneous pain, although pain can often be elicited in an asymptomatic subject by a mechanical stimulus.

The exact mechanism of myofascial trigger points is still unclear. They can develop after trauma, overuse, or prolonged spasm of muscles. The "energy crisis" hypothesis states that overload of the muscle causes increase of calcium release, which stimulates prolonged contractility and increased metabolic activity causing localized ischemia. Another hypothesis states that prolonged nociceptive input from muscles can produce central nervous system sensitization (6). The motor component is attributable to dysfunctional endplates, which are responsible for taut band formation as a result of excessive acetylcholine. Excessive acetylcholine release, sarcomere shortening, and release of sensitizing substances are three essential features that seem to relate to one another in a positive feedback cycle.

History should include the characteristics of pain (pain drawing can be very helpful), initiating event, and aggravating/alleviating factors. Pain is usually worse with activity and stretching, muscle overload (eccentric more than concentric), stress, and temperature changes; pain is often described by the patient as "stiffness." Evaluation should include assessment for sleep and/or psychological disturbances.

Key elements of the physical examination include evaluation of posture (symmetry, stance, and scoliosis), palpation, ROM of the lumbar spine and restrictions due to pain, neurological examination, and palpation (flat or pincer palpation) of superficial and deep soft tissue looking for: tenderness, taut bands, twitch responses, and referral patterns. Neurologic examination may identify sensory or motor deficits associated with radiculopathy, which often coexists and can be the primary and undiagnosed condition (4,6,7).

The diagnosis is usually made with clinical findings and essentially is a diagnosis of exclusion. Studies like x-rays and MRIs are used to rule out other possible causes for symptoms. Electromyography of the trigger point can exhibit spontaneous electrical activity with endplate noise. Potential tools for diagnosis under study include measurement of biochemicals associated with pain and inflammation in the trigger point region, sonographic studies, magnetic resonance elastography for taut band imaging, and infrared thermography (7–9).

Many methods have been used to treat myofascial pain, including stretching, massage, ischemic compression, laser therapy, heat, ultrasound, transcutaneous electrical nerve stimulation (TENS), biofeedback, pharmacological treatments, trigger point injections with local anesthetic and/or steroid solutions, shockwave therapy, and botulinum toxin type A injection (9,10). In this chapter, we will focus on the rehabilitation, or non-interventional and nonpharmacologic component of treatment.

NONSPECIFIC CHRONIC LOW BACK PAIN

Nonspecific LBP is defined as pain not attributable to a specific, recognizable, known pathology. CLBP is a non-diagnostic term, often described as pain that has persisted for at least 3 months. The lifetime prevalence of LBP is reported to be as high as 84%, and the prevalence of CLBP is about 23%, with 12% of the population being disabled by LBP (11). CLBP may originate from traumatic injury or spine disease. An important risk factor for developing CLBP a previous history of LBP. Pain intensity is strongly associated with disability. "Yellow flags" have been described as psychosocial factors that act as barriers to recovery and increase the risk of developing or perpetuating pain and long-term disability. These include emotional problems, attitudes and beliefs about back pain, inappropriate pain behavior, and work-related problems or compensation issues. Factors such as depression, anxiety, emotional lability, and sleep disturbance have been associated with inactivity, work loss, and long-term disability (12).

History should include assessment for "red flags" like weight loss, previous history of cancer or spine disease, night pain, age more than 50 years, violent trauma, fever, saddle anesthesia, difficulty with micturition, intravenous drug use, progressive neurological disturbances, and use of systemic steroids to rule out serious disease (13). It is also necessary to inquire about psychosocial factors and employment status.

Key elements of the physical examination include ROM of the lumbar spine, palpation of the lumbar region to assess for areas of localized tenderness, manual muscle testing may or may not reveal weakness in a myotomal distribution, and assessment of sensation and deep tendon reflexes. The examination is often limited due to pain. Specialized tests are often used to rule out other spine conditions, including blood tests, X-rays, MRI, and electromyography. The most common functional outcome measures used for CLBP are the Oswestry Disability Index and the Roland Morris Disability Questionnaire, which have been validated with proven reliability. These tests are useful in assessing patients within the CLBP population. Most common pain outcome measures include the numeric pain rating scale and the Visual Analog Scale (14). Most guideline recommendations for management of CLBP include use of brief education about the problem, advice to stay active, nonsteroidal anti-inflammatory drugs, weak opioids (short-term use), exercise therapy, and spinal manipulation. Some patients may also benefit from cognitive behavioral therapy, acupuncture, multidisciplinary rehabilitation, and adjunctive or strong opioid analgesics (15). A helpful tip with this patient population is to focus on making functional progress as opposed to focusing on numeric pain scores, as the latter can lead to a frustrating relationship between patient and provider.

FAILED BACK SURGERY SYNDROME

Failed back surgery syndrome (FBSS) is defined as LBP persisting at the same location as the original pain despite operative interventions or with a post-surgery onset (1). A more functional definition states that FBSS results when the outcome of lumbar spinal surgery does not meet the presurgical expectations of the patient and surgeon (16). The incidence of patients who will develop FBSS following lumbar spinal surgery is in the range of 10% to 40%. Studies suggest that failure rate for microdiscectomy is less than that of spinal fusion. Classification for possible etiologies for FBSS includes preoperative, intraoperative and postoperative factors. Preoperative etiology might include psychological factors (anxiety, depression), worker's compensation case, revision surgery, candidate selection (e.g., microdiscectomy for axial pain), surgery selection (e.g., inadequate decompression in multilevel pathology). Intraoperative factors include poor technique, incorrect level of surgery, and inability to achieve the aim of surgery. Postoperative factors include progressive disease (e.g., recent disc herniation, spondylolisthesis), epidural fibrosis, surgical complications (e.g., nerve injury, infection, and hematoma), new spinal instability, and myofascial pain development (17).

History taking should include assessment of symptoms prior to surgery (including radicular symptoms), history of previous spine surgery, and history of psychiatric disorders and/or psychosocial factors. *Key elements of the physical examination* include inspection of posture, gait, surgical incision, ROM, and paravertebral muscle spasm. Also to be completed are palpation of localized points of tenderness and step-offs, soft tissue indentation along the midline of the spine caused by high-grade spondylolisthesis, manual muscle strength testing, and neurological examination. Physical examination should also include specialized tests, such as the seated and supine straight leg raise tests and dural tension tests. Imaging studies, such as MRI and CT scan/myelogram, are helpful in identifying recurrent disc herniation, fibrosis and infection. Nerve root blocks with local anesthetics or epidural steroid injections can relieve pain and serve as diagnostic tests to determine whether surgery will be of benefit and to identify the levels in the spine that require surgery. For patients with FBSS, an interdisciplinary care model for pain control is very important. The role of medications and conservative management should be within a model of care where the major aim is to facilitate an improvement in function and, when possible, a return to the patient's premorbid social role. Some patients will not improve with these measures, and may require interventional procedures. Nerve root blocks have been found to be effective in pain relief and have been included in the evidence-based practice guidelines for the management of chronic spinal pain (18). Other studies have suggested that spinal cord stimulators provide sustained, long-term pain reduction. The rate of pain relief using spinal cord stimulator in FBSS can be up to 50% to 60% (19), but has also been associated with complications including infection. The overall success rate after reoperation on FBSS patients is low and worsens with each additional surgery (17,20).

THE REHABILITATION PROGRAM

Most CLBP patients will have experienced significant pain, rated higher than a five using a numeric pain rating scale of 0 to 10, which has gone uninterrupted for greater than 3 months. Multiple factors affect the way a patient will respond to conservative management, including length of time with LBP, psychosocial factors, ethnicity/cultural beliefs, bodyweight/BMI, extent of physiological abnormalities, and radiating versus nonradiating pain. CLBP patients need to believe in the rehabilitation approach in order to reap the rewards of physical therapy (PT). Early on in therapy, patient education will be a crucial step in convincing the patient that compliance with their home exercise program (HEP) and staying consistent with PT 2 to 3 days a week for a minimum of 6 weeks will give them the best chance at a pain-free and functional lifestyle. It takes a multidisciplinary approach from multiple practitioners including but not limited to physical therapists, pain management physicians, family practitioners, neurologists, psychologists, chiropractors, and acupuncturists to provide the appropriate coordinated care to effectively treat this population. The goal of PT with these patients is to reduce disability and improve their quality of life.

Therapeutic Modalities

Superficial moist heat is a common modality used in the treatment of individuals with CLBP, although evidence is limited. There is moderate evidence that continuous heat wrap therapy reduces pain and disability in the short term for acute LBP (21). One of the most widely used modalities in PT for treating LBP is therapeutic ultrasound. Despite its common use, there is still inconclusive evidence to support its effectiveness in this group of patients (22). TENS may provide short term relief of LBP with little to no long term effect (23). Traction, although used in the clinic by therapists, has been proven ineffective for the treatment of CLBP in a systematic review (24,25).

Manual Therapy

Spinal manipulation/mobilization is widely used in PT and has become the standard of practice among physical therapists in outpatient clinics. Spinal manipulation is a high velocity, low amplitude movement to the vertebral segment at end range to help restore pain-free ROM. A recent review article that was published in *Spine* revealed that spinal manipulation was no more effective than other common interventions for reducing pain and improving function for patients with CLBP, although it is important to know that short term pain reduction was slightly in favor of spinal manipulation and no major adverse effects were reported (26). Mobilization is a back-and-forth oscillatory movement which can be divided into 4 grades. The clinician physically moves the joint within the available physiological joint ROM. It must be stated that the physical therapist needs to be properly trained in manual techniques prior to utilizing them in the work place. Each state has its own practice act on the use of manipulation/mobilization and the correct terminology to be used in documentation. Other forms of manual therapies include myofascial release, active release technique (ART), muscle energy technique, and Mulligan's movement with mobilization techniques. All of these treatment techniques offer the therapist at hand an alternative to more traditional treatments as stated above. When used in conjunction with one another, these treatments can release muscle tension, and soft-tissue restriction, improve flexibility, and reduce pain.

Massage therapy may be effective for treatment of chronic back pain, with benefits lasting at least 6 months (27). Massage (soft-tissue mobilization, effleurage, petrissage, etc.) has been used to improve soft-tissue extensibility, blood flow, flexibility, and ROM among other benefits. Individuals with CLBP have many psychological stressors that add to their disability. Massage can be beneficial by increasing blood flow to surrounding muscles and creating a relaxation effect (28). Additional studies are needed to evaluate the long-term effects of massage when combined with exercise and education for the treatment of CLBP. In addition, there are many available alternative therapies out on the market today including but not limited to acupuncture, Rolfing, Alexander technique, and Feldenkrais method that attempt to reduce symptoms and improve function through the use of manual treatments and exercise. To date, evidence best supports the use of acupuncture as an adjunctive treatment for CLBP.

Therapeutic Exercise

CLBP patients need to be managed differently than patients with acute LBP. With CLBP we must focus on restoring normal motion if stiff, normalizing neuromuscular control if unstable, and begin exercise in comfortable ranges. Exercise produces large reductions in pain and disability, a feature that suggests that exercise should play a major role in the management of CLBP (29,30). CLBP patients will often exhibit characteristics that include: poor kinesthetic awareness, poor transversus abdominis (TrA)/multifidus (MF) muscle activation, poor

body mechanics when moving and lifting, psychological distress, fear avoidance for reinjury, and generally lack of directional preference. The first step in treating these individuals is gaining their trust and confidence in you, in order to allow for maximal therapeutic benefit. Once a relationship has been established, the patient should be educated on long term self management which will include a comprehensive HEP.

The next step is to develop core awareness and focus on proper posture and spinal biomechanics, using both mechanical and verbal biofeedback tools. According to available research, individuals with CLBP exhibit decreased timing and activation of their postural muscles, specifically the erector spinae (25,31). Low load exercises to volitionally activate the TrA (Figure 47.1) should be introduced to restore trunk muscle activation patterns. Patients can progress by learning to perform gentle alternate limb movements during core muscle contraction (Figures 47.2a and 47.2b), especially contraction of the TrA (32). Exercise positions should start with the patient in gravity-eliminated position with the least amount of resistance, followed by progressing to performing them against gravity without external resistance, and then external resistance (e.g., ankle weights, dumbbells, body weight exercises). Utilizing a therapeutic stability ball has been shown to increase maximal volitional contraction (MVC) in the abdominal muscles in healthy patients (33). This therapeutic modality places a larger emphasis on the motor control system, which is lacking in the setting of CLBP.

As the patient begins to regain pre-morbid function with less pain, an emphasis on alternate strengthening regimens may be beneficial for the long term management of CLBP. Although research is limited on its efficacy, Yoga and Pilates have been gaining popularity over the last decade.

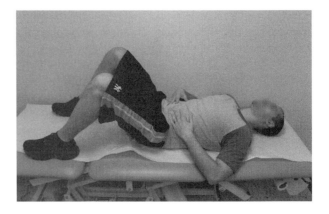

FIGURE 47.1: Abdominal bracing for recruitment of the transverse abdominis.

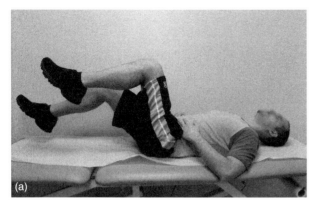

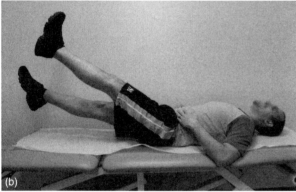

FIGURE 47.2: Core muscle activation with progressive lower limb movements.

Both Yoga and Pilates are mind-body exercise interventions that address both the physical and mental aspects of pain with core strengthening, flexibility, and relaxation as their central components. CLBP patients need both the physical and emotional aspects of their illness addressed, as well as improved kinesthetic awareness. This is what makes Yoga and/or Pilates such viable options to treat CLBP (34). As the patient gains improved control of his/her posture, total body strengthening and conditioning should be incorporated to encourage the patient to return to their pre-morbid functional level. Other therapeutic exercise options included in the treatment of CLBP are: balance training, manual perturbations in multiple positions, aerobic exercise, plate load equipment use, and quadruped exercises with resistance bands. A combination of the aforementioned modalities should be included in the treatment protocol to enhance recovery.

Specialized Techniques

Kinesiology taping has been gaining popularity in the United States over the last decade and is now used in professional sports. It is designed to facilitate the body's natural healing process while allowing support and stability to muscles and joints without restricting the body's ROM. Even though it's widely used in orthopedics and neurology, there is a lack of randomized controlled trials justifying the benefits with various populations.

Aquatic Therapy is an alternative therapeutic option for individuals who cannot tolerate land-based exercise or who may need that reduction in bodyweight in order to exercise successfully.

Orthotics/prosthetics should be recommended as needed based on a full gait analysis and evaluation. The use of lumbar corsets or supports for CLBP is not supported by the literature (35), and prolonged bracing may lead to abdominal and trunk musculature weakness due to disuse atrophy. Prolonged bracing may also lead to impaired proprioceptive awareness and may increase the risk of additional injury to the lumbar spine.

Complementary and Alternative Medicine

Patients with CLBP frequently utilize complementary and alternative medicine (CAM) therapies when traditional medical treatments fail to relieve their pain and suffering. In this chapter, acupuncture, massage therapy, alternative movement therapies such as Alexander technique, Feldenkrais method, yoga, and Pilates have already been discussed. Of course, chiropractic care is frequently sought and utilized by patients who suffer from CLBP. The available literature suggests that yoga is the most effective nonphysician directed treatment approach for nonspecific LBP, whereas acupuncture is a medical practitioner directed treatment shown to be a good adjunctive treatment for LBP (36). A thorough review of CAM therapies for CLBP is beyond the scope of this chapter, but those who provide healthcare to patients with CLBP need to be aware of these therapies and the available research to counsel their patients properly.

Home Exercise Program

A well-planned HEP is an essential part of the rehabilitation experience and is critical to the maintenance of long term flexibility, strength, and balance. Patient compliance at home continues to be an unresolved issue. Research has yet to outline what motivates people to do their exercises. Exercise demonstration and patient education into the proper technique of the exercise will help reinforce the importance of completing the HEP as prescribed. Patients should also be given paper handouts with the prescribed exercises and specific instructions that the therapist may deem appropriate. Exercise prescription including frequency, duration, and intensity of HEP all depend on the patient's current level of function and how they present objectively on physical examination.

Early on, the HEP will consist of stretching of the lower limb muscles (hamstrings, hip flexors, piriformis), strengthening exercises consisting of supine and prone TrA exercises including the draw-in maneuver and abdominal bracing (Figure 47.1), supine marching with TrA contraction, prone hip extensions with TrA contraction, isometric to isotonic strengthening for hip adduction/abduction/external rotation with resistance bands, and supine pelvic tilts if necessary (anterior/posterior). The goal of the initial HEP is TrA contraction, improved flexibility, and pelvic mobility if needed.

If the patient can exhibit good control of TrA with the above exercises, he or she is ready for an updated HEP. The next phase of the HEP will be contracting TrA against gravity while moving the limbs on a fixed surface. Some exercises may include quadruped TrA contraction with prolonged holds, quadruped TrA with alternating UE movements, isotonic side lying hip abduction/external rotation, supine straight leg raise with TrA, modified side raise/plank, and modified forward plank with knees flexed, just to name a few. This phase is focusing on the feed forward neuromuscular control mechanism. The goal of this phase is to improve muscle strength, endurance, and reduce pain through exercise.

The last phase of the HEP focuses on return to premorbid levels of function and perhaps a return to sport, if applicable. Some examples of exercises in this phase are dynamic balance activities on a single limb, single limb squatting, forward planks with lower limb movements, side planks with hip abduction, and sport-specific activities practiced with a team or coach. The patient should slowly progress back into sports in order to allow the body to adjust to this higher level of activity. This phase focuses on the feedback neuromuscular control mechanism which is critical for long term success.

Although patients may see a physical therapist three times per week, there is some evidence that low back exercises are most beneficial when performed daily (37). The HEP is extremely vital in helping patients attain a full or at least an improved recovery from their injury. Patients need to understand that they must take some responsibility for their own health, and actively participate in their recovery.

SUMMARY

The rehabilitation program for chronic (>3 months), long-standing LBP should be comprehensive. CLBP is generally defined as pain that persists for more than 3 months in the lower back region. Whether you're treating myofascial pain syndrome, nonspecific CLBP, or FBSS, this evidence-based treatment plan will assist you in helping your patients. The approach that harvests the best results includes utilizing a multidisciplinary approach with healthcare practitioners from different services. Proper evaluation of all tissues for dysfunction including muscle, joint, connective tissue, and nerve must be addressed first. Educating the patient on the functionality of his/her condition and the multifaceted treatment they will receive is essential. Keep in mind that any rehabilitation program must be individualized to each patient's clinical picture, and should follow a logical progression through the phases of rehabilitation. Lastly, continued compliance with the HEP is a critical part of the rehabilitation program for the treatment of nonspecific CLBP, myofascial pain syndrome, and failed back surgery syndrome.

REFERENCES

1. Mersky H, Bogduk N. Classification of chronic pain. In: Mersky H, Bogduk N, Eds. *Descriptions of Chronic Pain Syndromes and Definition of Pain Terms*. 2nd ed. Seattle, WA: IASP Press; 1994:47.
2. *Simons DG, Travell JG, Simons LS*. Travell and Simons' Myofascial Pain and Dysfunction: The Trigger Point Manual. *Volume 1, 2nd ed. Baltimore, MD: Williams & Wilkins;* 1999.
3. Mense S, Simmons DG. *Muscle Pain. Understanding Its Nature, Diagnosis, and Treatment*. Philadelphia, PA: Lippincott Williams and Wilkins; 2001.
4. Childers MK, Feldman JB, Guo HM. Myofascial pain syndrome. In: Frontera WR, Silver JK, Rizzo TD Jr, Eds. *Essentials of Physical Medicine and Rehabilitation*, 2nd ed. Philadelphia, PA: Saunders Elsevier; 2008: Chapter 96.
5. Scheneider MJ. Tender points/fibromyalgia vs. trigger points/myofascial pain syndrome: a need for clarity in terminology and differential diagnosis. *J Manipulative Physiol Ther*. 1995;18(6):398–406.
6. Robinson JP, Arendt-Nielsen L. Muscle pain syndromes. In: Braddom RL, Ed. *Physical Medicine and Rehabilitation,* 3rd ed. Philadelphia, PA: Saunders Elsevier; 2007:989–1020.

7. Jay GW. Myofascial pain syndrome. In: *Chronic Pain (Pain Management Series)*; 2007:Chapter 4.
8. Rha DW, Shin JC, Kim YK, Jung JH, Kim YU, Lee SC. Detecting local twitch responses of myofascial trigger points in the lower-back muscles using ultrasonography. *Arch Phys Med Rehabil*. 2011;92(10):1576–1580.e1.
9. Kuan TS. Current studies on myofascial pain syndrome. *Current Pain & Headache Reports*. 2009;13:365–369.
10. Kalichman L, Vulfsons S. Dry needling in the management of musculoskeletal pain. *J Am Board Fam Med*. 2010;23(5):640–646. Review.
11. Balagué F, Mannion AF, Pellisé F, et al. Non-specific low back pain. *Lancet*. 2012;379(9814):482–491.
12. Cedraschi C, Allaz AF. How to identify patients with a poor prognosis in daily clinical practice. *Best Pract Res Clin Rheumatol*. 2005;19(4):577–591. Review.
13. Greenhalgh S, Selfe J. A qualitative investigation of Red Flags for serious spinal pathology. *Physiotherapy*. 2009;95:224–227.
14. Chapman JR, Norvell DC, Hermsmeyer JT, et al. Evaluating common outcomes for measuring treatment success for chronic low back pain. *Spine*. 2011;36(Suppl 21):S54–68. Review.
15. Dagenais S, Tricco AC, Haldeman S. Synthesis of recommendations for the assessment and management of low back pain from recent clinical practice guidelines. *Spine J*. 2010;10:514–529.
16. Waguespack A, Schofferman J, Slosar P, Reynolds J. Etiology of long-term failures of lumbar spine surgery. *Pain Med*. 2002;3:18–22.
17. Chan CW, Peng P. Failed back surgery syndrome. *Pain Med*. 2011;12(4):577–606.
18. Boswell MV, Trescot AM, Datta S, et al. Interventional techniques: evidence-based practice guidelines in the management of chronic spinal pain. *Pain Phys*. 2007;10(1):7–111.
19. Carter ML. Spinal cord stimulation in chronic pain: a review of the evidence. *Anesth Intensive Care* 2004;32(1):11–21.
20. Ragab A, Deshazo RD. Management of back pain in patients with previous back surgery. *Am J Med*. 2008;121(4):272–278.
21. Chou R, Huffman LH. American Pain Society; American College of Physicians. Nonpharmacologic therapies for acute and chronic low back pain: a review of the evidence for an American Pain Society/American College of Physicians clinical practice guideline. *Ann Intern Med*. 2007;147(7):492–504.
22. Ebadi S, Ansari NN, Henschke N, Naghdi S, van Tulder MW. The effect of continuous ultrasound on chronic low back pain: protocol of a randomized controlled trial. *BMC Musculoskelet Disord*. 2011;12:59.
23. Bloodworth DM, Nguyen BN, Garver W, et al. Comparison of stochastic vs. conventional transcutaneous electrical stimulation for pain modulation in patients with electromyographically documented radiculopathy. *Am J Phys Med Rehabil*. 2004;83(8):584–591.
24. Clarke JA, van Tulder MW, Blomberg SE, et al. Traction for low-back pain with or without sciatica. *Cochrane Database Syst Rev*. 2007;(2):CD003010.
25. Jacobs JV, Henry SM, Nagle KJ. People with chronic low back pain exhibit decreased variability in the timing of their anticipatory postural adjustments. *Behav Neurosci*. 2009;123(2):455–458.
26. Rubinstein SM, van Middelkoop M, Assendelft WJ, de Boer MR, van Tulder MW. Spinal manipulative therapy for chronic low-back pain: an update of a Cochrane review. *Spine (Phila Pa 1976)*. 2011;36(13):E825–846.
27. Cherkin DC, Sherman KJ, Kahn J, et al. A comparison of the effects of 2 types of massage and usual care on chronic low back pain: a randomized, controlled trial. *Ann Intern Med*. 2011;155(1):1–9.
28. Sliz D, Smith A, Wiebking C, Northoff G, Hayley S. Neural correlates of a single-session massage treatment. *Brain Imaging Behav*. 2012;6:77–87.
29. Maher CG. Effective physical treatment for chronic low back pain. *Orthop Clin North Am*. 2004;35(1):57–64.
30. Murtezani A, Hundozi H, Orovcanec N, Sllamniku S, Osmani T. A comparison of high intensity aerobic exercise and passive modalities for the treatment of workers with chronic low back pain: a randomized, controlled trial. *Eur J Phys Rehabil Med*. 2011;47(3):359–366.
31. Thomas JS, France CR, Sha D, Vander Wiele N, Moenter S, Swank K. The effect of chronic low back pain on trunk muscle activations in target reaching movements with various loads. *Spine (Phila Pa 1976)*. 2007;32(26):E801–808.
32. Barr KP, Griggs M, Cadby T. Lumbar stabilization: a review of core concepts and current literature, part 2. *Am J Phys Med Rehabil*. 2007;86(1):72–80.
33. Vera-Garcia FJ, Grenier SG, McGill SM. Abdominal muscle response during curl-ups on both stable and labile surfaces. *Phys Ther*. 2000;80(6):564–569.
34. Sorosky S, Stilp S, Akuthota V. Yoga and pilates in the management of low back pain. *Curr Rev Musculoskelet Med*. 2008;1(1):39–47.
35. Jellema P, van Tulder MW, van Poppel MN, Nachemson AL, Bouter LM. Lumbar supports for prevention and treatment of low back pain: a systematic review within the framework of the Cochrane Back Review Group. *Spine (Phila Pa 1976)*. 2001;26(4):377–386.
36. Carneiro KA, Rittenberg JD. The role of exercise and alternative treatments for low back pain. *Phys Med Rehabil Clin N Am*. 2010;21(4):777–792.
37. Mayer TG, Gatchel RJ, Kishino N, et al. Objective assessment of spine function following industrial injury: a prospective study with comparison group and one-year follow-up. *Spine*. 1985;10:482–493.

48

Sacroiliac Joint Dysfunction

Janel B. Solano, Michael A. Romello, Ruihong Yao, and Asal Sepassi

INTRODUCTION

The sacroiliac (SI) joint should be considered as a potential source of pain during the systematic approach to diagnosis and treatment of low back pain (LBP). It commonly involves pain in the lower back and upper buttock region and should be considered in the differential diagnosis of pain in both regions. It has been found to be the pain generator in 13% to 30% of those with chronic LBP (1), although these high percentages remain controversial. The SI joint is composed of both fibrocartilage and hyaline cartilage and is C or L shape with anterior and posterior components (Figure 48.1). It is 1 to 2 mm wide with joint space decreasing with age. The joint does not truly fuse with normal aging, despite what has previously been taught (2). The exact nerve innervation is unclear; however Bernard proposed that the innervation posteriorly is through L4-S3 and anteriorly by L2-S2 (3). Therefore, SI joint pain may present in a variety of locations.

The biomechanics of the SI joint are complex. SI joint motion is affected by motion of the spine, ilium, pubic symphysis, and hip. During activities, movement does not usually exceed 2 to 3 degrees in the transverse or longitudinal planes (4). Contraction of the transverse abdominis significantly decreases the laxity of SI joint and those with SI joint pain have been found to actually fire muscles differently than those without pain (5).

On history, patients can indicate the presence of LBP, groin pain, thigh pain, or posterior pelvic pain. In addition, numbness, popping, or clicking with transitional activities (e.g., sit to stand) can be reported. Activities that involve asymmetric loading through the lower limb such as use of the elliptical trainer, step aerobics, golfing, or bowling have also been implicated (6). Pain usually does not present above the beltline and is usually unilateral or paramidline as opposed to midline LBP (7). History of trauma or pregnancy or even lumbar fusion should be identified, as SI joint pain tends to be more commonly associated with this history.

Key elements of the physical examination include inspection, palpation, lumbar spine and hip examinations, neurological examination, and SI joint provocative maneuvers. Inspection and palpation can identify pelvic asymmetries and if present, leg length discrepancies should also be assessed for. Palpation of the SI joint is usually considered over the region of the posterior superior iliac spine (PSIS).

A comprehensive lumbar spine and neurologic evaluation is necessary to rule out other potential causes of pain in this region such as referred facetogenic pain, discogenic pain, or lumbosacral radiculopathy. Examination of the hip joint to evaluate range of motion (ROM) and to rule out intra-articular hip pathology as a potential pain generator should be included. Provocative maneuvers have been described previously and by themselves have demonstrated little sensitivity and specificity. However, although still debatable, the usefulness of a confluence of physical examination maneuvers may improve specificity of the diagnosis of SI joint mediated pain. This has been described in an article by van der Wurff et al in which a multi test regimen of five SI joint provocation tests were compared to results of fluoroscopically guided double local anesthetic blocks. A combination of three or more positive tests was deemed to be a reliable indicator that showed fair to good specificity for SI joint pain (8). This includes FABER's or Patrick's maneuver, Gaenslen's maneuver, compression test, distraction test, and femoral shear test. However, Dreyfuss and colleagues studied 12 SI joint tests and found that no specific examination technique or groupings of techniques were particularly sensitive or specific for SI joint pain (9).

Other elements to consider during physical examination are flexibility testing particularly of the hamstrings, quadriceps (especially the rectus femoris), the iliopsoas, and piriformis muscles. These muscles play a significant role in the biomechanics of the hip and pelvis. An assessment of core strength should be done and an evaluation of pelvic floor musculature should also be considered. The abdominal muscles affect motion at the ilium, pubis, and

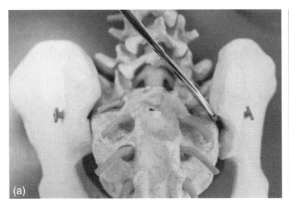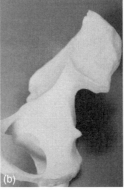

FIGURE 48.1: Sacroiliac joint anatomy: (a) Posterior view of sacroiliac joint articulation. (b) Articular surface on the iliac side.

lumbar spine. Abdominals firing in a lengthened position do not efficiently absorb forces that affect stability at the lumbar spine and pubic symphysis (6).

Imaging studies of the SI joint are fairly limited and usually are not particularly helpful. However, plain films would evaluate for arthropathy, degenerative changes, or erosions. If suspicion for inflammatory arthropathy is high, then more detailed examination with CT scan to better evaluate the joint could be considered. MRI has also been described as an imaging modality for evaluating spondyloarthropathy. Of note, the dorsocaudal synovial part of the joint is involved significantly more often than the ventral portion early in the disease (10).

While there is no true "gold standard" for the diagnosis of SI joint pain, administration of intra-articular lidocaine injection with pre and post injection pain evaluation is often used and considered by many to be the closest currently available gold standard (11).

THE REHABILITATION PROGRAM

Initial management involves a comprehensive physical examination of the lumbar spine, hips, and pelvis by the treating physical therapist. Muscle imbalances and poor flexibility can be appropriately identified and incorporated into the rehabilitation program. In general the phases of rehabilitation should be followed.

For acute SI joint pain the typical rehabilitation principles should be applied early on including decreasing pain and swelling through relative rest, use of modalities for symptomatic treatment, joint protection, and the use of pain medication on an as needed basis. The goal of this phase is pain management and restoration of mobility and ROM. In general avoidance of activities that require single leg stance such as skating, running, and stair stepping is recommended.

A gait analysis including examination of ankle/foot posture and alignment should be performed. Asymmetric foot pronation may result in genu valgus at the knee, internal rotation at the hip resulting in an iliac crest that appears lower than the opposite side with subsequent altered load transmission.

Lastly, if leg length discrepancy (LLD) is detected, particularly if it is anatomic, consider correcting this early on. In the case of functional leg length discrepancies, correction may be considered during the acute phase. Beyond this it may be detrimental since it may promote adaptive muscle imbalances leading to a shift in force transmission and a change in wear patterns.

SACROILIAC JOINT PAIN

- ▪ Should be considered in the differential diagnosis of LBP, buttock, groin, or lateral hip pain

- ▪ Etiology can be acute or part of chronic LBP, with a higher incidence in trauma, pregnancy, and after lumbar fusion

- ▪ Key historical elements: pain usually below the L5 level, often unilateral, worse with transitional movements

- ▪ Physical examination can be unreliable, however, should include a comprehensive neurologic examination, lumbar spine and hip examination, and a detailed musculoskeletal evaluation to assess for asymmetries in flexibility, muscle firing patterns, and strength (e.g., core strength) and even a pelvic floor examination

Functional LLD is better approached by correction of muscle imbalance (6).

Therapeutic Modalities

The use of ice can be considered in cases of acute SI joint pain or in cases of inflammatory arthropathy, particularly in the first 72 hours. Ice should be applied 15 to 20 minutes to the affected area every 2 hours as needed. Superficial and deep heating modalities can be considered as part of the rehabilitation program. Heat may be used for pain relief and to promote active and passive stretching as well as mobilization of the pelvis. Keep in mind that the research is limited and hasn't determined the efficacy of specific therapeutic modalities, nor have comparison studies been done in the setting of SI joint pain.

Manual Therapy

The use of manual medicine including chiropractic manipulation, and osteopathic manipulative treatment as well as myofascial techniques has been described in the treatment of SI joint pain.

Myofascial release can be applied to the soft tissues and ligaments surrounding the SI joint. Regions of restrictions can be detected at the dorsal SI ligament, iliolumbar ligaments, sacrospinous ligaments, and sacrotuberous ligaments. The chiropractic treatments include use of high velocity low amplitude (HVLA) thrusting procedures, and mechanical force manually assisted (MFMA) techniques, which are probably the most widely used of the chiropractic adjustment modalities (12). In a study comparing these two modalities, there were no differences in treatment response outcomes between groups, with both groups resulting in significant improvement from baseline in pain and disability (13).

A full discussion of the diagnosis and treatment of SI joint dysfunction with regards to osteopathic manipulation is beyond the scope of this chapter. However, one of the common treatment approaches for SI dysfunction is muscle energy. Muscle energy techniques employ a contract-relax pattern to encourage movement through a barrier of motion by isometric contraction of affected muscles (e.g., tight iliopsoas in the case of an anteriorly rotated ilium). This is to promote reflex relaxation via the Golgi tendon organ to move further through the barrier of motion (i.e., posterior rotation of the ilium in this case)

(14). A case report describes the use of muscle energy to correct somatic dysfunction of the SI joint in the context of compensated Trendelenburg gait in a person with multiple sclerosis. Post treatment gait analysis noted objective improvement in gait pattern, as well as increased velocity of gait (15).

Although it is felt that joint manipulation and mobilization does not induce lasting SI joint positional changes, it may still have clinical efficacy because of its effect on soft tissues (16); the pain relief provided by these treatments allows for a better response to therapeutic exercise.

Therapeutic Exercise

Once the patient emerges from the acute phase (phase I) of treatment in which pain is well controlled, then the next remaining phases (phases II–V) can be started and progressed through. This will gradually move the patient through ROM and flexibility exercises to strength training, proprioceptive and balance training, and then functional retraining (if applicable, sport-specific rehabilitation will be included).

The goal during the next phase of rehabilitation is to restore ROM, and flexibility, identify and correct biomechanical deficits, and reduce tissue overload. Evaluation for shortening or poor flexibility involving the iliopsoas, rectus femoris, tensor fascia lata, adductors, quadratus lumborum, latissimus dorsi, and obturator internus should be performed. These muscles commonly are found to be working in a "shortened" position, which does not permit optimal biomechanical advantage. Once length is restored, then strengthening of muscles that are inhibited can be started. Weak muscles typically include the gluteus medius, gluteus maximus, lower abdominals, and hamstrings.

Careful evaluation for subtle examination findings such as imbalances between muscle length and strength and asymmetric muscle recruitment patterns should be noted. Subjects with SI joint pain have been shown to have delayed firing of the multifidus and internal abdominal obliques as well as the gluteus maximus, while activating the biceps femoris earlier (17).

Evaluation of abdominal strength and incorporation of a strengthening program is essential. Targeted therapy of the transversus abdominus has been described as a method of stabilization of the SI joint. The act of "drawing in" of the abdominal wall has been shown to specifically activate the transversus abdominus muscle as opposed to the so-called "bracing pattern" in which all of the abdominal

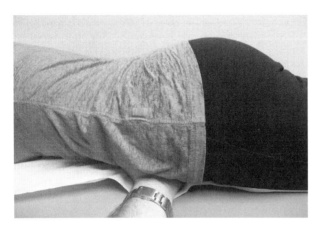

FIGURE 48.2: Transversus abdominis facilitation: Patient is prone, therapist places hand under the abdomen and below the navel. Ask the patient to maintain a pelvic floor contraction and gently draw the abdomen upwards to lift pressure off of examiner's hand. Observe for compensatory patterns. Hold for goal of 10 seconds.

wall muscles are isometrically contracted (Figure 48.2). The "drawing in" exercise also results in co-contraction of the multifidus that has previously been shown to be effective in the treatment of acute idiopathic LBP resulting in decrease in clinical recurrence of LBP from 75% to 35% (5). In contrast to this belief or approach, recent studies have shown that when assessed bio-mechanically, bracing of the abdominal muscles provides greater stability to the lumbar spine than hallowing or "drawing in." Activation of the transversus abdominis in isolation is unlikely to provide increased stability compared to activation of other core muscles; therefore, bracing enhances stability (18).

Neuromuscular reeducation with facilitation techniques and proprioceptive training (phase IV of rehabilitation) should start with closed kinetic chain strengthening and then can be incorporated into a lumbopelvic stabilization program. This is often a key component in the prevention of recurrent SI joint or LBP along with maintaining the balance of flexibility and strength across the pelvis that was acquired during previous rehabilitation phases (6). There should also be a thorough ergonomic evaluation including work, daily, and recreational activities. Functional re-training wraps up the final phase of rehabilitation and may be geared toward work and/or sport.

Specialized Techniques

The use of the McKenzie method of mechanical diagnosis and therapy (MDT) has been described in the literature. While often recognized as a method of centralization of discogenic pain and radiculopathy, a case report by Horton and Franz (19) demonstrated how the McKenzie method could be used in the case of SI joint pain. The MDT method emphasizes the use of patient self-generated loading strategies in the assessment and management of musculoskeletal problems. Repeated movement is crucial and helps the clinician to identify and further classify mechanical presentations of the spine. The term *directional preference* is used to describe a decrease in pain with movements in one direction with worsening of pain in the other direction (19). In the context of the SI joint, use of anterior and posterior pelvic rotation with or without the application of overpressure, as well as flexion, extension, and side bending while standing, seated, and supine is used to identify the posture or position that alleviates their usual pain (Figure 48.3).

To briefly mention complementary and alternative (CAM) treatments, acupuncture has been studied as a treatment for pregnancy associated pelvic girdle pain including SI region pain. In a randomized single blind controlled trial of 386 pregnant women with pelvic girdle pain, standard treatment was compared to either acupuncture or stabilizing exercises. Results demonstrated that the acupuncture group experienced decreased pain both subjectively reported (Visual Analogue Scale) as well as on assessment by an independent examiner (20).

Supportive Devices

A trial of an SI belt may be considered. It usually encircles the waist from the iliac crest to the greater trochanter, and extends anteriorly to the symphysis pubis. Some versions include a moldable plastic insert for LBP (21). They work by providing compression and proprioceptive feedback to gluteal muscles. This may be particularly helpful in cases of hypermobility or weakness such as in the case of pregnancy induced SI joint dysfunction. In cadaveric studies, use of an SI belt was found to decrease rotation by 30% (22).

Home Exercise Program

The home exercise program (HEP) should be instituted early in the rehabilitation program. Incorporating the patient as an active participant in his/her rehabilitation is essential to long term outcomes. In addition it also empowers the patient to be armed with the ability to treat themselves during episodes of acute or recurrent pain.

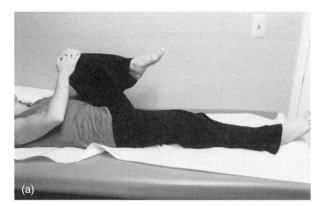
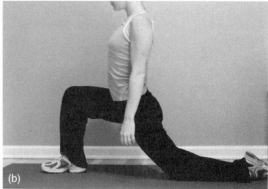
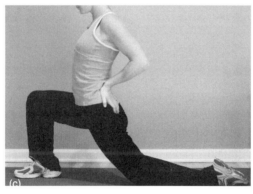

FIGURE 48.3: Pelvic rotations: (a) Posterior pelvic rotation for the left SI joint. (b) Anterior pelvic rotation for the left SI joint. (c) Anterior pelvic rotation with overpressure of the left SI joint.

Flexibility deficits should have been identified, and instruction in an appropriate stretching program for regions affected should be instituted. As previously mentioned, the iliopsoas, hamstrings, rectus femoris, hip adductors, latissimus dorsi, and quadratus lumborum are frequently involved in SI joint pain.

Stretching of the SI joint region can be incorporated into the HEP as well. This can be performed in both the right and left side lying position, preferably on a firm surface. The upper hip is flexed 70 to 80 degrees and the knee is flexed about 90 degrees. The trunk is then rotated toward the upper side as far as is comfortable (Figure 48.4). Isometric resistance can be incorporated into this stretch as well by the patient themselves or with help from another to create a contract-relax type of stretch. This involves gently attempting to abduct and internally rotate the top leg against resistance (23).

Core stabilization exercises including hip lift bridges (Figure 48.5) and isometric hip adduction ball squeezes should also be included. In addition, exercises specific to the SI joint including anterior and posterior pelvic rotation can be included as directed by the therapist.

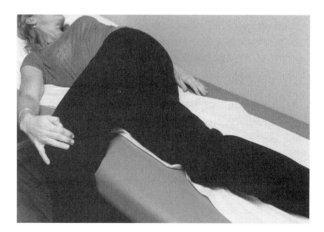

FIGURE 48.4: SI joint stretch: Patient is positioned in side lying with upper hip flexed 70 to 80 degrees and the knee flexed 90 degrees. Trunk is rotated toward the upper side as far as possible. If done on a table, the goal is to allow the leg to drop toward the floor with the use of breathing, isometric contractions followed by relaxation, and/or overpressure applied by therapist or patient.

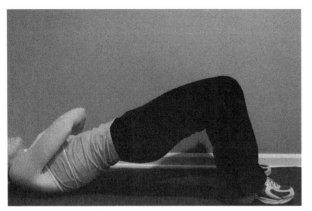

FIGURE 48.5: Hip lift bridging for core stabilization.

SUMMARY

Diagnosis and treatment of SI joint pain can pose a challenge to both the treating physician and therapist. Usually it does not present as an isolated problem, but rather as part of a complex, particularly in chronic LBP. It can be difficult to discern pain arising from the SI joint versus other spinal structures including the facet joints, discs, or lumbopelvic muscles. In addition, hip joint pathology itself can manifest similarly. Rehabilitation of SI joint pain should involve a comprehensive approach including therapeutic modalities, manual therapy, stretching, core strengthening, neuromuscular reeducation, corrections in the kinetic chain, if applicable, and instruction in an effective HEP.

SAMPLE CASE

A 29-year-old female who is 4 weeks postpartum from uncomplicated delivery presents with worsening right-sided posterior pelvic pain. She reports symptoms presented 2 to 3 weeks prior to delivery but have progressively worsened since returning to the gym where she does primarily step aerobics classes for conditioning. Her pain is worse with getting out of the car and she often feels like she is "getting stuck." She denies numbness, tingling, weakness, bowel or bladder symptoms, or polyarthralgia. An MRI of the lumbar spine was ordered by her primary care physician and was negative for disc herniation or facet pathology. Examination is notable for tenderness at the PSIS and gluteal muscles, full ROM in the lumbar spine and hip; normal neurologic examination, positive FABERS's, Gaenslen's, and thigh thrust test, and positive Ely's test on the right.

 SAMPLE THERAPY PRESCRIPTION

Discipline: Physical therapy.

Diagnosis: Right SI joint pain and dysfunction.

Precautions: Universal.

Frequency of visits: 2 to 3x/week.

Duration of treatment: 3 to 4 weeks; or an alternative would be to provide a total of 8 to 12 visits (used at the therapist's discretion).

Treatment:

1. *Modalities:* cryotherapy (ice pack, ice massage) after treatment if needed

2. *Manual therapy:* SI joint mobilization, trial of muscle energy techniques

3. *Therapeutic exercise:* Stretching of iliopsoas, hamstrings, and piriformis; based on the PT's evaluation of muscle lengths. Core strengthening program including targeted transversus abdominus strengthening. Strengthening of gluteus medius, maximus, and lower abdominals, and hamstrings if found to be weak. Neuromuscular reeducation, aerobic and conditioning

4. *Specialized treatments:* biomechanical analysis of gait and the kinetic chain, trial of McKenzie's techniques for centralization including evaluation for directional preference for anterior and posterior pelvic rotation

5. *Patient education:* instruction in effective HEP. Avoidance of single leg stance activities

Goals: Decrease pain; restore normal lumbopelvic motion, correct biomechanics, safely return to functional activities (e.g., sport, hobbies, work).

Reevaluation: In 4 weeks by referring physician.

REFERENCES

1. Schwarzer AC, April CN, Bogduk N. The sacroiliac joint in chronic low back pain. *Spine*. 1995;20:30–37.
2. Kampen WU, Tillman B. Age-related changes in the articular cartilage of human sacroiliac joint. *Anat Embryol (Berl)*. 1998;198:505–513.
3. Bernard TN, Jr. The sacroiliac joint syndrome: Pathophysiology, diagnosis, and management, In: Frymoyer JW, Eds. *The Adult Spine Principles and Practice*. New York, NY: Raven; 1991:2107–2130.
4. Harrison DE, Harrison DD, Troyanovich SJ: The sacroiliac joint: A review of anatomy and biomechanics with clinical implications. *Journal Manipulative Physiol Ther*. 1997;20:607–661.
5. Richardson CA, Snijders CJ, Hides JA, et al: The relation between the transversus abdominis muscles, sacroiliac joint mechanics and low back pain. *Spine*. 2002;27:399–405.
6. Prather H, Hunt D. Sacroiliac joint pain. *Disability Monthly*. 2004;50:670–683.
7. Depalma MJ, Ketchum JM, Trussell BS, Saullo TR, Slipman CW. Does the location of low back pain predict its source? *PMR*. 2011;3(1):33–39.
8. van der Wurff P, Meyne W, Hagmeijer RH. Clinical tests of the sacroiliac joint. *Man Ther*. 2000;5:89–96.
9. Dreyfuss P, Michaelsen M, Pauza K, et. al. The value of history and physical examination in diagnosing sacroiliac joint pain: A prospective study. *Spine*. 1996;21(22):2594–2602.
10. Muche B, Bollow M, Francois RJ, et al. Anatomic structures involved in early and late stage sacroiliitis in spondyloarthritis. Arthritis Rheum. 2003;48:1374–1384.
11. Foley BS, Buschbacher RM. Sacroiliac joint pain anatomy, biomechanics, diagnosis and treatment. *Am J Phys Med Rehabil*. 2006;85(12):997–1006.
12. Christensen MG, Kerkoff D, Kollach MQ. Job Analysis of Chiropractic 2000. Greeley, CO: National Board of Chiropractic Examiners; 2000.
13. Shearer KA, Colloca CJ, White HL. A randomized clinical trial of manual versus mechanical force manipulation in the treatment of sacroiliac joint syndrome. J Manipulative Physiol Ther. 2005;28(7):493–501.
14. Dowling DJ. Principles of osteopathic manipulative techniques. In: DiGiovanna EL, Schiowitz S. Eds. An Osteopathic Approach to Diagnosis and Treatment. Philadelphia, PA: Lippincott Williams & Wilkins; 1997:86–88.
15. Gilliss AC, Swanson RL, Janora D, et al. Use of osteopathic manipulative treatment to manage compensated Trendelenburg gait caused by sacroiliac somatic dysfunction. JAOA. 2010;110(2):81–86.
16. Tullberg T, Blomberg S, Branth B, et al. Manipulation does not alter the position of the sacroiliac joint. A Roentgen stereophotogrammetric analysis. Spine. 1998;23:1124–1128.
17. Hungerford B, Gilleard W, Hodges P. Evidence of altered lumbopelvic muscle recruitment in the presence of sacroiliac joint pain. Spine. 2003;28:1593–1600.
18. Grenier SG, McGill SM. Quantification of lumbar stability by using 2 different abdominal activation strategies. Arch Phys Med Rehabil. 2007;88:54–62.
19. Horton SJ, Franz A. Mechanical diagnosis and therapy approach to assessment and treatment of derangement of the sacro-iliac joint. Man Ther. 2007;12:126–132.
20. Elden H, Ladfors L, Olsen MF, Ostgaard H, Hagberg H. Effects of acupuncture and stabilizing exercises as adjunct to standard treatment in pregnant women with pelvic girdle pain: randomized single blind controlled trial. BMJ. 2005;330(7494):761.
21. Gailey R. Orthotics in rehabilitation. In: Voight ML, Hoogenboom BJ, Prentice WE. Eds. Musculoskeletal Interventions. Techniques for Therapeutic Exercise. New York, NY: McGraw Hill Medical; 2007:424–425.
22. Vleeming A, Buyruk HM, Stoeckart R, et.al. Towards an integrated therapy for peripartum pelvic instability: a study of the biomechanical effects of pelvic belts. Am J Obs Gynecol. 1992;166:1243–1247.
23. Hooker DN, Prentice WE. Rehabilitation of injuries to the spine. In Voight ML, Hoogenboom BJ, Prentice WE. Eds. Musculoskeletal Interventions. Techniques for Therapeutic Exercise. New York, NY: McGraw Hill Medical; 2007:743–770.

Piriformis Syndrome

Jonathan S. Kirschner, Ron S. Ben-Meir, and Jonathan Diamond

INTRODUCTION

Piriformis syndrome is buttock pain radiating in a sciatic distribution due to a tight, tender piriformis muscle irritating or compressing the sciatic nerve. This can be differentiated from piriformis mediated muscle pain, which typically only causes buttock pain, although rehabilitation programs for both conditions are similar. Piriformis syndrome is relatively uncommon, and often confused with other disorders such as lumbar disc disease, radiculopathy, or pain originating from the sacroiliac joint. Although symptoms are similar to these other disorders, piriformis syndrome rarely presents with neurologic deficits and is typically a diagnosis of exclusion.

The piriformis is a flat, pear-shaped muscle that originates from the anterior border of the second through fourth sacral segments, the superior margin of the greater sciatic notch, and the sacrotuberous ligament. It shares fibers with the anterior capsule of the sacroiliac joint and the biceps femoris tendon, and can become taut when these structures are mobilized (Figure 49.1) (1). The piriformis extends inferolaterally through the greater sciatic foramen to attach to the superior margin of the greater trochanter. The piriformis is intimately related to the sciatic nerve. The ventral rami of L4 through S3 normally converge at the inferior border of the piriformis to form the sciatic nerve, which then emerges through the greater sciatic foramen inferior to the piriformis, therefore, any pathology of the piriformis can affect the sciatic nerve causing the classic lower limb referred pain and dysesthesia. The cause of piriformis syndrome may be due to anatomical variations in the muscle-nerve relationship; however it most commonly is a result of direct trauma to the muscle, overuse, or an imbalance between the hip flexors/extensors and external rotators and/or an imbalance between the hip adductors and abductors. Patients with piriformis syndrome typically describe deep aching ipsilateral buttock pain with variable referred pain down the posterolateral thigh and calf. Pain can be aggravated by climbing stairs, prolonged sitting, standing or walking, or placing the affected limb in an internally rotated position. The pain is often mitigated by external rotation of the leg in a position of comfort.

Key elements of the physical examination include inspection, palpation, range of motion (ROM) testing, neuromuscular evaluation, and provocative maneuvers. The examination may reveal tenderness to direct superficial palpation at the greater sciatic notch, or lateral pelvic wall pain on rectal examination. Deep palpation may reveal piriformis muscle spasm or a "sausage shaped mass" as originally described by Robinson in 1947 (2). Gluteal atrophy may be appreciated. If weakness or sensory loss is noted, other diagnoses such as lumbar radiculopathy or pelvic mass should be considered, although these may on rare occasion be present in chronic cases of piriformis syndrome. Functional movement screen or kinetic chain evaluation should be performed to evaluate for biomechanical deficits that may lead to compensatory movement patterns and repetitive strain on the piriformis muscle. Provocative tests should be performed, although sensitivity and specificity values have not been determined (3). Pain may be provoked by placing the hip of the affected side in flexion, adduction, and internal rotation (FAIR maneuver). The Lasegue test (straight leg raise) is considered positive with pain at 45 degrees. Freiberg's maneuver involves forcefully internally rotating the affected leg while the patient is supine in an attempt to stretch the irritated piriformis and provoke sciatic nerve compression. The Pace maneuver elicits pain by abducting the hip in the seated position, activating the piriformis rather than stretching it. The Beatty test involves having the patient lie on the unaffected side with the knee and hip flexed, abducting the thigh to raise the knee off the table. This has been shown to elicit deep buttock pain in those with PS, but back and leg pain in those with lumbar disk disease (4).

Piriformis syndrome is largely a clinical diagnosis. Diagnostic modalities such as CT, MRI, ultrasound, and electromyography (EMG) are useful mainly in excluding other conditions. Magnetic resonance neurography is an emerging technology that has been shown to accurately identify patients with piriformis syndrome who respond to surgery (5). Lumbosacral MRI is recommended to evaluate for herniated discs, spinal stenosis, and mass lesions that may cause lumbosacral nerve root compression. Standard hip or pelvic MRI is not sensitive in identifying cases of piriformis syndrome but can be used to evaluate for piriformis asymmetry, but more importantly evaluate the surrounding structures that can cause pain such as the ischial bursa, proximal hamstring tendons, bursopathies or tendinopathies at the greater trochanter, or even intrinsic hip joint pathology. CT and ultrasound are less sensitive than MRI, but can be useful in identifying aberrant structures such as tumors, hematomas, and abscesses that may cause sciatic nerve compression. Electrodiagnostic studies are typically normal, although Fishman has shown ipsilateral prolongation of the H-reflex latency greater than 1.86 msec when limbs affected by piriformis syndrome are placed in the FAIR position. However, his results have not been validated by others (3). These diagnostic studies are often ordered, but not reliable; therefore the history and physical examination should be the mainstay of diagnosis.

THE REHABILITATION PROGRAM

Rehabilitation and selected injection therapies continue to be the mainstay of treatment (6). The rehabilitation program should focus on piriformis stretching, which aims to relax a tight, spastic muscle to relieve nerve compression. The stretching program can be performed standing, sitting, or supine. If the hip is flexed less than 90 degrees the patient is stretched in the FAIR position, however many therapists recommend stretching in a position of abduction and external rotation with the hip flexed greater than 90 degrees. Reproduction of pain in these positions notifies the therapist that the muscle has been localized and is ready for stretching. In addition to stretching, core strengthening, lumbosacral stabilization, and hip strengthening exercises should be incorporated along with deep tissue massage and heating modalities. In fact, there is evidence to support that this approach is effective (7). As with any therapy program, it should initially be a structured program supervised by a physical

PIRIFORMIS SYNDROME

- Piriformis syndrome is a controversial diagnosis, but likely both an overdiagnosed and underdiagnosed cause of sciatic pain

- The mechanism of injury is direct trauma to the muscle, overuse, muscle group imbalance, or anatomic variations causing compression of the sciatic nerve

- Piriformis mediated muscle pain is characterized by a focal pain in the buttock, whereas piriformis syndrome presents with referred pain down the posterior calf and thigh on the ipsilateral side

- The physical examination should include inspection, palpation, ROM testing, neuromuscular evaluation, and provocative maneuvers. The examination may demonstrate tenderness to palpation over the greater sciatic notch or over the muscle belly and reproduction of sciatic pain with provocative maneuvers.

- Diagnostic modalities used to exclude other pathologies include MRI, CT, ultrasound, and EMG, however history and physical examination provide the greatest diagnostic yield

therapist to maximize safety and efficacy, and eventually transitioned to a home exercise program (HEP). The rehabilitation program should again follow the five phases of rehabilitation discussed throughout this book.

Therapeutic Modalities

Initially, in an acute case or with patients who have significant pain or loss of function, modalities may be employed to increase comfort and allow pain free activities of daily living. Ultrasound or moist heat can be utilized to increase tissue temperature, blood flow, and tissue extensibility and decrease pain. At the end of each session, ice or cold packs may be applied as tolerated. Electrical stimulation and transcutaneous electrical nerve stimulation (TENS) can be used to address pain and reduce muscle spasms, although long-term reliance on modalities should be avoided and long term efficacy is not well established in the literature.

Manual therapy

Foam rollers can also be used to improve flexibility, break down soft tissue adhesions, and decrease scar tissue formation. Tissue tightness, as in the case of piriformis syndrome, results in blood flow changes leading to altered biomechanics and loss of flexibility in a muscle group. Loss of flexibility can result in tissue strain and scar tissue formation (8). This repetitive strain injury cycle results in pain and loss of ROM and function. In a patient with piriformis syndrome the foam roller is an effective way to perform self-massage and address any trigger points. These manual treatments are reasonable adjunctive treatments but remain unproven in the literature.

Osteopathic manipulation can be a useful adjunct in the treatment of piriformis syndrome. The osteopathic technique employed is an indirect technique that involves taking the dysfunctional muscle in a direction away from the restricted motion barrier until a state of balance or change in the tissue is obtained (9). In piriformis syndrome, if a muscle is restricted in the adducted position, the indirect approach would place the muscle in the abducted position when treating. Conversely a direct approach involves taking the dysfunctional muscle or tissue in a direction toward the restricted barrier. If the muscle is restricted in the flexed adducted internally rotated position (FAIR), then the direct approach would further place that muscle in the FAIR position. The two indirect techniques employed for the treatment of piriformis syndrome are facilitated positional release and counterstrain (10). The goals of both techniques are to decrease pain and restore normal ROM.

▓ Counterstrain is a soft-tissue technique where the physician identifies tender points in myofascial structures and positions the patient so that the dysfunctional tissue is at a point of balance and tenderness is relieved

▓ Facilitated positional release is an indirect myofascial release treatment method where the point of dysfunction is gradually moved until a neutral position is realized on all planes; an activating influence (either torsion or compression) is then applied in order to release joint restriction and remove tension from the tissue

Active Release Technique (ART) can also be used to treat piriformis syndrome. ART is a system of soft tissue mobilizations that can be utilized to treat repetitive strains, adhesions, and tissue hypoxia. Constant tension on a tissue, as in the case of piriformis syndrome, leads to adhesions in the muscle and fibrosis. This fibrosis leads to friction, pressure and tension on the sciatic nerve. To treat piriformis syndrome via ART, the patient is positioned in side lying with the involved side up, hip in anatomical position or abducted. The therapist contacts the distal portion of the muscle and draws tension medially. Tension is maintained or increased as the hip is moved into flexion adduction and external rotation. This technique should be performed repetitively in an attempt to localize discomfort and restriction of movement.

Therapeutic Exercise

After ROM and flexibility is improved or even restored with stretching and soft tissue mobilization, hip strengthening and lumbar stabilization exercises are performed. Tonley et al suggested that weakness of the gluteus medius leads to excessive medial femoral rotation and adduction in weight bearing tasks (11). This places greater strain on the piriformis muscle due to overloading and eccentric demand. Others have suggested L5 radiculopathies can cause weakness in the piriformis and other hip external rotators, increasing demand on the muscle. Excessive strain and microtrauma can lead to scar tissue formation and muscle shortening. This may cause intrinsic piriformis muscle pain or referred sciatic pain from nerve compression. Strengthening the hip abductors, extensors, and external rotators can help normalize femoral alignment and decrease this strain. Correction of deficits in the kinetic chain can decrease femoral rotation forces and also decrease strain on the piriformis.

Strength training exercises in a non-weight bearing position, such as the side lying clamshell (Figure 49.2) and supine bridge (Figure 49.3), are recommended initially. The weight bearing progression of these exercises focuses on squatting and lunging with emphasis on neutral femoral alignment in the transverse plane.

Lumbopelvic stabilization exercises that address the transversus abdominus, multifidi, and internal and external obliques are very important in treating piriformis syndrome. Plank and side plank exercises (Figures 49.4 and 49.5) are maneuvers that minimize rectus abdominus contraction while targeting gluteus medius and external oblique muscles (12).

Core exercises have recently been described as those involving the lumbopelvic hip complex (13). The

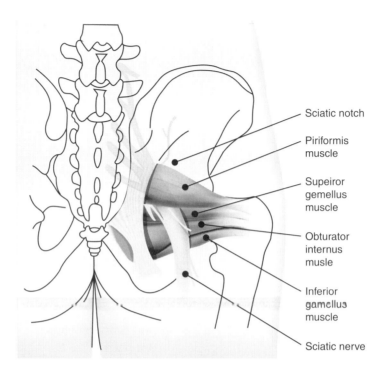

FIGURE 49.1: Piriformis anatomy. The sciatic nerve travels through the sciatic notch, anterior to the piriformis muscle. In a small percentage of patients, the sciatic nerve bifurcates at this level.

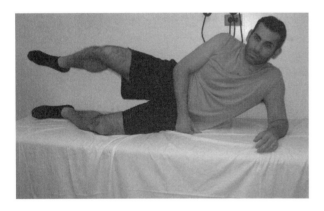

FIGURE 49.2: Modified clamshell.

Lie on side with shoulder and head supported and knees bent. Slightly raise top leg and rotate your hip/knee toward the ceiling without rotating pelvis. Repeat 10 times.

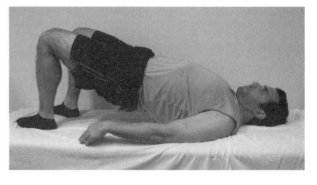

FIGURE 49.3: Bridging.

Slowly raise buttocks from floor, keeping stomach tight. Repeat 10 times per set. Do two sets per session. Do two sessions per day.

lumbopelvic hip complex, or core as it is commonly referred, is the integral link in the functional ability of the lower kinetic chain to normalize lower limb biomechanics. This group of muscles controls pelvic tilt, which, if excessive, can lead to femoral rotation and adduction. Tight hamstrings and iliopsoas, weak hip extensors, and tight iliotibial bands can also aggravate anterior pelvic tilt and femoral rotation and should be addressed. With efficient functionality of the entire hip complex, one can maintain a stable base for all

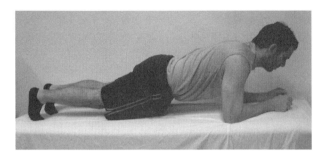

FIGURE 49.4: Plank.

Start lying on stomach. Lift your body up onto forearms and toes. Keep your back flat and your pelvis tucked in. Hold 20 seconds. Repeat three times.

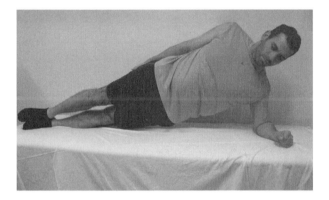

FIGURE 49.5: Side plank.

Start by lying on your side and propped up onto your elbow. Raise your hips up so your body is in a straight line. Try to raise your free arm overhead. Hold 20 seconds. Repeat two times each side.

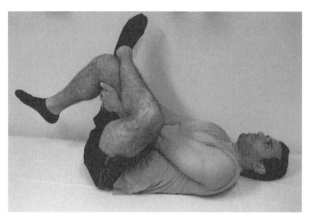

FIGURE 49.6: Piriformis stretch.

To stretch the left leg cross legs, left on top. Gently pull other knee toward chest until stretch is felt in buttock/hip of top leg. Hold 30 seconds. Repeat two times per set. Do two sets per session. Do two sessions per day.

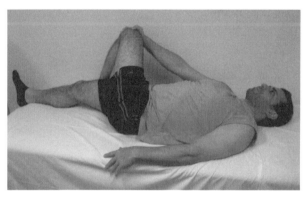

FIGURE 49.7: Supine piriformis stretch in the FADIR position.

movements and prevent excessive strain on the piriformis muscle.

Home Exercise Program

The exercises discussed in the prior section are eventually incorporated into the HEP. In addition, the patient may sit on top of the foam roller, with the hands behind them for balance, positioning the roller over the affected buttock. The involved foot is crossed over the opposite knee in the FABER position. Once in this position, the patient transfers their body weight onto the involved hip and slowly rolls to find a tender spot. The patient should localize three tender spots and hold each one for 30 seconds. The tenderness in the muscle itself denotes decreased extensibility which can lead to nerve adhesion and pain.

After utilizing the foam roller, the piriformis muscle is primed to be stretched. The rationale for stretching the piriformis is to elongate the muscle, thus decreasing compressive forces on the sciatic nerve (14). While lying supine with both knees bent, the involved hip should be flexed and externally rotated so that the ankle rests on the opposite knee (Figure 49.6). In this position, the patient then uses their hands to pull the involved leg toward the chest into greater hip flexion. This stretch should be held for 30 seconds. Alternative positions may also be utilized for piriformis stretching and the choice of stretch may be based on the comfort and effectiveness of each one (Figures 49.7 and 49.8).

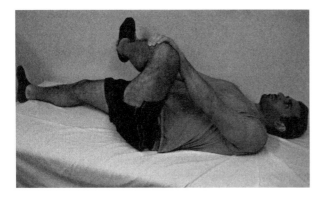

FIGURE 49.8: Alternative supine piriformis stretch.

SUMMARY

Piriformis syndrome is a contentious and both an under and over diagnosed condition in different healthcare settings, however with a thorough history, and physical examination and with the aid of diagnostic modalities and injections, the diagnosis has become clearer. Conservative methods have remained the mainstay of treatment for piriformis syndrome. Activity modification and stretching are most effective in relieving a tight, spastic muscle. Core strengthening, modalities, lumbopelvic stability exercises, and correction of deficiencies in the kinetic chain are important adjuncts. The use of osteopathic treatments and ART can be effective as well but require providers with advanced, specialized training. The HEP is the key to maintaining functional gains and minimizing recurrent symptoms.

SAMPLE CASE

A 35-year-old female runner slipped on ice and fell on her right buttock 1 week ago while running. She has a history significant for pes planus with hyper-pronation and iliotibial band (ITB) syndrome. She is taking Ibuprofen as needed for pain and applying ice with no relief. She works full time and is training for her local half marathon. Review of systems is negative for weakness but she feels numbness and tingling in the dorsum of her right foot. She has no back pain. X-rays of the lumbar spine and right hip are negative. Examination is significant for antalgic gait, normal lumbar ROM, normal strength and reflexes, dysesthesias in the right dorsum of the foot, tenderness to palpation over the sciatic notch with a palpable sausage shape mass noted. There is pain with straight leg raising on the right at 45 degrees, and reproduction of her usual pain with the FAIR, Pace, and Beatty maneuvers. She has a tight ITB and hip flexors, mild femoral anteversion, and popliteal angles of 35 degrees bilaterally. Right hip ROM is limited due to pain. There is mild paraspinal spasm and tenderness.

 SAMPLE THERAPY PRESCRIPTION

Discipline: Physical therapy.

Diagnosis: Right piriformis syndrome.

Problem list: Abnormality of gait, poor lower limb flexibility, history of ITB syndrome.

Precautions: Weight bearing as tolerated (WBAT).

Frequency of visits: 2 to 3x/week.

Duration of treatment: 4 weeks; or an alternative would be to provide a total of 8 to 12 visits used at the therapist's discretion.

Treatment:

1. *Modalities:* cryotherapy (ice pack, ice bath, ice massage) in the acute phase or following therapy. Moist heat and/or therapeutic ultrasound 2.0 W cm² to the right piriformis muscle prior to stretching

2. *Manual therapy:* Myofascial release to the right piriformis and lumbar paraspinals

3. *Therapeutic exercise:* Active/active-assisted/passive range of motion (A/AA/PROM) to restore normal hip ROM. Self-stretching, therapist assisted stretching of the hip flexors, hip external rotators, ITB, hamstrings, and gastroc/soleus. Specific attention to the

piriformis muscle. Progressive resistive exercise (PRE) including core strengthening, hip external rotator and extension strengthening, neuro-muscular reeducation, aerobic/conditioning exercises

4. *Specialized treatments:* ART and/or facilitated positional release to the right piriformis. Kinetic chain evaluation/functional movement screening

5. *Patient education:* HEP with handouts

Goals: Decrease pain and swelling; restore hip ROM/flexibility then restore strength, safely return to functional activities (e.g., sport, hobbies, work) and prevent recurrent injury.

Reevaluation: In 4–6 weeks by referring physician.

REFERENCES

1. Freiberg AH, Vinke TH. Sciatica and the sacro-iliac joint. *J Bone Joint Surg Am*. 1934;16:126–136.
2. Robinson D. Piriformis muscle in relation to sciatic pain. *Am J Surg*. 1947;73:355–358.
3. Kirschner JS, Foye PM, Cole JL. Piriformis syndrome, diagnosis and treatment. *Muscle Nerve*. 2009;40:10–18.
4. Beatty RA: The piriformis muscle syndrome: a simple diagnostic maneuver. *Neurosurg*. 1994;34:512–514.
5. Filler AG, Haynes J, Jordan SE, et al. Sciatica of non disc origin and piriformis syndrome: diagnosis by magnetic resonance neurography and interventional magnetic resonance imaging with outcome study of resulting treatment. *J Neurosurg Spine*. 2005;2:99–115.
6. Fishman LM, Dombi GW, Michaelson C, et al. Piriformis syndrome: diagnosis, treatment and outcome—a 10-year study. *Arch Phys Med Rehabil*. 2002;83:295–301.
7. Fishman LM, Zybert PA: Electrophysiologic evidence of piriformis syndrome. *Arch Physical Medicine and Rehabilitation* 1992;73:359–364.
8. Scarpelli DG, Chiga M. Cell injury and errors of metabolism. In: Anderson WAD, Kissane JM, Eds. *Pathology*, 7th ed. St Louis, MO: C.V. Mosby; 1977: 90–147.
9. Savarese RG. *OMT Review*. 3rd ed. New York, NY: Kaplan Medical; 2003:8–9.
10. DiGiovanna EL, Schiowitz S, Dowling DJ, eds. *An Osteopathic Approach to Diagnosis and Treatment*. 3rd ed. Philadelphia, PA: Lippincott Williams & Wilkins; 2005.
11. Tonley J, Yun SM, Kochevar RJ, et al. Treatment of an individual of Piriformis Syndrome focusing on hip muscle strengthening and movement reeducation: a case report. *J Orthop Sports Phys Ther*. 2010;40(2):103–111.
12. Ekstrom RA, Donatelli RA, Carp KC. Electromyographic analysis of core trunk, hip and thigh musculature during 9 rehabilitation exercises. *J Orthop Sports Phys Ther*. 2007;37(12):754–762.
13. Oliver GD, Dwelly PM, Sarantis ND, Helmer RA, Bonacci JA. Muscle activation of different core exercises. *J. Strength Cond*. 2010;24(11):3069–3074.
14. Gail D. Differential diagnosis and conservative treatment for piriformis syndrome: A review of the literature. *Current Orthopedic Practice*. 2009;20(3):313–319.

Pelvic Dysfunction: Diagnosis Directs Treatment

Jeffrey L. Cole and Marilyn Freedman

INTRODUCTION

Recognition of the cause of a problem is the most important determinant in directing the most efficacious treatment. Pelvic pain and any related genitourinary dysfunction is too often illusive or underdiagnosed because of the extreme difficulty in tracking any particular injury site. All we can monitor is the peripheral muscle tone and strength or its reflexive contraction (or lack thereof). Almost everything else is subjective.

The most common musculoskeletal, fascial, or nerve entrapment treatments involve stretching muscle, nerves, and related connective tissue if it feels "tight" or strengthening the muscles if the tone and reflexive responses feel too weak. The stretching is performed manually or with mechanical devices and strengthening is performed with some variation of the Kegel exercises and/or biofeedback. Fortunately, this approach works for the majority of clinical presentations; however, there are many who do not respond to this logical but empirical approach. For these individuals, further diagnostics are indicated.

An illustrative case is of a very athletic gentleman in his early 60s who had a past medical history of bilateral inguinal hernia repairs and right Achilles tendon repair who presented with 10 months of scrotum and perineal region pain. His hobbies include piano and he was an avid fencer. He was in good health until he sat on a very long airplane trip without pain but thereafter began to experience some urinary urgency that increased over the following two days. The default diagnosis was prostatitis and he was prescribed Flomax, Pyridium, and Bactrim. He reported "aching" perineal, penile tip, and testicular pains that are worst post-ejaculation, and urinary urgency. The symptoms resolved slightly but after four more antibiotic courses, despite negative or nonspecific cultures, persisted. Transrectal prostate sonogram, pelvic and lumbar CT scans, and conventional electrodiagnostics only revealed a mild asymmetric prostatic enlargement suggesting a chronic bladder outlet obstruction, severe bilateral L5-S1 facet hypertrophy, a suggestion of left greater than right osteitis condensans ilii, and asymmetrical piriformis muscles, left appeared 50% thicker than on the right.

With no other diagnosis, he was referred for pelvic floor PT (PFPT) and for a lumbosacral MRI that showed a large L3-L4 broad-based herniation with significant central canal stenosis, small L4-L5 and L5-S1 ventral herniations, left L4-L5 facet effusion and bilateral L5-S1 facet arthritis, and L3-L4 ligamentum flavum hypertrophy at the L3-L4 level. He underwent an L4-L5 facet injection and then tried yoga, acupuncture, and chiropractic treatment without improvement.

His physical examination: lumbar spine right lateral bending produced pain radiating down the lateral aspect of the right leg down to the foot and the left lateral bending produced pain radiation into his buttock; positive left Kemp's sign associated with radiation of pain down the right leg; no rectal-pelvic, Alcock's, genitofemoral, or lumbosacral tenderness; no inguinal hernias; but right gastrocnemius muscle atrophy. In other words, despite repeated extensive medical work-ups, nothing suggested any localizing diagnosis beyond the lumbar imaging findings.

He was then given a comprehensive electrodiagnostic examination, which showed normal lower extremity motor and sensory nerves, normal cremasteric reflexes, and normal H-reflex studies (Figure 50.1) (1,2). The electrical bulbocavernosus reflexes (see Figure 50.2) showed a low-normal right latency (34.7 ms) and a normal left latency (30.0 ms) with preservation of bilaterally normal response amplitudes. The bulbocavernosus muscles' EMG examination was normal. The pudendal nerve somatosensory evoked potential studies (Figure 50.3) and the terminal motor latencies (Figure 50.4) revealed a relatively low-normal right latency (3.63 ms) with low-amplitude responses (0.8 mV) with

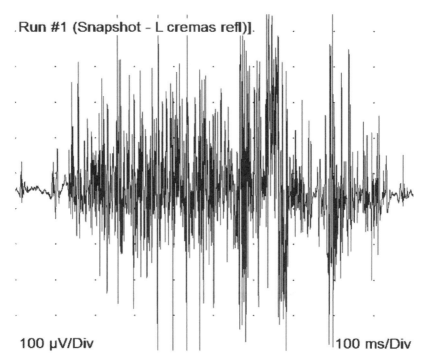

FIGURE 50.1: Left cremasteric reflex elicited by a downward stroke along the ipsilateral proximal-medial thigh and recorded from intramuscular electrodes.

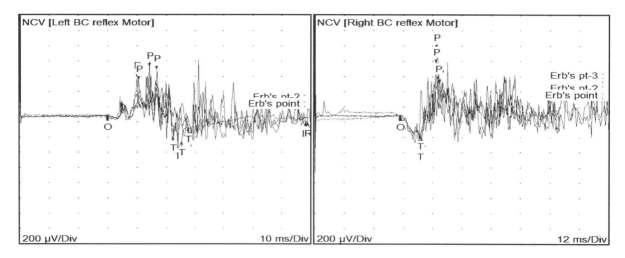

FIGURE 50.2: Left (recorded at 10 ms/div) and right (recorded at 12 ms/div) electrical bulbocavernosus reflex studies recorded from stimulation of the dorsal nerve of the penis to individual intramuscular electrodes.

preservation of a normal left latency (2.70 ms) with normal-amplitude responses (3.5 mV) (3,4). The EMG showed right and left L4 and left S1 paraspinal denervation and bilateral L4-L5-S1 polyphasic motor units, while the bilateral lower extremities, internal and external rectal sphincters levator ani, and piriformis muscles were normal (3). These findings were consistent with a mild chronic bilateral lumbosacral polyradiculitis and a

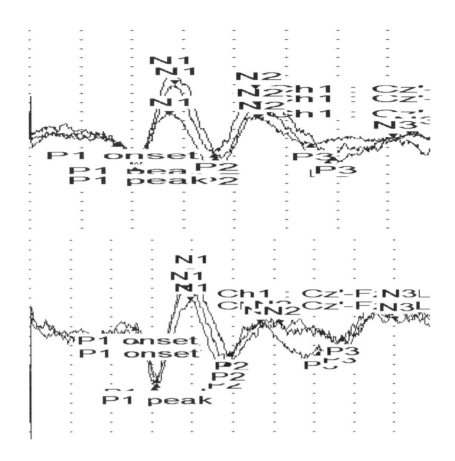

FIGURE 50.3: Top (recorded at 12 ms/div) and bottom (recorded at 10 ms/div) pudendal nerve somatosensory evoked potential studies recorded from unilateral stimulation of the dorsal nerve of the penis to scalp electrodes from Cz' to Fz.

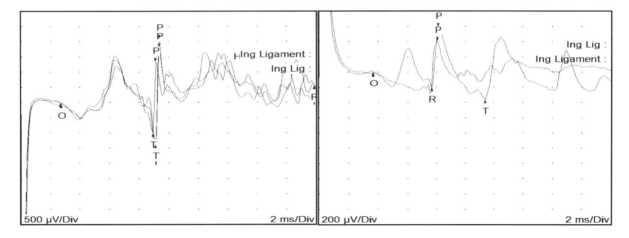

FIGURE 50.4: Left (500 µV/div) and right (200 µV/div) pudendal nerve terminal motor latencies were evoked for percutaneous stimulation at Alcock's canal and recorded from ipsilateral intramuscular (flexible wire) electrodes in the rectal sphincter muscles.

mild-chronic demyelinating right pudendal nerve segmental injury or entrapment at Alcock's canal as evidenced by the symmetrical bulbocavernosus reflex and pudendal nerve terminal motor latencies. He was then successfully treated with right pudendal nerve (Alcock canal level) and caudal epidural steroid injections.

He also benefitted from a comprehensive PFPT approach addressing the neuromuscular-fascial and visceral pelvic pain with normalization of skeletal range of motion (ROM) and strength with first treating the external myofascial trigger points (TP), then the internal TP, then mobilization of the restricted visceral fascia, patient education on physiological relaxation, restore muscle dysfunctions, reeducate visceral function, teach core stabilization, reeducate posture and body mechanics, and address functional life specific training (5,6). Any needed therapeutic modalities are taught to allow independent use. These would include: analgesics, ice or heat applications; TENS-IF; biofeedback training (BFB) for internal vaginal or anal use; electrical stimulation (ES) for internal vaginal or anal use; manual therapy; skin rolling; external and internal myofascial release; external and internal sphincter, levator ani, and obturator TP release; muscle energy technique; lumbar-pelvic skeletal mobilization; visceral mobilization; muscle energy/therapeutic exercises to restore lumbosacral spine, pelvis, and lower extremity passive range of motion (LE PROM) and active range of motion (AROM); proprioceptive training; aerobic exercise; education in self (digital or assistive device) release internally; paradoxical and physiological relaxation training; acupuncture; seating alternatives; and any other specialized techniques as needed. By following a logical progression through the rehabilitation phases to an independent self-treatment through essential independent exercises and neuromuscular and proprioceptive training, with the goal of return to active participation in all premorbid activities and an understanding that flares are common. With the correct diagnosis, reasonable response to self and professional treatment, and follow-up care, most can expect good outcomes.

In spite of the best attempt to corroborate and correlate presenting complaints with diagnostic and laboratory findings, sometimes a diagnosis is clinically defined.

An example of this musculoskeletal approach is a 32-year-old male presenting with perineal and anal pain of 9 months duration, exacerbated by sitting. He lifts weights and engages in long distance bicycle riding. He reports slight "burning pain" with ejaculation followed by significant post-ejaculatory penile tip pain lasting

up to 36 hours, post-bowel movement discomfort lasting several hours, and mild suprapubic pain and urinary urgency. He consulted three urologists and was given three courses of broad-spectrum antibiotics; he also consulted a colorectal surgeon. Radiographs, cultures, serologies, and imaging were negative. His examination was significant for: myofascial restrictions over the entire abdomen, particularly suprapubic tissues; tenderness and restrictions over the medial ischial tuberosities bilaterally; active trigger points palpated bilaterally over the pubis; ischiopubic rami (both medial and lateral borders); rectus abdominus; internal and external abdominal obliques; psoas; hip adductors (especially pectineus); external and internal anal sphincters, puborectalis; levator ani anterior (most acute with reproduction of all his symptoms), medius (referred to anus) and posterior (also referring to anus), and urethral tenderness with poor motility throughout. He was started on a program of stretching that he immediately incorporated into a home exercise program (HEP). The early HEP included stretching, self external myofascial, trigger point release, and diaphragmatic breathing. Modalities (hot bath twice daily, cryotherapy over perineum after treatment), TENS (or low- to mid-frequency interferential current therapy [IFC]), antispasmodics (benzodiazepines, etc.), manual therapy (myofascial release over pubis and suprapubic, ischio-pubic rami, abdominal tissue, ischial tuberosities, sacrum, and puborectalis areas), TP release to abdominal obliques, rectus abdominus, hip adductors, perineum, and levator ani (anterior, middle, and posterior) muscles, and visceral mobilization to urethra and prostate are included. The therapeutic stretching (self and/or therapist assisted) exercises including abdominals, hip adductors, hip flexors, pelvic floor and rectal muscles, followed by neuromuscular reeducation (mainly down-training) of the pelvic floor, muscles and appropriate contraction and/or moment to moment relaxation of core abdominal and pelvic floor muscles with activities of daily living (ADL). Then instruction in pelvic diaphragm respiratory movement of pelvic diaphragm, i.e., one uses diaphragmatic breathing to inhale, pelvic diaphragm descends, and with exhalation it returns to neutral with a cadence of pelvic floor recruitment and relaxation during tonic (5 second) and phasic (1 second) contraction cycles. Then instruction in conventional aerobic and conditioning exercise, to ensure core stabilization, as the final component.

When objective physical findings and laboratory, imaging, and electrodiagnostic studies fail to define the problem, the default is "chronic pelvic pain syndrome" as in the above example. All that means is that the problem needs to be addressed with clinical expertise and education about the problem. The teaching for the cited case should include: avoid ejaculation, bicycle riding or calisthenics (especially abdominal exercise), and weight lifting during early phase of treatment while, aerobics, including walking, and elliptical trainer, and stretching are encouraged.

The goals include: decrease spasm with hot baths; elevation of the pelvis in anti-gravity position; release painful tight soft tissue and TP; stretch tight tissue; bring attention to awareness of pelvic muscle function with neuromuscular training; using core stabilization training, posture, and bio-mechanics to safely return to functional activities, for example, sport, work, ejaculation, and sex (which are often the last to return pain free); and prevent recurrent flare-ups with regular follow-ups; and restore normal functional contraction and relaxation of pelvic floor.

REFERENCES

1. Cole JL, Gottesman L. Anal electrophysiology and pudendal nerve evoked potentials. In: Smith L, Ed. *Practical Guide to AnoRectal Testing*. 2nd ed. New York, NY: Igaku-Shoin; 1995:207–220.
2. Ertekin C, Bademkiran F, Yildiz N, et al. Central and peripheral motor conduction to cremasteric muscle. *Muscle Nerve.* 2005;31:349–354.
3. Cole JL, Goldberg G. Central nervous system electrodi agnostics. In: DeLisa JA, Ed. *Rehabilitation Medicine: Principles and Practice*. 4th ed. Philadelphia, PA: Lippincott; 2004:105–137.
4. Niu X, Shao B, Ni P, et al. Bulbocavernosus reflex and pudendal nerve somatosensory evoked potentials responses in female patients with nerve system diseases. *J Clin Neurophysiol.* 2010;27:207–211.
5. Groysman V. Vulvodynia: new concepts and review of the literature. *Dermatol Clin.* 2010;28(4):681–696.
6. Glazer H, Rodke G. *The Vulvodynia survival Guide.* Retrieved from www.amazon.com/Vulvodynia-Survival-Guide-Overcome-Lifestyle/dp/1572242914. Consumer information site on vulvodynia, http://www.vulvodynia.com

Index

Note: Page numbers following by "*f*" and "*t*" refer to figures and tables, respectively.